OSTEOPOROSIS

OSTEOPOROSIS

Edited by

John C. Stevenson

Wynn Department of Metabolic Medicine
Imperial College School of Medicine
London
UK

and

Robert Lindsay

Helen Hayes Hospital
West Haverstraw
New York
USA

CHAPMAN & HALL MEDICAL
London · Weinheim · New York · Tokyo · Melbourne · Madras

Published by Chapman & Hall,
an imprint of Thomson Science, 2–6 Boundary Row, London SE1 8HN, UK

Thomson Science, 2–6 Boundary Row, London SE1 8HN, UK

Thomson Science, 115 Fifth Avenue, New York, NY 10003, USA

Thomson Science, Suite 750, 400 Market Street, Philadelphia, PA 19106, USA

Thomson Science, Pappelallee 3, 69469 Weinheim, Germany

First edition 1998

Thomson Science is a division of International Thomson Publishing I(T)P®

Typeset in 10/12pt Palatino by Cambrian Typesetters, Frimley, Surrey

Printed in Great Britain at the University Press, Cambridge

ISBN 0 412 48870 1

A catalogue record for this book is available from the British Library

Library of Congress Catalog Card Number: 97–76818

∞ Printed on acid-free text paper, manufactured in accordance with ANSI/NISO Z39.48–1992 (Permanence of Paper).

CONTENTS

Colour plates appear between pages 104 and 105

CONTRIBUTORS

P.R. ALLEN,
Department of Trauma and Orthopaedics,
Bromley Hospitals NHS Trust,
Farnborough Hospital,
Farnborough Common,
Orpington BR6 8ND, UK

L.V. AVIOLI,
Division of Bone and Mineral Diseases,
Department of Internal Medicine,
Washington University School of Medicine,
216 South Kingshighway Boulevard,
St Louis,
MO 63110–1072, USA

L.M. BANKS,
X-ray Academic Unit,
Imperial College School of Medicine,
Hammersmith Campus,
London W12 0NN, UK

F.J. BONNER,
Department of Physical Medicine in Rehabilitation,
Graduate Hospital,
1 Graduate Plaza, Philadelphia,
PA 19146, USA

C. CHRISTIANSEN,
Center for Clinical and Basic Research,
Ballerup Byvej 222,
DK-2750 Ballerup,
Denmark

J. COMPSTON,
Department of Medicine,
Level 5,
University of Cambridge Clinical School,
Addenbrooke's Hospital,
Hills Road,
Cambridge CB2 2QQ, UK

C. COOPER,
MRC Environmental Epidemiology Unit
(University of Southampton),
Southampton General Hospital,
Tremona Road,
Southampton SO9 4XY, UK

F. COSMAN,
Helen Hayes Hospital,
Route 9W, West Haverstraw,
New York 10993, USA

P.D. DELMAS,
Pavillon F,
Service de Rhumatologie et de Pathologie Osseuse,
Hopital Edouard Herriot,
Place d'Arsouval,
69437 Lyon, France

D. DEMPSTER,
Regional Bone Center,
Helen Hayes Hospital,
Route 9W, West Haverstraw,
NY 10993–1195, USA

H.A. FLEISCH,
Department of Pathophysiology,
University of Bern,
Murtenstrasse 35,
Bern 3010, Switzerland

R.M. FRANCIS,
Musculoskeletal Unit,
Bone Clinic, Freeman Hospital,
High Heaton,
Newcastle on Tyne NE7 7DN, UK

J.C. GALLAGHER,
Bone Metabolism Unit,
St Joseph Hospital,
601 N 30th Street,
Suite 5730, Omaha,
NE 68131, USA

P. GARNERO,
INSERM Research Unit 403,
Pavillon F,
Services de Rhumatologie et de Pathologie Osseuse,
Hopital Edouard Herriot,
Place d'Arsonval,
69437 Lyon, France

C.C. JOHNSTON JR,
Emerson Hall 421,
Indiana University,
Department of Medicine,
545 Barnhill Drive,
Indianapolis,
IN 46202–5124, USA

J.A. KANIS,
Department of Human Metabolism and Clinical Biochemistry,
University of Sheffield Medical School,
Beech Hill Road,
Sheffield S10 2RX, UK

B.J. KIRATLI,
Spinal Cord Injury Service,
Veterans Affairs Medical Center,
Palo Alto,
CA 94304, USA

M. KLEEREKOPER,
Wayne State University,
Division of Endocrinology,
4201 St Antoine,
Detroit,
MI 48201, USA

B. LEES,
Wynn Department of Metabolic Medicine,
Imperial College School of Medicine,
21 Wellington Road,
London NW8 9SQ, UK

R. LINDSAY,
Internal Medicine Department,
Helen Hayes Hospital,
Route 9W, West Haverstraw,
NY 10993, USA

R. MARCUS,
GRECC 182–B,
Veterans Affairs Medical Center,
Palo Alto,
CA 94304, USA

T.J. MARTIN,
St Vincent's Institute of Medical Research,
41 Victoria Parade,
Melbourne 3065,
Australia

L.J. MELTON III,
Department of Clinical Epidemiology,
Mayo Clinic,
200 First Street SW,
Rochester,
MN 55905, USA

G.R. MUNDY,
Endocrinology in Metabolism UTHSC,
7703 Floyd Curl Drive,
San Antonio,
TX 78284–7877, USA

D.A. NELSON,
Wayne State University,
Division of Rheumatology,
4707 St Antoine,
Detroit,
MI 48201, USA

A.C. SCANE,
Department of Medicine,
North Tees General Hospital,
Hardwick
Stockton on Tees, TS19 8PE, UK

C.W. SLEMENDA (deceased)

J.C. STEVENSON,
Wynn Department of Metabolic Medicine,
Imperial College School of Medicine,
21 Wellington Road,
London NW8 9SQ, UK

A.M. SUTCLIFFE,
Musculoskeletal Unit,
Bone Clinic,
Freeman Hospital,
High Heaton,
Newcastle on Tyne NE7 7DN, UK

PREFACE

Osteoporosis is a condition characterized by low bone density which increases the risk of fragility fractures. The incidence of the disease has increased steadily in the latter half of this century, and will continue to do so into the millennium as the number of elderly people increases. Thus osteoporosis represents a major challenge to public health and will continue to do so. The purpose of this book is to review the many different aspects of osteoporosis with particular respect to the practical management of the disease.

The first few chapters deal with bone tissue, the factors which affect it to result in low bone mass and in fractures, and the epidemiology of osteoporosis. An understanding of bone structure and cellular activity is necessary to help understand both the pathogenesis and treatment modalities of the disease. Many different factors can affect bone mass and bone remodelling, thereby resulting in low bone mass, but in addition there are factors responsible for the clinical endpoint of the disease – namely fracture. The review of the epidemiology of low bone mass and fractures highlights the widespread nature of the disease and the enormity of the problem which confronts us.

There are then chapters on the assessment of the skeleton by histomorphometric means, by biochemical markers of bone turnover and by direct measurements of bone mass. All these techniques have helped in the understanding of the disease process, the way that different treatments produce their effects, and the early diagnosis of osteoporosis before the clinical end-point of fracture has been reached.

The next few chapters review the various therapeutic options currently available, including the anti-resorptive and anabolic agents as well as nutritional and lifestyle modalities. The role of physical medicine and orthopaedic management in the rehabilitation of osteoporotic patients is also discussed. Finally, a prediction of the future in terms of therapeutic strategies concludes the book. Studies of the genetic basis of osteoporosis are still in their infancy but will doubtless continue to stimulate interest. However, it seems that we are a long way from gene therapy in this common and multifactorial disease.

We are fortunate in having persuaded such a number of eminent international experts to contribute to this book, and hope that it will be of help and interest to both clinicians and scientists in the field of metabolic bone disease.

John C. Stevenson
Robert Lindsay
1998

BONE STRUCTURE AND CELLULAR ACTIVITY

1

T.J. Martin and D.W. Dempster

The adult human skeleton weighs approximately 1 kg and contains 99% of the body's calcium and four-fifths of its phosphorus. The mammalian skeleton evolved to serve two functions: to provide a gravity-resisting structural and protective framework and to act as an extracellular reservoir for key ions, such as calcium, phosphorus, magnesium, sodium, citrate and bicarbonate. There are two types of bony tissue. *Compact or cortical bone* makes up 80% of the skeleton. It is hard and dense and forms the outer casing of most bones and the tubular shafts of the long bones. The remaining 20% of the skeleton is composed of *cancellous or spongy bone*, which consists of a honeycomb-like network of plates and rods called *trabeculae* (Figure 1.1). Cancellous bone is found primarily in the vertebral bodies and at the ends of the long bones.

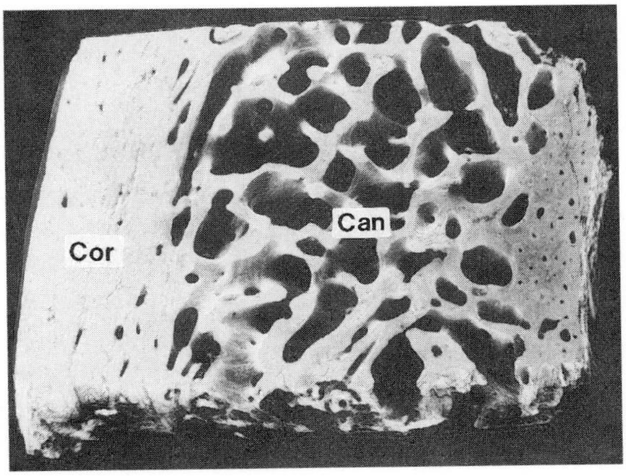

Figure 1.1 Scanning electron micrograph of a sample of human iliac crest illustrating the structural differences between cortical bone (Cor) and cancellous bone (Can). Reproduced with permission from Dempster, D.W. In: (1989) *Clinical Disorders of Bone and Mineral Metabolism*, (eds Kleerekoper, M. and Krane, S.), Mary Ann Liebert, New York, pp. 247–52.

BONE MATRIX

Bone owes its impressive mechanical properties to the fact that its matrix is a composite material. The organic component bestows elasticity and the mineral component rigidity (Currey, 1984). The organic and mineral components are closely associated at the ultrastructural and molecular levels (Weiner, 1986). About 60–70% of mature bone is made up of inorganic mineral salts, with the balance consisting of organic matrix and water (Doty *et al.*, 1976; Glimcher, 1981). The major component of the mineral phase is a poorly crystalline, non-stoichiometric analog of the naturally occurring mineral hydroxyapatite,

Osteoporosis. Edited by John C. Stevenson and Robert Lindsay. Published in 1998 by Chapman & Hall, London.
ISBN 0 412 48870 1

$Ca_{10}(PO_4)_6(OH)_2$ (Posner, 1987; Glimcher, 1992). Compared to the stoichiometric formula for hydroxyapatite, bone mineral has about a 5–10% deficit in calcium. This deficiency is balanced by the presence of fewer hydroxyl ions and by hydrogen bonds between the oxygen atoms of the orthophosphate groups. Furthermore, approximately 3–4% of the PO_4 ions present in true hydroxyapatite are substituted by CO_3 ions in bone apatite. There is also a separate phase of calcium carbonate on the surface of the apatite cystals. This is in readily exchangeable form (Neuman and Mulryan, 1967) and is probably involved in the buffering of extracellular fluids in acidotic states (Lemann *et al.*, 1966; Bushinsky *et al.*, 1986).

The organic phase of bone matrix is predominantly (90%) composed of collagen with the balance consisting of a range of other substances, such as lipids, glycoproteins and proteoglycans (Tracy *et al.*, 1987; Robey *et al.*, 1988). Bone collagen is almost exclusively type I with only trace amounts of types II, V and XI, which may be derived from vascular tissue rather than from the matrix itself (Leushner, 1983; Veis and Sabsay, 1987; Robey *et al.*, 1992).

A large number of different non-collagenous peptides have been identified in bone matrix. Their function is not well understood and their levels decline as the matrix matures. Two classes of such peptides are worthy of mention here: the γ-carboxylated proteins, osteocalcin (bone Gla protein) and matrix Gla protein, and the RGD sequence-containing proteins, such as osteopontin and fibronectin (see below). Osteocalcin is the most abundant of the non-collagenous peptides (Price, 1985, 1987; Hauschka, 1986). The peptide, which is synthesized and secreted by the osteoblast (Nishimoto and Price, 1980), accounts for about 15% of the extractable non-collagenous bone proteins. The complete amino acid sequence and cDNA structure are now available. Osteocalcin is a 50-residue protein, three of which are the calcium-binding amino acid γ-carboxyglutamic acid (Gla). The incorporation of these residues is necessary for secretion of the peptide and requires the presence of vitamin K. Its secretion is also regulated by 1,25-dihydroxyvitamin D (Price and Baukol, 1980). Despite its relative abundance, the function of osteocalcin remains uncertain. It was initially thought to affect mineralization (Price, 1985, 1987) but probably appears in matrix too late to play a significant role in this process. Moreover, warfarin treatment, which severely depresses bone BGP levels, does not interfere with mineralization (Price, 1987). It does, however, render bone matrix less resorbable (Lian *et al.*, 1984) leading to speculation that osteocalcin is involved in the recruitment and activation of osteoclasts (Lian *et al.*, 1986). Although the function of osteocalcin is not yet defined, the circulating concentration of the peptide has nonetheless become a widely used and useful biochemical marker of bone turnover when resorption and formation are coupled and a specific marker of bone formation when it is uncoupled from resorption (Delmas, 1993).

BONE CELL BIOLOGY

Optimum skeletal function is maintained by a continuous process of removal and replacement of bony tissue. This process, called bone remodeling, is achieved by teams of different bone cell types which work together in bone remodeling units. Simply put, the bone remodeling units consist of osteoclasts, which remove old bone, and osteoblasts, which deposit new bone in place of that removed. In reality this is a very complex process involving co-operation between not only osteoclasts and osteoblasts but also many other different cell types, including osteocytes, bone-lining cells, macrophages, marrow stromal cells and, almost certainly, several others whose role is not yet defined. The process of bone remodeling is the subject of several recent reviews (Parfitt, 1988; Dempster, 1992) and is discussed in detail in Chapter 2.

The remainder of this chapter will focus on recent advances in our understanding of bone cell biology with particular emphasis on the osteoclast and the osteoblast, which understandably, but also for reasons of technical feasibility, have received the most attention.

OSTEOCLAST FUNCTION AND REGULATION

Although Kolliker recognized osteoclasts as early as 1873 (Kolliker, 1873) and, furthermore, knew what their function was, detailed knowledge of how osteoclasts accomplish the formidable task of removing both the organic and inorganic components of bone matrix has only been obtained relatively recently. Slow progress in this area can be explained in large part by difficulties in retrieving sufficient quantities of viable osteoclasts for *in vitro* study. However, about 10 years ago methods were developed to overcome this problem (Osdoby *et al.*, 1982; Boyde *et al.*, 1984; Chambers *et al.*, 1984; Zambonin-Zallone *et al.*, 1984) and this has led directly to a dramatic expansion in our understanding of the osteoclast.

OSTEOCLAST ATTACHMENT

Prior to initiating resorption, the osteoclast must first recognize and then bind firmly to the bone matrix. This is achieved by means of integrin receptors located in the osteoclast membrane (Davies *et al.*, 1989; Lakkakorpi *et al.*, 1991) (Figure 1.2). A number of members of the VLA (very late activation) family of integrin receptors have been recognized in osteoclasts. These include α_2, α_v, β_1, β_3, the integrin complex, $\alpha_v\beta_3$, which is the classic vitronectin receptor, and possibly also $\alpha_5\beta_1$ (VLA-5), the fibronectin receptor (Horton and Davies, 1989; Clover *et al.*, 1992; Hughes, *et al.*, 1993). There are a number of probable ligands for these receptors in the organic matrix of bone, including the most abundant protein, collagen, which is recognized by β_1. The ligand for the $\alpha_v\beta_3$ integrin in bone is not vitronectin but the RGD-containing sequence present in several of the non-collagenous matrix proteins, including fibronectin, thrombospondin, osteopontin and bone sialoprotein II (BSP II) (Oldberg *et al.*, 1986; Reinholt *et al.*, 1990; Teti and Zambonin-Zalone, 1992; Helfrich *et al.*, 1992). Osteoclasts apparently also synthesize BSP II and are therefore capable of producing at least one of their own putative adhesive substrates (Bianco *et al.*, 1991).

While there is still debate over the exact role of individual integrins in matrix recognition and in sealing the osteoclast to bone (Oursler and Spellsberg, 1993), the functional importance of these receptors in osteoclastic bone resorption is confirmed by the observation that receptor expression is regulated by factors, such as 1,25-dihydroxyvitamin D and transforming growth factor β, that are important in osteoclast differentiation (Horton and Davies, 1989; Teitelbaum, 1993). Moreover, both monoclonal antibodies against $\alpha_v\beta_3$ and

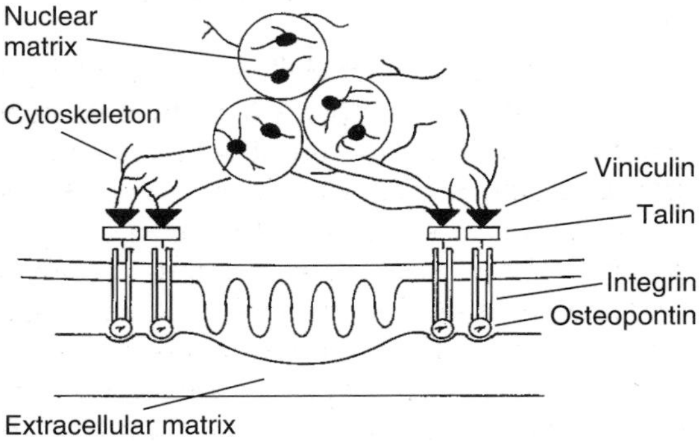

Figure 1.2 The binding of osteoclasts to bone matrix via interaction of integrin receptors with RGD-containing peptides, such as osteopontin. The integrin receptors are in turn linked to the osteoclast's cytoskeleton by means of the attachment proteins talin and vinculin. Reproduced with permission from Donahue, H.J. In (1992) *Biology and Physiology of the Osteoclast*, (eds Rifkin, B.R. and Gay, C.), CRC Press, Boca Raton, pp. 207–22.

peptides containing the RGD sequence inhibit adhesion to and resorption of bone by isolated osteoclasts (Chambers *et al.*, 1986; Sato *et al.*, 1990; Horton *et al.*, 1991). These observations are not only of theoretical interest but open the door for the development of pharmaceutical agents that could inhibit bone resorption by interfering with osteoclast integrin expression or integrin-matrix adhesion (Oursler and Spellsberg, 1993).

MECHANISMS OF MINERAL AND MATRIX REMOVAL

Once the osteoclast has recognized bone matrix, it forms an annular 'sealing zone' (also called the 'clear zone') which enables it to create a unique extracellular environment between itself and the bone surface (Figure 1.3). This microenvironment, which has been likened to that in a secondary lysosome (Baron *et al.*, 1985), is acidic, enabling dissolution of bone mineral, and rich in proteolytic enzymes, which degrade the organic matrix. Osteoclastic acid production is under hormonal control (Anderson *et al.*, 1986; Hunter *et al.*, 1988) and is achieved by the conversion of glucose to lactic or citric acid and by the carbonic anhydrase-catalyzed conversion of $CO_2 + H_2O$ to H_2CO_3 (Delaisse and Vaes, 1992). The latter mechanism is quantitatively the most important source of

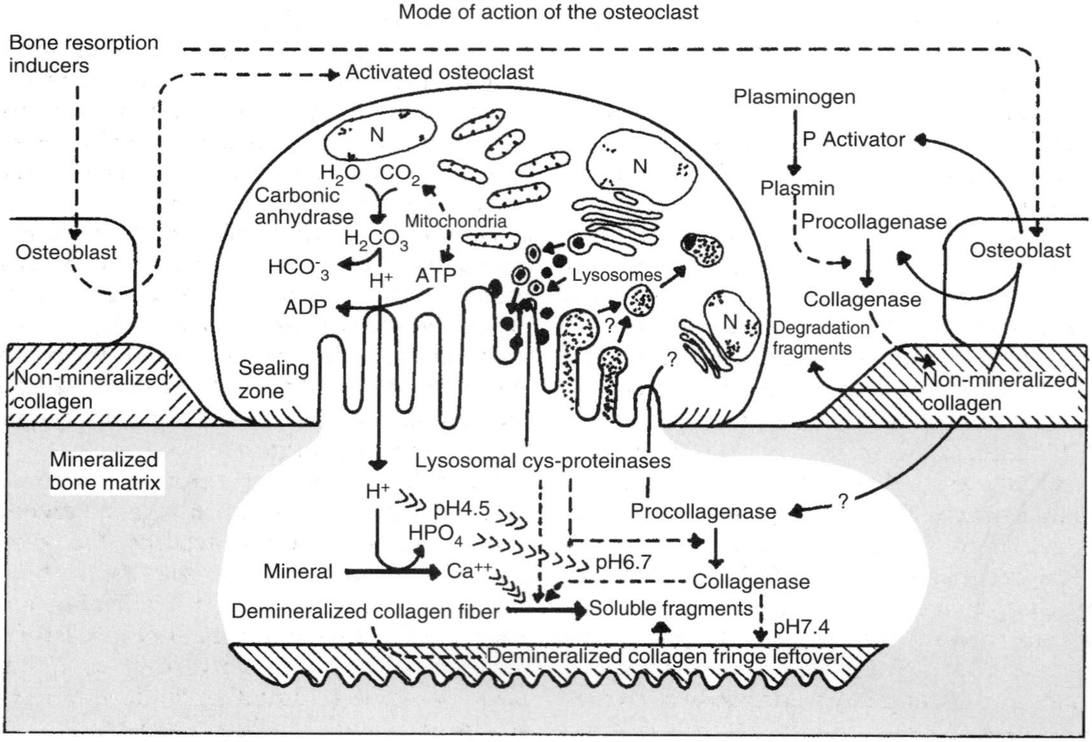

Figure 1.3 Some hypothetical mechanisms employed by the osteoclast to remove the extracellular matrix of bone. The solubilization of bone mineral and the degradation of organic matrix is achieved in the resorption hemivacuole that the osteoclast creates between itself and the bone matrix by means of the annular sealing zone. See text for further details. Reproduced with permission from Delaisse and Vaes (1992).

hydrogen ions. Involvement of carbonic anhydrase has been confirmed both by the fact that carbonic anhydrase inhibitors, such as acetazolamide, decrease osteoclast acidification and inhibit resorption both *in vivo* and *in vitro* (e.g. Waite *et al.*, 1970; Hunter *et al.*, 1988, 1991) and by the observation that carbonic anhydrase II deficiency is the primary defect in the autosomal recessive syndrome of osteopetrosis, a disorder in which the osteoclasts are effete (Sly *et al.*, 1985).

Protons generated by either carbonic anhydrase activity or glucose metabolism are transported to the extracellular space by means of a proton pump located on the cytosolic side of the osteoclast's ruffled border. While early immunoelectron microscopical and functional studies suggested that the osteoclast proton pump was similar to the gastric H^+,K^+-ATPase (Baron *et al.*, 1985; Anderson *et al.*, 1986; Tuukkanen and Vaananen, 1986), later work by several independent groups has provided convincing evidence that the pump shares more common features with the vacuolar type of electrogenic H^+ATPase found in lysosomes and renal tubular epithelium (Blair *et al.*, 1989; Bekker and Gay, 1990; Vaananen *et al.*, 1990).

There are, however, some recent data which suggest that, although the osteoclast proton pump belongs to this general family of V-ATPases, at least in the chicken it may exhibit some novel and unique pharmacological and structural features, such as sensitivity to inhibitors of both V-ATPases and P-ATPases (Chatterjee *et al.*, 1992). The possibility that both types of proton pump are present in the ruffled border also cannot be rejected (Gay, 1992). The proton pump is capable of shifting large quantities of hydrogen ions to the extracellular resorption space but, at the same time, the osteoclast must maintain neutral cytoplasmic pH and charge and is therefore required to transport equivalent amounts of acid and base and of anions and cations. Blair and his colleagues have constructed a simple yet elegant hypothesis that explains how the osteoclast could achieve net HCl transport which is electrically balanced, does not alter cytoplasmic pH and requires only one energy (ATP)-consuming process, i.e. the proton pump (Blair and Schlessinger, 1992). In this model, carbonic acid dissociates rapidly in the presence of carbonic anhydrase to produce H^+ ions and HCO_3^-. The protons are exported to the resorbing space by the ATPase, while the HCO_3^- ions are exchanged passively for Cl^- ions at the basolateral membrane, a step that is driven by the inward Cl^- gradient. The imported Cl^- ions are transferred to the resorbing space, this time against the Cl^- gradient, but the transfer is still passive because it is coupled electrostatically to the proton transporter (Figure 1.4).

This body of new information on the intracellular mechanisms involved in osteoclast acidification affords another opportunity for the rational design of drugs to inhibit excessive bone resorption in osteoporosis and other skeletal diseases, such as Paget's disease, osteoarthritis and bone tumors. If it transpires that the mammalian osteoclast proton pump possesses a unique pharmacological profile (Chatterjee *et al.*, 1992), it may be possible to deliver an agent systemically that will specifically inhibit osteoclast acid production, but will not affect vital proton transport in other organs.

Degradation of the organic matrix is achieved by a battery of proteolytic enzymes that are secreted or activated by the osteoclast. Chief among these are the cysteine proteases, cathepsins B and L (Delaisse and Vaes, 1992). These enzymes have pH optima between pH 4 and 5 (Delaisse *et al.*, 1991a). Thus osteoclast acidification of the extracellular space is not only important for mineral dissolution but also for matrix degradation. Experimental evidence for the important role of the cysteine proteases in bone resorption comes from the observations that resorption *in vitro* is correlated with the accumulation of

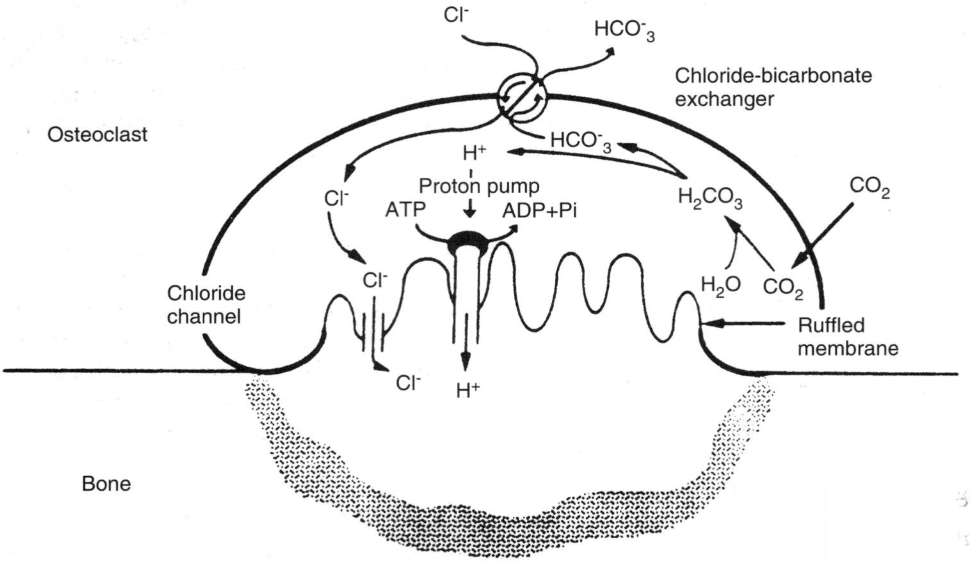

Figure 1.4 A proposed mechanism for the efficient production and transport of protons to the resorbing space. See text for further details. Reproduced with permission from Blair and Schlessinger (1992).

cathepsin B in the culture medium and that specific inhibitors of this class of enzyme reversibly inhibit bone resorption both *in vivo* and *in vitro* (Delaisse *et al.*, 1980, 1984, 1986). Blair *et al.* (1993) have recently purified a 31 kDa proteinase from enriched populations of avian osteoclasts. This enzyme was shown to be 77% identical to mammalian cathepsin Bs by cDNA cloning. An antibody to a fragment of the enzyme inhibited the ability of osteoclast lysates to degrade collagen and the enzyme was immunolocalized to osteoclasts *in situ*. Osteoclast-derived cathepsins are not only capable of degrading collagen but also non-collagenous proteins, such as osteocalcin, osteonectin and α_2HS-glycoprotein, that are present in the matrix (Page *et al.*, 1993).

There is also growing evidence that collagenase plays a role in matrix degradation. Thus, bone resorption, stimulated by a variety of agents, is accompanied by accumulation of procollagenase (Delaisse *et al.*, 1988; Delaisse and van Ngoc, 1990) and specific inhibitors of collagenase decrease bone resorption *in vivo* and *in vitro* (Delaisse *et al.*, 1985, 1991b). Osteoblasts synthesize and secrete procollagenase and production is increased by bone resorption stimulators (Heath *et al.*, 1984; Partridge *et al.*, 1987; Meikle *et al.*, 1992). Given the osteoblastic source of collagenase, Chambers has speculated that this enzyme may be involved in the removal of the thin organic layer that is purported to line free bone surfaces and, in so doing, allow osteoclasts access to the underlying mineralized matrix (Chambers *et al.*, 1985). But collagenase may also play a role in the breakdown of more mature matrix. Vaes and colleagues have hypothesized that collagenase previously incorporated in the matrix by osteoblasts, or derived from other cells, may be activated by cysteine proteases secreted by the osteoclast (Figure 1.4) (Delaisse and Vaes, 1992). Indeed, the osteoclast may not have to rely on other cells as a source of collagenase as work by Delaisse *et al.* (1992) has localized collagenase not only to the resorption space but also within the osteoclast itself. The argument that neutral collagenase would be inactive at the acidic pH of the subosteoclastic resorption space is easily circumvented by speculating that close to the bone surface the pH will be higher due to the neutralizing effect of the dissolving bone salts or that collagenase is activated when the osteoclast breaks its seal with bone and moves on to another location (Delaisse and Vaes, 1992).

REGULATION OF OSTEOCLAST ACTIVITY AND RECRUITMENT

The amount of bone resorbed by a bone remodeling unit depends on three factors:

1. the *number* of osteoclasts recruited at the site of resorption;
2. the *rate* at which each osteoclast works;
3. the *lifespan* of the osteoclasts.

Our knowledge of how the first two of these factors are regulated is growing steadily, but the last one remains a virtual mystery. As a general rule agents that stimulate osteoclast *activity* also enhance osteoclast *recruitment* (e.g. parathyroid hormone) and, conversely, agents that decrease activity also depress recruitment (e.g. calcitonin) (Holtrop, 1977; Baron and Vignery, 1977). However, there are exceptions to this rule. For example, the bisphosphonate 3-amino-1-hydroxypropylidene-1,1-bisphosphonate (APD) decreases osteoclast activity but, apparently, enhances recruitment (Marshall *et al.*, 1993). Effects on osteoclast activity are more rapid (minutes) than those on recruitment (hours), but recruitment effects are longer lasting and quantitatively more important in terms of net bone resorption. A second generalization, discussed in more detail later, is that agents that stimulate osteoclastic bone resorption do so indirectly via initial interaction with cells of the osteoblast lineage, whereas agents that inhibit osteoclast function act directly on the osteoclast itself (Rodan and Martin, 1981). Again, however, there are exceptions to this. For example, recent data suggest that one mechanism whereby bisphosphonates inhibit osteoclast activity is by decreasing osteoblastic production of osteoclast stimulatory factor(s) (Fleisch, 1993; Sahni *et al.*, 1993). Conversely, hydrogen peroxide is thought to stimulate resorptive activity by a direct action on the osteoclast itself (Zaidi *et al.*, 1993). The following section contains a brief description of the effects of four hormones on osteoclast recruitment and function. The list is not intended to be exhaustive, but rather to include those agents which may play a role in the pathogenesis and treatment of osteoporosis.

Parathyroid hormone (PTH)

PTH stimulates both the recruitment and activity of osteoclasts. The enhancement of activity is apparently mediated by cells of the osteoblast lineage (McSheehy and Chambers, 1986) (see below). While PTH increases the activation frequency of bone remodeling units, there is evidence that the net amount of bone resorbed in each unit is reduced under the influence of PTH. Thus, the resorption depth is decreased in patients with primary hyperparathyroidism (Eriksen, 1986) and cancellous bone volume and trabecular connectivity are both higher than in control subjects, despite the increase in bone turnover rate (Parisien *et al.*, 1990, 1992, 1993). Such an effect can also be demonstrated *in vitro*. Using the bone slice assay, Murrills *et al.* (1990) found that, while PTH activated quiescent osteoclasts and increased the number of resorption lacunae on the slice, the plan area of the lacunae was significantly reduced. These observations add support to the theoretical basis for the use of PTH in the treatment of osteoporosis, alleviating concerns that a PTH-mediated increase in remodeling activation frequency may lead to trabecular perforation before the positive effect of the hormone on bone formation can be realized (Dempster *et al.*, 1993a,b).

Parathyroid-related protein (PTHrP) also stimulates osteoclast activity but, interestingly, a carboxyl terminal fragment (PTHrP[107-139]) of this peptide is a potent inhibitor of osteoclast activity (Fenton *et al.*, 1991). Like calcitonin, PTHrP[107-139] appears to act directly on the osteoclast but, unlike calcitonin, it has a prolonged inhibitory effect without evidence of the 'escape' phenomenon (Fenton *et al.*, 1993). Also unlike calcitonin, PTHrP[107-139] appears to affect osteoclast differentiation of 'maturation', even in short-term cultures, as opposed to a direct inhibitory effect on the mature osteoclast.

Calcitonin (CT)

Calcitonin decreases the number of osteoclasts in bone as well as their activity. Mammalian osteoclasts possess high affinity receptors for the hormone with an estimated receptor density of over 106 copies/cell in neonatal rats, which is the highest density recorded so far for a peptide receptor (Nicholson *et al.*, 1986). Consequently, neonatal rat osteoclasts are exquisitely sensitive to the hormone with concentrations as low as 1 pg/ml causing almost complete inhibition of resorption (Dempster *et al.*, 1987). Human osteoclasts appear to be less sensitive to CT with only 70% inhibition of resorption at a concentration of 1 μg/ml of human CT (Murrills *et al.*, 1989). Human osteoclasts also fail to display the contractile response that is a characteristic feature of the CT response in neonatal rat osteoclasts (Murrills *et al.*, 1989). At the opposite end of the spectrum from rats, embryonic chick osteoclasts do not respond to CT and lack receptors for the hormone (Arnett and Dempster, 1987; Dempster *et al.*, 1987; Nicholson *et al.*, 1987), although some effects have been reported in adult birds (Belanger and Copp, 1972; Anderson *et al.*, 1982; Eliam *et al.*, 1988). As noted above, the inhibitory effect of continuous exposure to calcitonin on mammalian osteoclasts 'wears off' after several days in culture (Wener *et al.*, 1972). Moreover, Fenton *et al.* (1993) have recently shown that during the escape period, isolated osteoclasts display a 'rebound' phenomenon in which they resorb bone at a rate that is 6–80 times faster than in control cultures. The authors have suggested that this may not be due to downregulation of CT receptors but to the differentiation of CT receptor-deficient clones of osteoclasts in cultures continuously exposed to CT.

1,25 dihydroxyvitamin D [1,25(OH)$_2$D]

The active metabolite of vitamin D is a potent stimulator of bone resorption *in vitro* and *in vivo*, increasing both the number and activity of osteoclasts (Tanaka and DeLuca, 1971; Raisz *et al.*, 1972; Reynolds *et al.*, 1976; Holtrop and Raisz, 1979; Tinkler *et al.*, 1981). The *in vivo* effects of 1,25(OH)$_2$D on resorption are independent of PTH as they can be elicited in thyroparathyroidectomized animals (Reynolds *et al.*, 1976). 1,25(OH)$_2$D stimulates osteoclast activity indirectly via osteoblasts (McSheehy and Chambers, 1987). Receptors for the hormone are present in bone cells, including osteoprogenitor cells, osteoblasts, chondroblasts and chondrocytes, but have consistently been shown to be absent from osteoclasts (Stumpf and DeLuca, 1981; Merke *et al.*, 1986; Clemens *et al.*, 1988). Receptors are present, however, in circulating monocytes (Merke *et al.*, 1986) and, consistent with this observation, 1,25(OH)$_2$D appears to play an important role in the formation and differentiation of osteoclasts from hemopoietic precursors as its presence is necessary for the appearance of osteoclast-like cells in long-term cultures of bone marrow or spleen cells (Takahashi *et al.*, 1988a,b; Hattersley and Chambers, 1989). This effect appears to be mediated by transforming growth factor β (TGFβ) and prostaglandins as antibodies to TGFβ and indomethacin both inhibit the generation of osteoclast-like cells in response to 1,25(OH)$_2$D (Shinar and Rodan, 1990).

Estrogen

Estrogen plays a pivotal role in the regulation of bone resorption. Declining estrogen levels following menopause lead to an increase in the activation frequency of bone remodeling units with a resultant increase in bone resorption and formation rates (Delmas *et al.*, 1983; Fogelman *et al.*, 1984; Seibel *et al.*, 1993), which can be reversed by estrogen treatment (Riggs *et al.*, 1969; Lindsay *et al.*, 1976; Steiniche *et al.*, 1989; Seibel *et al.*, 1993). Moreover, estrogen also protects the skeleton against the resorptive effects of parathyroid hormone as directly demonstrated by Cosman *et al.* (1993). Until recently, lack of evidence of estrogen receptors in bone necessitated the construction of indirect mechanisms for estrogen's action on the skeleton. However, in 1988 two independent groups documented the presence of biologically responsive estrogen receptors in osteoblasts (Eriksen *et al.*, 1988; Komm *et al.*, 1988) and a number of authors have reported direct effects of estrogen on osteoblast or osteoblast-like cell replication and/or function (Gray *et al.*, 1987; Ernst *et al.*, 1989) (see below). More recently, convincing evidence has been obtained for the presence of estrogen receptors in avian osteoclasts (Oursler *et al.*, 1991) and somewhat less compelling evidence for their presence in human osteoclasts (Pensler *et al.*, 1990).

Despite the evidence for receptors in bone, direct effects of estrogen on bone resorption have been variable and generally difficult to demonstrate *in vitro*, at least in mammalian systems (Caputo *et al.*, 1976). Using cultures of neonatal mouse calvariae, Pilbeam *et al.* (1989) reported that 17β-estradiol in the pM to nM range inhibited prostaglandin E_2 release by 50–70%, but PTH-stimulated resorption was only inhibited by 10–20% with no dose dependency. Moreover, resorption was inhibited to a similar degree by 17α-estradiol, which has substantially less affinity for the estrogen receptor. Using the bone slice assay, Tobias and Chambers (1991) found that, in the presence of added osteoblasts, 17β-estradiol inhibited osteoclastic resorption by 25% at a concentration of 1 nmol/l, but not at higher or lower concentrations. Surprisingly, these authors also reported that, in the absence of added osteoblasts, 17β-estradiol had a **stimulatory** effect on resorption.

Recent work suggests that estrogen may depress bone resorption by enhancing the elaboration of a factor that inhibits osteoblast-derived resorption stimulating activity (BRSA) (Ishii *et al.*, 1993). Using isolated avian osteoclasts, Oursler *et al.* have demonstrated a 70% reduction in resorption pit number with 10^{-8}M 17β-estradiol and an unexpected increase in pit formation with 10^{-8}M 17α-estradiol (Oursler *et al.*, 1993). The reduction in resorption was accompanied by a reversible, dose-dependent decrease in lysosomal protein mRNA levels.

Perhaps one reason why the effects of estrogen on mammalian bone resorption have been difficult to demonstrate *in vitro* is that the hormone primarily affects osteoclast recruitment rather than the activity of the mature cell. Another reason could be the involvement of local factors in mediating estrogen action. Pacifici and his colleagues have implicated interleukin-1 and other cytokines (tumor necrosis factor and granulocyte-macrophage colony stimulating factor) in this regard, based on their observations that monocytic production of these resorption stimulators is increased following menopause and in osteoporotic women and, furthermore, that the increase can be reversed by hormone replacement therapy (Pacifici *et al.*, 1987, 1989) (Figure 1.5). Jilka and colleagues have obtained more definitive evidence, albeit in an animal model, implicating interleukin-6 (Figure 1.6) (Jilka *et al.*, 1992). They quantified osteoclasts in the cancellous bone of the rat tibia. As expected, ovariectomy increased the number of osteoclasts and this could be reversed not only by treatment with 17β-estradiol but also by a neutralizing

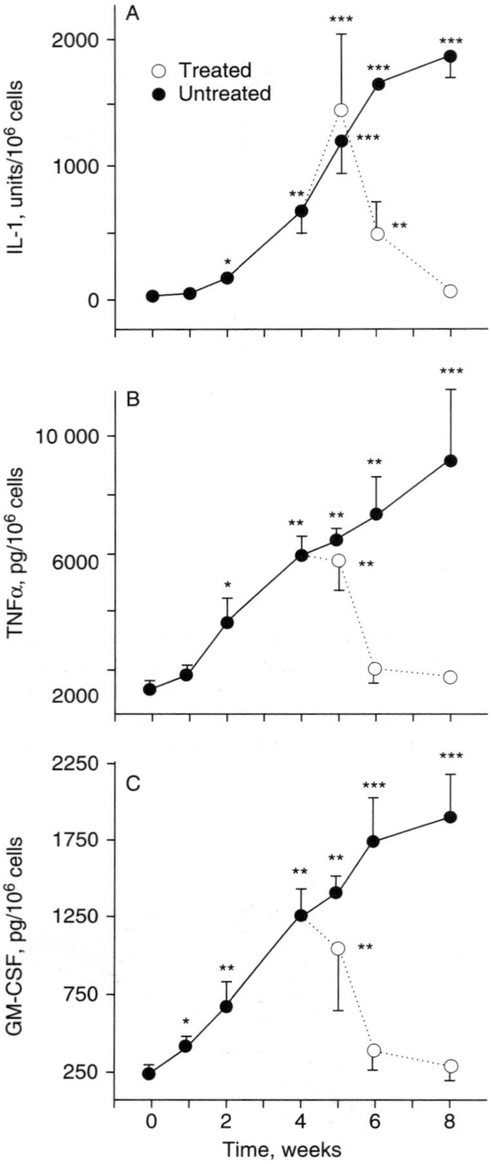

Figure 1.5 Effect of surgical menopause (closed circles) and subsequent estrogen therapy (open circles) on cytokine release from human blood mononuclear cells. IL-1 = interleukin-1; TNFα = tumor necrosis factor α; GM-CSF = granulocyte-macrophage colony-stimulating factor. $^*p = 0.05$, $^{**}p < 0.005$; $^{***}p < 0.0005$ compared to baseline. Reproduced with permission from Pacifici *et al.* (1991) *Proc Natl Acad Sci USA* **88**: 5134–8.

monoclonal antibody to IL-6. Another neutralizing antibody (to β-glactosidase) of the same isotype had no effect. Similar results were obtained when the investigators studied osteoclast formation in long-term cultures of bone marrow from the treated animals. The authors hypothesize that bone and bone marrow cells produce cytokines, such as IL-6, which promote osteoclast development. In the estrogen-replete state, the production and/or action of these cytokines is inhibited by estrogen. In the estrogen-deficient state, this inhibition is removed, leading to enhanced osteoclast formation and increased bone loss (Figure 1.7).

ORIGIN AND PROPERTIES OF THE OSTEOBLAST LINEAGE

The term 'osteoblast' has been used mainly to describe those cells in bone which are responsible for the synthesis of the components of the organic matrix of bone. These can be recognized as plump, cuboidal cells lying on the matrix which they have synthesized. It is important to recognize, however, that cells with many different functions comprise the osteoblast lineage. The latter derives from a multipotential pluripotent stem cell (review by Owen, 1988), products of which appear as osteogenic cells in the stromal compartment of marrow. They appear also as preosteoblasts in bone, as osteocytes, trapped behind the advancing mineralization front, and as 'lining cells' or 'resting' osteoblasts, which line trabecular and endosteal surfaces in very large numbers, having completed their synthetic functions. There are many phenotypic properties associated with the osteoblast lineage, varying combinations of which will be expressed by the different members of the osteoblast lineage, depending on stage of differentiation and most likely upon location in bone. It is not appropriate to consider that expression of all or even the majority of these properties is required in order for a cell to be called an osteoblast.

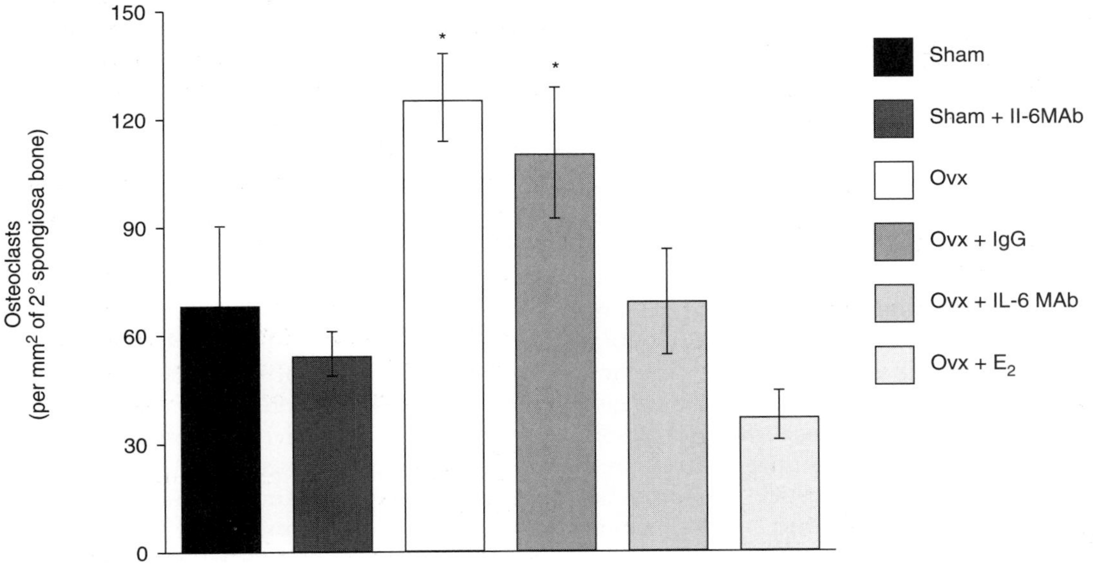

Figure 1.6 Effects of ovariectomy followed by treatment with a monoclonal antibody to interleukin-6 on the number of osteoclasts in rat cancellous bone. From left to right, the treatments are sham operation, sham operation + IL-6 antibody, ovariectomy, ovariectomy + IgG (antibody control), ovariectomy + IL-6 antibody, ovariectomy + estrogen. Ovariectomy caused a significant increase in osteoclast number, which could be reversed by treatment with the antibody to IL-6 or estrogen. Drawn from data presented in Jilka *et al.* (1992).

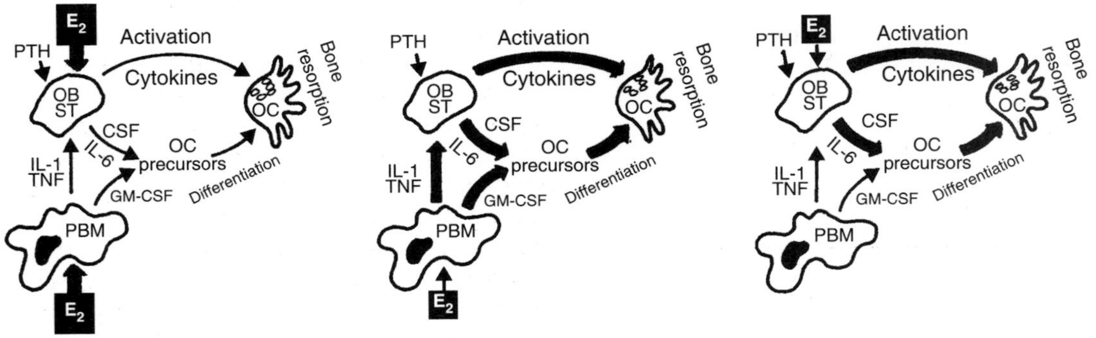

Figure 1.7 Proposed mechanisms for the role of cytokines in mediating the effect of estrogen on bone resorption. The left-hand panel illustrates that when estrogen levels are high, production of cytokines by peripheral blood monocytes and marrow stromal cells or osteoblasts is low. As a result differentiation of osteoclasts from precursors is kept in check. The middle and right-hand panels illustrate that when estrogen levels decline, peripheral blood monocytes (middle panel) and marrow stromal cells secrete more cytokines, leading to enhanced osteoclast differentiation and activity. OB = osteoblasts; ST = stromal cells; OC = osteoclast. Other abbreviations as in legend to Figure 1.5. Reproduced with permission from Horowitz (1993).

The pluripotent nature of osteogenic stem cells was proposed from the work of Friedenstein (1976), in studies of stromal cell differentiation in which diffusion chambers were implanted into rabbits. Bone marrow cells processed in this way after *in vitro* culture were able to form several tissues *in vivo*, including bone. These observations were extended by Ashton *et al.* (1984) and Bab *et al.* (1984), who showed that if cells taken from close to the endosteal surface of rabbit long bones were treated in this way, this population was clearly more osteogenic. In these and other early experiments, the bulk of evidence suggested that the mesenchymal precursors were capable of differentiation by four distinct pathways: myocytic, chondrocytic, adipocytic and osteogenic. More recent evidence in support of this has been provided in studies of clonal populations from fetal rat bones (Grigoriadis *et al.*, 1988; Aubin *et al.*, 1990). It is particularly intriguing to note the close inverse relationship between adipocytic and osteogenic development observed in marrow cultures (Beresford *et al.*, 1992), an observation which may be relevant to the increased amount of adipose tissue in bone marrow in the elderly and in osteoporotics at all ages (Meunier *et al.*, 1971; Minaire *et al.*, 1984; Burckhardt *et al.*, 1987).

Clearly it will be of great interest to define the mechanisms by which the mesenchymal stem cell system provides mature members of four diverse tissue types. The processes of commitment might be analogous to those mapped through the hemopoietic pathway. The interdependence of osteogenic and adipocytic development might provide useful clues to begin this search. In the meantime, studies of osteoblast differentiation have been confined to observations on isolated cells. Such work will provide a very useful guide to investigation of states of osteoblast differentiation in bone as an organ, using various *in situ* methods now that these are becoming available.

The stromal fibroblast of bone marrow is rich in rough endoplasmic reticulum, microtubules and microfilaments, consistent with its ability to synthesize macromolecules. The progression to cells which are overtly osteogenic can be demonstrated readily in appropriate experiments, but even the unselected marrow stromal cell shares certain properties with osteoblasts – most strikingly the ability to promote osteoclast formation. This property of the lineage will be discussed in detail later, but it was suggested by certain of the experiments of Friedenstein (1981), in which single stromal cell colonies, transplanted under the renal capsule of mice, formed bone in which hemopoiesis established and a marrow colony was excavated. Stromal cells are essential for the formation of osteoclasts in long-term murine bone marrow cultures (Suda *et al.*, 1992) and osteoclast formation from spleen cells can be promoted in contact-dependent cocultures with either osteoblasts (Takahashi *et al.*, 1988a) or clonal stromal cells (Udagawa *et al.*, 1989).

Of the three 'mature' members of the osteoblast lineage, the best recognized are the active synthetic osteoblasts. Their capacity for protein synthesis is evident from their prominent Golgi apparatus and basophilic cytoplasm rich in endoplasmic reticulum. They possess gap junctions connecting them to their neighbors and to adjacent bone-lining cells (Doty, 1981). They also communicate with osteocytes beneath the bone surface through a network of canaliculi (Figure 1.8) and synthesize the components of the ground substance of bone. These include type I collagen, osteopontin, osteonectin, osteocalcin, matrix Gla protein, biglycan and decorin (see above). They are rich in alkaline phosphatase, the function of which may be to contribute to the mineralization process. Several hormones act directly upon osteoblasts, including parathyroid hormone (PTH), 1,25-dihydroxycholecalciferol, glucocorticoids and growth hormone. The cells have receptors for and respond to certain growth factors whose local production and action are vital determinants

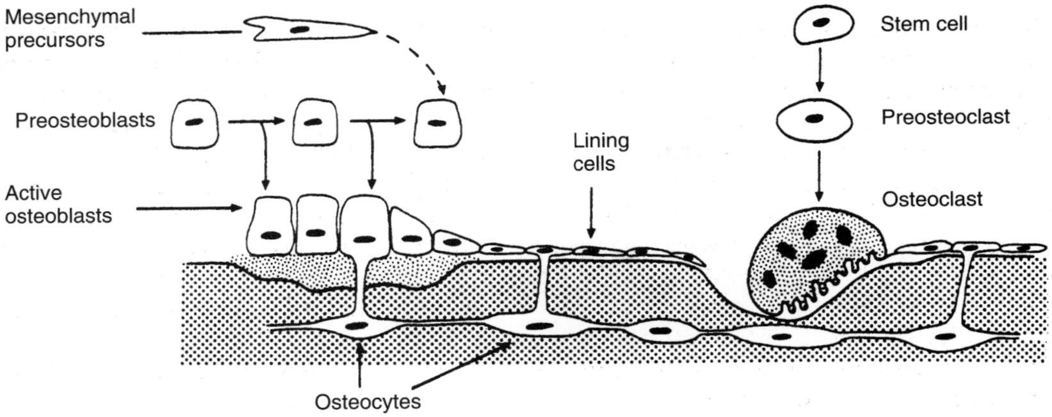

Figure 1.8 The developing and mature cells of bone, illustrating the connections between osteocytes and surface cells.

of bone growth and development. The most important of these, transforming growth factor β (TGFβ), insulin-like growth factor 1 (IGF-1) and bone morphogenetic proteins (BMPs) will be discussed in detail later.

Bone-lining cells, having largely lost their synthetic function, have little cytoplasm or endoplasmic reticulum and somewhat less cytoplasmic basophilia and alkaline phosphatase staining. Numerically they are the most abundant cells of the osteoblast lineage in bone, lining as they do the endosteal surfaces and trabeculae (Miller and Jee, 1987). Although they no longer contribute to the synthesis of structural macromolecules of bone, they nevertheless share several phenotypic properties with synthetic osteoblasts, including receptors for hormones, cytokines and growth factors and the ability to produce certain cytokines and growth factors with important local functions. The lining cells provide a barrier which might serve to prevent access of osteoclasts to the bone surface, a barrier removed with the onset of cellular contraction in response to bone-resorbing hormones or cytokines (Jones and Boyde, 1976; Rodan and Martin, 1981). This is one of several possible roles of lining cells in intercellular communication in bone. Others include the production of factors which promote osteoclast formation or activity (Martin *et al.*, 1979; Chambers, 1980; Rodan and Martin, 1981), the production of cytokines acting locally upon other members of the osteoblast lineage and the production of proteases which contribute to tissue turnover and growth factor activation. There is little doubt that lining cells and synthetic osteoblasts are closely related cells. Although we have spoken of the lining cell as an osteoblast which has completed its synthetic functions, we cannot be certain that lining cells and synthetic osteoblasts do not follow divergent pathways at a late stage of differentiation or even whether synthetic osteoblasts can be formed from lining cells.

The third mature member of the osteoblast lineage is the osteocyte. The osteocytes are osteoblasts which have become embedded in bone after being trapped behind the advancing mineralization front. They are located at lacunae and are connected with each other and with the osteoblasts and lining cells on the surface by means of intercellular processes which extend along canaliculi. It seems likely that this physical arrangement equips osteocytes to take an active part in intercellular communication in bone, for example by sensing pressure changes, and transmitting chemical messengers to surface cells, programming formation or resorption responses as appropriate. Many of our views of osteocyte function are speculative, because with all the bone cell culture systems which have been used, it is difficult to appreciate what properties might be those of osteocytes. The recent advent of the reagents and methods for the study of protein and mRNA synthesis by *in situ* methods in sections of bone from organ culture and *in vivo* experiments will surely advance our understanding of osteocyte function.

DIFFERENTIATION OF OSTEOBLASTS

Studies of osteoblast differentiation in a number of rodent cell culture systems have provided a clear indication of the heterogeneity of the cells within the osteoblast lineage. They have also focused attention upon the potent ability of several hormones and cytokines to influence progression of cells through the differentiation pathways. Among the most studied of these agents are retinoic acid (RA), 1,25-dihydroxyvitamin D_3, the BMP and TGFβ. Interesting though these studies have been, their greatest use is likely to be in the background information which they provide for the studies beginning now, of *in situ* properties of bone cells in different locations in bone and at different stages of development.

Concepts of the 'osteoblast phenotype' have arisen from these investigations of primary cell cultures, osteogenic sarcoma cell lines, certain stable and transformed cell lines and organ culture (Majeska *et al.*, 1980; Aubin *et al.*, 1982; Partridge *et al.*, 1983; Ng *et al.*, 1985, 1988, 1989a,b; Bellows *et al.*, 1986; Yoon *et al.*, 1987; Heath *et al.*, 1989; Stein *et al.*, 1989; Owen *et al.*, 1990; Strauss *et al.*, 1990; Yamaguchi *et al.*, 1991). Clonal cell lines, whether transformed or not, have provided useful model systems for study, representing as they might osteoblasts arrested at a particular point in the developmental sequence (e.g. as proposed by Greaves (1986) for other lineages). Certain of these clonal lines undergo dramatic changes in phenotype with treatments promoting differentiation, e.g. RA, TGFβ or BMPs (Ng *et al.*, 1989a,b; Heath *et al.*, 1989, 1992).

Retinoic acid, known for many years to affect bone formation and resorption (Mellanby, 1944), has been implicated recently as the natural morphogen responsible for pattern formation in chick limb buds (Thaller and Eichele, 1987; Wagner *et al.*, 1990). Treatment of osteogenic sarcoma cells or preosteoblasts with RA inhibits proliferation and confers a more differentiated phenotype (Thein and Lotan, 1982; Livesey *et al.*, 1985; Ng *et al.*, 1985, 1989a,b; Heath *et al.*, 1989; Zhou *et al.*, 1991). Of the three receptor subtypes of the RA receptor (RARα, β and γ), all were found in rat osteogenic sarcoma cells (UMR 106-06) and preosteoblasts (UMR 201) and it is interesting to note that the γ-RAR has been shown to be located specifically in the developing limb buds during mouse embryogenesis (Dolle *et al.*, 1990; Ruberte *et al.*, 1990). Some of the effects of RA on gene expression in preosteoblasts are likely to be the result of transcriptional effects (Ng *et al.*, 1989a,b; Heath *et al.*, 1992), but an interesting alternative control mechanism is suggested by evidence for RA regulation of maturation of alkaline phosphatase and osteopontin mRNA as a post-transcriptional event in the nucleus (Zhou *et al.*, 1993b). Other evidence shows that cytokines of bone or marrow origin can modify differentiation effects of agents as RA (Noda and Rodan, 1987; Ng *et al.*, 1989a; Allan *et al.*, 1990). Such interactions reinforce the view that differentiation results from co-operative effects of many humoral and local agents. Although RA has striking effects on expression of certain osteoblast genes, including those for osteopontin and matrix Gla protein (MGP) (Zhou *et al.*, 1991), in addition to alkaline phosphatase, it is likely to be only one of many possible contributors to the overall process *in vivo*. It has also been shown to promote expression of mRNA for bone morphogenetic protein 1 (BMP-1), raising the possibility of a developmental cascade proceeding after an initiating event.

Of the growth factors of bone, TGFβ and the BMPs are attracting most interest for their role as agents of osteoblast differentiation. TGFβ promotes synthesis of components of bone matrix, which most likely reflects its importance in the normal bone formation process. It also has transcriptional effects on certain genes, in preosteoblasts (Zhou *et al.*, 1991, 1993a) and modifies phenotypic effects of RA (Zhou *et al.*, 1993a), all of which are consistent with a role in osteoblastic differentiation. This is reinforced by the demonstration that local injection of TGFβ into the subperiosteal region of newborn rat bone results in localized intramembranous bone formation (Noda and Camilliere, 1989; Marcelli *et al.*, 1990) and chondrogenesis followed by endochondral ossification when the cartilage is replaced by bone (Joyce *et al.*, 1990).

The BMPs belong to a group of proteins which act to induce the differentiation of mesenchymal-type cells into chondrocytes and osteoblasts before initiating bone formation (Urist, 1989). Several members of this family have been isolated, cloned and expressed as recombinant proteins (Wang *et al.*, 1988, 1990; Wozney *et al.*, 1988; Celeste *et al.*, 1990). BMP is a novel protein but the remaining BMPs have been included in the TGFβ superfamily, based on homology of protein structure. In studies of the actions of TGFβ and BMP-4 on preosteoblasts, unique effects of the two have been clearly shown, but some actions overlap.

The differences between their actions support the concept that co-ordinated expression of different members of the TGFβ superfamily is required to control the progression of different cell types through their differentiation pathways. Overlapping but temporally and spatially distinct patterns of BMP-2, Vgr-1 (BMP-6) (Celeste *et al.*, 1990), TGFβ1 and TGFβ2 mRNAs were found to be expressed in different populations of mesenchymal cells in the developing skeletal system (Lyons *et al.*, 1989). During the development of long bones, BMP-2 was first expressed and localized in condensing precartilaginous mesenchyme, but was undetectable in chondrocyte and osteoblast lineages, all of which were shown to contain TGFβ transcripts (Pelton *et al.*, 1989). BMP-6 transcripts were expressed at the final stage of chondroblast differentiation in the form of hypertrophic chondrocyte cells. The model proposed by Lyons *et al.* (1989) postulated that different members of the TGFβ superfamily are expressed as the mesenchyme progresses down the differentiation pathway. The newly induced growth factors may then regulate the proliferation and differentiation of the cells in which they are produced in an autocrine manner. In addition, they may also act on additional cell types in the differentiation pathway in a paracrine manner to ensure a co-ordinated progression through the lineage. The same pattern of sequential regulation by members of the TGFβ superfamily in the control of the progression of specific cell types through their differentiation pathways may also apply to osteoblast differentiation.

Future studies are likely to consider the regulation of osteoblast differentiation by BMPs as autocrine factors. For example, the production of BMPs and their actions upon cells at a very early stage of differentiation may prime them for the co-operative effects of cytokines, growth factors or hormones (Urist, 1989). Evidence for such a mechanism is obtained from experiments in which treatment of osteoblast precursors with BMP-2 led to striking induction of osteocalcin expression by 1,25-dihydroxyvitamin D_3 (Yamaguchi *et al.*, 1991).

1,25-dihydroxyvitamin D_3 is a further

major influence on osteoblastic differentiation, which modulates expression in osteoblasts of several genes, including type I collagen, alkaline phosphatase, osteopontin, osteocalcin and MGP (Majeska and Rodan, 1982; Canalis and Lian, 1985; Prince and Butler, 1987; Fraser *et al.*, 1988; Lian *et al.*, 1989). A notable feature of its pleiotropic effects is that these genes are expressed at different stages of progression of the osteoblast through the differentiation pathway. The effects of the vitamin D hormone on expression of specific genes are dependent on the differentiation stage and apparently conflicting data are explained by this (Manolagas *et al.*, 1981; Majeska and Rodan, 1982; Owen *et al.*, 1991). Such differing responses could result from transcription factors changing throughout differentiation (Owen *et al.*, 1990) or from a variety of effects of matrix components on hormone responses (Owen *et al.*, 1991). The vitamin D role is probably one of a hormonal regulator of differentiation, which can either enhance or decrease expression of osteoblastic properties, depending on the stage of differentiation and the nature of the matrix.

Such a model of the vitamin D role could easily apply to other hormonal influences on osteoblast differentiation – for example, parathyroid hormone. In this discussion we have considered only a few examples of differentiating agents and mechanisms to illustrate the co-operative interactions which must occur and to emphasize the importance of understanding the molecular mechanisms operating in the differentiation processes. The renewal of osteoblast populations from precursors is a vital physiological process and defects are likely to provide the basis of several forms of osteoporosis (Marie *et al.*, 1991).

BONE FORMATION

The ordered formation of bone requires that osteoblasts synthesize a type I collagen-rich matrix which mineralizes to form mature bone. A number of non-collagenous proteins influence the mineralization process, either individually or collectively in the extracellular matrix. Replication of osteoblast precursors is obviously important, in addition to their faithful differentiation. The several growth factors of bone are mitogenic for osteoblasts and these events can also be influenced by hormones, e.g. PTH. However, it is likely that the most important effects of hormones on the bone formation process are the result of their ability to influence formation and/or activation of focal growth factors. Some of the more obvious examples of this will be discussed in some detail, because they can convey the idea of the importance of local regulation in bone cell function.

RECEPTORS FOR HORMONES AND CYTOKINES IN OSTEOBLASTS

The evidence for PTH receptors and direct actions upon cells of the osteoblast lineage is overwhelming. It comes from studies of hormonal responses in normal and malignant osteoblasts (Luben and Cohn, 1976; Martin *et al.*, 1976; Partridge *et al.*, 1981) and from direct demonstration of specific binding by autoradiography to osteoblasts *in vitro* (Silve *et al.*, 1982; Evely *et al.*, 1991) and *in vivo* (Rouleau *et al.*, 1986). There is no convincing evidence that PTH binds specifically to osteoclasts. The few claims to the contrary (Teti *et al.*, 1991; Agarwala and Gay, 1992) have either not been confirmed or applied inadequate controls for specificity (Rao *et al.*, 1983). Subsequent actions of PTH upon osteoblasts include stimulation of production of plasminogen activator (PA) activity through inhibition of PAI-1 formation (Fukumoto *et al.*, 1992a) and promotion of collagenase and tissue inhibitor of metalloproteinase (TIMP) production (Sakamoto *et al.*, 1975; Heath *et al.*, 1984; Partridge *et al.*, 1987) (Figure 1.3). The actions of PTH-related protein on osteoblasts are essentially identical to those of PTH and although receptors for PGE_2 have not been demonstrated directly on osteoblasts, its specific actions closely resemble those of PTH. Thus each of these bone-resorbing factors acts directly upon osteoblasts. It was this realization that resorbing hormones specifically act upon osteoblasts, but not osteoclasts, that led to the proposal that the initial hormonal step in bone resorption is through cells of the osteoblast lineage, which are in turn responsible for the formation and activation of osteoclasts (Martin *et al.*, 1979; Chambers, 1980; Rodan and Martin, 1981).

Osteoblasts also exhibit specific receptors for 1,25-dihydroxyvitamin D_3, as they do for the bone-resorbing cytokines interleukin 1 (IL-1), tumor necrosis factor α (TNFα) and leukemia inhibitory factor (LIF) (Thomson *et al.*, 1986, 1987; Allan *et al.*, 1990). In the case of PTH and each of these bone-resorbing agents, ample evidence has been produced that osteoblasts, most likely lining cells, are responsible for the activation of existing osteoclasts and probably also the generation of new osteoclasts (Chambers and Fuller, 1985; Chambers, 1985; Thomson *et al.*, 1986, 1987; Takahashi *et al.*, 1988a; Evely *et al.*, 1991).

One of the most striking hormonal influences on bone *in vivo* is that of estrogen, withdrawal of which results in substantial bone loss due to increased bone resorption. The action of estrogen on bone has never been adequately explained but, as noted above, recent evidence has revealed the presence of low numbers of estrogen receptors in osteoblasts (Eriksen *et al.*, 1988; Komm *et al.*, 1988). Furthermore, estrogen treatment of osteoblasts has resulted in increased production of mRNA and protein for IGF-1 (Ernst *et al.*, 1989), most likely through a transcriptional effect. Growth hormone has also been shown to have specific receptors on osteoblasts (Barnard *et al.*, 1991), although it has not been shown in these cells that growth hormone causes an increased production of IGF-1. The data with regard to direct oestrogen effects on osteoblasts are tantalizing for their suggestion that estrogen may positively influence bone formation. On the other hand, these results have been obtained in cultures of either transformed or neonatal osteoblasts. Estrogen was found to have no detectable effect on parameters of growth or differentiation of osteoblast-rich cell cultures of normal adult human origin (Keeting *et al.*, 1991). These workers point to the lack of evidence for a stimulating effect of estrogen on bone formation *in vivo* and propose that the antiresorptive effect of the hormone might be mediated through the osteoblast (lining cell).

Several peptide growth factors have receptors on or evoke responses from osteoblasts (reviewed in Martin *et al.*, 1989). Epidermal growth factor (EGF) receptors are located in normal and malignant osteoblasts and EGF treatment results in increased DNA synthesis and cell division. Similar effects are produced by TGFα and both of these peptides are promoters of bone resorption. Two of the most abundant growth factors in bones are TGFβ and IGF-1, both of which act directly on osteoblasts to influence the synthesis of a number of the organic components of bone.

OSTEOBLAST LINEAGE AND BONE RESORPTION

In the foregoing discussion, we have drawn attention to the considerable evidence that cells of the osteoblast lineage are central mediators of bone resorption. The implication is that they produce activators of existing osteoclasts and promoters of osteoclast formation from precursors.

The nature of the putative osteoclast resorption stimulating activity (ORSA) is unknown. Its unequivocal demonstration seems to require experiments in which osteoclasts are co-cultured with osteoblasts, although there were some early reports that conditioned medium from osteoblast cultures could stimulate highly purified osteoclasts to resorb bone.

In addition to this role in osteoclast activation, there is considerable evidence (reviewed by Suda *et al.*, 1992) that the formation of osteoclasts is also mediated by cells of the osteoblast lineage. This has been demonstrated by using spleen cells as a source of osteoclasts in co-cultures with osteoblasts (Takahashi *et al.*, 1988a) or with marrow-derived stromal cells (Udagawa *et al.*, 1989). An important aspect of this work is the evidence that cell–cell contact is necessary for the promotion of osteoclast formation by osteoblasts or stromal cells. Although the data in these experiments are convincing, it has been shown by two groups that osteoclast development from precursors can in some circumstances proceed apparently without participation of stromal cells or osteoblasts (Kurihara *et al.*, 1990; Hiura *et al.*, 1991). In each case the precursors were used after enrichment by colony formation. Our current view is that stromal cells/osteoblasts are required for osteoclast formation. Osteoclastogenesis might therefore be likened to myelopoiesis and lymphopoiesis, where in each case the progenitors lie in intimate association with stromal cells, and this micro-environment is essential for normal hemopoiesis to proceed (Dexter, 1982).

COUPLING OF RESORPTION TO FORMATION

The processes of bone resorption and formation are coupled, in that once osteoclastic resorption has occurred, osteoblasts respond by making the amount of bone that had been lost. This remodeling process in the skeleton is required for normal bone formation and proceeds throughout life. Balance must be achieved between resorption and formation and any change in one parameter results in a change in the other. For some time it was considered that resorbing bone might produce a particular factor which would influence the amount of bone laid down in response and indeed, some evidence was obtained for the existence of such a factor (Howard *et al.*, 1981). With increasing knowledge of local products in bone and their regulation, it is now possible to provide some explanations of the coupling process, without the need for a discrete coupling factor.

The bone-resorbng hormone, PTH, promotes the synthesis by osteoblasts of IGF-1 (Canalis *et al.*, 1989), an important bone growth factor which stimulates the formation of type I collagen and other matrix components. The biological activity of IGF-1 is determined by its association with IGF binding proteins (IGF BPs), several of which are secreted by osteoblasts. PTH has been shown to influence IGF BP production by osteoblasts (Schmid *et al.*, 1990; Torring *et al.*, 1991) and IGF BP3 production was increased in response to 1,25-dihydroxyvitamin D_3 in human osteogenic sarcoma cells (Moriwake *et al.*, 1992). The discussion of IGF-1 from its BPs plays a key role in its local bioavailability. A local control mechanism suggested for this is through the regulated production of plasmin, by control of the plasminogen activator (PA) system (Campbell *et al.*, 1992) (see below). Such a local mechanism of protease control, superimposed on the dual regulation of IGF-1 and IGF BP synthesis, could contribute to the coupling mechanism. It should be noted also that there is evidence for estrogen stimulation of IGF-1 production by osteoblasts (Ernst *et al.*, 1989). Glucocorticoids, on the other hand, inhibit IGF-1 production by osteoblasts (Canalis *et al.*, 1989) and incidentally, inhibit PA activity by promoting PAI-1 synthesis (Fukumoto *et al.*, 1992a). These actions together would favor uncoupling of formation from resorption and decrease in bone formation, effects that are a feature of glucocorticoid treatment.

A second and related mechanism which could be part of the coupling process involves another major growth factor of bone, TGFβ, and its relationship to the PA-plasmin system. The PA-plasmin system is tightly regulated in osteoblasts. Several bone-resorbing hormones and cytokines promote PA activity in osteoblast-like cells (Hamilton *et al.*, 1985) by inhibiting production of PAI-1 (Fukumoto *et al.*, 1992b). The targeted and controlled regulation of plasmin formation can lead to changes in protease activity in spatial and temporal arrangements which lead to appropriate growth factor activation. Osteoblasts synthesize TGFβ, which is stored in bone matrix in a latent, inactive form (Carrington *et al.*, 1988) capable of activation by acid or proteases, including plasmin (Allan *et al.*, 1991). We have proposed that plasmin, generated in a targeted manner through PA activation, may be responsible for the local activation of TGFβ, making it available for its stimulatory effects on synthesis of collagen and other proteins by osteoblasts (Allan *et al.*, 1990, 1991; Yee *et al.*, 1993). Such a regulated mechanism of TGFβ activation is susceptible to both humoral and local control and because of the latter, can respond to physical stimuli. Given the very large amount of latent TGFβ stored in bone matrix, it is likely that local activation mechanisms are the most important means of controlling its bioavailability. Humoral control of TGFβ synthesis, while important in terms of replenishing supply, is less likely to be significant in this respect.

NOTE IN PROOF

Published literature up to and including 1993 was reviewed for this chapter.

REFERENCES

Agarwala, N. and Gay, C.V. (1992) Specific binding of parathyroid hormone to living osteoclasts. *J Bone Miner Res* **7**: 531.

Allan, E.H., Hilton, D.J., Brown, M.A. *et al.* (1990) Osteoblasts display receptors for and responses to leukemia inhibitory factor. *J Cell Physiol* **145**: 110–19.

Allan, E.H., Zeheb, R., Gelehrter, T.D. *et al.* (1991) Transforming growth factor beta stimulates production of urokinase-type plasminogen activator mRNA and plasminogen activator inhibitor-1 mRNA and protein in rat osteoblast-like cells. *J Cell Physiol* **149**: 34.

Anderson, A.E., Schraer, H. and Gay, C.V. (1982) Ultrastructural immunocytochemical localization of carbonic anhydrase in normal and calcitonin-treated chick osteoclasts. *Anat Rec* **204**: 9.

Anderson, R.E., Woodbury, D.M. and Jee, W.S.S. (1986) Humoral and ionic and osteoclast acidity. *Calcif Tissue Int* **39**: 252.

Arnett, T.R. and Dempster, D.W. (1987) A comparative study of disaggregated chick and rat osteoclasts in vitro: effects of calcitonin and prostaglandins. *Endocrinology* **120**: 602–8.

Ashton, B.A., Eaglesome, C.C., Bab, I. and Owen, M.E. (1984) Distribution of fibroblast colony-forming cells in rabbit bone marrow and assay of their osteogenic potential by an *in vivo* diffusion chamber method. *Calcif Tissue Int* **36**: 83–6.

Aubin, J.E., Heersche, J.N.M. and Merrilees, M.J. (1982) Isolation of bone cell clones with differences in growth, hormone responses and extracellular matrix production. *J Cell Biol* **92**: 452–61.

Aubin, J.E., Heersche, J.N.M., Bellows, C.G. and Grigoriadis, A.E. (1990) Osteoblast lineage analysis in fetal rat calvarial cells. In: *Calcium Regulation and Bone Metabolism*, (eds Cohn, D.V., Glorieux, F.H. and Martin, T.J.), Elsevier Science Publishers, Amsterdam, pp. 362–70.

Bab, I., Ashton, B.A., Syftestad, G.T. and Owen, M.E. (1984) Assessment of an *in vivo* diffusion chamber method as a quantitative assay for osteogenesis. *Calcif Tissue Int* **36**: 77–82.

Barnard, R., Ng, K.W., Martin, T.J. and Waters, M.J. (1991) Growth hormone (GH) receptors in clonal osteoblast-like cells mediate a mitogenic response to GH. *Endocrinology* **128**: 1459–64.

Baron, R. and Vignery, A. (1977) Proceedings of the Second International Workshop on Bone Histomorphometry, (ed. Meunier, P.J.), pp. 147–56, Societe de la Nouvelle, Fournie.

Baron, R., Neff, L., Louvard, D. and Courtoy, P.J. (1985) Cell-mediated extracellular acidification and bone resorption: evidence for a low pH in resorbing lacunae and localization of a 100-kD lysosomal membrane protein at the osteoclast ruffled border. *J Cell Biol* **101**: 2210–22.

Bekker, P.J. and Gay, C.V. (1990) Biochemical characterization of an electrogenic vacuolar proton pump in purified chicken osteoclast plasma membrane vesicles. *J Bone Miner Res* **5**: 569.

Belanger, L.F. and Copp, D.H. (1972) In: *Calcium, Parathyroid Hormone and the Calcitonins*, (eds

Talmage, R.V. and Munson, P.L.), Excerpta Medica, Amsterdam, p. 41.

Bellows, C.G., Aubin, J.E., Heersche, J.N.M. and Antose, M.E. (1986) Mineralized nodules formed *in vitro* from enzymatically released rat calvaria populations. *Calcif Tissue Int* **38**: 143–54.

Beresford, J.N., Bennett, J.H., Devlin, C., Leboy, P.S. and Owen, M.E. (1992) Evidence for an inverse relationship between the differentiation of adipocytic and osteogenic cells in rat marrow stromal cell cultures. *J Cell Sci* **102**: 341–51.

Bianco, P., Fisher, L.W., Young, M.F., Termine, T.J. and Gehron-Robey, P. (1991) Expression of bone sialoprotein in developing human tissues. *Calcif Tissue Int* **49**: 421–6.

Blair, H.C. and Schlessinger, P.H. (1992) The mechanism of osteoclast acidification. In: *Biology and Physiology of the Osteoclast*, (eds Rifkin, B.R. and Gay, C.V.), CRC Press, Boca Raton, pp. 295–88.

Blair, H.C., Teitelbaum, S.L., Ghiselli, R. and Gluck, S. (1989) Osteoclastic bone resorption by a polarized vacuolar proton pump. *Science* **245**: 855.

Blair, H.C., Teitelbaum, S.L., Grosso, L.E. *et al.* (1993) Extracellular-matrix degradation at acid pH. *Biochem J* **290**: 873–84.

Boyde, A., Ali, A.A. and Jones, S.J. (1984) Resorption of dentine by isolated osteoclasts in vitro. *Br Dent J* **156**: 216.

Burckhardt, R., Kettner, G., Bohm, W. *et al.* (1987) Changes in trabecular bone, hematopoiesis and bone marrow vessels in aplastic anaemia, primary osteoporosis, and old age: a comparative histomorphometric study. *Bone* **8**: 157–64.

Bushinsky, D.A., Levi-Setti, R. and Coe, F.L. (1986) Ion microprobe determination of bone surface elements: effects of reduced medium pH. *Am J Physiol* **19**: F1090–F1097.

Campbell, P.G., Novak, J.F., Yanosick, T.B. and McMaster, J.H. (1992) Involvement of the plasmin system in dissociation of the insulin-like growth factor-binding protein complex. *Endocrinology* **130**: 1401–12.

Canalis, E. and Lian, J.B. (1985) 1,25-dihydroxyvitamin D3 effects on collagen and DNA synthesis in periosteum and periosteum-free calvaria. *Bone* **6**: 457–60.

Canalis, E., Centrella, M., Burch, W. and McCarthy, T.L. (1989) Insulin-like growth factor I mediates selective anabolic effects of parathyroid hormone in bone cultures. *J Clin Invest* **83**: 60–7.

Caputo, C.B., Meadow, D. and Raisz, L.G. (1976) Failure of estrogens and androgens to inhibit bone resorption in tissue culture. *Endocrinology* **98**: 1065–8.

Carrington, J.L., Roberts, A.B., Flanders, K.C., Roche, N.S. and Reddi, A.H. (1988) Accumulation, localization, and compartmentation of transforming growth factor-β during endochondral bone development. *J Cell Biol* **107**: 1969–75.

Celeste, A.J., Iannazzi, J.A., Taylor, R.C. *et al.* (1990) Identification of transforming growth factor b to family members present in bone-inductive protein purified from bovine bone. *Proc Natl Acad Sci USA* **87**: 9843–7.

Chambers, T.J. (1980) The cellular basis of bone resorption. *Clin Orthop Rel Res* **151**: 283–93.

Chambers, T.J. (1985) The pathobiology of the osteoclast. *J Clin Pathol* **38**: 241–52.

Chambers, T.J. and Fuller, K. (1985) Bone cells predispose endosteal surfaces to resorption by exposure of bone mineral to osteoclastic contact. *J Cell Sci* **76**: 155–63.

Chambers, T.J., Revell, P.A., Fuller, K. and Athanasou, N.A. (1984) Resorption of bone by isolated rabbit osteoclasts. *J Cell Sci* **66**: 383.

Chambers, T.J., Darby, J.A. and Fuller, K. (1985) Mammalian collagenase predisposes bone surfaces to osteoclastic resorption. *Cell Tissue Res* **241**: 671.

Chambers, T.J., Fuller, K., Darby, J.A, Pringle, J.A.S. and Horton, M.A. (1986) Monoclonal antibodies against osteoclasts inhibit bone resorption in vitro. *Bone Mineral* **1**: 127–35.

Chatterjee, D., Chakraborty, M., Leit, M. *et al.* (1992) The osteoclast proton pump differs in its pharmacology and catalytic subunits from other vacuolar H^+-ATPases. *J Exp Biol* **172**: 193–204.

Clemens, T.L., Garrett, K.P., Zhou, X-Y. *et al.* (1988) Immunocytochemical localization of the 1,25-dihydroxyvitamin D3 receptor in target cells. *Endocrinology* **122**: 1224–30.

Clover, J., Dodds, R.A. and Gowen, M. (1992) Integrin subunit expression by human osteoblasts and osteoclasts in situ and in culture. *J Cell Sci* **103**: 267–71.

Cosman, F., Shen, V., Xie, F. *et al.* (1993) Estrogen protection against bone resorbing effects of parathyroid hormone infusion. *Ann Intern Med* **118**: 337–43.

Currey, J. (1984) *The Mechanical Adaptations of Bones*. Princeton University Press.

Davies, J., Warwick, J., Totty, N., Philp, P., Helfrich, M. and Horton, M.A. (1989) The osteoclast functional antigen, implicated in the regulation of bone resorption, is biochemically related to the vitronectin receptor. *J Cell Biol* **109**: 1817–1826.

Delaisse, J.M. and Vaes, G. (1992) Mechanism of mineral solubilization and matrix degradation in osteoclastic bone resorption. In: *Biology and Physiology of the Osteoclast*, (eds Rifkin, B.R. and Gay, C.V.), CRC, Boca Raton, pp. 289–314.

Delaisse, J.M. and Van Ngoc, H. (1990) Induction of procollagenase in bone tissue under *in vivo* conditions. *Calcif Tissue Int* **2**: A17.

Delaisse, J.M., Eeckhout, Y. and Vaes, G. (1980) Inhibition of bone resorption in culture by inhibitors of thiol proteinase. *Biochem J* **192**: 365.

Delaisse, J.M., Eeckhout, Y. and Vaes, G. (1984) *In vivo* and *in vitro* evidence for the involvement of cysteine proteinase in bone resorption. *Biochem Biophys Res Commun* **125**: 441.

Delaisse, J.M., Eeckhout, Y., Sear, C. *et al.* (1985) A new synthetic inhibitor of mammalian tissue collagenase inhibits bone resorption in culture. *Biophys Res Commun* **133**: 483.

Delaisse, J.M., Ledent, P., Eeckhout, Y. and Vaes, G. (1986) Cysteine proteinases and bone resorption. In: *Cysteine Proteinases and Their Inhibitors*, (ed. Turk, V.), Walter de Gruyter, Berlin.

Delaisse, J.M., Eeckhout, Y. and Vaes, G. (1988) Bone-resorbing agents affect the production and distribution of procollagenase as well as the activity of collagenase in bone tissue. *Endocrinology* **123**: 264.

Delaisse, J.M., Ledent, P. and Vaes, G. (1991a) Collagenolytic cysteine proteinase of the bone tissue: cathepsin B (pro)cathepsin L and a cathepsin L-like 70 KDa proteinase. *Biochem J* **279**: 167.

Delaisse, J.M., Terlain, B., Cartwright, T., Lefebvre, V. and Vaes, G. (1991b) A collagenase inhibitor inhibits bone resorption *in vivo*, as evaluated by 3H-tetracycline retention in bones of prelabelled mice. *Bone* **12**: 289.

Delaisse, J.M., Neff, L., Eeckhout, Y. *et al.* (1992) Evidence for the presence of (Pro) collagenase in osteoclasts. *Bone Miner* **17**: 46.

Delmas, P.D. (1993) Biochemical markers of bone turnover for the clinical investigation of osteoporosis. *Osteoporosis Int* **3** (Suppl 1): s81–s86.

Delmas, P.D., Stenner, D, and Wahner, H.W. (1983) Increase in serum bone γ-carboxyglutamic acid protein with aging in women: implications for the mechanism of age-related bone loss. *J Clin Invest* **71**: 1316–21.

Dempster, D.W. (1992) Bone remodeling. In: *Disorders of Bone and Mineral Metabolism*, (eds Coe, F.L. and Favus, M.J.), Raven Press, New York, pp. 355–80.

Dempster, D.W., Murrills, R.J., Horbert, W.R. and Arnett, T.R. (1987) Biological activity of chicken calcitonin: effects of neonatal rat and embryonic chick osteoclasts. *J Bone Miner Res* **2**: 443.

Dempster, D.W., Cosman, F., Nieves, J., Shen, V. and Lindsay, R. (1993a) Proceedings of the Fourth International Symposium on Osteoporosis, (ed. Riis, B.), Osteopress, Rodovre, pp. 144–5.

Dempster, D.W., Cosman, F., Parisien, M., Shen, V. and Lindsay, R. (1993b) Anabolic actions of parathyroid hormone on bone. *Endocr Rev* **14**: 690.

Dexter, T.M. (1982) Stromal cell associated haemopoiesis. *J Cell Physiol* **1**: 87–94.

Dolle, P., Ruberte, E., Kastner, P. *et al.* (1990) Differential expression of genes encoding a, b and g retinoic receptors and CRABP in the development limbs of the mouse. *Nature* **342**: 702–5.

Doty, S.B. (1981) Morphological evidence of gap junctions between cells. *Calcif Tissue Int* **33**: 509–12.

Doty, S.B., Robinson, R.A. and Schofield, B. (1976) In: *Handbook of Physiology*, (eds Astwood, E.B. and Greep, R.O.), American Physiological Society, Washington, DC, p. 3.

Eliam, M.C., Basle, M., Bouizar, Z. *et al.* (1988) Influence of blood calcium on calcitonin receptors in isolated chick osteoclasts. *J Endocrinol* **119**: 243–8.

Eriksen, E.F. (1986) Normal and pathological remodeling of human trabecular bone: three dimensional reconstruction of the remodeling sequence in normals and in metabolic bone disease. *Endocr Rev* **7**: 379–408.

Eriksen, E.F., Colvard, D.S., Berg, N.J. *et al.* (1988) Evidence of estrogen receptors in normal human osteoblast-like cells. *Science* **241**: 84–7.

Ernst, M., Heath, J.K. and Rodan, G.A. (1989) Estradiol effects on proliferation messenger ribonucleic acid for collagen and infusion-like growth factor-I and parathyroid hormone-stimulated adenylate cyclase activity in osteoblastic cells from calvariae and long bones. *Endocrinology* **125**: 825–33.

Evely, R.S., Bonomo, A., Schneider, H-G. *et al.* (1991) Structural requirements for the action of parathyroid hormone-related protein (PTHrP) on bone resorption by isolated osteoclasts. *J Bone Miner Res* **6**: 85–94.

Fenton, A.J., Kemp, B.E., Kent, G.N. *et al.* (1991) A carboxyl-terminal peptide from the parathyroid hormone-related protein inhibits bone resorption by osteoclasts. *Endocrinology* **129**: 1762–8.

Fenton, A.J., Martin, T.J. and Nicholson, G.C. (1993) Long term culture of disaggregated rat osteoclasts: inhibition of bone resorption and reduction of osteoclast-like cell number by calcitonin and pthrp(107–139). *J Cell Physiol* **155**: 1–7.

Fleisch, H. (1993) New bisphosphonates in osteoporosis. *Osteoporosis Int* **2**: s15–s22.

Fogelman, I., Poser, J.W., Smith, M.L. *et al.* (1984) Alterations in skeletal metabolism following oophorectomy. In: Osteoporosis, Proceedings of Copenhagen International Symposium Stiftsbogtrykkery, 519–21.

Fraser, J.D., Otawara, Y. and Price, P.A. (1988) 1,25-dihydroxyvitamin D3 stimulates the synthesis of matrix γ-carboxyglutamic acid protein by osteosarcoma cells: mutually exclusive expression of vitamin K-dependent bone proteins by clonal osteoblastic cell lines. *J Biol Chem* **263**: 911–16.

Friedenstein, A.J. (1976) Precursor cells of mechanocytes. *Int Rev Cytol* **46**: 327–55.

Friedenstein, A.J. (1981) Stromal mechanisms of bone marrow: cloning *in vitro* and transplantation *in vivo*. *Haematol Bluttranofus* **25**: 19–29.

Fukumoto, S., Allan, E.H., Zeheb, R., Gelehrter, T.D. and Martin, T.J. (1992a) Glucocorticoid regulation of plasminogen activator inhibitor-1 mRNA and protein in normal and malignant osteoblasts. *Endocrinology* **130**: 797–804.

Fukumoto, S., Allan, E.H., Yee, J.A., Gelehrter, T.D. and Martin, T.J. (1992b) Plasminogen activator regulation in osteoblasts: parathyroid hormone inhibition of type-1 plasminogen activator inhibitor and its mRNA. *J Cell Physiol* **152**: 346–55.

Gay, C.V. (1992) Osteoclast ultrastructure and enzyme histochemistry: functional implications. In: *Biology and Physiology of the Osteoclast*, (eds Rifkin, B.R. and Gay, C.V.), CRC, Boca Raton, pp. 120–5.

Glimcher, M.J. (1981) On the form and function of bone: from molecules to organs. Wolff's law revisited. In: *The Chemistry and Biology of Mineralized Connective Tissues*, (ed. Veis, A.), Elsevier, North Holland, pp. 618–73.

Glimcher, M.J. (1992) The nature of the mineral component of bone and the mechanism of calcification. In: *Disorders of Bone and Mineral Metabolism*, (eds Coe, F.L. and Favus, M.J.), Raven Press, New York, pp. 265–86.

Gray, T.K., Flynn, T.C., Gray, K.M. and Nabell, L.M. (1987) 17-b estradiol acts directly on the clonal osteoblast cell line UMR 1006. *Proc Natl Acad Sci USA* **84**: 6267–71.

Greaves, M.F. (1986) Differentiation-linked leukemogenesis in lymphocytes. *Science* **234**: 697–704.

Grigoriadis, A.E., Heersche, J.N.M. and Aubin, J.E. (1988) Differentiation of muscle, fat, cartilage, and bone from progenitor cells present in a bone-derived clonal cell population: effect of dexamethasone. *J Cell Biol* **106**: 2139–51.

Hamilton, J.A., Lingelbach, S.R., Partridge, N.C. and Martin, T.J. (1985) Regulation of plasminogen activator production by bone resorbing hormones in normal and malignant osteoblasts. *Endocrinology* **116**: 2186–91.

Hattersley, G. and Chambers, T.J. (1989) Generation of osteoclastic function in mouse bone marrow culture: multinuclearity and tartrate-resistant acid phosphatase are unreliable markers for osteoclastic differentiation. *Endocrinology* **124**: 1689–96.

Hauschka, P.V. (1986) The vitamin K-dependent Ca^{2+} binding protein of bone matrix. *Haemostasis* **16**: 258–72.

Heath, J.K., Atkinson, S.J., Meikle, M.C. and Reynolds, J.J. (1984) Mouse osteoblasts synthesize collagenase in response to bone resorbing agents. *Biochim Biophys Acta* **802**: 151–4.

Heath, J.K., Rodan, S.B., Yoon, K. and Rodan, G.A. (1989) Rat calvarial cell lines immortalized with SV-40 large T antigen: constitutive and retinoic acid-inducible expression of osteoblastic features. *Endocrinology* **124**: 3060–8.

Heath, J.K., Suva, L.J., Kiledjian, M., Martin, T.J. and Rodan, G.A. (1992) Retinoic acid stimulates transcriptional activity from the alkaline phosphatase promoter in the immortalized rat calvarial cell line RCT-1. *Mol Endocrinol* **6**: 636–46.

Helfrich, M.H., Nesbitt, S.A. and Horton, M.A. (1992) Integrins on rat osteoclasts: characterization of two monoclonal antibodies (F4 and F11) to rat β3. *J Bone Miner Res* **7**: 345–51.

Hiura, K., Sumitani, D., Kawata, T. *et al.* (1991) Mouse osteoblastic cells (MC3T3-E1) at different stages of differentiation have opposite effects on osteoclastic cell formation. *Endocrinology* **128**: 1630–7.

Holtrop, M.E. (1977) In Proceedings of the Second International Workshop on Bone Histomorphometry, (ed. Meunier, P.J.), pp. 133–145, Societe de la Nouvelle, Fournie.

Holtrop, M.E. and Raisz, L.G. (1979) Comparison of the effects of 1,25-dihydroxycholecalciferol, prostaglandin E2 and osteoclast activating factor with parathyroid hormone on the ultrastructure of osteoclasts in cultural long bone of fetal rats. *Calcif Tissue Int* **29**: 201.

Horowitz, M.C. (1993) Cytokines and estrogen in bone: anti-osteoporotic effects. *Science* **260**: 626–7.

Horton, M.A. and Davies, J. (1989) Perspectives: adhesion receptors in bone. *J Bone Miner Res* **4**: 803–7.

Horton, M.A., Taylor, M.L., Arnett, T.R. and Helfrich, M.H. (1991) Arg-Gly-Asp (RGD) peptides and the anti vitronectin receptor antibody 23C6 inhibit dentine bone resorption and cell spreading by osteoclast. *Exp Cell Res* **195**: 368–75.

Howard, G.A., Bottemiller, B.L., Turner, R.T., Rader, J.I. and Byalink D.J. (1981) Parathyroid hormone stimulates bone formation and resorption in organ culture: evidence for a coupling mechanism. *Proc Natl Acad Sci USA* **78**: 3204–8.

Hughes, D.E., Salter, D.M., Dedhar, S. and Simpson, R. (1993) Integrin expression in human bone. *J Bone Miner Res* **8**: 527–32.

Hunter, S.J., Schraer, H. and Gay, C.V. (1988) Characterization of isolated and cultured chick osteoclasts: the effects of acetazolamid, calcitonin, and parathyroid hormone on acid production. *J Bone Miner Res* **3**: 297.

Hunter, S.J., Rosen, C.J. and Gay, C.V. (1991) *In vitro* resorptive activity of isolated chick osteoclast: effects of carbonic anhydrase inhibition. *J Bone Miner Res* **6**: 61.

Ishii, T., Saito, T., Morimoto, K. *et al.* (1993) Estrogen stimulates the elaboration of cell/matrix surface-associated inhibitory factor of osteoclastic bone resorption from osteoblastic cells. *Biochem Biophys Res Commun* **191**: 495–502.

Jilka, R., Hangoc, G., Girasole, G. *et al.* (1992) Increased osteoclast development after estrogen loss: mediation by interleukin-6. *Science* **257**: 88–91.

Jones, S.J. and Boyde, A. (1976) Experimental study of changes in osteoblast shape induced by calcitonin and parathyroid extract in an organ culture system. *Cell Tissue Res* **169**: 449–65.

Joyce, M.E., Roberts, A.B., Sporn, M.B. and Bolander, M.E. (1990) Transforming growth factor-b and the initiation of chondrogenesis and osteogenesis in the rat femur. *J Cell Biol* **110**: 2196–207.

Keeting, P.E., Scott, R.E., Colvard, D.S. *et al.* (1991) Lack of a direct effect of estrogen on proliferation and differentiation of normal human osteoblast-like cells. *J Bone Miner Res* **6**: 297–304.

Kolliker, A. (1873) *Die normale resorption des knochengewebes and ihre bedeutug fur die entsehung der typischen knochenformen*. Vogel, Leipzig.

Komm, B.S., Terpening, C.M., Benz, D.J. *et al.* (1988) Estrogen binding receptor mRNA, and biologic response in osteoblast-like osteosarcoma cells. *Science* **241**: 81–4.

Kurihara, N., Chenu, C., Miller, M., Civin, C. and Roodman, G.D. (1990) Identification of committed mononuclear precursors for osteoclast-like cells formed in long term human marrow cultures. *Endocrinology* **126**: 2733–41.

Lakkakorpi, P.T., Horton, M.A., Helfich, M.H., Karhukorpi, E.K. and Vaananen, H.K. (1991) Vitronectin receptor has a role in bone resorption but does not mediate tight sealing zone attachment of osteoclasts to the bone surface. *J Cell Biol* **115**: 1179–86.

Lemann, J., Litzow, J.R. and Lennon, E.J. (1966) The effect of chronic acid loads in normal man: further evidence for the participation of bone mineral in the defense against chronic metabolic acidosis. *J Clin Invest* **45**: 1608.

Leushner, J.R. (1983) Heterogeneity in the collagens extracted from human embryonic calvaria. *Can J Biochem Cell Biol* **61**: 1012–17.

Lian, J.B., Tassinari, M. and Glowacki, J.G. (1984) Resorption of implanted bone from normal and warfarin treated rats. *J Clin Invest* **73**: 1223.

Lian, J.B., Dunn, K. and Key Jr, L.L. (1986) *In vitro* degradation of bone particles by human monocytes is decreased with the depletion of the vitamin k-dependent bone protein from the matrix. *Endocrinology* **118**: 1636.

Lian, J.B., Stewart, C., Puchacz, E. *et al.* (1989) Structure of the rat osteocalcin gene and regulation of vitamin D-dependent expression. *Proc Natl Acad Sci USA* **84**: 1143–7.

Lindsay, R., Aitken, J.M., Anderson, J.B. *et al.* (1976) Long term prevention of postmenopausal osteoporosis by estrogen. *Lancet* **i**: 1038–41.

Livesey, S.A., Ng, K.W., Collier, G.R. *et al.* (1985) Effects of retinoids on cellular content and human parathyroid hormone activation of cyclic adenosine 3′:5′-monophosphate-dependent protein kinase isoenzymes in clonal rat osteogenic sarcoma cells. *Cancer Res* **45**: 5734–40.

Luben, R.A. and Cohn, C.V. (1976) Effects of parathormone and calcitonin on citrate and hyaluronate metabolism in cultured bone. *Endocrinology* **98**: 413–19.

Lyons, K.M., Pelton, R.W. and Hogan, B.L. (1989) Patterns of expression of murine Vgr-1 and BMP-2a RNA suggest that transforming growth factor-b-like genes coordinately regulate aspects of embryonic development. *Genes Dev* **3**: 1657–68.

Majeska, R.J. and Rodan, G.A. (1982) The effect of 1,25(OH)2D3 on alkaline phosphatase in osteoblastic osteosarcoma cells. *J Biol Chem* **257**: 3362–65.

Majeska, R.J., Rodan, S.B. and Rodan, G.A. (1980) Parathyroid hormone-responsive clonal lines from rat osteosarcoma. *Endocrinology* **107**: 1494–503.

Manolagas, S.C., Burton, D.W. and Deftos, L.J. (1981) 1,25-dihydroxyvitamin D3 stimulates the alkaline phosphatase activity of osteoblast-like cells. *J Biol Chem* **256**: 7115–17.

Marcelli, C., Yates, A.J. and Mundy, G.R. (1990) *In vivo* effects of human recombinant transforming growth factor b on bone turnover in normal mice. *J. Bone Miner Res* **5**: 1087–96.

Marie, P.J., de Vernejoul, M.-C., Connes, D. and Nott, M. (1991) Decreased DNA synthesis by cultured osteoblastic cells in eugonadal osteoporotic men with defective bone formation. *J Clin Invest* **88**: 1167–72.

Marshall, M.J., Holt, I. and Davie, M.W.J. (1993) Osteoclast recruitment in mice is stimulated by (3-amino-1-hydroxypropylidene)-1,1-bisphosphonate. *Calcif Tissue Int* **52**: 21–5.

Martin, T.J., Ingleton, P.M., Underwood, J.C.E. *et al.* (1976) Parathyroid hormone responsive adenylate cyclase in an induced transplantable osteogenic sarcoma in the rat. *Nature* **260**: 436–8.

Martin, T.J., Partridge, N.C., Greaves, M., Atkins, D. and Ibbotson, K.J. (1979) Prostaglandin effects on bone and role in cancer hypercalcemia. In: *Molecular Endocrinology*, (eds MacIntyre, I. and Szelke, M.), Elsevier, North Holland, pp. 251–64.

Martin, T.J., Ng, K.W. and Suda, T. (1989) Bone cell physiology. *Endocrinol Metab Clin North Am* **18**: 833–58.

McSheehy, P.M.J. and Chambers, T.J. (1986) Osteoblastic cells mediate osteclastic responsiveness to parathyroid hormone. *Endocrinology* **118**: 824.

McSheehy, P.M.J. and Chambers, T.J. (1987) 1,25-dihydroxyvitamin D_3 stimulates rat osteoblastic cells to release a soluble factor that increases osteoclastic bone resorption. *J Clin Invest* **80**: 425.

Meikle, M.C., Bord, S., Hembry, R.M. *et al.* (1992) Human osteoblasts in culture synthesize collagenase and other matix metalloproteinases in response to osteotropic hormones and cytokines. *J Cell Sci* **103**: 1093–9.

Mellanby, E. (1944) Croonian lecture. Nutrition in relation to bone growth and nervous system. *Proc R Soc Lond Ser B* **132**: 28–46.

Merke, J., Klaus, G., Hugel, U., Waldherr, R. and Ritz, E. (1986) No 1,25-dihydroxyvitamin D3 receptors on osteoclasts of calcium-deficient chicken despite demonstrable receptors on circulating monocytes. *J Clin Invest* **77**: 312.

Meunier, P.J., Aaron, J., Edouard, C. and Vignon, G. (1971) Osteoporosis and the replacement of cell populations of the marrow by adipose tissue: a quantitative study of 84 iliac crest bone biopsies. *Clin Orthop Rel Res* **80**: 147–54.

Miller, S.C. and Jee, W.S.S. (1987) The bone lining cell: a distinct phenotype? *Calcif Tissue Int* **41**: 1–5.

Minaire, P., Edouard, C., Arlot, M. and Meunier, P.J. (1984) Marrow changes in paraplegic patients. *Calcif Tissue Int* **36**: 338–40.

Moriwake, T., Tanaka, H., Kanzaki, S., Higuchi, J. and Seino, Y. (1992) 1,25-dihydroxyvitamin D3 stimulates the secretion of insulin-like growth factor binding protein 3 (IGF BP-3) by cultured human osteosarcoma cells. *Endocrinology* **130**: 1071–73.

Murrills, R.J., Shane, E., Lindsay, R. and Dempster, D.W. (1989) Bone resorption by isolated human osteoclasts in vitro: effects of calcitonin. *J Bone Miner Res* **4**: 259–68.

Murrills, R.J., Stein, L.S., Fey, C.P. and Dempster, D.W. (1990) The effects of parathyroid hormone (PTH) and PTH-related peptide on osteoclast resorption of bone slices in vitro: an analysis of pit size and the resorption focus. *Endocrinology* **127**: 2648–53.

Neuman, W.F. and Mulryan, B.J. (1967) Synthetic hydroxyapatite crystals. III The carbonate system. *Calcif Tissue Res* **1**: 94–104.

Ng, K.W., Livesey, S.A., Collier, F., Gummer, P.R. and Martin, T.J. (1985) Effect of retinoids on the growth, ultrastructure and cytoskeletal structures of malignant rat osteoblasts. *Cancer Res* **45**: 5106–13.

Ng, K.W., Gummer, P.A., Michelangeli, V.P. *et al.* (1988) Regulation of alkaline phosphatase expression in a neonatal rat clonal calvarial cell strain by retinoic acid. *J Bone Miner Res* **3**: 53–61.

Ng, K.W., Hudson, P.J., Power, B.E. *et al.* (1989a) Retinoic acid and tumour necrosis factor-a act in concert to control the level of alkaline phosphatase mRNA. *J Mol Endocrinol* **3**: 57–64.

Ng, K.W., Manji, S.S., Young, M.R. and Findlay, D.M. (1989b) Opposing influences of glucocorticoid and retinoic acid on transcriptional control in preosteoblasts. *Mol Endocrinol* **3**: 2079–85.

Nicholson, G.C., Moseley, J.M., Sexton, P.M., Mendelsohn, F.A.O. and Martin, T.J. (1986) Abundant calcitonin receptors in isolated rat osteoclasts: biochemical and autoradiographic characterization. *J Clin Invest* **78**: 355.

Nicholson, G.C., Moseley, J.M., Sexton, P.M. and Martin, T.J. (1987) Chicken osteoclasts do not possess calcitonin receptors. *J Bone Miner Res* **2**: 53.

Nishimoto, S.K. and Price, P.A. (1980) Secretion of the vitamin K-dependent protein of bone by rat osteosarcoma cells: evidence for an intracellular precursor. *J Biol Chem* **255**: 6579–83.

Noda, M. and Camilliere, J.J. (1989) *In vivo* stimulation of bone formation by transforming growth factor b. *Endocrinology* **124**: 2991–4.

Noda, M. and Rodan, G.A. (1987) Type b transforming growth factor (TGFβ) regulation of alkaline phosphatase expression and other phenotype-related mRNA's in osteoblastic rat osteosarcoma cells. *J Cell Physiol* **133**: 426–34.

Oldberg, A., Franzen, A. and Heingegard, D. (1986) Cloning and sequence analysis of rat bone sialoprotein (osteopontin) cDNA reveals an arg-gly-asp cell-binding sequence. *Proc Natl Acad Sci USA* **83**: 8819–23.

Osdoby, P., Martin, M.C. and Kaplan, A.I. (1982) Isolated osteoclasts and their presumed progenitor cells, the monocyte, in culture. *J Exp Zool* **224**: 331.

Oursler, M.J. and Spelsberg, T.C. (1993) Editorial: echistatin, a potential new drug for osteoporosis. *Endocrinology* **132**: 939–40.

Oursler, M.J., Osdoby, P., Pyfferoen, J., Riggs, B.L. and Spelsberg, T.C. (1991) Avian osteoclasts as estrogen target cells. *Proc Natl Acad Sci USA* **88**: 6613–17.

Oursler, M.J., Pederson, L., Pyfferoen, J. *et al.* (1993) Estrogen modulation of avian osteoclast lysosomal gene expression. *Endocrinology* **132**: 1373–80.

Owen, M.E. (1988) Marrow stromal stem cells. *J Cell Sci* **88** (Suppl 10): 63–76.

Owen, T.A., Aronow, M., Shalhoub, V. *et al.* (1990) Progressive development of the rat osteoblast phenotype in vitro: reciprocal relationships in expression of genes associated with osteoblast proliferation and differentiation during formation of the bone extracellular matrix. *J Cell Physiol* **143**: 420–30.

Owen, T.A., Aronow, M.S., Barone, L.M. *et al.* (1991) Pleiotropic effects of vitamin D on osteoblast gene expression are related to the proliferative and differentiated state of the bone cell phenotype: dependency upon basal levels of gene expression, duration of exposure and bone matrix competency in normal rat osteoblast cultures. *Endocrinology* **128**: 1494–504.

Pacifici, R., Rifas, L., Teitelbaum, S. *et al.* (1987) Spontaneous release of interleukin 1 from human blood monocytes reflects bone formation in idiopathic osteoporosis. *Proc Natl Acad Sci USA* **84**: 4616–20.

Pacifici, R., Rifas, L., McCracken, R. *et al.* (1989) Ovarian steroid treatment blocks a postmenopausal increase in blood monocyte interleukin 1 release. *Proc Natl Acad Sci USA* **86**: 2398–402.

Page, A.E., Hayman, A.R., Andersson, L.M.B., Chambers, T.J. and Warburton, M.J. (1993) Degradation of bone matrix protein by osteoclast cathepsins. *Int J Biochem* **25**: 545–50.

Parfitt, A.M. (1988) Bone remodeling: relationship to the amount and structure of bone and the pathogenesis and prevention of fractures. In: *Osteoporosis: Etiology, Diagnosis, and Management*, (eds Rigg, B.L. and Melton III, L.J.), Raven Press, New York, pp. 45–93.

Parisien, M., Silverberg, S.J., Shane, E. *et al.* (1990) The histomorphometry of bone in primary hyperparathyroidism: preservation of cancellous bone structure. *J Clin Endocrinol Metabol* **70**: 930.

Parisien, M., Mellish, R.W.E., Silverberg, S.J. *et al.* (1992) Maintenance of cancellous bone connectivity in primary hyperparathyroidism: trabecular strut analysis. *J Bone Miner Res* **7**: 913.

Parisien, M., Schnitzer, M., Nieves, J. *et al.* (1993) Proceedings of the Fourth International Symposium on Osteoporosis, (ed. Riis, B.), Osteopress, Rodovre.

Partridge, N.C., Alcorn, D., Michelangeli, V.P. *et al.* (1981) Functional properties of hormonally responsive cultured normal and malignant rat oestoblastic cells. *Endocrinology* **108**: 213–19.

Partridge, N.C., Alcorn, D., Michelangeli, V.P., Ryan, G.B. and Martin, T.J. (1983) Morphological and biochemical characterization of four osteogenic sarcoma cell lines of rat origin. *Cancer Res* **43**: 4308–14.

Partridge, N.C., Jeffrey, J.J., Ehlich, L.S. *et al.* (1987) Hormonal regulation of the production of collagenase and a collagenase inhibitor activity by rat osteogenic sarcoma cells. *Endocrinology* **120**: 1956–62.

Pelton, R.W., Nomura, S., Moses, H.L. and Hogan, B.L.M. (1989) Expression of transforming growth factor B2 mRNA during murine embryogenesis. *Development* **106**: 759–67.

Pensler, J.M., Radosevich, J.A., Higbee, R. and Langman, C.B. (1990) Osteoclasts isolated from membranous bone in children exhibit nuclear estrogen and progesterone receptors. *J Bone Miner Res* **5**: 797–802.

Pilbeam, C.C., Klein-Nulend, J. and Raisz, L.G. (1989) Inhibition by 17ß estradiol of PTH stimulated resorption and prostaglandin production in cultured neonatal mouse calvariae. *Biochem Biophys Res Commun* **183**: 1319–24.

Posner, A.S. (1987) In: *Bone and Mineral Research*, (ed. Peck, W.A.), Elsevier, Amsterdam, pp. 65–116.

Price, P.A. (1985) Vitamin K-dependent formation of bone Gla protein (osteocalcin) and its function. *Vitam Horm* **42**: 65–108.

Price, P.A., (1987) Vitamin K-dependent bone proteins. In: *Calcium Regulation and Bone Metabolism: Basic and Clinical Aspects, vol. 9*, (eds Cohn, D.V., Martin, T.J. and Meunier, P.J.), Elsevier Science Publishers, Amsterdam, pp. 419–25.

Price, P.A. and Baukol, S.A. (1980) 1,25-dihydroxyvitamin D3 increases synthesis of the vitamin k-dependent bone protein by osteosarcoma cells. *J Biol Chem* **225**: 11660–3.

Prince, C.W. and Butler, W.T. (1987) 1,25-dihydroxyvitamin D3 regulates the biosynthesis of osteopontin, a bone-derived cell attachment protein, in clonal osteoblast-like osteosarcoma cells. *Coll Relat Res* **7**: 305–15.

Raisz, L.G., Trummel, C.L., Holick, M.F. and DeLuca, J.F. (1972) 1,25-dihydroxycholecalciferol: a potent stimulator of bone resorption in tissue culture. *Science* **175**: 768.

Rao, L.G., Murray, T.M. and Heersche, J.N.M. (1983) Immunohistochemical demonstration of parathyroid hormone binding to specific cell types in fixed rat bone tissues. *Endocrinology* **113**: 805–10.

Reinholt, F.P., Hultenby, K., Oldberg, A. and Heinegard, D. (1990) Osteopontin – a possible anchor of osteoclasts to bone. *Proc Natl Acad Sci USA* 87: 4473–5.

Reynolds, J.J., Pavlovitch, H. and Balsan, S. (1976) 1,25-dihydroxycholecalciferol increases bone resorption in thyroparathyroidectomized mice. *Calcif Tissue Res* **21**: 207.

Riggs, B.L., Jowsey, J., Kelly, P.J., Jones, J.D. and Maher, F.T. (1969) Effect of sex hormones on bone in primary osteoporosis. *J Clin Invest* **48**: 1065–72.

Robey, P.G., Bianco, P. and Termine, J.D. (1992) The cellular biology and biochemistry of bone formation. In: *Disorders of Bone and Mineral Metabolism*, (eds Coe, F.L. and Favus, M.J.), Raven Press, New York, pp. 241–63.

Robey, P.G., Fisher, L.W., Young, M.F. and Termine, J.D. (1988) The biochemistry of bone. In: *Osteoporosis: Etiology, Diagnosis, and Management*, (eds Riggs, B.L. and Melton III, L.J.), Raven Press, New York, pp. 95–109.

Rodan, G.A. and Martin, T.J. (1981) Role of osteoblasts in hormonal control of bone resorption – a hypothesis. *Calcif Tissue Int* **33**: 349–51.

Rouleau, M.F., Warshawsky, H. and Goltzman, D. (1986) Parathyroid hormone binding *in vivo* to renal, hepatic and skeletal tissues of the rat using an autoradiographic approach. *Endocrinology* **118**: 919–28.

Ruberte, E., Dolle, P., Krust, A. *et al.* (1990) Specific spatial and temporal distribution of retinoic acid receptor gamma transcripts during mouse embryogenesis. *Development* **108**: 213–22.

Sahni, M., Guenther, H.L., Fleisch, H., Collin, P. and Martin, T.J. (1993) Bisphosphonates act on rat bone resorption through the mediation of osteoblasts. *J Clin Invest* **91**: 2004–11.

Sakamoto, S., Sakamoto, M., Goldhaber, P. and Glimcher, M.J. (1975) Collagenase and bone resorption: isolation of collagenase from culture medium containing serum after stimulation of bone resorption by addition of parathyroid extract. *Biochem Biophys Res Commun* **63**: 172–8.

Sato, M., Sardana, M.K., Grasser, W.A. *et al.* (1990) Echistatin is a potent inhibitor of bone resorption in culture. *J Cell Biol* **111**: 1713–23.

Schmid, C., Schapfer, I., Boni-Schnetzler, M. *et al.* (1990) PTH and cAMP stimulate the expression of the growth hormone (GH)-dependent insulin-like growth factor binding protein (IGFBP-3) by rat osteoblasts in vitro. In: *Osteoporosis 1990*, (eds Christiansen, C. and Overgaard, K.), Osteopress, Copenhagen, p. 264–73.

Seibel, M.J., Cosman, F., Shen, V. *et al.* (1993) Urinary hydroxypyridinium crosslinks of collagen as markers of bone resorption and estrogen efficacy in postmenopausal osteoporosis. *J Bone Miner Res* **8**: 881–9.

Shinar, D.M. and Rodan, G.A. (1990) Biphasic effects of transforming growth factor-b on the production of osteoclast-like cells in mouse bone marrow cultures: the role of prostaglandins in the generation of these cells. *Endocrinology* **126:** 3153–8.

Silve, C.M., Hradek, G.T., Jones, A.L. and Arnaud, C.D. (1982) Parathyroid hormone receptor in intact embryonic chicken bone: characterization and cellular location. *J Cell Biol* **94**: 379–86.

Sly, W.S., Whyte, M.P., Sundaram, V. *et al.* (1985) Carbonic anhydrase II deficiency in 12 families with the autosomal recessive syndrome of osteopetrosis with renal tubular acidosis and cerebral calcification. *N Engl J Med* **313**: 139–45.

Stein, G.S., Lian, J.B., Gerstenfeld, L.G. *et al.* (1989) The onset and progression of osteoblast differentiation is functionally related to cellular proliferation. *Connective Tissue Res* **20**: 3–13.

Steiniche, T., Hasling, C., Charles, P. *et al.* (1989) A randomized study on the effects of estrogen/gestagen or high dose oral calcium on trabecular bone remodeling in postmenopausal osteoporosis. *Bone* **10**: 313–20.

Strauss, P.G., Closs, E.I., Schmidt, J. and Erfle, V. (1990) Gene expression during osteogenic differentiation in mandibular condyles in vitro. *J Cell Biol* **116:** 1369–79.

Stumpf, W.E. and DeLuca, S.M. (1981) Sites of action of 1,25$(OH)_2$-D_3 identified by thaw-mount autoradiography. In: *Hormonal Control of Calcium Metabolism*, (eds Cohn, D.V., Talmage, R.V. and Matthew, J.L.), Excerpta Medica, Amsterdam, p. 222.

Suda, T., Takahashi, N. and Martin, T.J. (1992) Modulation of osteoclast differentiation. *Endocr Rev* **13**: 66–80.

Takahashi, N., Akatsu, T., Udagawa, N. *et al.* (1988a) Osteoblastic cells are involved in osteoclast formation. *Endocrinology* **123**: 2600–2.

Takahashi, N., Yamana, H., Yoshiki, S. *et al.* (1988b) Osteoclast-like cell formation and its regulation by osteotropic hormones in mouse bone marrow cultures. *Endocrinology* **122**: 1373–82.

Tanaka, Y. and DeLuca, H.F. (1971) Bone mineral mobilization of 1,25 (OH)2D3, a metabolic of vitamin d. *Arch Biochem Biophys* **146**: 574.

Teitelbaum, S.L. (1993) Proceedings of the Fourth International Symposium on Osteoporosis, (eds Christiansen, C. and Riis, B), Osteopress, Rodovre, pp. 265–6.

Teti, A. and Zambonin-Zallone, A. (1992) Osteoclast cytoskeleton and attachment proteins. In: *Biology and Physiology of the Osteoclast*, (eds Rifkin, B.R. and Gay, C.V.), CRC Press, Boca Raton, pp. 245–57.

Teti, A., Rizzoli, R. and Zambonin-Zallone, A. (1991) Parathyroid hormone binding to cultured avian osteoclasts. *Biochem Biophys Res Commun* **174**: 1217–22.

Thaller, C. and Eichele, G. (1987) Identification and spatial distribution of retinoids in the developing chick limb bud. *Nature* **327**: 625–8.

Thein, R. and Lotan, R. (1982) Sensitivity of cultured human osteosarcoma and chondrosarcoma cells to retinoic acid. *Cancer Res* **42**: 4771–5.

Thomson, B.M., Saklatvala, J. and Chambers, T.J. (1986) Osteoblasts mediate interleukin 1 responsiveness of bone resorption by rat osteoclasts. *J Exp Med* **164**: 104–12.

Thomson, B.M., Mundy, G.R. and Chambers, T.J. (1987) Tumour necrosis factors a and b induce osteoblastic cells to stimulate osteoclastic bone resorption. *J Immunol* **138**: 775–9.

Tinkler, S.M.B., Williams, D.M. and Johnson, N.W. (1981) Osteoclast formation in response to intraperitoneal injection of 1α-hydroxycholecalciferol in mice. *J Anat* **133**: 91.

Tobias, J.H. and Chambers, T.J. (1991) The effects of sex hormones on bone resorption by rat osteoclasts. *Acta Endocrinol* **124**: 121–7.

Torring, O., Firek, A.F., Heath, J. and Conover, C.A. (1991) Parathyroid hormone and parathyroid hormone-related peptide stimulate insulin-like growth factor-binding protein secretion by rat osteoblast like cells through an adenosine 3′,5′-monophosphate-dependent mechanism. *Endocrinology* **128**: 1006–14.

Tracy, R.P., Stenner, D.D., Mintz, K.P. *et al.* (1987) In: *Calcium Regulation and Bone Metabolism: Basic and Clinical Aspects*, (eds Cohn, D.V., Martin, T.J. and Meunier, P.J.), Elsevier, Amsterdam, pp. 401–8.

Tuukkanen, J. and Vaananen, H.K. (1986)

Omeprazole, a specific inhibitor of H+ K–ATPase, inhibits bone resorption *in vitro*. *Calcif Tissue Int* **38**: 123.

Udagawa, N., Takahashi, N., Akatsu, T. *et al.* (1989) The bone marrow-derived stromal cell lines MC3T3-G2/PA6 and ST2 support osteoclast-like cell differentiation in co-cultures with mouse spleen cells. *Endocrinology* **125**: 1805–13.

Urist, M.R. (1989) Bone morphogenetic protein, bone regeneration, heterotopic ossification and the bone-bone-marrow consortium. In: *Bone and Mineral Research 6*, (ed. Peck, W.A.), Elsevier, Amsterdam, pp. 57–112.

Vaananen, H.K., Karhukorpi, E.K., Sundquist, K. *et al.* (1990) Evidence for the presence of a proton pump of the vacuolar H+-ATPase type in the ruffled borders of osteoclast. *J Cell Biol* **111**: 1305.

Veis, A. and Sabsay, B. (1987) In: *Bone and Mineral Research*, (ed. Peck, W.A.), Elsevier, Amsterdam, pp. 1–63.

Wagner, M., Thaller, C., Jessell, T. and Eichele, G. (1990) Polarizing activity and retinoid synthesis in the floor plate of the neural tube. *Nature* **345**: 819–22.

Waite, L.C., Volkert, W.A. and Kenny, A.D. (1970) Inhibition of bone resorption by acetazolamide in the rat. *Endocrinology*, **87**: 1129.

Wang, E.A., Rosen, V., Cordes, P. *et al.* (1988) Purification and characterization of other distinct bone-inducing factors. *Proc Natl Acad Sci USA* **85**: 9484–88.

Wang, E.A., Rosen, V., D'Alessandro, J.S. *et al.* (1990) Recombinant human bone morphogenetic protein induces bone formation. *Proc Natl Acad Sci USA* **87**: 220–4.

Weiner, S. (1986) Organization of extracellularly mineralized tissues: a comparative study of biological crystal growth. *Crit Rev Biochem* **20**: 365–408.

Wener, J.A., Gorton, S.J. and Raisz, L.G. (1972) Escape from inhibition of resorption in cultures of fetal bone treated with calcitonin and parathyroid hormone. *J Endocrinol* **90**: 752–9.

Wozney, J.M., Rosen, V., Celeste, A.J. *et al.* (1988) Novel regulators of bone formation: molecular clones and activities. *Science* **242**: 1528–34.

Yamaguchi, A., Katagiri, T., Ikeda, T. *et al.* (1991) Recombinant human bone morphogenetic protein-2 stimulates osteoblast maturation and inhibits myogenic differentiation in vitro. *J Cell Biol* **113**: 681–7.

Yee, J.A., Yan, Y.L., Dominguez, J.C., Allan, E.H. and Martin T.J. (1993) Plasminogen-dependent activation of latent transforming growth factor beta by growing cultures of osteoblast-like cells. *J Cell Physiol* **157**: 528–34.

Yoon, K., Buenaga, R. and Rodan, G.A. (1987) Tissue specificity and development expression of rat osteopontin. *Biochem Biophys Res Commun* **148**: 1129–36.

Zaidi, M., Alam, A.S.M.T., Bax, B.E. *et al.* (1993) Role of the endothelial cell in osteoclast control: new perspectives. *Bone* **14**: 97–102.

Zambonin-Zallone, A., Teti, A. and Primavera, M.V. (1984) Resorption of vital and devitalized bone by isolated osteoclasts in vitro. *Cell Tissue Res* **235**: 561.

Zhou, H., Findlay, D.M., Hammonds, R.G., Martin, T.J. and Ng, K.W. (1993a) Differential effects of transforming growth factor-β1 and bone morphogenetic protein 4 on gene expression and differentiated function of preosteoblasts. *J Cell Physiol* **155**: 112–19.

Zhou, H., Findlay, D.M., Heath, J.K., Martin, T.J. and Ng, K.W. (1993b) Novel action of retinoic acid: stabilization of newly synthesized alkaline phosphatase and osteopontin transcripts. *J Bone Miner Res* **8**: S119.

Zhou, H., Hammonds Jr, R.G., Findlay, D.M. *et al.* (1991) Retinoic acid-induced gene expression in malignant, non-transformed and immortalized osteoblasts. *J Bone Miner Res* **6**: 767–75.

PATHOGENESIS OF OSTEOPOROSIS 2

R.M. Francis, A.M. Sutcliffe and A.C. Scane

BONE REMODELLING

Bone is a living tissue which continuously remodels throughout life. This allows the skeleton to increase in size during growth, respond to physical stresses and repair structural damage due to fatigue failure or trauma. The skeleton comprises 80% cortical and 20% trabecular bone. Cortical bone is predominantly found in the shafts of the long bones, whilst trabecular bone is mainly located in the vertebrae, pelvis and the ends of long bones.

The major cells involved in bone remodelling are osteoclasts, osteoblasts and osteocytes. Osteoclasts are multinucleate cells derived from macrophage-monocyte precursors which resorb bone and remove degraded organic material. Osteoblasts are derived from fibroblast precursors and synthesize bone matrix or osteoid, which is subsequently mineralized around foci of crystal formation known as matrix vesicles. Osteocytes are mature osteoblasts trapped within calcified bone, which are interconnected by long dendritic processes. These may provide a communication network to transmit information about mechanical forces, which can then be used to modify bone resorption and formation.

Bone remodelling is initiated by a period of resorption lasting about two weeks, when osteoclasts erode an area of bone. Osteoblasts are then attracted to the resorption cavity where, over the subsequent three months, new bone matrix is deposited and mineralized. Resorption and formation are usually closely coupled, probably through local humoral factors, though bone formation exceeds resorption during skeletal growth, while resorption outstrips bone formation in later life. Bone remodelling may be influenced by mechanical forces applied to the skeleton, by local humoral factors such as interleukins 1 and 6, transforming growth factor β and tumour necrosis factor and by circulating hormones like oestrogens, testosterone, calcitonin, parathyroid hormone (PTH) and 1,25-dihydroxyvitamin D ($1,25(OH)_2D$).

BONE MASS THROUGHOUT LIFE

Bone mass changes throughout life during skeletal growth, consolidation and involution. About 90% of the peak bone mass is deposited during skeletal growth, which lasts until the closure of the epiphyses. This is then followed by a phase of skeletal consolidation lasting for up to 15 years, when bone mass increases further until the peak bone mass is achieved. Cortical and trabecular bone is lost with advancing age in both sexes, though the rate of bone loss varies according to bone type and anatomical site. Women lose 35–50% of trabecular and 25–30% of cortical bone mass with age, whilst men lose 15–45% of

Osteoporosis. Edited by John C. Stevenson and Robert Lindsay. Published in 1998 by Chapman & Hall, London.
ISBN 0 412 48870 1

trabecular and 5–15% of cortical bone (Riggs and Melton, 1986; Francis, 1990).

Genetic factors account for as much as 80% of the variance in peak bone mass (Slemenda *et al.*, 1991). Negroid populations have a higher bone mass than Caucasians or Asians and men have bigger, denser skeletons than women (Cohn *et al.*, 1977; Mazess, 1982). There is also greater concordance of bone mass between monozygotic than dizygotic twins, whilst the daughters of osteoporotic women have a lower than expected bone density (Smith *et al.*, 1973; Seeman *et al.*, 1989). Recent work suggests that polymorphism of the vitamin D receptor gene may have an important effect on bone density in women (Morrison *et al.*, 1994). Other potential determinants of peak bone mass include exercise, diet, smoking, alcohol consumption and hormonal factors. Bone mass is greater in young adults who exercise regularly than in more sedentary individuals, emphasizing the importance of mechanical factors in the determination of bone mass (Nilsson and Westlin, 1971). Several studies suggest that a high dietary calcium intake during skeletal growth and consolidation may also be beneficial to the skeleton (Sandler *et al.*, 1985; Kanders *et al.*, 1988; Johnston *et al.*, 1992). The combination of regular exercise and high dietary calcium intake may act together to produce an optimal peak bone mass (Kanders *et al.*, 1988). In contrast, smoking and alcohol consumption during adolescence and early adult life may have an adverse effect on peak bone mass (Stevenson *et al.*, 1989). Endocrine factors also affect peak bone mass, as early menarche, pregnancy and the use of the oral contraceptive pill are associated with higher bone mass (Goldsmith and Johnston, 1975).

Bone loss starts between the ages of 35 and 40 in both sexes, possibly related to impaired new bone formation, due to declining osteoblast function. The onset of bone loss is likely to be genetically predetermined and the subsequent rate of bone loss may also be influenced by genetic factors, as there is a greater concordance of bone loss, $1,25(OH)_2D$, PTH, calcium absorption and biochemical markers of bone remodelling in monozygotic than dizygotic twins (Eisman *et al.*, 1992; Peacock *et al.*, 1992). Bone loss increases at the menopause, due to the marked reduction in the circulating concentrations of oestradiol and progesterone. Other causes of age-related bone loss include low body weight, smoking, excess alcohol consumption, physical inactivity, nutritional factors and declining calcium absorption (Riggs and Melton, 1986; Francis, 1990; Compston, 1992).

Body weight is an important determinant of bone mass, as the loss of bone is more rapid in women with low body weight. The protective effects of high body weight on the skeleton may be due to the mechanical effects of body weight on bone formation and the increased production of oestrone in fat (Davidson *et al.*, 1982; Christiansen *et al.*, 1987).

Smoking increases bone loss by hastening the menopause by several years, increasing the catabolism of oestrogens thereafter and depressing osteoblast function (Jick *et al.*, 1977; De Vernejoul *et al.*, 1983; Jensen *et al.*, 1985). The deleterious effect of smoking on the skeleton may also be related to the associated reduction in body weight. Modest alcohol consumption may have an adverse effect on the skeleton, though it is uncertain if this is due to an effect on peak bone mass or the subsequent rate of bone loss (Stevenson *et al.*, 1989).

The decline in physical activity with advancing age is also likely to cause further bone loss. Physical activity is important to the skeleton, as the associated weight-bearing and muscular activity stimulates bone formation and increases bone mass. In contrast, immobilization leads to rapid bone loss (Krolner and Toft, 1983; Krolner *et al.*, 1983). The importance of physical activity is underlined by several case control studies, which show that patients with femoral fracture are habitually less active than control subjects (Cooper *et al.*, 1988; Lau *et al.*, 1988).

The role of dietary calcium intake in the pathogenesis of bone loss remains controversial. Metabolic balance studies suggest that the dietary requirement for calcium increases at the menopause from 1000 to 1500 mg/day (Heaney *et al.*, 1978). Nevertheless, there is little relationship between dietary calcium intake and bone mass or bone loss at this time of life (Riggs *et al.*, 1987; Stevenson *et al.*, 1988). The risk of femoral fracture may be lower in subjects with a higher dietary intake of calcium, but this is not a universal finding and may be due to an effect on peak bone mass rather than the subsequent rate of bone loss (Wooton *et al.*, 1979; Holbrook *et al.*, 1988; Matkovic *et al.*, 1979).

The efficiency of calcium absorption from the gut declines with age in both sexes, which if uncompensated may cause further bone loss (Bullamore *et al.*, 1970). The reduction in calcium absorption is due in part to the age-related fall in plasma 25 hydroxyvitamin D (25OHD), secondary to reduced sunlight exposure. There is also impaired metabolism of 25OHD to $1,25(OH)_2D$ in later life, because of declining renal function (Baker *et al.*, 1980; Francis *et al.*, 1984). Recent studies suggest that low circulating 25OHD concentrations may lead to elevation of the serum PTH and bone loss (Krall *et al.*, 1989; Khaw *et al.*, 1992). Renal function may also be a significant determinant of bone mass, presumably through its effects on $1,25(OH)_2D$ and calcium absorption (Buchanan *et al.*, 1988).

OSTEOPOROSIS

Osteoporosis is characterized by a reduction in the amount of bone in the skeleton, associated with increased fragility and risk of fracture. The mechanical properties of bone are closely related to its mineral content and architectural structure, so a reduction in bone mass is inevitably associated with an increased susceptibility to fracture. The major osteoporotic fractures are those of the forearm, vertebral body and femoral neck. By the age of 60, about 7% of women and 3% of men have sustained a fracture at one of these sites, rising to 25% and 8% respectively at the age of 80 (Francis, 1990).

Osteoporosis may be classified into primary or secondary osteoporosis, depending on the absence or presence of an underlying condition known to cause osteoporosis. Underlying secondary causes of osteoporosis are present in 20–35% of women and 40–55% of men with vertebral crush fractures. There are a large number of causes of secondary osteoporosis which are described later in this chapter (Table 2.1).

Table 2.1 Causes of secondary osteoporosis

Endocrine
Male hypogonadism
Hyperthyroidism
Hyperparathyroidism
Hypercortisolism
Diabetes
Amenorrhoea
Amenorrhoeic athletes
Anorexia nervosa
Hyperprolactinaemia
Drugs
Steroids
Anticonvulsants
Heparin
Neoplasms
Myelomatosis
Skeletal metastases
Other conditions
Gastric surgery
Alcoholism
Pregnancy
Immobilization
Osteogenesis imperfecta
Homocystinuria
Systemic mastocytosis
Transplantation

MALE OSTEOPOROSIS

As mentioned earlier, men lose 15–45% of trabecular and 5–15% of cortical bone with advancing age (Francis, 1990). This leads to an increased incidence of fractures of the vertebral body and femoral neck, but not the forearm (Riggs and Melton, 1986; Obrant *et al.*, 1989). In contrast to women, there is no increase in the frequency of falls in middle age in men, which may explain the protection against forearm fractures (Winner *et al.*, 1989). Swedish data suggest that the annual incidence of vertebral crush fractures in men increases from 8/10 000 in the seventh decade to 45/10 000 in the ninth decade, whilst the prevalence rises from 1% in the sixth decade to 7% in the ninth decade (Obrant *et al.*, 1989). The annual incidence of femoral neck fractures in men in Oxford in 1983 increased from 6.3/10 000 between the ages of 55 and 64 to 131.6/10 000 over the age of 85 (Boyce and Vessey, 1985). Using current age-specific incidence rates for England and Wales, it has been estimated that 5% of men will have sustained a femoral neck fracture by the age of 85 (Royal College of Physicians of London, 1989). The number of men with osteoporotic fractures is rising, because of the demographic trend towards an ageing population and an increase in the age-specific incidence of fractures (Boyce and Vessey, 1985; Royal College of Physicians of London, 1989; Obrant *et al.*, 1989).

The risk of fracture is influenced by bone mass and architecture and the frequency and severity of trauma applied to the skeleton. Bone mass at any age is determined by the peak bone mass, the age at which bone loss starts and the rate at which it proceeds. Peak bone mass is higher in men than women, although peak bone density is similar in both sexes. Peak bone mass is influenced in men as in women by race, heredity, hormonal factors, physical activity and calcium intake during childhood and adolescence (Francis, 1990; Compston, 1992). It has recently been reported that young men with constitutionally delayed puberty have reduced bone density in the forearm and lumbar spine, when compared to normal men matched for duration of exposure to postpubertal levels of testosterone (Finkelstein *et al.*, 1992). There was a correlation between radial and spinal bone mineral measurements in normal men, but this was not present in those with delayed puberty, suggesting that cortical and trabecular bone may respond differently to testosterone in this situation.

Age-related bone loss in men is characterized by a reduction in bone formation rather than an increase in resorption (Aaron *et al.*, 1987; Francis *et al.*, 1989). Furthermore, there is greater preservation of trabecular architecture during bone loss in men than in women (Aaron *et al.*, 1987; Francis *et al.*, 1989). There is no endocrine counterpart of the menopause in middle-aged men, though some workers have shown a fall in testosterone levels in men over the age of 70, which may cause bone loss in later life (Vermeulen *et al.*, 1972; Baker *et al.*, 1976). Other factors which may be implicated in the pathogenesis of age-related bone loss in men include tobacco and alcohol consumption, nutrition, physical activity and decreased calcium absorption (Francis *et al.*, 1990; Compston, 1992). In a group of 48 men with a median age of 44, Kelly and colleagues (1990) demonstrated that weight and free testosterone index (ratio of serum testosterone to sex hormone-binding globulin) correlated with bone mineral density (BMD) in the distal and ultradistal radius. They also showed that dietary calcium intake was a significant predictor of BMD in the lumbar spine and femoral neck, but not in the forearm. Preliminary results from a cross-sectional study suggest that short stature, alcohol consumption, reduced muscle bulk, physical inactivity and malabsorption of calcium are all significant determinants of bone mass in normal elderly men (Francis *et al.*, 1992).

In a case control study of men presenting

with vertebral crush fractures, smoking, alcohol consumption and medical conditions known to affect bone or calcium metabolism were shown to be significant risk factors, with a relative risk of 2.3, 2.4 and 5.5 respectively (Seeman *et al.*, 1983). In contrast, obesity was marginally protective, with a relative risk of 0.3 (Seeman *et al.*, 1983). An underlying secondary cause of osteoporosis may be detected in up to 55% of men with vertebral fractures (Seeman *et al.*, 1983; Francis *et al.*, 1989; Baillie *et al.*, 1992). The major causes of secondary osteoporosis in men are steroid therapy, hypogonadism, skeletal metastases, multiple myeloma, gastric surgery and anticonvulsant treatment, with more than one cause being detected in about 10% of cases (Figure 2.1).

Men with vertebral crush fractures due to primary osteoporosis have reduced cortical and trabecular bone mass, decreased trabecular number and biochemical evidence of increased bone turnover compared with age-matched controls (Francis *et al.*, 1989). Other histological studies suggest that bone

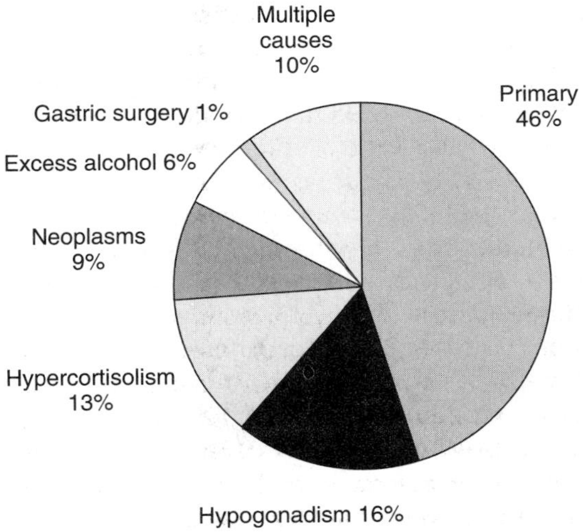

Figure 2.1 Causes of osteoporosis in men with vertebral crush fractures. Data from Baillie *et al.* (1992).

formation is reduced in men with primary osteoporosis (De Vernejoul *et al.*, 1983; Jackson *et al.*, 1987). In a series of men with primary osteoporosis presenting with veterbral crush fractures, the plasma sex steroid concentrations were similar to those of age-matched control subjects (Francis *et al.*, 1989). Calcium absorption was, however, reduced in osteoporotic men, apparently due to a reduction in plasma 1,25$(OH)_2D$ concentration (Jackson *et al.*, 1987; Francis *et al.*, 1989). The increased bone resorption in these men with osteoporosis was slight and probably not enough to account for the observed reduction in plasma 1,25$(OH)_2D$ (Francis *et al.*, 1989). Osteoporosis in men may also be associated with hypercalciuria, with or without renal stone disease, though the cause of the increased urinary calcium remains uncertain (Perry *et al.*, 1982; Zerwekh *et al.*, 1992). A recent study suggests that the hypercalciuria is due to increased calcium absorption, which also appears to be associated with impaired bone formation, though the cause for this is not apparent (Zerwekh *et al.*, 1992).

A case control study of femoral neck fractures in men suggested that physical inactivity and low dietary calcium intake were significant risk factors, though the effect of calcium intake disappeared when allowance was made for confounding variables (Cooper *et al.*, 1988). Other studies suggest that reduction in serum testosterone may be a risk factor for femoral fracture in men (Jackson and Spiekerman, 1989; Stanley *et al.*, 1991).

SECONDARY OSTEOPOROSIS

Secondary osteoporosis accounts for 20–35% of women and 40–55% of men presenting with two or more vertebral crush fractures (Francis, 1990). Of the causes noted in Table 2.1, the most frequently encountered are steroid therapy, skeletal metastases, myeloma, gastric surgery, anticonvulsant therapy, thyrotoxicosis and male hypogonadism.

Cushing's syndrome

The association between Cushing's syndrome and osteoporosis has been recognized since 1932, when Harvey Cushing first described the clinical features of endogenous hypercortisolism. He recognized that the majority of patients with this condition have spinal osteoporosis, which has been confirmed in subsequent studies (Howland *et al.*, 1958; Soffer *et al.*, 1961; Ross and Linch, 1982). In a review of 70 patients with Cushing's syndrome, Ross and Linch (1982) found that osteoporosis was present in 50% of cases. The reduction in bone mass is more marked in the trabecular bone of the spine, ribs and femoral neck than in the cortical bone of the appendicular skeleton (Genant *et al.*, 1982; Pocock *et al.*, 1987). The decrease in trabecular bone density in Cushing's syndrome is of the order of 20% (Pocock *et al.*, 1987; Manning *et al.*, 1992), and is associated with an increased risk of fractures of the ribs and vertebrae (Sprague *et al.*, 1956; Howland *et al.*, 1958; Soffer *et al.*, 1961). Successful treatment of Cushing's syndrome appears to lead to a gradual increase in bone density (Pocock *et al.*, 1987; Manning *et al.*, 1992), such that the bone density may be normal 10 years later (Manning *et al.*, 1992). Although this suggests that the osteoporosis of Cushing's syndrome may be reversible, this has yet to be confirmed in a longitudinal study.

Corticosteroid therapy

Since corticosteroids were first used therapeutically in 1948, it has become apparent that exogenous hypercortisolism is also associated with the development of osteoporosis. Although Cushing's syndrome is a relatively rare cause of osteoporosis, corticosteroid therapy is the commonest cause of secondary osteoporosis, occurring in up to 20% of patients with vertebral crush fractures (Baillie *et al.*, 1992). Up to 50% of patients on oral corticosteroids have osteoporosis (Lukert and Raisz, 1990), though inhaled steroids also appear to affect bone remodelling and decrease bone mass (Reid *et al.*, 1986; Toogood *et al.*, 1991).

The extent of bone loss seen with corticosteroid therapy depends on skeletal site, underlying disease, dose and duration of treatment (Reid, 1990). Corticosteroid therapy has a greater effect on trabecular than cortical bone, so that the reduction in bone density is more marked in the spine and proximal femur than in the forearm or femoral shaft (Seeman *et al.*, 1982; Schaadt and Bohr, 1984). The decrease in bone density ranges from 4% to 19.5% in the spine and 9% to 12% in the femoral neck (Reid, 1990). The reduction in bone mass associated with corticosteroids appears to be greater in rheumatoid arthritis than asthma or polymyalgia rheumatica (Hahn *et al.*, 1974; Mueller, 1976), possibly because of the effect of rheumatoid arthritis on bone loss (Reid *et al.*, 1986). Reid and colleagues (1982) have shown a correlation between bone loss and corticosteroid dose in rheumatoid arthritis, but not with duration of therapy or total dose. Other studies, however, suggest that total cumulative dose or duration of therapy may be the most important determinant of bone loss or fracture risk (Crilly *et al.*, 1983; Dykman *et al.*, 1985). Nevertheless, biochemical, histological and densitometric studies indicate that bone loss occurs early with corticosteroid therapy. There is biochemical evidence of decreased bone formation within a week of starting treatment (Ekenstam *et al.*, 1986), whilst histomorphometric studies show dramatic loss of trabecular bone in the first seven months of therapy, which then slows down subsequently (Lo Cascio *et al.*, 1984, 1987). Single photon absorptiometry of the distal forearm demonstrates significant bone loss after only three months, with no further loss over the next three months (Rickers *et al.*, 1982). Dual photon absorptiometry of the spine shows rapid bone loss in the first year of treatment, with less bone loss subsequently (Gennari and Civitelli, 1986). The reduction in bone mass observed with corticosteroid treatment is associated with an increased risk of fractures, particularly of the vertebrae, ribs and pelvis (Curtiss *et al.*, 1954; Rosenberg, 1958; Murray, 1960). The prevalence of fractures in patients treated with oral corticosteroids has been reported to be between 11% and 20% (Reid, 1990).

The effects of corticosteroids on calcium metabolism and bone remodelling are complex, but have been extensively reviewed elsewhere (Reid, 1989, 1990; Smith, 1990). High-dose corticosteroid therapy (>10 mg prednisolone daily) decreases calcium absorption by a direct effect on the bowel mucosa (Kimberg, 1969; Klein *et al.*, 1977), resulting in secondary hyperparathyroidism and elevation of the plasma $1,25(OH)_2D$ (Fucik *et al.*, 1975; Hahn *et al.*, 1981). Exogenously administered corticosteroids also suppress the adrenal production of androgens, which in turn leads to a reduction in plasma oestrone levels (Crilly *et al.*, 1979a). The release of calcitonin in response to increases in plasma calcium is also decreased by corticosteroid therapy (Gennari and Civitelli, 1986). As a result of these changes, plasma PTH and $1,25(OH)_2D$ may rise, whilst plasma concentrations of oestrone and calcitonin fall, leading to increased bone resorption. In addition to these indirect actions on bone resorption, cell culture techniques suggest that corticosteroids may also increase bone resorption by a direct effect on the osteoclast (Bar-Shavit *et al.*, 1984). The attachment of bone-resorbing cells to bone appears to be mediated by cell surface oligosaccharides (Bar-Shavit *et al.*, 1983). Corticosteroids alter the expression of these cell surface sugars, thereby enhancing the attachment of the resorbing cells to bone and stimulating its degradation (Bar-Shavit *et al.*, 1984). Corticosteroid therapy commonly causes hypercalciuria, but it is unclear if this is due to the increased bone resorption or decreased tubular reabsorption of calcium.

In addition to the stimulation of bone resorption, corticosteroids also suppress bone formation and collagen production (Hall, 1977; Aaron *et al.*, 1989). Corticosteroid therapy leads to a reduction of serum osteocalcin within one week, suggesting a rapid decline in bone formation (Ekenstam *et al.*, 1986). The effects of corticosteroids on bone formation may be mediated by $1,25(OH)_2D$, as glucocorticoids downregulate $1,25(OH)_2D$ receptors, whilst treatment with $1,25(OH)_2D_3$ stimulates collagen synthesis and the production of alkaline phosphatase and osteocalcin (Beresford *et al.*, 1986; Jowell *et al.*, 1987). The reduction in bone formation with corticosteroid treatment may also be due to decreased androgen levels in both men and women (Crilly *et al.*, 1979a; MacAdams *et al.*, 1986). Adrenal suppression leads to low androstenedione and testosterone levels in women (Crilly *et al.*, 1979b), whilst reduction in testosterone levels may also occur in men, because of impaired secretion of gonadotrophin-releasing hormone (Reid *et al.*, 1985; MacAdams *et al.*, 1986). Corticosteroid therapy may have a direct effect on the production of sex steroids by the ovaries and testes (Smith, 1990).

Myeloma

Myeloma is characterized by extensive bone destruction, with multiple osteolytic lesions or a diffuse osteopenia, and is associated with vertebral crush fractures and pathological fractures elsewhere. The condition may present with osteoporosis (Dolan *et al.*, 1989; Baillie *et al.*, 1992) and is found in 5% of patients with vertebral crush fractures (Baillie *et al.*, 1992). The increased bone resorption is due to the production of an osteoclast-activating factor by the myeloma cells (Mundy *et al.*, 1974), which has been identified as lymphotoxin (Garrett *et al.*, 1987). A diagnosis of myeloma should be suspected in osteoporotic patients with anaemia, raised ESR, hypercalcaemia or radiological evidence of osteolytic lesions. Further investigations might include serum and urine immunoelectrophoresis and bone marrow examination. Serum and urine immunoelectrophoresis should probably be performed in all osteoporotic patients with vertebral crush fractures, as myeloma is not uncommon in such patients, even in the absence of other abnormalities on investigation. Non-secretory myeloma may also present with osteoporosis and although no paraprotein band is detected on serum and urine electrophoresis, there may be evidence of immunosuppression with low immunoglobulin levels (Dolan *et al.*, 1989). Treatment of myeloma with melphalan and steroids may improve the prognosis, particularly when given early in the course of the disease. Radiotherapy may also be helpful in patients with localized bone pain. Hypercalcaemia should be managed along conventional lines including bisphosphonates. Dichloromethylene bisphosphonate (Clodronate) reduces bone pain and the incidence of fracture in myeloma patients even in the absence of hypercalcaemia (Delmas *et al.*, 1982).

Skeletal metastases

The skeleton is one of the most common sites of metastases and the bones most frequently involved are the vertebrae, femur, pelvis, ribs, sternum and humerus (Krane and Schiller, 1987). The tumours which most commonly metastasize to bone are carcinomas of the prostate, breast, lung, kidney, thyroid and bladder. Skeletal metastases may be either osteolytic or osteoblastic, with carcinoma of the thyroid, kidney and large bowel usually producing osteolytic metastases, whilst carcinoma of the prostate, carcinoid tumours and Hodgkin's lymphoma are associated with osteoblastic metastases (Krane and Schiller, 1987). Breast carcinoma may produce either osteolytic or osteoblastic metastases. The bone destruction associated with skeletal metastases may be due to the stimulation of osteoblast activity by local humoral factors released by tumour cells or to direct resorption of bone by tumour cells (Galasko, 1976; Eilon and Mundy, 1978). The osteoblastic response seen with some metastases is probably due to the production of specific mitogens for osteoblasts from the metastatic tumour cells (Koutsilleris *et al.*, 1987). The possibility of skeletal metastases should be considered in osteoporotic patients with severe bone pain, other clinical features of malignancy, anaemia, elevated ESR, raised plasma alkaline phosphatase or hypercalcaemia. Radiology may then demonstrate osteolytic or osteoblastic lesions and isotope bone scan may show multiple areas of increased isotope uptake. The presence of such 'hot spots' confined to the sites of crush fracture only neither confirms nor refutes the diagnosis of metastatic disease, as any crush fracture may be associated with an osteoblastic response and therefore appear as an area of increased isotope uptake (Hordon *et al.*, 1986). Biopsy of bone which appears radiologically abnormal may also occasionally be useful in the diagnosis of skeletal metastases.

Gastric surgery

Although gastrectomy has long been considered a cause of osteomalacia, the precise role of gastric surgery in the pathogenesis of osteoporosis is unclear. Osteoporosis is encountered more frequently than would be expected by chance in men and women following gastric surgery (Nordin *et al.*, 1984) and in one series of men with crush fractures, 9% had a past history of gastric surgery (Francis *et al.*, 1989). Possible factors in the pathogenesis of bone loss after gastric surgery include decreased absorption of vitamin D, the reduced food intake which commonly follows gastric surgery and malabsorption of calcium due to marginal vitamin D deficiency, the absence of gastric acid and intestinal hurry.

Anticonvulsant therapy

Bone densitometry indicates that bone mass in epileptic patients on anticonvulsant drugs is 70–90% of the expected value (Hahn, 1980) and up to 8% of osteoporotic men with crush fractures are on anticonvulsant therapy, suggesting that it is a genuine risk factor for the development of osteoporosis (Francis *et al.*, 1989). Anticonvulsant drugs increase the hepatic microsomal metabolism of vitamin D, leading to the formation of polar biologically inactive metabolites of vitamin D and to low plasma 25OHD levels (Hahn, 1980). This, together with evidence of a direct effect of certain anticonvulsant drugs on bowel mucosa, may account for the observed decrease in calcium absorption seen in patients taking anticonvulsant drugs. Anticonvulsant treatment during bone growth and consolidation may also potentially reduce the peak bone mass and therefore lead to osteoporotic fractures in early adult life. It is also important to appreciate that vertebral crush fractures may result from the trauma of convulsions rather than any underlying osteoporosis.

Male hypogonadism

Hypogonadism is a well-established cause of osteoporosis in males and is found in up to 20% of men with vertebral crush fractures (Baillie *et al.*, 1992). Low serum testosterone levels have also been reported in 58% of elderly men presenting with hip fracture after minimal trauma, compared with 18% in control subjects (Stanley *et al.*, 1991). The reported causes of hypogonadal osteoporosis in men include Klinefelter's syndrome, idiopathic hypogonadotropic hypogonadism, hyperprolactinaemia, haemochromatosis and primary testicular failure (Jackson and Kleerekoper, 1990).

There is a reduction in cortical and trabecular bone density in hypogonadal osteoporosis and histological studies have demonstrated increased bone resorption and decreased mineralization (Winks and Felts, 1980; Delmas and Meunier, 1981; Francis *et al.*, 1986; Jackson *et al.*, 1987). The pathogenesis of bone loss in hypogonadal men remains uncertain, though it has been suggested that it may be due to the direct effects of androgen or oestrogen deficiency (Smith and Walker, 1977), low plasma 1,25$(OH)_2$D concentrations (Francis *et al.*, 1986), malabsorption of calcium (Francis *et al.*, 1986) and reduced circulating calcitonin levels (Foresta *et al.*, 1983). These abnormalities may be reversed by treatment with testosterone, which decreases bone resorption and stimulates bone mineralization (Francis *et al.*, 1986). This leads to an increase in bone density in the forearm and lumbar spine, although the increase in vertebral bone density is confined to patients with open epiphyses (Finkelstein *et al.*, 1989). Furthermore, restoration of gonadal function in patients with hyperprolactinaemia by medical or surgical treatment significantly increases radial bone density, with only a minimal rise in lumbar spine bone mass. No change in bone mass is seen at either site in patients who remain hypogonadal despite the correction of hyperprolactinaemia (Greenspan *et al.*, 1986). The diagnosis of hypogonadism may not always be clinically apparent in men with osteoporosis (Baillie *et al.*, 1992), so routine measurement of serum testosterone and gonadotrophins may be worthwhile, particularly as treatment with testosterone may partly reverse the bone loss.

Hyperthyroidism

The effects of severe hyperthyroidism on bone were first described by von Recklinghausen in 1891, when he reported a 23-year-old woman with a five-year history of severe thyrotoxicosis. She had a severe kyphoscoliosis and complained of constant pain in the back and limbs. At post-mortem seven years later, she had osteoporosis with evidence of increased osteoclastic activity and fibrosis. Although it is now unusual to see such florid thyroid-induced bone disease, the association between hyperthyroidism and osteoporosis is now well established. Fraser and colleagues (1971) demonstrated an overall reduction in the bone mass of the metacarpal and distal radius of 7% and 5% in women with hyperthyroidism, though greater bone loss was present in women over the age of 50. Hyperthyroidism may present with osteoporotic fractures (Adams *et al.*, 1967; Francis *et al.*, 1982), though the diagnosis may not always be apparent as elderly osteoporotic patients with thyrotoxicosis may have no other clinical features of hyperthyroidism (Francis *et al.*, 1982). A recent case control study indicates that hyperthyroidism is associated with a 2.5-fold increase in the risk of hip fracture (Wejda *et al.*, 1995). Women with untreated multinodular goitre and subclinical hyperthyroidism, as confirmed by normal T4 and suppressed TSH, also have reduced forearm bone density (Mudde *et al.*, 1992). The magnitude of the reduction in bone mass is related more closely to the duration of subclinical hyperthyroidism than the severity of thyroid hormone excess (Mudde *et al.*, 1992), as shown previously in hyperthyroidism (Meunier *et al.*, 1972). The exogenous administration of thyroxine may also reduce bone density (Ross *et al.*, 1987; Paul *et al.*, 1988), which is also related to duration of treatment rather than dose or serum thyroid hormone levels (Ross *et al.*, 1987). The potentially adverse effect of exogenous thyroxine on the skeleton may be offset by concurrent treatment with oestrogen (Schneider *et al.*, 1994).

Hyperthyroidism is associated with an increase in bone formation and resorption, though resorption usually exceeds formation such that bone is lost from the skeleton (Adams *et al.*, 1967). Increased bone resorption in thyrotoxicosis leads to suppression of PTH production, low plasma $1,25(OH)_2D$ and malabsorption of calcium (Adams *et al.*, 1967; Francis and Peacock, 1987). Treatment of thyrotoxicosis reverses these effects, decreasing bone resorption and increasing plasma $1,25(OH)_2D$ and calcium absorption (Francis and Peacock, 1987). Treatment also leads to biochemical evidence of a further increase in bone formation, which closely parallels the rise in plasma $1,25(OH)_2D$, suggesting that the initial disparity between bone formation and resorption may be due to low plasma $1,25(OH)_2D$ levels (Francis and Peacock, 1987). The uncoupling of bone resorption and formation during treatment of thyrotoxicosis lasts for up to a year and might be expected to lead to an increase in bone mass and at least a partial reversal of the osteoporosis. Fraser and colleagues showed in 1971 that young hyperthyroid patients treated with drugs or surgery appear to increase bone mass back to normal, though osteoporosis persists in older women and in women treated with ^{131}I. They subsequently showed increases in bone density of 21.5% in women below the age of 50 and 16.7% in older women (Smith *et al.*, 1973).

Hyperparathyroidism

Primary hyperparathyroidism is associated with the development of three types of bone disease: osteitis fibrosa cystica, osteomalacia and osteoporosis (Davies, 1992). Hyperparathyroidism increases bone remodelling and therefore magnifies the imbalance between bone formation and resorption seen after the menopause, leading to the development of osteoporosis (Parfitt, 1976; Davies, 1992). Histological data suggest that primary hyperparathyroidism is associated with loss of cortical bone, though trabecular bone is conserved (Parisien *et al.*, 1990). Bone density measurements, however, show reduction of forearm and lumbar spine bone mass (Pak *et al.*, 1975; Seeman *et al.*, 1982; Martin *et al.*, 1986). The reduction in forearm bone density may be as great as 26% and is more marked in postmenopausal women than in younger women or men (Pak *et al.*, 1975; Martin *et al.*,

1986). Several studies suggest that primary hyperparathyroidism is associated with an increased risk of vertebral crush fractures, which may occur in up to 20% of cases (Peacock *et al.*, 1984; Martin *et al.*, 1986; Kochersberger *et al.*, 1987). These findings were not confirmed in a later study, when the authors suggested that the apparent increase in crush fractures reported in the earlier papers may have been due to selection bias and the use of inappropriate controls (Wilson *et al.*, 1988). Surgical treatment of primary hyperparathyroidism has been shown to increase bone density by up to 6.9%, leading to a partial correction of osteoporosis (Martin *et al.*, 1986).

Amenorrhoeic athletes

Exercise is considered to have beneficial effects on the skeleton and athletes tend to have a higher bone mass than more sedentary individuals (Nilsson and Westlin, 1971). Nevertheless, female athletes who become amenorrhoeic have a lower than expected bone mass (Drinkwater *et al.*, 1984; Marcus *et al.*, 1985) and sustain stress fractures as a result (Heath, 1985; Riggs and Eastell, 1986). Amenorrhoea occurs in up to 50% of competitive runners and ballet dancers (Nelson *et al.*, 1986), probably due to hypothalamic-pituitary dysfunction secondary to low body weight. It is therefore likely that amenorrhoeic athletes develop osteoporosis because of increased bone resorption, due to low circulating oestrogen levels, in an analogous manner to that seen in young women after bilateral oophorectomy (Aitken *et al.*, 1973). In addition to any effect on bone loss, amenorrhoeic athletes may also have a reduced peak bone mass, as many start training before the cessation of linear bone growth and experience a later than expected menarche (Frisch *et al.*, 1981). The osteopenia observed in amenorrhoeic athletes may be partly reversible, as a reduction in training leads to weight gain, increase in circulating oestrogens, resumption of menses and improvement in bone mass (Drinkwater *et al.*, 1986).

Anorexia nervosa

Anorexia nervosa is associated with a lower than expected bone mass and an increased risk of fractures, which may occur early in adult life (Rigotti *et al.*, 1984; Szmukler *et al.*, 1985). A review of the published literature shows that anorexia nervosa is associated with reduced bone density in the forearm, spine and femur (Salisbury and Mitchell, 1991). Spine bone density may be as much as 30% below the expected value, particularly where the anorexia nervosa has developed during adolescence (Biller *et al.*, 1989). Factors implicated in the pathogenesis of osteoporosis in this condition include poor nutrition, low dietary calcium intake, decreased body weight, early onset and long duration of amenorrhoea, reduced physical activity and hypercortisolism (Salisbury and Mitchell, 1991). It has been suggested that bulimia nervosa is also associated with osteoporosis, though the reduction in bone mass is less marked than that seen in anorexia nervosa (Joyce *et al.*, 1990). Another study showed normal bone density in bulimia nervosa compared with low values seen in anorexia nervosa, despite similar circulating oestradiol levels (Newman and Halmi, 1989). The 24-hour urine free cortisol excretion is considerably higher in anorexia nervosa than bulimia nervosa, suggesting that hypercortisolism may contribute to bone loss in anorexia nervosa (Newman and Halmi, 1989; Biller *et al.*, 1989).

Successful treatment of the anorexia nervosa is associated with an increase in bone mass (Treasure *et al.*, 1987), though this is likely to lead to only a partial correction of the deficit in bone mass. Follow-up of 27 women with anorexia nervosa for a median of 25 months suggests that although treatment prevents further bone loss, the increased risk of fracture persists (Rigotti *et al.*, 1991).

Hyperprolactinaemia

Amenorrhoea is a common problem in young women (Bachmann and Kemmann, 1982) and is due to hyperprolactinaemia in up to 30% of cases. Women with hyperprolactinaemia and amenorrhoea have a reduction in radial and vertebral bone mass (Klibanski *et al.*, 1980; Cann *et al.*, 1984), which is most severe in those with the lowest circulating oestradiol concentrations (Klibanski *et al.*, 1980), suggesting that the bone loss is due to oestrogen deficiency. Men with hyperprolactinaemic hypogonadism also have a low radial and vertebral bone mass (Jackson *et al.*, 1986; Greenspan *et al.*, 1986) and may present with vertebral fractures (Jackson *et al.*, 1986). Treatment of the hyperprolactinaemia with either surgery or bromocriptine increases bone mass in both sexes, though appears to only partially correct the osteopenia (Greenspan *et al.*, 1986; Klibanski and Greenspan, 1986). It is therefore important that hyperprolactinaemia is diagnosed and treated early, to limit the loss of bone and hopefully prevent osteoporotic fractures.

Amenorrhoea

In a cross-sectional study of 200 women aged 16–40 with a history of amenorrhoea, spine bone density was 15% lower than expected (Davies *et al.*, 1990). The reduction in bone mass was related to the duration of amenorrhoea and the severity of oestrogen deficiency, rather than the nature of the underlying disease (Davies *et al.*, 1990). Women who had sustained fractures after minimal trauma had significantly lower bone density than those without fractures. A higher than expected rate of bone loss from the lumbar spine has also been reported in women without amenorrhoea, but with anovulatory cycles or cycles with short luteal phases (Prior *et al.*, 1990). Together with the observations of the effects of hyperprolactinaemia, anorexia nervosa and amenorrhoea in athletes, it would appear that amenorrhoea is an important cause of bone loss and osteoporosis in women.

Diabetes mellitus

Osteoporosis is not generally considered to be a major complication of diabetes mellitus, though bone mass is reduced in insulin-dependent diabetic subjects by about 10% compared to age-matched controls and this is associated with an increased risk of fracture (Selby, 1988). In a small group of insulin-dependent diabetics, a longitudinal study over 11 years suggested that continued bone loss only occurred in those patients who had developed microvascular complications of their diabetes. Furthermore, this group had elevated urinary excretion of calcium and hydroxyproline. A negative correlation was observed between serum osteocalcin and haemoglobin A1c for all patients, suggesting that poor diabetic control may lead to impaired bone formation (Mathiassen *et al.*, 1990). In non-insulin-dependent diabetics, the confounding effects of obesity on bone density have led to conflicting reports of increased and decreased bone mass. Bone loss may develop soon after the onset of diabetes (Selby, 1988), though its pathogenesis is unclear. Histomorphometry has shown decreased bone turnover, with a decrease in osteoblast number and osteoid formation, whilst bone resorption appears to be reduced only slightly. Relative insulin resistance in both type I and type II diabetes produces osteoporosis through a variety of mechanisms including hypercalciuria, decrease in osteoblast number and a reduction in growth factor and vitamin D synthesis. Bone fragility may also be increased due to excess glycosylation of collagen (Bouillon, 1991).

Alcoholism

Alcoholism has long been recognized as a cause of osteoporosis (Saville, 1965), though it has recently become apparent that even modest alcohol consumption may have a deleterious effect on bone mass (Nordin and Polley, 1987; Stevenson *et al.*, 1989). Bone density is low in alcoholics (Saville, 1965; Nilsson and Westlin, 1973), with reductions in bone mass as much as 42% in the lumbar spine and 10% in appendicular cortical sites (Bikle *et al.*, 1985). The rate of bone loss in alcoholics is also 2% higher than in control subjects (Dalen and Lamke, 1976). There may be radiological evidence of osteoporosis with vertebral crush fractures in 50% of alcoholics (Spencer *et al.*, 1986; Crilly *et al.*, 1988), whilst between 5% and 10% of men with vertebral crush fractures may be alcoholic (Saville, 1973, Francis *et al.*, 1989).

Alcoholism is associated with a decreased bone formation (Bikle *et al.*, 1985), which may be due to a direct effect of ethanol on osteoblast function (Farley *et al.*, 1985). Serum osteocalcin levels are low in alcoholics (Diamond *et al.*, 1989; Labib *et al.*, 1989) reflecting decreased bone formation, but a similar reduction also occurs in normal subjects given alcohol acutely (Nielsen *et al.*, 1990). Long-standing alcoholics have evidence of low formation and resorption, despite normal or high PTH levels. Other studies show low formation but less inhibition of resorption (Crilly *et al.*, 1988; Diamond *et al.*, 1989). Acute alcohol intoxication causes transient hypoparathyroidism, hypocalcaemia and hypercalciuria (Laitinen and Valimaki, 1991). The transient suppression of PTH after alcohol ingestion may be followed by a rebound increase in PTH above the normal range, which may then stimulate bone resorption (Laitinen and Valimaki, 1991). Other possible causes of bone loss in alcoholism include poor diet, malabsorption of calcium due to vitamin D deficiency, alcohol-induced loss of calcium in the urine, alcohol-related liver disease and pseudo-Cushing's syndrome. Although alcohol-induced hypogonadism has been implicated in the pathogenesis of bone loss in alcoholics, a recent study shows normal testosterone levels (Bikle *et al.*, 1985). The diagnosis of alcoholism may be overlooked (Spencer *et al.*, 1986) and should be particularly considered in osteoporotic male subjects who have a raised MCV, abnormal liver function tests or rib fractures on chest X-ray (Lindsell *et al.*, 1982).

Immobilization

As mentioned earlier, physical activity and weight-bearing exercise are essential for the maintenance of skeletal mass and declining physical activity probably contributes to age-related bone loss. Immobilization leads to rapid bone loss of about 1% per week (Krolner *et al.*, 1983), which continues for about six months, when bone loss slows down and the bone mass reaches a new steady state (Minaire *et al.*, 1974). Bone loss in immobilization is due to a stimulation of bone resorption and a decrease in bone formation (Minaire *et al.*, 1974) and this is associated with an increase in plasma calcium, hypercalciuria and possibly suppression of PTH, $1,25(OH)_2D$ and calcium absorption (Anon, 1983). Immobilization leads to more rapid bone loss in weight-bearing bones, suggesting that bone loss is due to local mechanical factors, rather than changes in systemic factors such as thyroxine or cortisol (Anon, 1983). Therapeutic agents such as calcium and phosphate supplements, bisphosphonates and thiazide diuretics have been given to prevent further bone loss in immobilization, though the results have so far been disappointing (Anon, 1983; Mazess and Whedon, 1983). Where practical, remobilization should be encouraged, as this appears to increase trabecular bone mass by 0.25% per week and may at least in part correct the osteoporosis (Krolner *et al.*, 1983).

Osteogenesis imperfecta

Osteogenesis imperfecta is a rare and heterogeneous group of disorders, caused by mutations within the genes coding for type I collagen. Type I collagen comprises a triple helix of two α_1 chains and one α_2 chain. The production of the α_1 chains is controlled by the COL1A1 gene on chromosome 17, whilst the α_2 chain is regulated by the COL1A2 gene on chromosome 7. Over 70 mutations of the COL1A1 gene have now been identified and about 30 have been discovered to affect the COL1A2 gene. The exact nature of the mutation and its site profoundly influence the phenotype which results. Alterations in the gene leading to decreased production of normal collagen will result in a mildly affected individual, whilst those causing a structural change in the helices give rise to more serious clinical effects. In order for the collagen chains to form a triple helix, every third residue should be glycine. Patients with glycine substitutions occurring nearer to the carboxy terminus of the molecule are more severely affected, as are those involving the α_1 chains compared to the α_2 and those in which the substituting amino acid has a large side chain (Byers *et al.*, 1991).

Osteogenesis imperfecta therefore leads to abnormal collagen synthesis, composition, crosslinking and stability. This is characterized clinically by osteoporosis, multiple fractures, skeletal deformity, blue sclerae, deafness, dental abnormalities, thin skin, cardiac abnormalities and joint laxity. Osteogenesis imperfecta may be classified clinically into four main types (Table 2.2). Type I is characterized by mild bone disease, blue sclerae and early onset of deafness. Type II leads to perinatal or intrauterine fetal death (IUFD), though the distinct radiological appearances lead to a subclassification into types IIa, IIb and IIc. Type III is associated with progressive deformity with short stature and dentinogenesis imperfecta, though the sclerae appear normal. Type IV is typified by moderate bone deformity and short stature but normal sclerae.

Homocystinuria

Homocystinuria is an inborn error of methionine metabolism, most commonly due to cystathionine synthase deficiency, which leads to accumulation of methionine and homocystine and low levels of cystathionine and cystine. It has an autosomal recessive inheritance and an incidence of 1 in 200 000 live births (Mudd and Levy, 1983). Clinical features include osteoporosis, skeletal abnormality, lens dislocation, epilepsy, mental retardation, thrombotic tendency and a malar flush. The osteoporosis particularly affects the

Table 2.2 Clinical patterns of osteogenesis imperfecta (after Sillence *et al.*, 1979)

	Inheritance	*Fractures*	*Sclerae*	*Dentinogenesis*	*Hearing loss*
IA	Autosomal dominant	+	Blue	-	+
IB	Autosomal dominant	+	Blue	+	+
II	Autosomal recessive	+++	Blue	Often intrauterine fetal death	
III	Autosomal recessive	++	Blue at birth, less with age	+	Rare
IVA	Autosomal dominant	+	White	-	Rare
IVB	Autosomal dominant	+	White	+	Rare

spine and is classically associated with vertebral biconcavity, though the biconcavity tends to be posterior rather than central (Brenton *et al.*, 1972). The long bones are also osteoporotic, with a tendency to pathological fractures which are slow to heal (Mudd and Levy, 1983). Other skeletal features include arachnodactyly, high-arched palate, scoliosis, sternal deformity, widening of the metaphyses and enlargement of the epiphyses of the long bones, genu valgum and pes vacus (Brenton *et al.*, 1972; Mudd and Levy, 1983). The skeletal features of homocystinuria may be due to abnormal collagen crosslinking caused by excess homocysteine (Mudd and Levy, 1983) and to the somatomedin-like effect of homocystine (Dehnel and Francis, 1972). Treatment with pyridoxine may reverse the biochemical abnormalities in a proportion of patients with homocystinuria, though it is uncertain if this will improve the clinical state or prevent its progression.

Osteoporosis of pregnancy

Although the onset of osteoporosis during pregnancy is a rare phenomenon, it presents an important clinical problem. Nordin and Roper initially suggested the possibility of a syndrome of pregnancy-associated osteoporosis in 1955 and since then about 65 cases have been reported in the literature (Smith *et al.*, 1985; Dunne *et al.*, 1993). The incidence and aetiology remain poorly defined and it is uncertain whether the association is coincidental or causal (Khastgir and Studd, 1994).

Vertebral collapse with severe back pain and loss of height are the commonest features of the condition. These symptoms usually develop during the third trimester of pregnancy or in the postpartum period (Smith *et al.*, 1985; Dunne *et al.*, 1993). The pathogenesis is still unknown, but histological findings suggest that it is not due to increased resorption (Smith *et al.*, 1985). In a series of eight women investigated by Smith and colleagues (1985), plasma concentrations of $1,25(OH)_2D$ tended to be low. This suggests a transient failure of the usual changes in calcium-regulating hormones which normally prepare the maternal skeleton for the demands of pregnancy and lactation (Smith *et al.*, 1985). In the series of 35 women with pregnancy-associated osteoporosis collected by Dunne, there was a higher than expected incidence of fractures in the mothers of the women, suggesting that genetic factors may be involved (Dunne *et al.*, 1993).

Transitory osteoporosis of the hip during pregnancy has also been described (Curtiss and Kincaid, 1959; Beaulieu *et al.*, 1976). Curtiss and Kincaid (1959) speculated that this may be caused by mechanical compression of the obturator nerve with selective demineralization of the hip. Rosen (1970) considered that obstruction of venous return during pregnancy might be a causative factor, whilst Beaulieu and colleagues (1976) postulated that microfractures of the femoral neck might be responsible for the condition. In general, osteoporosis of pregnancy is transitory, stabilizes and appears not to recur in subsequent pregnancies (Smith *et al.*, 1985).

Heparin therapy

Osteoporosis in association with heparin therapy was first reported by Griffith and colleagues (1965) in seven patients receiving long-term heparin for ischaemic heart disease. Subsequently there have been reports following heparin in other medical conditions and also during pregnancy, when heparin is preferable to warfarin because of teratogenic side effects of the latter. In 70 pregnant women treated with heparin, there was radiological osteopenia present in 17% of cases at one week postpartum, with no osteopenia amongst 30 control pregnancies. Re-examination 6–12 months later suggested the changes were reversible (Dahlman *et al.*, 1990). Ginsberg *et al.* (1990), using dual photon absorptiometry of the lumbar spine and single photon absorptiometry of the wrist, showed a significantly higher proportion of individuals with low bone density (more than two standard deviations below the mean) in a cohort of 61 premenopausal women previously treated with heparin compared to controls.

The suggested mechanisms of the pathogenesis of heparin-associated osteoporosis include: potentiation of parathyroid effect on osteoclast activity; decreased osteoblast activity; increased bone resorption due to heparin-related collagenase activity; and abnormalities in vitamin D metabolism (Avioli, 1975).

In most cases of heparin-associated osteoporosis, the daily dose was between 15 000 and 20 000 units and the duration of treatment exceeded six months (Levine and Anderson, 1990). It would therefore seem that short-term treatment (less than 14 days) is unlikely to be associated with osteoporosis and in patients requiring medium or long-term heparin the dose should be kept below 20 000 units daily if possible.

Systemic mastocytosis

Systemic mastocytosis (SM) is a multiorgan disease characterized by an abnormal increase in mast cells, predominantly affecting the skin and skeleton. Back pain due to osteoporosis may be the presenting symptom in some patients with SM. Chines *et al.* (1991) reported 10 patients with SM who presented with osteoporosis; in nine cases there were multiple vertebral compression fractures. Histomorphometric parameters of bone formation showed an increase in osteoid volume and osteoid and osteoblast surfaces, and indices of bone resorption were also increased.

One postulated mechanism for osteoporosis in SM is that mast cells release substances which affect bone metabolism and in particular heparin (see above). They also release several prostaglandins, predominantly PGD_2 which is weakly resorptive, but this in turn may stimulate production of the more potent bone-resorbing PGE_2. Mast cells may also interfere with coupling of bone formation and resorption (Harvey *et al.*, 1989). The role of mast cells in bone resorption remains to be fully established.

Transplantation

With increasing survival after organ transplantation, osteoporosis is now seen as a significant complication of renal, liver, cardiac and bone marrow transplants. Patients with liver disease such as primary biliary cirrhosis have lower bone density and higher rates of bone loss than age-matched controls. Bone density increases further after liver transplantation, resulting in atraumatic fractures in up to 65% of cases (Eastell *et al.*, 1991). In the longer term, bone density increases again, suggesting that osteoporosis may become less severe. In a series of 40 patients studied after cardiac transplantation, reduced bone density was present in 28% at the lumbar spine and in 20% at the hip, whilst vertebral fractures were found in 35% (Shane *et al.*, 1993). Patients undergoing cardiac transplantation tend to have low spine bone density before surgery, which may be due to immobility, poor nutrition and the use of loop diuretics. After cardiac transplantation, the spine bone density falls to values up to 50% lower than normal at six months, possibly due to treatment with steroids and cyclosporin A (Muchmore *et al.*, 1991; Shane *et al.*, 1993).

REFERENCES

Aaron, J.E., Makins, N.B. and Sagreiya, K. (1987) The microanatomy of trabecular bone loss in normal aging men and women. *Clin Orthop* **215**: 260–71.

Aaron, J.E., Francis, R.M., Peacock, M. and Makins, N.B. (1989) Contrasting microanatomy of idiopathic and corticosteroid-induced osteoporosis. *Clin Orthop* **243**: 294–305.

Adams, P.H., Jowsey, J., Kelly, P.J. *et al.* (1967)

Effect of hyperthyroidism on bone and mineral metabolism. *Q J Med* **36**: 1–15.

Aitken, J.M., Hart, D.M., Anderson, J.B. *et al.* (1973) Osteoporosis after oophorectomy for malignant disease in premenopausal women. *Br Med J* **2**: 325–8.

Anon (1983) Osteoporosis and activity. *Lancet* **i**: 1365–6.

Avioli, L.V. (1975) Heparin induced osteoporosis: an appraisal. *Adv Exp Med Biol* **52**: 375–87.

Bachmann, G.A. and Kemmann, E. (1982) Prevalence of oligomenorrhea and amenorrhea in a college population. *Am J Obstet Gynecol* **144**: 98–102.

Baillie, S.P., Davison, C.E., Johnson, F.J. and Francis, R.M. (1992) Pathogenesis of vertebral crush fractures in men. *Age Ageing* **21**: 139–41.

Baker, H.W.G., Burger, H.G., De Kretser, D.M. *et al.* (1976) Changes in the pituitary-testicular system with age. *Clin Endocrinol* **5**: 349–72.

Baker, M.R., Peacock, M. and Nordin, B.E.C. (1980) The decline in vitamin D status with age. *Age Ageing* **9**: 249–52.

Bar-Shavit, Z., Teitelbaum, S.L. and Kahn, A.J. (1983) Saccharides mediate the attachment of rat macrophages to bone in vitro. *J Clin Invest* **72**: 516–25.

Bar-Shavit, Z., Kahn, A.J., Pegg, L.E., Stone, K.R. and Teitelbaum, S.L. (1984) Glucocorticoids modulate macrophage surface oligosaccharides and their bone binding activity. *J Clin Invest* **73**: 1277–83.

Beaulieu, J.G., Razzano, C.D. and Levine, R.B. (1976) Transient osteoporosis of the hip in pregnancy. *Clin Orthop* **115**: 165–8.

Beresford, J.N., Gallagher, J.A. and Russell, R.G.G. (1986) 1,25 Dihydroxyvitamin D_3 and human bone derived cells in vitro. Effects on alkaline phosphatase, type I collagen and proliferation. *Endocrinology* **119**: 1776–85.

Bikle, D.D., Genant, H.K., Cann, C. *et al.* (1985) Bone disease in alcohol abuse. *Ann Intern Med* **103**: 42–8.

Biller, B.M., Saxe, V., Herzog, D.B. *et al.* (1989) Mechanisms of osteoporosis in adult and adolescent women with anorexia nervosa. *J Clin Endocrinol Metabol* **68**: 548–54.

Bouillon, R. (1991) Diabetic bone disease. *Calcif Tissue Int* **49**: 155–160.

Boyce, W.J. and Vessey, M.P. (1985) Rising incidence of fracture of the proximal femur. *Lancet* **i**: 150–1.

Brenton, D.P., Dow, C.J., James, J.I.P., Hay, R.L. and Wynne-Davies, R. (1972) Homocystinuria and Marfan's syndrome. A comparison. *J Bone Joint Surg* **54B**: 277–98.

Buchanan, J.R., Myers, C.A. and Greer, R.B. III (1988) Effect of declining renal function on bone density in aging women. *Calcif Tissue Int* **43**: 1–6.

Bullamore, J.R., Gallagher, J.C., Wilkinson, R., Nordin, B.E.C. and Marshall, D.H. (1970) Effect of age on calcium absorption. *Lancet* **ii**: 535–7.

Byers, P.H., Wallis, G.A. and Willing, M.C. (1991) Osteogenesis imperfecta: translation of mutation to phenotype. *J Med Genet* **28**: 433–42.

Cann, C.E., Martin, M.C., Genant, H.K. and Jaffe, R.B. (1984) Decreased spinal mineral content in amenorrheic women. *J Am Med Assoc* **251**: 626–9.

Chines, A., Pacifici, R., Avioli, L.V., Teitelbaum, S.L. and Korenblat, P.E. (1991) Systemic mastocytosis presenting as osteoporosis: a clinical and histomorphomometric study. *J Clin Endocrinol Metabol* **72**: 140–4.

Christiansen, C., Riis, B.J. and Rodbro, P. (1987) Prediction of rapid bone loss in postmenopausal women. *Lancet* **i**: 1105–8.

Cohn, S.H., Abesamis, C., Yasumura, S. *et al.* (1977) Comparative skeletal mass and radial bone mineral content in black and white women. *Metabolism* **26**: 171–8.

Compston, J.E. (1992) Risk factors for osteoporosis. *Clin Endocrinol* **36**: 223–4.

Cooper, C., Barker, D.J.P. and Wickham, C. (1988) Physical activity, muscle strength, and calcium intake in fracture of the proximal femur in Britain. *Br Med J* **297**: 1443–6.

Crilly, R.G., Marshall, D.H. and Nordin, B.E.C. (1979a) Metabolic effects of corticosteroid therapy in postmenopausal women. *J Steroid Biochem* **11**: 429–33.

Crilly, R.G., Marshall, D.H. and Nordin, B.E.C. (1979b) Effect of age on plasma androstenedione concentration in oophorectomized women. *Clin Endocrinol* **10**: 199–201.

Crilly, R.G., Marshall, D.H., Horsman, A., Nordin, B.E.C. and Peacock, M. (1983) Corticosteroid osteoporosis. In: *Osteoporosis: A Multidisciplinary Problem*, (eds Dixon, A.StJ., Russell, R.G.G. and Stamp, T.C.B.), Royal Society of Medicine International Congress and Symposium Series No 55. Academic Press, London, pp.153–9.

Crilly, R.G., Anderson, C., Hogan, D. and Delaquerriere-Richardson, L. (1988) Bone histomorphometry, bone mass, and related parameters in alcoholic males. *Calcif Tissue Int* **43**: 269–76.

Curtiss, P.H. Jr and Kincaid, W.E. (1959) Transitory demineralization of the hip in pregnancy. *J Bone Joint Surg* **41A**: 1327–32.

Curtiss, P.H. Jr, Clark, W.S. and Herndon, C.H. (1954) Vertebral fractures resulting from prolonged cortisone and corticotrophin therapy. *J Am Med Assoc* **156**: 467–9.

Dahlman, T., Lindvall, N. and Hellgren, M. (1990) Osteopaenia in pregnancy during longterm heparin treatment: a radiological study postpartum. *Br J Obstet Gynaecol* **97**: 221–8.

Dalen, N. and Lamke, B. (1976) Bone mineral loss in alcoholics. *Acta Orthop Scand* **47**: 469–71.

Davidson, B.J., Ross, R.K., Paganini-Hill A. *et al.* (1982) Total and free estrogens and androgens in postmenopausal women with hip fractures. *J Clin Endocrinol Metab* **54**: 115–20.

Davies, M. (1992) Primary hyperparathyroidism: aggressive or conservative treatment? *Clin Endocrinol* **36**: 325–32.

Davies, M.C., Hall, M.L. and Jacobs, H.S. (1990) Bone mineral loss in young women with amenorrhoea. *Br Med J* **301**: 790–3.

Dehnel, J.M. and Francis, M.J.O. (1972) Somatomedin (sulphation factor)-like activity of homocystine. *Clin Sci* **43:** 903–6.

Delmas, P. and Meunier, P.J. (1981) L'osteoporose au cours du syndrome de Klinefelter. *Nouv Presse Med* **10**: 687–90.

Delmas, P.D., Charhon, S., Chapuy, M.C. *et al.* (1982) Long term effects of dichloromethylene diphosphonate (Cl_2MDP) on skeletal lesions in multiple myeloma. *Metab Bone Dis Relat Res* **4**: 163–8.

De Vernejoul, M.C., Bielakoff, J., Herve, M. *et al.* (1983) Evidence for defective osteoblastic function. A role for alcohol and tobacco consumption in osteoporosis in middle-aged men. *Clin Orthop* **179**: 107–15.

Diamond, T., Stiel, D., Lunzer, M., Wilkinson, M. and Posen, S. (1989) Ethanol reduces bone formation and may cause osteoporosis. *Am J Med* **86**: 282–8.

Dolan, A.L., Wheeler, T.K., Jones, D.H. and Crisp, A.J. (1989) Osteoporosis and immunosuppression in multiple myeloma. *Br Med J* **299**: 718–19.

Drinkwater, B.L., Nilson, K., Chesnut, C.H. III. *et al.* (1984) Bone mineral content of amenorrheic and eumenorrheic athletes. *N Engl J Med* **311**: 277–81.

Drinkwater, B.L., Nilson, K., Ott, S. and Chesnut, C.H. III. (1986) Bone mineral density after resumption of menses in amenorrheic athletes. *J Am Med Assoc* **256**: 380–2.

Dunne, F., Walters, B., Marshall, T. and Heath, D.A. (1993) Pregnancy associated osteoporosis. *Clin Endocrinol* **39**: 497–90.

Dykman, T.R., Gluck, O.S., Murphy, W.A., Hahn, T.J. and Hahn, B.H. (1985) Evaluation of factors associated with glucocorticoid induced osteopenia in patients with rheumatic diseases. *Arthritis Rheum* **28**: 361–8.

Eastell, R., Dickson, E.R., Hodgson, S.F *et al.* (1991) Rates of vertebral bone loss before and after liver transplantation in women with primary biliary cirrhosis. *Hepatology* **14**: 296–300.

Eilon, G. and Mundy, G.R. (1978) Direct resorption of bone by human breast cancer cells *in vitro*. *Nature* **276**: 726–8.

Eisman, J.A., Kelly, P.J., Morrison, N.A *et al.* (1992) Genetic and environmental interactions on bone mass. *Bone Miner* **17** (Suppl 1): 72 (abstract).

Ekenstam, E.A.F., Ljunghall, S. and Hallgren, R. (1986) Serum osteocalcin in rheumatoid arthritis and other inflammatory arthritides: relation between inflammatory activity and the effect of glucocorticoids and remission inducing drugs. *Ann Rheum Dis* **45**: 484–90.

Farley, J.R., Fitzsimmons, R., Taylor, A.K., Jorch, U.M. and Lau, K-HW. (1985) Direct effects of ethanol on bone resorption and formation in vitro. *Arch Biochem Biophys* **238**: 305–14.

Finkelstein, J.S., Klibanski, A., Neer, R.M. *et al.* (1989) Increases in bone density during treatment of men with idiopathic hypogonadotrophic hypogonadism. *J Clin Endocrinol Metabol* **69**: 776–83.

Finkelstein, J.S., Neer, R.M., Biller, B.M.K., Crawford, J.D. and Klibanski, A. (1992) Osteopenia in men with a history of delayed puberty. *N Engl J Med* **326**: 600–4.

Foresta, C., Busnardo, B., Ruzza, G., Zanatta, G. and Mioni, R. (1983) Lower calcitonin levels in young hypogonadic men with osteoporosis. *Horm Metab Res* **15**: 206–7.

Francis, R.M. (1990) Pathogenesis of osteoporosis. In: *Osteoporosis: Pathogenesis and Management*, (ed. Francis, R.M.), Kluwer, Lancaster, pp.51–80.

Francis, R.M. and Peacock, M. (1987) The pathogenesis of osteoporosis in thyrotoxicosis. In: *Osteoporosis 1987*, (eds Christiansen, C., Johansen, J.S. and Riis, B.J.) Osteopress, Copenhagen, pp.166–7.

Francis, R.M., Barnett, M.J., Selby, P.L. and Peacock, M. (1982). Thyrotoxicosis presenting as fracture of femoral neck. *Br J Med* **285**: 97–8.

Francis, R.M., Peacock, M. and Barkworth, S.A. (1984) Renal impairment and its effects on calcium metabolism in elderly women. *Age Ageing* 13: 14–20.

Francis, R.M., Peacock, M., Aaron, J.E *et al.* (1986) Osteoporosis in hypogonadal men: role of decreased plasma 1,25-dihydroxyvitamin D, calcium malabsorption and low bone formation. *Bone* **7**: 261–8.

Francis, R.M., Peacock, M., Marshall, D.H., Horsman, A. and Aaron, J.E. (1989) Spinal osteoporosis in men. *Bone and Mineral* **5:** 347–57.

Francis, R.M., Johnson, F.J. and Rawlings, D. (1992) The determinants of bone mass in normal elderly men. In: *Current Research in Osteoporosis and Bone Mineral Measurement II*: 1992, (ed. Ring, E.F.J.), British Institute of Radiology, London, pp.54–5.

Fraser, S.A., Anderson, J.B., Smith, D.A. and Wilson, G.M. (1971) Osteoporosis and fractures following thyrotoxicosis. *Lancet* **i**: 981–3.

Frisch, R.E., Gotz-Welbergen, A.V., McArthur, J.W. *et al.* (1981) Delayed menarche and amenorrhea of college athletes in relation to age of onset of training. *J Am Med Assoc* **246**: 1559–63.

Fucik, R.F., Kukreja, S.C., Hargis, G.K. *et al.* (1975) Effect of glucocorticoids on function of the parathyroid glands in man. *J Clin Endocrinol Metab* **40**: 152–5.

Galasko, C.S.B. (1976) Mechanisms of bone destruction in the development of skeletal metastases. *Nature* **263**: 507–8.

Garrett, I.R., Durie, B.G.M., Nedwin, G.E. *et al.* (1987) Production of lymphotoxin, a bone-resorbing cytokine, by cultured human myeloma cells. *N Engl J Med* **317**: 526–32.

Genant, H.K., Cann, C.E. and Foul, D.D. (1982) Quantitative computed tomography for assessing vertebral bone mineral. In: *Non-Invasive Bone Measurements*, (eds Dequeker, J. and Johnston, C.C.), IRL Press, Oxford, pp. 215–49.

Gennari, C. and Civitelli, R. (1986) Glucocorticoid-induced osteoporosis. *Clin Rheum Dis* **12**: 637–54.

Ginsberg, J.S., Kowalchuk, G., Hirsh, J. *et al.* (1990) Heparin effect on bone density. *Thromb Haemost* **64**: 286–9.

Goldsmith, N.F. and Johnston, J.O. (1975) Bone mineral: effects of oral contraceptives, pregnancy and lactation. *J Bone Joint Surg* **57A**: 657–68.

Greenspan, S.L., Neer, R.M., Ridgway, E.C. and Klibanski, A. (1986) Osteoporosis in men with hyperprolactinemic hypogonadism. *Ann Intern Med* **104**: 777–82.

Griffith, G.C., Nicholas, G. Jr, Asher, J.D. and Flanagan, B. (1965) Heparin osteoporosis. *J Am Med Assoc* **193**: 91–4.

Hahn, T.J. (1980) Drug-induced disorders of vitamin D and mineral metabolism. *Clin Endocrinol Metab* **9**: 107–29.

Hahn, T.J., Boisseau, V.C. and Avioli, L.V. (1974) Effect of chronic corticosteroid administration on diaphyseal and metaphyseal bone mass. *J Clin Endocrinol Metab* **39**: 274–82.

Hahn, T.J., Halstead, L.R. and Baran, D.T. (1981) Effects of short-term corticosteroid administration on intestinal calcium absorption and circulating vitamin D metabolite concentrations in man. *J Clin Endocrinol Metab* **52**: 111–15.

Hall, D.H. (1977) Synergistic effect of age and corticosteroid treatment on connective tissue metabolism. *Ann Rheum Dis* **36**s: 58–62.

Harvey, J.A., Anderson, H.C., Borek, D., Morris, D. and Lukert, B.P. (1989) Osteoporosis associated with mastocytosis confined to bone: Report of two cases. *Bone* **10**: 237–41.

Heaney, R.P., Recker, R.R. and Saville, P.D. (1978) Menopausal changes in calcium balance performance. *J Lab Clin Med* **92**: 953–63.

Heath, H. (1985) Athletic women, amenorrhea and skeletal integrity. *Ann Intern Med* **102**: 258–60.

Holbrook, T.L., Barrett-Connor, E. and Wingard, D.L. (1988) Dietary calcium and risk of hip fracture: 14-year prospective population study. *Lancet* **ii**: 1046–9.

Hordon, L.H., Francis, R.M., Marshall, D.H., Smith, A.H. and Peacock, M. (1986) Are scintigrams of the spine useful in verterbral osteoporosis? *Clin Radiol* **37**: 487–9.

Howland, W.J., Pugh, D.C. and Sprague, R.G. (1958) Roentgenologic changes in the skeletal system in Cushing's syndrome. *Radiology* **71**: 69–78.

Jackson, J.A. and Kleerekoper, M. (1990) Osteoporosis in men: diagnosis, pathophysiology and prevention. *Medicine* **69**: 137–52.

Jackson, J.A. and Spiekerman, A.M. (1989) Testosterone deficiency is common in men with hip fractures after simple falls. *Clin Res 37*: **131** (abstract).

Jackson, J.A., Kleerekoper, M. and Parfitt, A.M. (1986) Symptomatic osteoporosis in a man with hyperprolactinemic hypogonadism. *Ann Intern Med* **105**: 543–5.

Jackson, J.A., Kleerekoper, M., Parfitt, A.M. *et al.* (1987) Bone histomorphometry in hypogonadal and eugonadal men with spinal osteoporosis. *J Clin Endocrinol Metabol* **65**: 53–8.

Jensen, J., Christiansen, C. and Rodbro, P. (1985) Cigarette smoking, serum estrogens and bone loss during hormone-replacement therapy early after menopause. *N Engl J Med* **313**: 973–5.

Jick, H., Porter, J. and Morrison, A.S. (1977) Relation between smoking and the age of natural menopause. *Lancet* **i**: 1354–5.

Johnston, C.C. Jr, Miller, J.Z., Slemenda, C.W. *et al.* (1992) Calcium supplementation and increases in bone mineral density in children. *N Engl J Med* **327**: 82–7.

Jowell, P.S., Epstein, S., Fallon, M.D., Reinhardt, T.A. and Ismail, F. (1987) 1,25-Dihydroxyvitamin D_3 modulates glucocorticoid-induced alteration in serum GLA protein and bone histomorphometry. *Endocrinology* **120**: 531–8.

Joyce, J.M., Warren, D.L., Humphries, L.L., Smith, A.J. and Coon, J.S. (1990) Osteoporosis in women with eating disorders: comparison of physical parameters, exercise, and menstrual status with SPA and DPA evaluation. *J Nucl Med* **31**: 325–31.

Kanders, B., Dempster, D.W. and Lindsay, R. (1988) Interaction of calcium nutrition and physical activity on bone mass in young women. *J Bone Miner Res* **3**: 145–9.

Kelly, P.J., Pocock, N.A., Sambrook, P.N. and Eisman, J.A. (1990) Dietary calcium, sex hormones, and bone mineral density in men. *Br Med J* **300**: 1361–4.

Khastgir, G. and Studd, J. (1994) Pregnancy-associated osteoporosis. *Br J Obstet Gynaecol* **101**: 836–8.

Khaw, K-T., Sneyd, M-J. and Compston, J. (1992) Bone density, parathyroid hormone and 25-hydroxyvitamin D concentrations in middle aged women. *Br Med J* **305**: 273–7.

Kimberg, D.V. (1969) Effects of vitamin D and steroid hormones on the active transport of calcium by the intestine. *N Engl J Med* **280**: 1396–405.

Klein, R.G., Arnaud, S.B., Gallagher, J.C., De Luca, H.F. and Riggs, B.L. (1977) Intestinal calcium absorption in exogenous hypercortisolism. *J Clin Invest* **60**: 253–9.

Klibanski, A. and Greenspan, S.L. (1986) Increase in bone mass after treatment of hyperprolactinemic amenorrhea. *N Engl J Med* **315**, 542–6.

Klibanski, A., Neer, R.M., Beitins, I.Z. *et al.* (1980) Decreased bone density in hyperprolactinemic women. *N Engl J Med* **303**: 1511–14.

Kochersberger, G., Buckley, N.J., Leight, G.S. *et al.* (1987) What is the clinical significance of bone loss in primary hyperparathyroidism? *Arch Intern Med* **107**: 1951–3.

Koutsilleris, M., Rabbani, S.A., Bennett, H.P.J. and Goltzman, D. (1987) Characteristics of prostate-derived growth factors for cells of the osteoblast phenotype. *J Clin Invest* **80**: 941–6.

Krall, E.A., Sahyoun, N., Tannenbaum, S., Dallal, G.E. and Dawson-Hughes, B. (1989) Effect of vitamin D intake on seasonal variations in parathyroid hormone secretion in post-menopausal women. *N Engl J Med* **321**: 1777–83.

Krane, S.M. and Schiller, A.L. (1987) Hyperostosis, neoplasms and other disorders of bone and cartilage. In: *Harrison's Principles of Internal Medicine*, 11th edn, (eds Braunwald, E., Isselbacher, K.J., Petersdorf, R.G. *et al.*), McGraw-Hill, New York, pp. 1902–10.

Krolner, B. and Toft, B. (1983) Vertebral bone loss: an unheeded effect of therapeutic bed rest. *Clin Sci* **64**: 537–40.

Krolner, B., Toft, B., Pors Nielsen, S. and Tondevold, E. (1983) Physical exercise as prophylaxis against involutional bone loss: a controlled trial. *Clin Sci* **64**: 541–6.

Labib, M., Abdel-Kader, M., Ranganath, L., Teale, D. and Marks, V. (1989) Bone disease in chronic alcoholism: the value of plasma osteocalcin measurement. *Alcohol Alcohol* **24**: 141–4.

Laitinen, K. and Valimaki, M. (1991) Alcohol and bone. *Calcif Tissue Int* **49**: S70–S73.

Lau, E., Donnan, S., Barker, D.J. and Cooper, C. (1988) Physical activity and calcium intake in fracture of the proximal femur in Hong Kong. *Br Med J* **297**: 1441–3.

Levine, M.N. and Anderson, D.R. (1990) Side-effects of antithrombotic therapy. *Baillière's Clin Haematol* **3**: 815–29.

Lindsell, D.R.M., Wilson, A.G. and Maxwell, J.D. (1982). Fractures on chest radiograph in detection of alcoholic liver disease. *Br J Med* **285**: 597–9.

Lo Cascio V., Bonucci, E., Imbimbo, B. *et al.* (1984) Bone loss after glucocorticoid therapy. *Calcif Tissue Int* **36**: 435–8.

Lo Cascio, V., Bonucci, E., Ballanti, P. *et al.* (1987) Glucocorticoid osteoporosis: a longitudinal study. In: *Osteoporosis 1987*, (eds Christiansen, C., Johansen, J.S. and Riis, B.J.), Osteopress, Copenhagen, pp.1062–4.

Lukert, B.P. and Raisz, L.G. (1990) Glucocorticoid induced osteoporosis; pathogenesis and management. *Ann Intern Med* **112**: 353–64.

MacAdams, M.R., White, R.H. and Chipps, B.E. (1986) Reduction of serum testosterone levels during chronic glucocorticoid therapy. *Ann Intern Med* **104**: 648–51.

Manning, P.J., Evans, M.C. and Reid, I.R. (1992) Normal bone mineral density following cure of Cushing's syndrome. *Clin Endocrinol* **36**: 229–34.

Marcus, R., Cann, C., Madvig, P. *et al.* (1985) Menstrual function and bone mass in elite women distance runners. *Ann Intern Med* **102**: 158–63.

Martin, P., Bergmann, P., Gillet, C. *et al.* (1986) Partially reversible osteopenia after surgery for primary hyperparathyroidism. *Arch Intern Med* **106**: 689–91.

Mathiassen, B., Nielsen, S., Johansen, J.S. *et al.* (1990) Long-term bone loss in insulin-dependent diabetic patients with microvascular complications. *J Diabetic Complications* **4**: 145–9.

Matkovic, V., Kostial, K., Simonovic, I. *et al.* (1979) Bone status and fracture rates in two regions of Yugoslavia. *Am J Clin Nutr* **32**: 540–9.

Mazess, R.B. (1982) On aging bone loss. *Clin Orthop* **165**: 239–52.

Mazess, R.B. and Whedon, G.D. (1983) Immobilization and bone. *Calcif Tissue Int* **35**: 265–7.

Meunier, P.J., Bianchi, G.G.S., Edouard, C.M. *et al.* (1972) Bony manifestations of thyrotoxicosis. *Orthop Clin North Am* **3**: 745–74.

Minaire, P., Meunier, P., Edouard, C. *et al.* (1974) Quantitative histological data on disuse osteoporosis. *Calcif Tissue Res* **17**: 57–73.

Morrison, N.A., Qui, J.C., Tokita, A. *et al.* (1994) Prediction of bone density from vitamin D receptor alleles. *Nature* **367**: 284–7.

Muchmore, J.S., Cooper, D.K.C., Ye, Y., Schlegel, U.T. and Zuhdi, N. (1991) Loss of vertebral bone density in heart transplant patients. *Transplant Proc* **23:** 1184–5.

Mudd, S.H. and Levy, H.L. (1983) Disorders of transsulfuration. In: *The Metabolic Basis of Inherited Disease*, 5th edn, (eds Stanbury, J.B., Wyngaarden, J.B., Fredrickson, D.S. *et al.*), McGraw-Hill, New York, pp. 522–59.

Mudde, A.H., Reijnders, F.J.L. and Nieuwenhuijzen Kruseman, A.C. (1992) Peripheral bone density in women with untreated multinodular goitre. *Clin Endocrinol* **37**, 35–9.

Mueller, M.N. (1976) Effects of corticosteroids on bone mineral in rheumatoid arthritis and asthma. *Am J Roentgenol* **126**: 1300.

Mundy, G.R., Raisz, L.G., Cooper, R.A., Schechter, G.P. and Salmon, S.E. (1974) Evidence for the secretion of an osteoclast stimulating factor in myeloma. *N Engl J Med* **291**, 1041–6.

Murray, R.O. (1960) Radiological bone changes in Cushing's syndrome and steroid therapy. *Br J Radiol* **33**: 1–19.

Nelson, M.E., Fischer, E.C., Catsos, P.D. *et al.* (1986) Diet and bone status in amenorrheic runners. *Am J Clin Nutr* **43**: 910–16.

Newman, M.M. and Halmi, K.A. (1989) Relationship of bone density to estradiol and cortisol in anorexia nervosa and bulimia. *Psychiatry Res* **29**: 105–12.

Nielsen, H.K., Lundby, L., Rasmussen, K., Charles, P. and Hansen, C. (1990) Alcohol decreases serum osteocalcin in a dose-dependent way in normal subjects. *Calcif Tissue Int* **46**: 173–8.

Nilsson, B.E. and Westlin, N.E. (1971) Bone density in athletes. *Clin Orthop* **77**: 179–82.

Nilsson, B.E. and Westlin, N.E. (1973) Changes in bone mass in alcoholics. *Clin Orthop* **90**: 229–32.

Nordin, B.E.C. and Polley, K.J. (1987) Metabolic consequences of the menopause. *Calcif Tissue Int* **41** (Suppl 1): 1–59.

Nordin, B.E.C. and Roper, A. (1955) Post-pregnancy osteoporosis – a syndrome? *Lancet* **i**: 431–4.

Nordin, B.E.C., Crilly, R.G. and Smith, D.A. (1984) Osteoporosis. In: *Metabolic Bone and Stone Disease*, 2nd edn, (ed. Nordin, B.E.C.) Churchill Livingstone, Edinburgh, pp. 1–70.

Obrant, K.J., Bengner, U., Johnell, O., Nilsson, B.E. and Sernbo, I. (1989) Increasing age-adjusted risk of fragility fractures: a sign of increasing osteoporosis in successive generations? *Calcif Tissue Int* **44**: 157–67.

Pak, C.Y.C., Stewart, A., Kaplan, R. *et al.* (1975) Photon absorptiometric analysis of bone density in primary hyperparathyroidism. *Lancet* **ii**: 7–8.

Parfitt, A.M. (1976) The action of parathyroid hormone on bone. Relation to bone remodelling and turnover, calcium homeostasis and metabolic bone disease. Part III. *Metabolism* **25**: 1033–69.

Parisien, M., Silverberg, S.J., Shane, E. *et al.* (1990) The histomorphometry of bone in primary hyperparathyroidism: preservation of cancellous bone structure. *J Clin Endocrinol Metab* **70**: 930–8.

Paul, T.P., Kerrigan, J., Kelly, A.M., Braverman,

L.E. and Baran, D.T. (1988) Long-term L-thyroxine therapy is associated with decreased hip bone density in premenopausal women. *J Am Med Assoc* **259**: 3137–41.

Peacock, M., Horsman, A., Aaron, J.E. *et al.* (1984) The role of parathyroid hormone in bone loss. *Proceedings of the Copenhagen International Symposium on Osteoporosis, 3–8 June 1984*, (eds Christiansen, C., Arnaud, C.D., Nordin, B.E.C. *et al.*), Aalborg Stiftsbogtrykkeri, Copenhagen, pp. 463–8.

Peacock, M., Johnston, C.C. Jr and Christian, J. (1992) Inheritance of calcium absorption. *Bone Miner* **17** (Suppl 1): 92 (abstract).

Perry, H.M., Fallon, M.D., Bergfeld, M., Teitelbaum, S.L. and Avioli, L.V. (1982) Osteoporosis in young men: a syndrome of hypercalciuria and accelerated bone turnover. *Arch Intern Med* **142**: 1295–8.

Pocock, N.A., Eisman, J.A., Dunstan, C.R. *et al.* (1987) Recovery from steroid-induced osteoporosis. *Ann Intern Med* **107**: 319–23.

Prior, J.C., Vigna, Y.M., Schechter, M.T. and Burgess, A.E. (1990) Spinal bone loss and ovulatory disturbances. *N Engl J Med* **323**: 1221–7.

Reid, D.M. (1990) Corticosteroid osteoporosis. In: *Osteoporosis: Pathogenesis and Management*, (ed. Francis, R.M.), Kluwer, Lancaster, pp. 103–44.

Reid, D.M., Kennedy, N.S.J., Smith, M.A., Tothill, P. and Nuki, G. (1982) Total body calcium in rheumatoid arthritis: effects of disease activity and corticosteroid treatment. *Br Med J* **285**: 330–2.

Reid, D.M., Nicoll, J.J., Smith, M.A. *et al.* (1986) Corticosteroids and bone mass in asthma: comparisons with rheumatoid arthritis and polymyalgia rheumatica. *Br Med J* **293**: 1463–4.

Reid, I.R. (1989) Steroid osteoporosis. *Calcif Tissue Int* **45**: 63–7.

Reid, I.R., France, J.T., Pybus, J. and Ibbertson, H.K. (1985) Plasma testosterone concentrations in asthmatic men treated with glucocorticoids. *Br Med J* **291**: 574.

Rickers, H., Deding, A., Christiansen, C., Rodbro, P. and Naestoft, J. (1982) Corticosteroid-induced osteopenia and vitamin D metabolism. Effect of vitamin D_2, calcium, phosphate and sodium fluoride administration. *Clin Endocrinol* **16**: 409–15.

Riggs, B.L. and Eastell, R. (1986) Exercise, hypogonadism and osteopenia. *J Am Med Assoc* **256**: 392–3.

Riggs, B.L. and Melton, L.J. III (1986) Involutional osteoporosis. *N Engl J Med* **314**: 1676–84.

Riggs, B.L., Wahner, H.W., Melton, L.J. III *et al.* (1987) Dietary calcium intake and rates of bone loss in women. *J Clin Invest* **80**: 979–82.

Rigotti, N.A., Nussbaum, S.R., Herzog, D.B. and Neer, R.M. (1984) Osteoporosis in women with anorexia nervosa. *N Engl J Med* **311**: 1601–6.

Rigotti, N.A., Neer, R.M., Skates, S.J., Herzog, D.B. and Nussbaum, S.R. (1991) The clinical course of osteoporosis in anorexia nervosa. A longitudinal study of cortical bone mass. *J Am Med Assoc* **265**: 1133–8.

Rosen, R.A. (1970) Transitory demineralisation of the femoral head. *Radiology* **94**: 509–12.

Rosenberg, E.F. (1958) Rheumatoid arthritis. Osteoporosis and fractures related to steroid therapy. *Acta Med Scand* **341**s: 211–24.

Ross, E.J. and Linch, D.C. (1982) Cushing's syndrome – killing disease: discriminatory value of signs and symptoms aiding early diagnosis. *Lancet* **ii**: 646–9.

Ross, D.S., Neer, R.M., Ridgway, E.C. and Daniels, G.H. (1987) Subclinical hyperthyroidism and reduced bone density as a possible result of prolonged suppression of the pituitary-thyroid axis with L-thyroxine. *Am J Med* **82**: 1167–72.

Royal College of Physicians of London (1989) *Fractured Neck of Femur: Prevention and Management*, Royal College of Physicians of London, London.

Salisbury, J.J. and Mitchell, J.E. (1991) Bone mineral density and anorexia nervosa in women. *Am J Psychiatry* **148**: 768–74.

Sandler, R.B., Slemenda, C.W., LaPorte, R.E. *et al.* (1985) Postmenopausal bone density and milk consumption in childhood and adolescence. *Am J Clin Nutr* **42**: 270–4.

Saville, P.D. (1965) Changes in bone mass with age and alcoholism. *J Bone Joint Surg* **47B**: 492–9.

Saville, P.D. (1973) The syndrome of spinal osteoporosis. *Clin Endocrinol Metabol* **2**: 177–85.

Schaadt, O. and Bohr, H. (1984) Bone mineral in lumbar spine, femoral neck and femoral shaft measured by dual photon absorptiometry with 153-gadolinium in prednisone treatment. *Adv Exp Med Biol* **171**: 201–8.

Schneider, D.L., Barrett-Connor, E.L. and Morton, D.J. (1994) Thyroid hormone use and bone mineral density in elderly women. Effect of estrogen. *J Am Med Assoc* **271**: 1245–9.

Seeman, E., Wahner, H.W., Offord, K.P. *et al.* (1982) Differential effects of endocrine dysfunction on the axial and appendicular skeleton. *J Clin Invest* **69**: 1302–9.

Seeman, E., Melton, L.J. III, O'Fallon, W.M. and Riggs, B.L. (1983) Risk factors for spinal osteoporosis in men. *Am J Med* **75**: 977–83.

Seeman, E., Hopper, J.L., Bach, L.A. *et al.* (1989) Reduced bone mass in daughters of women with osteoporosis. *N Engl J Med* **320**: 554–8.

Selby, P.L. (1988) Osteopenia and diabetes. *Diabetic Med* **5**: 423–8.

Shane, E., Rivas, M.C., Silverberg, S.J. *et al.* (1993) Osteoporosis after cardiac transplantation. *Am J Med* **94**: 257–64.

Sillence, D.O., Senn, A. and Danks, D.M. (1979) Genetic heterogeneity in osteogenesis imperfecta. *J Med Genet* **16**: 101–16.

Slemenda, C.W., Christian, J.C., Williams, C.J., Norton, J.A. and Johnston Jr, C.C. (1991) Genetic determinants of bone mass in adult women: a reevaluation of the twin model and the potential importance of gene interaction on heritability estimates. *J Bone Miner Res* **6**: 561–7.

Smith, D.A., Fraser, S.A. and Wilson, G.M. (1973) Hyperthyroidism and calcium metabolism. *Clin Endocrinol Metab* **2**: 333–54.

Smith, D.A.S. and Walker, M.S. (1977) Changes in plasma steroids and bone density in Klinefelter's syndrome. *Calcif Tissue Res* **22S**: 225–8.

Smith, D.M., Nance, W.E., Kang, K.W., Christian, J.C. and Johnston Jr, C.C. (1973) Genetic factors in determining bone mass. *J Clin Invest* **52**: 2800–8.

Smith, R. (1990) Corticosteroids and osteoporosis. *Thorax* **45**: 573–8.

Smith, R., Stevenson, J.C., Winearls, C.G., Woods, C.G. and Wordsworth, B.P. (1985) Osteoporosis of pregnancy. *Lancet* **i**: 1178–80.

Soffer, L.J., Iannaccone, A. and Gabrilove, J.L. (1961) Cushing's syndrome. A study of fifty patients. *Am J Med* **30**: 129–46.

Spencer, H., Rubio, N., Rubio, E., Indreika, M. and Seitam, A. (1986) Chronic alcoholism. Frequently overlooked cause of osteoporosis in men. *Am J Med* **80**: 393–7.

Sprague, R.G., Randall, R.V., Scilassa, R.M. *et al.* (1956) Cushing's syndrome. A progressive and often fatal disease. *Arch Intern Med* **98**: 389–98.

Stanley, H.L., Schmitt, B.P., Poses, R.M. and Deiss, W.P. (1991) Does hypogonadism contribute to the occurrence of a minimal trauma hip fracture in elderly men? *J Am Geriatr Soc* **39**: 766–71.

Stevenson, J.C., Whitehead, M.I., Padwick, M. *et al.* (1988) Dietary intake of calcium and postmenopausal bone loss. *Br Med J* **297**: 15–17.

Stevenson, J.C., Lees, B., Devenport, M., Cust, M.P. and Ganger, K.F. (1989) Determinants of bone density in normal women: risk factors for future osteoporosis. *Br Med J* **298**: 924–8.

Szmukler, G.I., Brown, S.W., Parsons, V. and Darby, A. (1985) Premature loss of bone in chronic anorexia nervosa. *Br Med J* **290**: 26–7.

Toogood, J.H., Jennings, B., Hodsman, A.B., Baskerville, J. and Fraher, L.J. (1991) Effects of dose and dosing schedule of inhaled budesonide on bone turnover. *J Allergy Clin Immunol* **88:** 572–80.

Treasure, J.L., Russell, G.F.M., Fogelman, I. and Murby, B. (1987) Reversible bone loss in anorexia nervosa. *Br Med J* **295**: 474–5.

Vermeulen, A., Rubens, R. and Verdonck, L. (1972) Testosterone secretion and metabolism in male senescence. *J Clin Endocrinol Metab* **34**: 730–5.

Wejda, B., Hintze, G., Katschinski, B. *et al.* (1995) Hip fracture and the thyroid: a case control study. *J Intern Med* **273**: 241–7.

Wilson, R.J., Rao, D.S., Ellis, B., Kleerekoper, M. and Parfitt, A.M. (1988) Mild asymptomatic primary hyperparathyroidism is not a risk factor for vertebral fractures. *Ann Intern Med* **109**: 959–62.

Winks, C.S. and Felts, W.J.L. (1980) Effects of castration on the bone structure of male rats: a model of osteoporosis. *Calcif Tissue Int* **32**: 77–82.

Winner, S.J., Morgan, C.A. and Evans, J.G. (1989) Perimenopausal risk of falling and incidence of distal forearm fracture. *Br Med J* **298**: 1486–8.

Wooton, R., Brereton, P.J., Clark, M.B. *et al.* (1979) Fractured neck of femur in the elderly: an attempt to identify patients at risk. *Clin Sci* **57**: 93–101.

Zerwekh, J.E., Sakhaee, K., Breslau, N.A., Gottschalk, F. and Pak, C.Y.C. (1992) Impaired bone formation in male idiopathic osteoporosis: further reduction in the presence of concomitant hypercalciuria. *Osteoporosis Int* **2**: 128–34.

PATHOGENESIS OF POSTMENOPAUSAL OSTEOPOROTIC FRACTURES 3

*C.C. Johnston Jr and C.W. Slemenda**

Osteoporosis has been defined as a disease characterized by low bone mass and microarchitectural deterioration of bone tissue, leading to enhanced bone fragility and a consequent increase in fracture risk (Consensus Development Conference, 1991). This definition applies equally to the disease as it occurs in the postmenopausal woman, although the mechanisms responsible for bone loss occurring in this population may differ from others that also develop osteoporotic fractures.

Fractures which have been attributed to osteoporosis include those of the spine, hip and distal radius and these are more common among women than men. However, most fractures occurring in the aging population are associated with low bone mass and are thus likely due to osteoporosis (Seeley *et al.*, 1991).

Low bone mass at the site of fracture is the major determinant of fracture risk. Other factors also play a role in fracture pathogenesis and may provide opportunities for interventions to protect from fracture. Trauma, especially that associated with a fall, is important for the occurrence of many fractures. Hip fractures usually develop after a fall and how the fall occurs seems important in determining which fracture will occur. A fall to the side, landing upon the hip, is associated with a much greater risk of fracture than is a fall upon the buttocks (Hayes *et al.*, 1993). There is sufficient energy generated by a fall from standing height to fracture the proximal femur if the energy is not diffused by overlying tissue (Greenspan *et al.*, 1994). Many who fracture are thin and have poor tissue covering over the hip, resulting in inadequate energy diffusion. The importance of this factor has been shown by the studies of Lauritzen *et al.* (1993), who demonstrated that those wearing pads over the hip had markedly reduced fracture incidence. In fact,

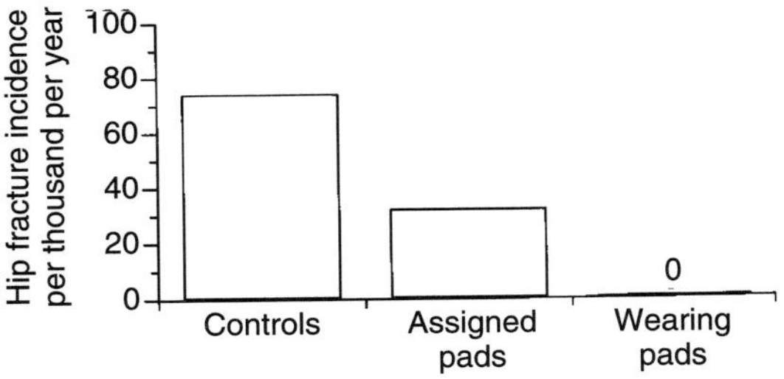

Figure 3.1 Hip fracture incidence in subjects assigned to hip protectors and a control group. Adapted from Lauritzen *et al.* (1991).

*Sadly, Charles Slemenda died in 1997.

Osteoporosis. Edited by John C. Stevenson and Robert Lindsay. Published in 1998 by Chapman & Hall, London. ISBN 0 412 48870 1

among those who fractured in the group assigned to wear hip pads, none was wearing the device when fractures occurred (Figure 3.1). These data accentuate the need for the development of protective devices which are both effective and likely to be worn, i.e. both comfortable and convenient.

The role of trauma in other osteoporotic fractures is now becoming better understood. It is probably uncommon for any fracture to be truly atraumatic (e.g. a hip collapsing under the force of body weight alone). Fractures of vertebral bodies probably result not only from reduced bone mass but also from the trauma associated with lifting, coughing, sneezing or similar events. It is also probable that those with low bone mass are more likely to fracture under the strain of higher levels of trauma, e.g. in falls from ladders or down stairs. A better understanding of the role of trauma in fracture etiology would be an important step in the prevention of such fractures.

Skeletal fragility plays an important role in fracture pathogenesis and low bone mass contributes substantially to the development of this fragility. However, other factors are also important. It has been clearly shown that architectural abnormalities occur in the cancellous bone of the aging skeleton (Parfitt, 1987). Trabecular connections are lost, especially horizontal connections between vertical trabeculae, and the loss of this support weakens the structure beyond that due to loss of bone tissue alone. Such abnormalities have been demonstrated to exist, but since they cannot be measured non-invasively, their contribution to the development of fractures is not known. Some studies (Kleerekoper *et al.*, 1985; Recker and Kimmel, 1989) have shown that trabecular discontinuity is more prominent in biopsies from patients with fractures than in subjects without fractures but with similar bone mass. It has also been shown that the presence of a fracture, either of the spine (Ross *et al.*, 1991) or elsewhere (Wasnich *et al.*, 1994), contributes to subsequent risk of spinal fracture even after adjustment for bone mass. Although it is clear that a fracture within the spine could produce greater strains on the remaining intact vertebrae through a change in the geometry of the spine, the predictive value of fractures elsewhere provides further information. One possibility is that structural (architectural) abnormalities, independent of bone mass, have predisposed a patient to fractures throughout the skeleton.

As with other materials subjected to stress and strain, fatigue or microdamage might be expected to occur. Such micro-cracks have been demonstrated in bone (Frost, 1981; Burr, 1993), but the extent to which these abnormalities contribute quantitatively to fracture risk has not been ascertained since they cannot be measured non-invasively. It has been suggested that ultrasound measurements of the heel or patella may provide information on such structural properties independent of bone mass. It has been shown that ultrasound measurements of the patella are significantly different between those with and without vertebral fractures (Heaney *et al.*, 1989), but this association was not shown to provide more information than bone mass alone. However, it has recently been shown that ultrasound measurements of the heel and bone mass measurements of the femoral neck are independent contributors to the prediction of fractures of the proximal femur (Cummings, personal communication; Turner *et al.*, 1995), suggesting that ultrasound measurements may indeed contain information that is not included in the usual measurements of bone mass. Further study will be necessary to clarify the role of ultrasound in the evaluation of microarchitectural abnormalities in osteoporosis.

The geometry of the bone at the fracture site might also be an important factor in determining fracture risk, especially for proximal femoral fractures. Hip axis length measured from DXA scans has been shown to contribute independently of bone mass to fracture risk (Faulkner *et al.*, 1993). Differences in femoral neck geometry may also account for a lower hip fracture incidence among Japanese when compared to Caucasians even though femoral neck bone mass is lower in the Japanese population (Nakamura *et al.*, 1994). In a retrospective study comparing hip fracture cases with similar controls, bone mass, a measurement of bone architecture (Singh Index) and a measurement of geometry (the distance from the superior aspect of the femoral neck to its center of mass) were each independently associated with fracture prevalence (Peacock *et al.*, 1995). Interestingly, it appears that many elements of femoral neck geometry and architecture may have genetic components. This is reflected not only by Japanese–American differences, but also by significantly higher correlations in monozygotic than dizygotic twin pairs (Slemenda *et al.*, 1996b) for many of these variables. The observation that the familial association in hip fracture incidence is not entirely attributable to inherited levels of bone mass (Cummings *et al.*, 1993) may be at least partly explained by the inheritance of geometric properties of the femoral neck (Slemenda *et al.*, 1996b), which also contribute to the susceptibility to fractures (Faulkner *et al.*, 1993; Peacock *et al.*, 1995).

All of these variables – trauma, architectural abnormalities, fatigue damage, geometrical differences – may contribute to fracture pathogenesis in postmenopausal women, but one major determinant is low bone mass at the site of fracture. In addition, most diagnostic procedures or therapeutic interventions are aimed at detecting low bone mass and preventing bone loss. It must be recognized, however, that the fracture risk associated with any level of bone mass is modified by the presence of other risk factors (e.g. a previous fracture or disadvantageous femur geometry) and, thus, the level of bone mass at which treatment would be initiated increases if other risk factors are present. For example, a history of fracture after age 50 appears to approximately double the risk of subsequent fractures (Cummings *et al.*, 1993; Wasnich *et al.*, 1994). Thus, a patient with a positive fracture history would have approximately the same risk of future fractures as someone with a negative fracture history but with a one standard deviation lower bone mass. The identification of other risk factors, independent of bone mass, is therefore, critical to clinical decision making.

Low bone mass occurring later in life at the time fracture rates increase may be due to either low peak bone mass (the maximum amount of bone attained before loss begins) or bone loss. It has been shown for a population followed longitudinally that each may contribute equally by the age of 70 (Hui *et al.*, 1990) (Figure 3.2), but this may vary among individuals.

Peak bone mass is primarily determined by genetic factors. This has been shown for all skeletal sites in a number of twin studies, where monozygotic and dizygotic twins were compared (Smith *et al.*, 1973; Pocock *et al.*, 1987; Slemenda *et al.*, 1991a). The intraclass correlation for monozygotic twins is usually 0.7 to 0.8 and for dizygotic twins approximately half of this. This suggests that up to

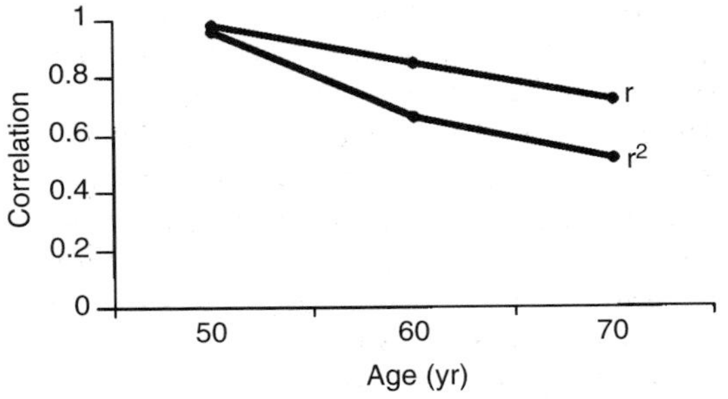

Figure 3.2 The estimated correlation (r) between midshaft radius bone mass measured at age 50 and at ages 60 and 70. r^2 represents the proportion of variability that can be accounted for by the initial bone mass measurement. These data do not imply that short-term measurements of bone loss will produce similar r^2 values because error in estimation diminishes these. From Hui *et al.* (1990).

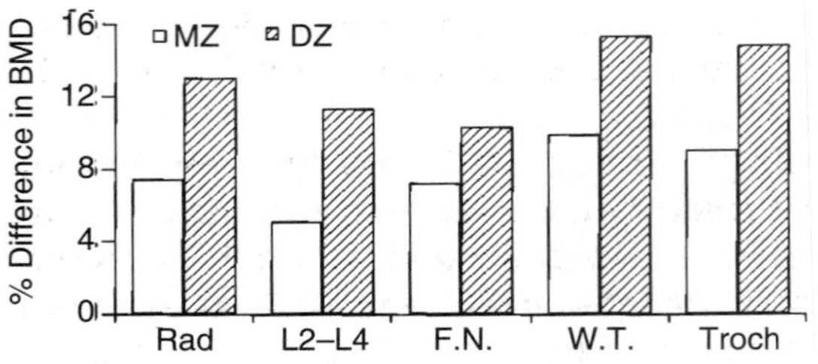

Figure 3.3 Within-pair differences in BMD expressed as a percentage of the group mean value. MZ < DZ ($p < 0.01$) for all skeletal sites. Adapted from Slemenda *et al.* (1991a).

80% of the variability in peak bone mass may be attributable to genetic factors (Figure 3.3). When heritabilities are calculated by the methods of Falconer, some are elevated (even above 1), suggesting that some of the assumptions of the model are incorrect (Slemenda *et al.*, 1991a). It has been shown that the means for the monozygotic and dizygotic twins are the same and when the effects of more similar environments of the monozygotic twins are removed, heritability estimates remain elevated above the monozygotic intraclass correlation, indicating additional violations of the assumption. We have suggested that this may be due to dominance or epistasis, implying that a few interacting, major genes are responsible for the determination of peak bone mass (Slemenda *et al.*, 1991a).

Recently, it has been reported that polymorphisms in the vitamin D receptor (VDR) gene could account for a substantial portion of the genetic variance (Morrison *et al.*, 1994). The strongest evidence for this large contribution was found in their studies of twins discordant for the VDR gene. Studies of similar polymorphisms in dizygotic twins in Indiana have not yielded similar results (Hustmyer *et al.*, 1994). Since these early studies a number of investigators have approached this issue with mixed results. It seems clear, however, that if the VDR gene is involved in determining the risk for osteoporosis, it accounts for only a few percent of the variation in peak bone mass and other genes are also as important or more so in the establishment of osteoporosis risk. The finding of a gene responsible for a large portion of the genetic variance awaits further study.

It is plausible that interactions between genes and environments will vary in different parts of the world. There have been numerous observations of geographic variability in fracture susceptibility (Kanis, 1990) and this may reflect differences in genetics or environment alone or their interaction or even non-skeletal influences on fracture incidence (e.g. falls). There are other candidates for genetic factors that may influence bone mass. A recent report described a young adult male with osteopenia and continued longitudinal growth (at age 28) associated with a defect in the estrogen receptor (Smith *et al.*, 1994). This suggests that estrogen may play a more important role in the development and maintenance of the male skeleton than previously appreciated.

Even though genetic determinants are important, environmental factors may account for 20–30% of the variability in peak bone mass. Since relatively small changes in peak bone mass could result in substantial reductions in fractures (Matkovic *et al.*, 1979), such environmental factors may be important in maximizing the genetic potential for peak bone mass. These factors include nutrition, especially calcium intake (Johnston *et al.*, 1992), exercise (Slemenda *et al.*, 1991b) and probably hormonal changes during the rapid acquisition of bone after puberty. Regarding nutrition, it is necessary to take a broad view of what this subject encompasses. Absolute quantity is rarely considered, but it is clear that anorexia nervosa is probably the most potent threat to skeletal integrity during growth (Crosby *et al.*, 1985). Only young women have been well studied in this regard and, thus, it is difficult to disentangle the effects of the nutritional deprivation and the accompanying hormonal disturbances, but the result is frequently a 20–40% reduction in bone mass. This deficit may be difficult or impossible to repair, although those who recover from anorexia do improve their skeletal status. Total caloric content of the diet may also be critical to maintaining normal gonadal function in female athletes (Snead *et al.*, 1992) and early dieting or dietary restrictions should be considered as potential threats to skeletal health, although further study in these areas is needed.

With regard to the role of specific nutrients in the development of peak skeletal mass, calcium has been best studied. Two randomized, controlled clinical trials have been completed (Johnston *et al.*, 1992; Lloyd *et al.*, 1993) and each has shown short-term benefits of calcium supplementation (500–1000 mg daily) in growing children. Each of these studies has shown 3–5% increases in the rate of skeletal mineralization over 2–3 years. With the cessation of supplementation in our study much of the benefit appears to be lost within one year (Slemenda *et al.*, 1993). It would appear that long-term increases in calcium intake during growth could be recommended since studies of subjects with high calcium intakes throughout growth have shown these people to have roughly 5–7% more skeletal mass as adults (Sandler *et al.*, 1985) than those with lower long-term intakes. Short-term supplementation is probably not valuable; after two years off supplement there is a convergence between the higher and lower calcium intake groups (Slemenda *et al.*, 1993), with only a non-significant difference remaining.

Protein has also been studied, albeit in observational studies. A study of growth in the third decade showed negative correlations between protein intake (or protein/calcium ratio) and rates of growth in women between the ages of 20 and 30 (Recker *et al.*, 1992). These data are consistent with the negative effect on calcium balance observed at higher protein intakes (Lutz, 1984) and suggest that the high-protein diets common in Western countries may not be ideal in skeletal terms.

Physical activity is clearly necessary for proper skeletal development. Beyond this simplistic statement, however, much is uncertain, including the intensity and duration of activity necessary to stimulate skeletal growth, the types of activity most likely to be beneficial and the potential for activity to yield negative effects. Children who are more active tend to have denser skeletons than those who are less so, even after adjustment for body size differences (Slemenda *et al.*, 1991b). Moreover, greater levels of weight-bearing physical activity are associated with more rapid skeletal growth, at least in prepubertal children (Slemenda *et al.*, 1996a). There is little evidence that non-weight-bearing activities, such as swimming, have beneficial skeletal effects, although it is important to recognize that improved muscle strength and other similar changes may have indirect benefits on skeletal health through the prevention of falls and the avoidance of other trauma. Despite the obvious positives with activity during growth there is the potential for high levels of exercise to have detrimental effects on normal gonadal function and hence on the skeleton. Initially, these observations were made in young women, for whom athletic amenorrhea has been associated with significant reductions in skeletal mass, especially in the spine (Drinkwater *et al.*, 1990). Recently, it has been observed that young men with extreme levels of activity (i.e. running more than 100 km weekly) have significantly less bone than inactive men of similar ages (Hetlund *et al.*, 1993). It is likely that precisely the same mechanism is involved in both men and women with high levels of activity, i.e. a reduction in the serum concentrations of sex steroids, which are probably necessary for the maintenance of skeletal integrity in both sexes.

Two additional observations further complicate the issue of activity and skeletal growth and development. First, there have been recent observations that even among young women with athletic amenorrhea certain types of activity seem to protect against bone loss (or failure to gain bone). National-level competitors in both figure skating and gymnastics have higher bone mass than inactive control groups despite a higher prevalence of amenorrhea (Slemenda and Johnston, 1993). This very likely represents the effects of activities which produce extreme strain rates in the areas of the skeleton used in these endeavors. Further supporting this concept is the observation that the skaters had increased bone densities in the legs and pelvis only, reflecting their training and competition, whereas the gymnasts had increased densities throughout the skeleton as would be expected for athletes whose training involves both legs and arms (Fehling *et al.*, 1993). Although not reported for the gymnasts, the skaters had negative correlations with total hours of training, suggesting that there may be limits to the skeleton's ability to respond to training. Physical activity is clearly necessary for proper skeletal development and maintenance, but further research is needed to better understand the quantity and type of activity needed.

Peak bone mass is reached in the late second (Theintz *et al.*, 1992) or third decades of life (Recker *et al.*, 1992). It is not entirely clear when bone loss begins. This may vary from site to site in the skeleton. In a recent cross-sectional study, it appeared that bone gain in the radius and spine might even persist until the age of 50, although loss appeared to occur in the hip (Matkovic *et al.*, 1994). Cross-sectional data from NHANES III indicate lower femoral neck BMD in each decade after the 20–30-year-old cohort (Looker *et al.*, 1995a, b). Some of these observed differences may be due to cohort effects and must be confirmed in prospective studies. In our own prospective studies, no loss from the spine or radius was found before the perimenopausal period, although loss did occur from the hip. This loss may be due to lower androgen concentrations (Slemenda *et al.*, 1994), but other potential explanations exist. Diminished physical activity, for example, may play a role.

As noted, bone loss from some sites may begin before menopause but it has been shown that loss is accelerated from most sites at the time of menopause. The association between menopause and osteoporosis has been known for many years (Albright *et al.*, 1941), but the development of methods for measuring bone mass and changes in bone mass precisely and accurately has led to a better understanding of the relationship between menopause and bone loss.

Oophorectomy is associated with the onset of bone loss from both the axial and appendicular skeletons (Lindsay *et al.*, 1976; Ettinger *et al.*, 1985) and this loss can be prevented in most women by the administration of estrogen alone (Lindsay *et al.*, 1976; Writing Group, 1996), thus establishing the clear link between estrogen insufficiency and bone loss. Studies of women going through a natural menopause have also documented accelerated bone loss which is significantly correlated with estrogen and androgen concentrations and production rates (Johnston *et al.*, 1985; Slemenda *et al.*, 1987). Bone loss begins in the perimenopausal period when irregular bleeding is still occurring. However, this does not occur until concentrations of FSH have increased and the estrogens have decreased, increasing the rate of skeletal remodeling (Table 3.1). Androgen concentrations also contribute to the preservation of bone mass during the early postmenopausal period (the higher the androgen concentrations, the slower the loss) and this is independent of the estrogen effect (Slemenda *et al.*, 1987). Bone loss is more rapid immediately after menopause and then slows at most measured sites (Harris and Dawson-Hughes, 1992). Later in life, the relationship between estrogen concentration and loss becomes weaker or is no longer found. Bone loss

Table 3.1 Rates of change in radial bone mass and concentrations of serum estrogens and osteocalcin (BGP) in 84 peri- and postmenopausal women followed for 3.5 years. Adapted from Slemenda *et al.* (1987)

	Early perimenopause (FSH < 40 mIU)	*Late perimenopause (FSH > 40 mIU)*	*Postmenopause (<1 year)*	*Postmenopause (1–3 years)*
Midshaft radius change g/cm/yr	+0.005	-0.006*	-0.006*	-0.010*
Distal radius change g/cm/yr	+0.007	-0.010*	-0.016*	-0.011*
Estrone pg/ml	88	46*	40*	38*
Estradiol pg/ml	107	48*	32*	25*
BPG ng/ml	4.8	6.8*	7.0*	7.5*

* Significantly different from early perimenopausal women.

continues, however, indicating that other variables may play an increasingly important role in controlling the rate of change. However, women in the seventh and eighth decades still respond to administration of exogenous estrogen (Lindsay and Tohme, 1990; Lufkin *et al.*, 1992), indicating that the skeletal receptors are still intact, but concentrations of hormones are probably too low to be effective.

Men are also losing bone at these same ages. Rates of loss in men are slower than in women, perhaps by half, and are more rapid in smokers and in those who consume larger amounts of alcohol (Slemenda *et al.*, 1992). It is also clear that older women who smoke lose bone more rapidly than non-smokers (Krall and Dawson-Hughes, 1991). Activity may also play a role in rates of bone loss in older people. It is likely that the non-hormonal component of bone loss in the elderly relates in large part to factors such as these. Genetic influences, although critical in growth, have yet to be shown to have an important role in bone loss. In men there are slightly stronger correlations in monozygotic than dizygotic pairs, but these are attributable to shared environmental factors (Slemenda *et al.*, 1992). In women there have been no published reports examining populations experiencing substantial bone loss. In one report a genetic component to changes in bone mass was reported (Kelly *et al.*, 1993), but the majority of these subjects were gaining rather than losing bone. It remains to be shown that genetic influences play a major role in bone loss, although this may yet be shown when studies of older women are completed.

Certainly, the evidence is strong for a relationship of estrogen deficiency to postmenopausal bone loss, but the mechanism of action of estrogen to produce this effect is less clear. Bone remodeling, as indicated by increases in indices of bone turnover (Fogelman *et al.*, 1984) and as seen in bone biopsies (Recker *et al.*, 1988), is increased. This increase in remodeling is primarily due to an increase in activation of osteoclastic resorption. However, an increase in remodeling, if resorption is balanced by formation at the basic unit of remodeling, would not lead to bone loss. Thus, the balance between resorption and formation at the site must be perturbed by estrogen deficiency (Parfitt, 1988). This concept is further supported by studies of long-term replacement of estrogen in estrogen-deficient women, which result in restored balance between formation and resorption, and essentially no bone loss for up to 10 years (Nachtigall *et al.*, 1979; Abdalla *et al.*, 1984).

Heaney has suggested that estrogen deficiency is associated with an increased sensitivity to the stimulation of bone resorption by parathyroid hormone (Heaney, 1965) and parathyroid hormone may be responsible for stimulation of new remodeling sites (McGuire and Marks, 1974). In addition, infusion of an active parathyroid hormone fragment produces less of an effect in estrogen-replete than estrogen-deficient women (Cosman *et al.*, 1993). Thus, parathyroid hormone may play a role in postmenopausal bone loss.

Estrogen receptors have been found in osteoblasts (Komm *et al.*, 1988; Eriksen *et al.*, 1988) and perhaps in osteoclasts (Oursler *et al.*, 1991) so that the effect of the hormone is presumably directly upon bone cells. However, the mechanism by which the local effects of the hormone on bone cells is produced remains to be elucidated. A number of cytokines which have effects upon bone resorption (Mundy, 1993) may be affected by estrogen. These include prostaglandins (Feven and Raisz, 1987), interleukin 1 (Pacifici *et al.*, 1991), interleukin 6 (Jilka *et al.*, 1992) and TGFβ (Pfeilschifter *et al.*, 1988). The local control of bone resorption is complex and resembles the cascade of factors which are responsible for blood clotting. In addition to estrogen's effect on bone resorption, some evidence also suggests an effect upon stimulation of bone formation (Chow *et al.*, 1992). Elucidation of the control of bone formation and resorption at the remodeling unit may lead to new interventions to treat or prevent postmenopausal osteoporosis.

Bone loss continues at most skeletal sites throughout the remainder of life and the factors responsible in women in addition to estrogen deficiency are not clear but a range of variables could be responsible. Many postmenopausal women have a low intake of calcium and studies have shown that calcium supplementation in postmenopausal women, especially in those greater than five years after menopause, slows or stops bone loss (Heaney, 1993). In a very large clinical trial of institutionalized elderly, supplementation with both vitamin D and calcium significantly reduced the incidence of hip fractures over a period of several years (Chapuy *et al.*, 1992). Parathyroid hormone concentrations increase with age (Wiske *et al.*, 1979; Gallagher *et al.*, 1980) and may play a role in accelerated bone loss. Whether the cited reductions in hip fracture with vitamin D and calcium reflected a reduction in the parathyroid hormone-mediated bone loss is not clear. However, PTH was clearly reduced in the supplemented group. Immobilization and the sedentary lifestyle could be important (Prince *et al.*, 1988) and with aging and intercurrent illness, individuals become less active. All of these variables require further study, for they present opportunities for interventions to reduce the frequency of fracture in postmenopausal women.

Postmenopausal osteoporosis has been addressed as if fractures which occur in the postmenopausal woman at any age are due to similar conditions. However, some have previously considered the disorder under two categories – postmenopausal and senile osteoporosis (Albright and Reifenstein, 1948) or type I and type II osteoporosis (Riggs and Melton, 1986). Type I osteoporosis is said to occur primarily in women, is associated with decreases in cancellous bone and results primarily in crush fractures of the spine and fractures of the distal radius. Type II osteoporosis occurs in older individuals, is more common in women than in men (but this discrepancy is not as marked as for type I osteoporosis), is associated with a loss of both cortical and cancellous bone and results in wedge fractures of the spine and fractures of the hip. These distinctions are based to a large extent on the patterns of different fracture types with age. There is considerable overlap between the syndromes and it is not clear whether they are distinct entities from an etiologic standpoint. Perhaps early spinal crush and distal radial fractures occur in those women who have low peak bone mass or lower peak bone mass and accelerated cancellous bone loss. Since all individuals are losing bone, all will be at variable risk of fracture depending on their individual peak bone mass and rate of loss. It has been shown that most fractures which occur in the aging population are associated with low bone mass (Seeley *et al.*, 1990). There are preliminary data that suggest crush fractures may be associated not only with low bone mass but with more rapid menopausal bone loss (Christiansen *et al.*, 1993). It is certainly plausible that rapid bone loss might lead to perforation of trabeculae and a greater weakness in primarily trabecular bone than is reflected by lower bone mass alone, but these observations await confirmation.

The etiology of postmenopausal osteoporosis is complex and although the predisposition to fractures becomes almost universal among the very old, fractures usually occur in those who suffer trauma. Peak bone mass in healthy children appears amenable to interventions which might increase it, although the public health would probably be best served by the prevention of early life events which substantially diminish peak bone mass, notably long periods of amenorrhea, immobilization or inactivity and serious dietary deficiencies. Bone loss can also be prevented later in life, particularly in estrogen-deficient women, and the protection afforded by estrogen replacement probably reduces the subsequent risk of fracture by nearly half. The effectiveness of such therapies depends primarily on the duration of use; numerous studies have shown durations of use of five or more years to be associated with significant reductions in fracture risk, whereas there are no data to support the necessity of beginning therapy at any specific point in postmenopausal life. With aging, other therapies also appear to be beneficial, including calcium alone or with vitamin D. Investigations into the prevention of trauma, especially at the hip, may include both the prevention of falls and the reduction of impact forces. Padding to reduce forces appears to offer the greatest promise, although there are clearly circumstances where more appropriate medications and perhaps balance training can reduce the occurrence of falls. The most effective prevention of osteoporotic fractures will require efforts in all of these areas.

REFERENCES

Abdalla, H., Hart, D.M. and Lindsay, R. (1984) Differential bone loss and effects of long-term estrogen therapy according to time of introduction of therapy after oophorectomy. In: *Osteoporosis 2*, (eds Christiansen, C. *et al.*) Aalborg Stifsbogtrykkeri, Copenhagen, pp. 621–4.

Albright, F. and Reifenstein Jr, E.C. (1948) *The Parathyroid Glands and Metabolic Bone Disease – Selected Studies*, Williams and Wilkins, Baltimore.

Albright, F., Smith, P.H. and Richardson, A.M. (1941) Postmenopausal osteoporosis. *J Am Med Assoc* **116**: 2465–74.

Burr, D.B. (1993) Remodeling and the repair of fatigue damage. *Calfic Tissue Int* **53(1)**: S75–S81.

Chapuy, M.C., Arlot, M.E., Duboef, F. *et al.* (1992) Vitamin D_3 and calcium to prevent hip fractures in elderly women. *N Engl J Med* **327**: 1637–42.

Chow, J., Tobias, J.H., Colston, K.W. *et al.* (1992) Estrogen maintains trabecular bone volume in rats not only by suppression of bone resorption but also by stimulation of bone formation. *J Clin Invest* **89**: 74–8.

Christiansen, C., Hansen, M.A., Overgaard, K. *et al.* (1993) Prediction of future fracture risk. Proceedings of the 4th International Symposium on Osteoporosis, Hong Kong, pp. 52–4.

Consensus Development Conference (1991) Prophylaxis and treatment of osteoporosis. *Am J Med* **90**: 107–10.

Cosman, F., Shen, V., Zie, F. *et al.* (1993) Estrogen protection against bone resorbing effects of parathyroid hormone infusion. Assessment by use of biochemical markers. *Ann Intern Med* **118**: 337–43.

Crosby, L.O., Kaplan, F.S., Pertschuk, M.J. *et al.* (1985) The effect of anorexia nervosa on bone morphometry in young women. *Clin Orthop Rel Res* **201**: 271–7.

Cummings, S.R., Browner, W.S., Black, D.M. *et al.* (1993) Risk factors for hip fracture: new findings, new questions. Proceedings of the 4th International Symposium on Osteoporosis, Hong Kong, pp. 73–4.

Drinkwater, B.L., Breumner, B. and Chesnut, C.H. (1990) Menstrual history as a determinant of current bone density in young athletes. *J Am Med Assoc* **263**: 545–8.

Eriksen, E.F., Colvard, D.S., Berg, N.J. *et al.* (1988) Evidence of estrogen receptors in normal human osteoblast-like cells. *Science* **241**: 84–6.

Ettinger, B., Genant, H.K. and Cann, C.E. (1985) Long-term estrogen therapy prevents bone loss fracture. *Ann Intern Med* **102**: 319–24.

Faulkner, K.G., Cummings, S.R., Black, D. *et al.* (1993) Simple measurement of femoral geometry predicts hip fracture: the study of osteoporotic fractures. *J Bone Miner Res* **8**: 1211–17.

Fehling, P.C., Alekel, L., Clasey, J. *et al.* (1993) A comparison of bone mineral densities among female athletes in impact loading and active loading sports. *Bone* **17**: 205–10.

Feven, J.H.M. and Raisz, L.G. (1987) Prostaglandin production by calvariae from sham-operated and oophorectomized rats: effect of 17β-estradiol in vivo. *Endocrinology* **121**: 819–21.

Fogelman, I., Poser, J.W., Smith, M.L. *et al.* (1984) Alterations in skeletal metabolism following oophorectomy. In: *Osteoporosis 2*, (eds Christiansen, C. *et al.*), Aalborg Stifsbogtrykkeri, Copenhagen, p.519.

Frost, H.M. (1981) Mechanical microdamage, bone remodeling, and osteoporosis: a review. In: *Osteoporosis: Recent Advances in Pathogenesis and Treatment*, (eds Deluca, H.F., Frost, H.M., Jee, W.S.S. *et al.*), University Park Press, Baltimore.

Gallagher, J.C., Riggs, B.L., Jerpbak, C.M. *et al.* (1980) The effect of age on serum immunoreactive parathyroid hormone in normal and osteoporotic women. *J Lab Clin Med* **95**: 373–85.

Greenspan, S.L., Myers, E.R., Maitland, L.A. *et al.* (1994) Fall severity and bone mineral density as risk factors for hip fracture in ambulatory elderly. *J Am Med Assoc* **271**(2): 128–34.

Harris, S. and Dawson-Hughes, B. (1992) Rates of change in bone mineral density of the spine, heel, femoral neck and radius in healthy postmenopausal women. *Bone Miner* **17**: 87–95.

Hayes, W.C., Myers, E.R., Morris, J.N. *et al.* (1993) Impact near the hip dominates fracture risk in elderly nursing home residents who fall. *Calcif Tissue Int* **52**: 192–8.

Heaney, R.P. (1965) A unified concept of osteoporosis. *Am J Med* **39**: 377–80.

Heaney, R.P. (1993) Nutritional factors in osteoporosis. *Annu Rev Nutr* **13**: 287–316.

Heaney, R.P., Avioli, L.V., Chesnut, C.H. *et al.* (1989) Osteoporotic bone fragility: detection by ultrasound transmission velocity. *J Am Med Assoc* **261**: 2986–90.

Hetland, M.L., Haarbo, J. and Christiansen, C. (1993) Low bone mass and high bone turnover in male long distance runners. *J Clin Endocrinol Metab* **77**: 770–5.

Hui, S., Slemenda, C.W. and Johnston Jr, C.C. (1990) The contribution of rapid bone loss to postmenopausal osteoporosis. *Osteoporosis Int* **1**: 30–4.

Hustmyer, F.G., Peacock, M., Hui, S., Johnston Jr, C.C. and Christian, J. (1994) Bone mineral density in relation to polymorphism at the vitamin D receptor gene locus. *J Clin Invest* **94**: 2130–4.

Jilka, R.L., Hangoc, G., Girasole, G. *et al.* (1992) Increased osteoclast development after estrogen loss: mediation by interleukin-6. *Science* **257**: 88–91.

Johnston Jr, C.C., Hui, S.L., Witt, R.M. *et al.* (1985) Early menopausal changes in bone mass and sex steroids. *J Clin Endocrinol Metab* **61**: 905–11.

Johnston Jr, C.C., Miller, J.Z., Slemenda, C.W. *et al.* (1992) Calcium supplementation and increases in bone mineral density in children. *N Engl J Med* **327**: 82–87.

Kanis, J.A., on behalf of the Medos Study Group (1990) The epidemiology of hip fracture in Europe. Third International Symposium on Osteoporosis, Copenhagen, Denmark, pp. 42–7.

Kelly, P., Nguyen, T., Hopper, J. *et al.* (1993) Changes in axial bone density with age: a twin study. *J Bone Miner Res* **8**: 11–17.

Kleerekoper, M., Villanueva, A.R., Stanciu, J. *et al.* (1985) The role of three-dimensional trabecular microstructure in the pathogenesis of vertebral compression fractures. *Calcif Tissue Int* **37**: 594–7.

Komm, B.S., Terpening, C.M. and Benz, D.J. (1988) Estrogen binding, receptor mRNA, and biologic response in osteoblast-like osteosarcoma cells. *Science* **241**: 81–4.

Krall, E. and Dawson-Hughes, B. (1991) Smoking and bone loss among postmenopausal women. *J Bone Miner Res* **4**: 331–8.

Lauritzen, J.B., Petersen, M.M. and Lund, B. (1991) Effect of external hip protectors on hip fractures. *Lancet* **341**: 11–13.

Lindsay, R. and Tohme, L. (1990) Estrogen treatment of patients with established postmenopausal osteoporosis. *Obstet Gynecol* **76**: 1–6.

Lindsay, R., Hart, D.M., Aitken, J.M. *et al.* (1976) Long-term prevention of postmenopausal osteoporosis by oestrogen. *Lancet* **i**: 1038–41.

Lloyd, T., Andon, M.B., Rollings, N. *et al.* (1993) Calcium supplementation and bone mineral density in adolescent girls. *J Am Med Assoc* **270**: 841–4.

Looker, A.C., Wahner, H.W., Dunn, W.L. *et al.* (1995a) Proximal femur bone mineral levels of US adults. *Osteoporosis Int* **5**: 389–409.

Looker, A.C., Johnston Jr, C.C., Wahner, H.W. *et al.* (1995b) Prevalence of low femoral bone density in older US women from NHANES III. *J Bone Miner Res* **10**: 796–802.

Lufkin, E., Wahner, H.W., O'Fallon, W.M. *et al.* (1992) Treatment of postmenopausal osteoporosis with transdermal estrogen. *Ann Intern Med* **117**: 1–9.

Lutz, J. (1984) Calcium balance and acid-base status of women as affected by increased protein intake and by sodium bicarbonate ingestion. *Am J Clin Nutr* **39**: 281–8.

Matkovic, V., Kostial, K., Simonovic, I. *et al.* (1979) Bone status and fracture rates in two regions of Yugoslavia. *Am J Clin Nutr* **32**: 540–9.

Matkovic, V., Jelic, T., Wardlaw, G.M. *et al.* (1994) Timing of peak bone mass in caucasian females and its implication for the prevention of osteoporosis. *J Clin Invest* **93**: 799–808.

McGuire, J.L. and Marks, S.C. Jr (1974) The effects of PTH on bone cell structure and function. *Clin Orthop Rel Res* **100**: 392–405.

Morrison, N.A., Qi, J.C., Tokita, A. *et al.* (1994) Prediction of bone density from vitamin D receptor alleles. *Nature* **367**: 284–7.

Mundy, G.R. (1993) Role of cytokines in bone resorption. *J Cell Biochem* **53**: 296–300.

Nachtigall, L.E., Nachtigall, R.H. and Nachtigall, R.D. (1979) Estrogen replacement therapy I: a 10-year prospective study in the relationship to osteoporosis. *Obstet Gynecol* **53**: 277–83.

Nakamura, T., Turner, C.H., Yoshikawa, T. *et al.* (1994) Do variations in hip geometry explain differences in hip fracture risk between Japanese and white Americans? *J Bone Miner Res* **9**: 1071–6.

Oursler, M.J., Osdoby, P., Pyfferoen, J. *et al.* (1991) Avian osteoclasts as estrogen target cells. *Proc Natl Acad Sci USA* **88**: 6613–17.

Pacifici, R., Brown, C., Pusek, E. *et al.* (1991) Effects of surgical menopause and estrogen replacement on cytokin release from human blood mononuclear cells. *Proc Natl Acad Sci USA* **88**: 5134–8.

Parfitt, A.M. (1987) Trabecular bone architecture in the pathogenesis and prevention of fracture. *Am J Med* **82**: 68–72.

Parfitt, A.M. (1988) Bone remodeling: relationship to the amount and structure of bone, and the pathogenesis and prevention of fractures. In: *Osteoporosis: Etiology, Diagnosis, and Management*, (eds Riggs, B.L. and Melton, L.J.), Raven Press, New York, pp.45–93.

Peacock, M., Turner, C.H., Liu, G. *et al.* (1995) Better discrimination of hip fracture using bone density, geometry and architecture. *Osteoporosis Int* **5**: 167–73.

Pfeilschifter, J.P., Seyedin, S. and Mundy, G.R. (1988) Transforming growth factor beta inhibits bone resorption in fetal rat long bone cultures. *J Clin Invest* **82**: 680–5.

Pocock, N.A., Eisman, J.A., Hopper, J.L. *et al.* (1987) Genetic determinants of bone mass in adults: a twin study. *J Clin Invest* **80**: 706–10.

Prince, R.L., Price, R.I. and Ho, S. (1988) Forearm bone loss in hemiplegia: A model for the study of immobilization osteoporosis. *J Bone Miner Res* **3**: 305–10.

Recker, R.R. and Kimmel, D.B. (1989) Changes in trabecular microstructure in osteoporosis occur with normal bone remodeling dynamics. *J Bone Miner Res* **4** (Suppl. 1): (abstract) 563.

Recker, R.R., Kimmel, D.B. and Parfitt, A.M. (1988) Static and tetracycline-based bone histomorphometric data from 34 normal postmenopausal females. *J Bone Miner Res* **3**: 133–44.

Recker, R.R., Davies, K.M., Hinders, S.M. *et al.* (1992) Bone gain in young adult women. *J Am Med Assoc* **268**: 2403–8.

Riggs, B.L. and Melton III, J.L. (1986) Involutional osteoporosis. *N Engl J Med* **314**: 1676–86.

Ross, P.D., Davis, J.W., Epstein, R.S. *et al.* (1991) Pre-existing fractures and bone mass predict vertebral fracture incidence in women. *Ann Intern Med* **114**: 919–23.

Sandler, R.B., Slemenda, C.W., LaPorte, R.E. *et al.* (1985) Postmenopausal bone density and milk consumption in childhood and adolescence. *Am J Clin Nutr* **40**: 270–4.

Seeley, D.G., Browner, W.S., Nevitt, M.C. *et al.* (1991) Which fractures are associated with low appendicular bone mass in elderly women? *Ann Intern Med* **115**: 837–42.

Slemenda, C.W. and Johnston, C.C. (1993) High intensity activities in young women: site specific bone mass effects among female figure skaters. *Bone Miner* **20**: 125–32.

Slemenda, C.W., Hui, S.L., Longcope, C. *et al.* (1987) Sex steroids and bone mass. *J Clin Invest* **80**: 1261–9.

Slemenda, C.W., Christian, J.C., Williams, C.J. *et al.* (1991a) Genetic determinants of bone mass in adult women: a reevaluation of the twin model and the potential importance of gene interaction of heritability estimates. *J Bone Miner Res* **6**: 561–7.

Slemenda, C.W., Miller, J.Z., Hui, S.L. *et al.* (1991b) Role of physical activity in the development of skeletal mass in children. *J Bone Miner Res* **6**: 1227–33.

Slemenda, C.W., Christian, J.C., Reed, T. *et al.* (1992) Long-term bone loss in men: effects of genetic and environmental factors. *Ann Intern Med* **117**: 286–91.

Slemenda, C.W., Reister, T.K. *et al.* (1993) Bone growth in children following the cessation of calcium supplementation. *J Bone Miner Res* **8**: S1–151.

Slemenda, C.W., Reister, T.K., Hui, S.L. *et al.* (1994) Influences on skeletal mineralization in children and adolescents: evidence for varying effects of sexual maturation and physical activity. *J Pediatr* **125**: 201–7.

Slemenda, C., Longcope, C., Peacock, M., Hui, S. and Johnston Jr, C.C. (1996a) Sex steroids, bone mass and bone loss: a prospective study of pre-, peri-, and postmenopausal women. *J Clin Invest* **97**: 14–21.

Slemenda, C.W., Turner, C.H., Peacock, M. *et al.* (1996b) Genetics of proximal femur geometry, distribution of bone mass and bone mineral density. *Osteoporosis Int* **6**: 178–82.

Smith, D.M., Nance, W.E. *et al.* (1973) Genetic factors in determining bone mass. *J Clin Invest* **52**: 2800–8.

Smith, E.P., Boyd, J., Frank, G.R. *et al.* (1994) Estrogen resistance caused by a mutation in the estrogen receptor gene in a man. *N Engl J Med* **331**: 1056–61.

Snead, D.B., Stubbs, C.C., Weltman, J.Y. *et al.* (1992) Dietary patterns, eating behaviors, and bone mineral density in women runners. *Am J Clin Nutr* **56**: 705–11.

Theintz, G., Buchs, B., Rizzoli, R. *et al.* (1992) Longitudinal monitoring of bone mass accumulation in healthy adolescents: evidence for a marked reduction after 16 years of age at the levels of lumbar spine and femoral neck in female subjects. *J Clin Endocrinol Metab* **75**: 1060–5.

Turner, C.H., Peacock, M., Timmerman, L., Neal, J.M. and Johnston Jr, C.C. (1995) Calcaneal ultrasonic measurements discriminate hip fracture independently of bone mass. *Osteoporosis Int* **5**: 130–5.

Wasnich, R.D., Davis, J.W. and Ross, P.D. (1994) Spine fracture risk is predicted by non-spine fractures. *Osteoporosis Int* **4**: 1–5.

Wiske, P.S., Epstein, S., Bell, N.S. *et al.* (1979) Increase of immunoreactive parathyroid hormone with age. *N Engl J Med* **300**: 1419–21.

Writing Group for PEPI Trial (1996) Effects of hormone therapy on bone mineral density: results from the postmenopausal estrogen/progestin interventions (PEPI) trial. *J Am Med Assoc* **276**: 1430–2.

EPIDEMIOLOGY 4

L.J. Melton III and C. Cooper

INTRODUCTION

How many people have osteoporosis? Who is at risk of the condition and why does it develop? How often does osteoporosis lead to adverse outcomes for the patient and what can be done to reduce the frequency of such events? What priority should be given to the development of programs to prevent or treat osteoporosis? These questions can be addressed, in part, through epidemiology (the study of disease in populations or groups of people). The scope of this discipline encompasses clinical issues relating to group experience, i.e. the findings that best define a particular disease, the characteristics of individuals at increased risk of acquiring the disease, the prognosis of patients with the disease and the usefulness of various means of preventing the disease or its complications. All of these applications of epidemiology are relevant to osteoporosis.

This chapter will review epidemiologic data concerning the frequency of osteoporosis and its related fractures in order to determine the impact that the condition has on society. The epidemiologic patterns of bone loss and of fractures in the community will be examined for clues to the etiology of osteoporosis and the natural history of the disorder will be assessed for guidance with regard to intervention strategies. This background will provide a context for the chapters that follow, which deal in greater detail with osteoporosis pathophysiology and therapy.

WHAT IS OSTEOPOROSIS?

Osteoporosis is a disease characterized by abnormalities in the amount and architectural arrangement of bone tissue which lead to impaired skeletal strength and an increased susceptibility to fractures (Kanis *et al.*, 1994). The term 'osteoporosis' was coined by a French pathologist over 170 years ago to describe porous bone (Schapira and Schapira, 1992) and the diagnosis fundamentally is a histological one, where bone tissue is normally mineralized but there is too little of it. Clinically, however, osteoporosis is recognized by the occurrence of characteristic fractures or, prior to the onset of fractures, by reduced bone mineral density. These two complementary notions of osteoporosis, as low bone mass or as fracture, have not been fully integrated nor has either been unequivocally defined. Because they have different implications for diagnosis and treatment and for understanding pathophysiology, the epidemiology of osteoporosis will be considered in both contexts.

OSTEOPOROSIS AS FRACTURE

Patients who experience characteristic fractures attributed to low bone mass are traditionally

Osteoporosis. Edited by John C. Stevenson and Robert Lindsay. Published in 1998 by Chapman & Hall, London.
ISBN 0 412 48870 1

said to have 'established osteoporosis' (Kanis *et al.*, 1994). Typically, this involves vertebral fractures, but patients with proximal femur or distal forearm fractures are sometimes included. The diagnosis of established osteoporosis is generally considered a highly specific one: whether it is measured or not, bone density is presumed to be low in such patients but this is not always so (Nordin, 1987). About one in six vertebral fractures (Cooper *et al.*, 1992a) and a comparable proportion of hip fractures (Madhok *et al.*, 1993) result from severe trauma; smaller proportions are due to malignancy and other specific lesions. These individuals may not have low bone mass. Even in the absence of significant trauma, a substantial minority of fracture patients will be found to have bone density levels above the 'fracture threshold' (see below).

More importantly, the diagnosis of established osteoporosis is very insensitive. Fractures at many sites besides the spine are attributable to low bone density (Table 4.1), but osteoporosis may not be diagnosed when they occur. Neither can this diagnosis be made in those who have not yet had a fracture though they may be at great risk by virtue of low bone mass. This leads to the awkward situation wherein a patient is normal one day and osteoporotic the next, when a fracture occurs, without any real change in the underlying status of the skeleton (Schapira and Schapira, 1992). The need to await the occurrence of fractures also restricts the diagnosis to more or less end-stage disease. While it is still important to treat such patients, so that additional fractures may be reduced, the opportunity to prevent the onset of fractures in the first place is missed.

OSTEOPOROSIS AS LOW BONE MASS

The concept of increased fracture risk is the basis for considering osteoporosis a disease, like hypertension or diabetes mellitus, that can be defined on the basis of a physiologic abnormality. At some low level of bone density as detected by bone biopsy or, more often, by non-invasive measures of bone mineral (Chapter 7), osteoporosis can be said to exist. Unlike hypertension and diabetes, however, consensus has not yet been reached regarding the exact level of bone density that should be considered presumptive evidence

Table 4.1 Standard hazard ratios* for specific fractures associated with low bone mass at two or more skeletal sites. Modified from Seeley *et al.* (1991)

	Measurement site		
Fracture site	*Calcaneus*	*Proximal radius*	*Distal radius*
Hand	1.63 (1.00 to 2.63)¶	1.69 (1.10 to 2.62)¶	1.87 (1.15 to 3.03)¶
Wrist	1.76 (1.49 to 2.09)‡	1.63 (1.39 to 1.90)‡	1.82 (1.53 to 2.16)‡
Humerus	1.85 (1.44 to 2.38)‡	1.96 (1.56 to 2.47)‡	2.04 (1.57 to 2.65)‡
Clavicle	1.10 (0.57 to 2.11)	1.96 (1.03 to 3.72)¶	2.63 (1.23 to 5.62)¶
Vertebra	1.70 (1.30 to 2.22)‡	1.40 (1.09 to 1.80)§	1.51 (1.15 to 1.98)§
Rib	1.53 (1.16 to 2.01)§	1.54 (1.19 to 2.00)§	1.80 (1.35 to 2.41)‡
Pelvis	2.44 (1.55 to 3.84)‡	1.61 (1.08 to 2.40)¶	1.30 (0.86 to 1.97)
Hip	1.70 (1.32 to 2.19)‡	1.42 (1.12 to 1.80)§	1.46 (1.13 to 1.88)§
Leg	1.73 (1.12 to 2.67)¶	1.52 (1.03 to 2.25)¶	1.97 (1.27 to 3.05)§
Foot	1.39 (1.11 to 1.75)§	1.29 (1.04 to 1.59)¶	1.43 (1.14 to 1.80)§
Toe	1.39 (1.04 to 1.85)¶	1.39 (1.06 to 1.82)¶	1.54 (1.15 to 2.05)§

*Hazard ratio (95% CI) associated with a one standard deviation decrease in bone mass, adjusted for age.
¶ $P < 0.05$, § $P < 0.01$, ‡ $P < 0.001$.

of osteoporosis. To increase the specificity of bone mineral measurements for predicting fractures, it has been proposed that very low levels be considered abnormal, such as three or four standard deviations below the mean of young normals (Mazess, 1987). This excludes many who ultimately will fracture, however. Alternatively, it has been recommended that the level be set at two standard deviations below the young normal mean (Nordin, 1987). When measured in the spine or hip, this value incorporates 90% or more of the patients with spine or hip fractures (Mazess, 1987) and thus corresponds to the empirical 'fracture threshold' (Riggs and Melton, 1986). A committee of the World Health Organization recently recommended a compromise cut-off level at 2.5 standard deviations below the mean for young normals (Kanis *et al.*, 1994).

Because currently available treatments can preserve existing bone mass but cannot restore osteoporotic bone to biomechanical normality (Riggs and Melton, 1992), there is also a clinical need to identify those at risk of osteoporosis and fractures before irreversible bone loss has occurred. Thus, perimeno-pausal women with bone density that is one standard deviation below the young normal mean might not have pathologically low bone mass today, but could still be at sufficiently high risk of fracture over their remaining lifetime that prophylactic therapy is indicated (Johnston *et al.*, 1989). This has led to increasing interest in defining osteoporosis on the basis of lifetime fracture risk (Melton and Wahner, 1989). In the World Health Organization scheme (Table 4.2), bone density between one and 2.5 standard deviations below young normal mean levels is considered low bone mass or 'osteopenia' and prophylaxis to prevent further bone loss is indicated for some of these individuals.

EPIDEMIOLOGY OF LOW BONE MASS

Emergence of the non-invasive assessment techniques delineated in Chapter 7 has made it possible to measure bone mass at various times during life. Although most studies have been cross-sectional, they suggest three skeletal phases: growth, consolidation and loss. The greatest gain in bone mass occurs during linear growth, which is completed by 20 years of age. For 5–15 years following the cessation of growth, mineral accretion continues in the absence of any appreciable change in skeletal size ('consolidation'). After a variable period that is still poorly defined, net bone loss commences. White women may lose a third of their cortical (or compact) bone, which forms the shafts of the limb bones and comprises up to 80% of the skeleton, and half of their cancellous (or trabecular) bone, which makes up the ends of the limb bones and most of the spine, pelvis and other flat bones of the skeleton; men lose about two-thirds of these amounts (Riggs and Melton, 1986). While much remains to be learned about the

Table 4.2 Diagnostic categories of bone mineral content (BMC) or bone mineral density (BMD) in women. From Kanis *et al.* (1994)

Normal. A value for BMD or BMC greater than 1 SD below the young adult reference range

Low bone mass (osteopenia). A value for BMD or BMC more than 1 SD below the young adult range but less than 2.5 SD below this range.

Osteoporosis. A value for BMD or BMC more than 2.5 SD below the young adult range.

Severe osteoporosis (established osteoporosis). A value for BMD or BMC more than 2.5 SD below the young adult range and the presence of one or more fragility fractures.

determinants of bone gain and loss, it is clear that this loss compromises the biomechanical integrity of the skeleton and increases the risk of fracture.

HOW MANY PEOPLE HAVE LOW BONE MASS?

A precise answer to this question is not possible pending final consensus on the definition of osteoporosis, as noted above. If defined, however, by the World Health Organization criteria, the prevalence is substantial. By this definition, an estimated 30% of postmenopausal white women might have osteoporosis of the hip, spine or distal forearm judging from extrapolations of population-based data on a small sample of women (Melton, 1995b). As shown in Figure 4.1, only 15% of women aged 50–59 years are affected but this rises dramatically with aging to include 70% of the women aged 80 years and over. The overall age-adjusted prevalence in the proximal femur alone was 16%. This is consistent with more extensive data from the National Health and Nutrition Examination Survey where an estimated 21% of postmenopausal white women had hip bone density that was more than 2.5 standard deviations below the young normal mean (Looker *et al.*, 1995). Comparable figures for African-American and Mexican-American women were 10% and 16%, respectively. As yet, comparable data have not been published for men.

Barring the widespread introduction of some effective intervention, these numbers will increase in the future as the population ages. In the United States, for example, the number of individuals aged 65 years and over is expected to rise from 32 to 69 million between 1990 and 2050, while the number aged 85 years and over will increase from 3 to 15 million. Because the prevalence of low bone mass rises with age and is quite high in elderly women, these demographic changes alone will eventually result in a doubling or

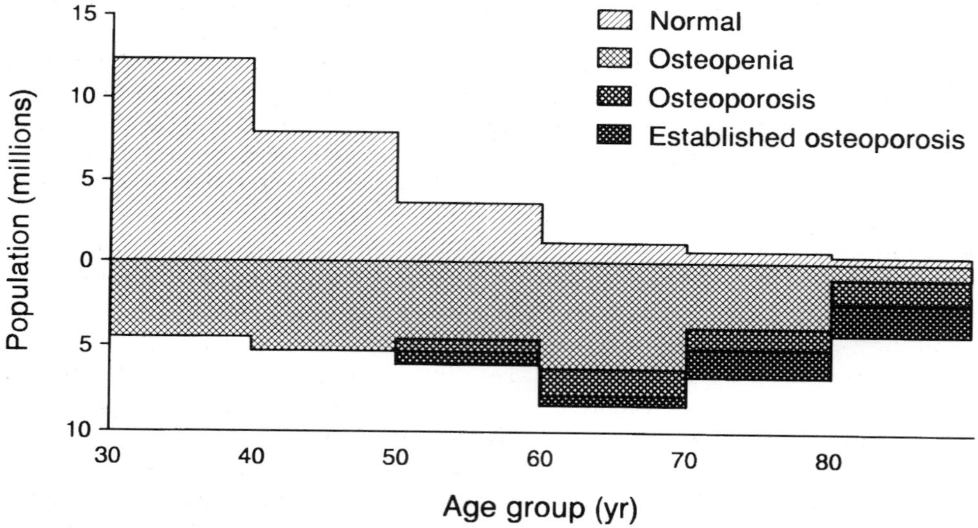

Figure 4.1 Estimated skeletal status of United States white women in 1990 by age group. Osteopenia is bone density of the hip, spine or distal forearm >1.0 but ≤2.5 SD below the young normal mean. Osteoporosis is bone density at one or more of these sites >2.5 SD below the mean and established osteoporosis indicates the additional presence of fragility fractures. From Melton (1995b).

tripling in the number of affected women. Thus, with these projected increases in the elderly population, the number of postmenopausal white women in the United States with bone mineral more than 2.5 standard deviations below the young normal mean could grow from 9 million now to 23 million by the year 2050. Even today, if one included non-white women and men as well as those with bone density in the osteopenic range, it is probably true that, altogether, 20–25 million Americans are at increased risk of fracture because of low bone mass (Peck *et al.*, 1988).

WHO IS AT RISK OF LOW BONE MASS?

Conceptually, at least, the risk factors for low bone mass are fairly straightforward. Each individual's bone mass in later life is dictated both by the peak bone mass that he or she achieves as a young adult and by the subsequent rate of bone loss; at age 70 years, these two determinants of bone mass are about equally important (Hui *et al.*, 1990). The factors that influence peak bone mass are not well understood at present, but it is recognized that skeletal size is inherited, accounting in part for the race and gender differences in osteoporosis risk. Although there are exceptions, bone mass is generally lower among people of Caucasian and Asian heritage than it is among other races and, within each ethnic group, it is lower in women than men (Melton, 1991). This suggests a strong genetic component, but environmental factors must also play a role (Eisman *et al.*, 1993). For example, increased calcium intake and exercise can augment bone mass in children (Slemenda *et al.*, 1991; Johnston *et al.*, 1992), while conditions that lead to amenorrhea reduce it (Cooper and Eastell, 1993). Most of the other risk factors that have been evaluated, such as pregnancy, lactation and oral contraceptive use, have weak or inconsistent effects (Melton *et al.*, 1993a). Indeed, the data available at present are insufficiently detailed to permit the design of a program to maximize peak bone mass. This is an important barrier to the development of effective public health measures to prevent osteoporosis.

More is known of the determinants of bone loss, which results from:

1. age-related factors that occur universally in the population;
2. an accelerated phase of bone loss associated with the menopause in women and hypogonadism in some men;
3. medical and surgical conditions that produce 'secondary' osteoporosis in particular individuals (Riggs and Melton, 1986).

Innumerable studies have shown that bone mass declines with age, in men as well as in women. The gradual decline of bone mass with aging is usually attributed to impaired calcium metabolism but could also relate to declining physical activity and fitness (Pocock *et al.*, 1989). Estrogen deficiency is another well-recognized cause of bone loss (Chapter 8). Bone mass decreases as a logarithmic function of years since menopause (Gallagher *et al.*, 1987) so that the accelerated phase of bone loss in perimenopausal women is superimposed upon the slower, age-related bone loss. Finally, bone loss is exacerbated by specific conditions that occur sporadically in the population, like corticosteroid excess, hyperthyroidism, multiple myeloma, etc. (Khosla and Melton, 1995). While medical or surgical conditions like these may be the predominant cause of osteoporosis in affected individuals, any resulting bone loss is additive to that from age-related factors and hypogonadism (Riggs and Melton, 1986).

Attempts to quantify these various risk factors for low bone mass have been less successful. In the most comprehensive study to date, the determinants of appendicular bone density were assessed in 9704 elderly women. Later age at menopause, estrogen or thiazide use, non-insulin-dependent diabetes and greater height, weight and strength were all positively associated with bone mass, while greater age, cigarette smoking, caffeine intake, prior gastric surgery and maternal history of fracture were negatively associated (Bauer *et al.*, 1993). Despite the large number of potential risk factors that were assessed and the enormous size of this study, with its corresponding ability to identify factors only weakly correlated with bone mass, models incorporating all of the independent predictors together explained only 20–35% of the variance in bone density at the radius or calcaneus. The same is true of earlier studies, where various risk factors have generally accounted for less than half of the variability in bone mass (Johnston *et al.*, 1989). Moreover, no unique set of risk factors has consistently been identified in the different studies.

As a result of these problems, no clinical index has been devised which can reliably identify high-risk patients. The futility of this approach was convincingly demonstrated by Slemenda and colleagues (1990), who identified predictors of bone mineral at various skeletal sites and then compared predicted values at those sites with the results actually observed among 124 perimenopausal women. For femoral neck bone mineral density, the best predictive model was 0.79 + (0.001 × height) + (0.0041 × weight) - (0.00018 × cigarette pack-years) - (0.00023 × urinary calcium/creatinine) + (0.00005 × dietary calcium). However, this model accounted for only 17% of the variability in bone mineral measurements at the hip and correctly classified only 65% of the women whose bone density was in the lowest tertile (Figure 4.2). Similar models correctly classified 68% of women with low midradius bone mineral content and only 61% of those with low bone density in the lumbar spine (Slemenda *et al.*, 1990). This is not adequate for patient care since bone mineral can be measured directly with less misclassification error.

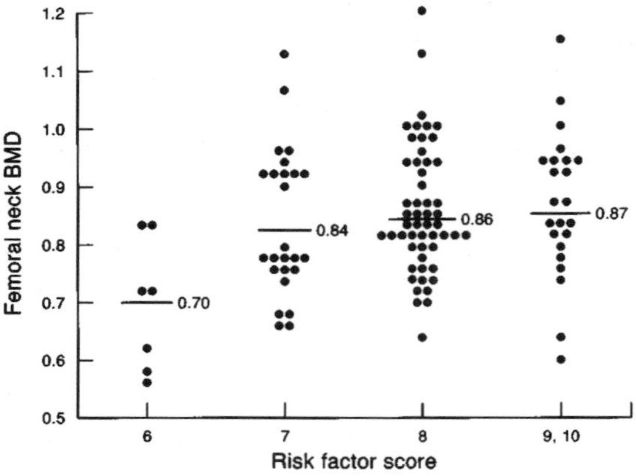

Figure 4.2 Observed femoral neck bone mineral density (BMD) plotted against risk factor score. From Slemenda *et al.* (1990).

WHAT ARE THE ADVERSE OUTCOMES OF LOW BONE MASS?

Bone loss in the jaw may lead to tooth loss and ill-fitting dentures (Anon., 1990), but reduced bone strength is the most important consequence of osteoporosis. Skeletal fragility is related not only to the amount of bone tissue present but also to its architectural arrangement, any abnormalities of bone matrix or mineralization and the presence or absence of microfractures. Defects in each of these areas may be present in osteoporosis (Melton *et al.*, 1988), leading to age-related reductions in bone strength that are greater in women than men. This is illustrated in Figure 4.3, where diminishing bone density and cross-sectional moment of inertia in the femur neck results in increased mechanical stresses with age. Although bone architecture and bone quality cannot be accurately assessed by non-invasive means for use in risk prediction, bone mineral measurements are very highly correlated with bone strength (Courtney *et al.*, 1995) and have been shown empirically to predict fractures (Ross *et al.*, 1990; Johnston and Melton, 1995). Most recently, it was shown that each standard deviation decrease in femoral neck bone density was associated with a 2.6-fold increase in the age-adjusted risk of hip fracture among 8134 women followed for 1.8 years (Cummings *et al.*, 1993). This short-term result was consistent with the 2.4-fold increase in age-adjusted hip fracture risk seen in a smaller group of 304 women followed for over eight years when bone mineral was measured at the same site (Melton *et al.*, 1993b). This relationship is stronger than that seen between serum cholesterol and coronary heart disease or between blood pressure and stroke mortality (Hui *et al.*, 1988; Browner *et al.*, 1991).

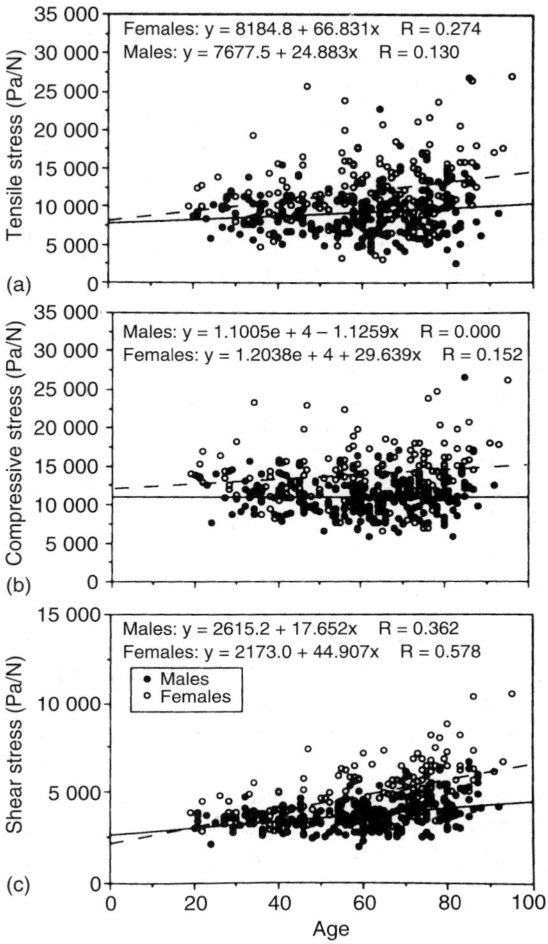

Figure 4.3 Computed femoral neck stresses at the narrowest section, as a function of age in the femoral necks of male and females in the BLSA sample. (a) Tensile stress at the superior-lateral margin of the section; (b) compressive stress at the inferior-medial margin of the section; (c) shear stress at the section centroid. Simple linear regressions are shown using a solid line for males and a dashed line for females. From Beck, T.J. *et al.* (1992) Sex differences in geometry of the femoral neck with aging: a structural analysis of bone mineral data. *Calcif Tissue Int*, **50**(1): 24–9.

WHAT ARE THE IMPLICATIONS FOR PATIENT MANAGEMENT?

Several important clinical principles derive from these epidemiological observations. First, there may be an irreversible component of bone loss. Available therapies are incapable of restoring structural elements of bone that have been completely lost (Riggs and Melton, 1992). Consequently, treatments that thicken existing bone structures, rather than re-establishing internal bone architecture, may not reduce subsequent fractures to the degree anticipated from observed increases in bone mineral. The same principle dictates early use of the regimens which are able to slow or prevent bone loss. However, a decision about the exact level of bone mass that requires intervention is necessarily somewhat arbitrary (Melton and Wahner, 1989) because the gradient of increasing fracture risk with decreasing bone mineral is continuous, with no true biological threshold at which fractures begin. None-theless, it is clear that large numbers of women are affected regardless of how low bone mass might be defined. This suggests that public health measures aimed at the general population will be needed to complement programs for identifying and treating high-risk individuals. Since osteoporosis may progress silently for decades, the only practical approach to diagnosis prior to the onset of fractures is on the basis of low bone mineral assessed *in vivo*. Even though bone mass is not strictly synonymous with skeletal fragility, most of the ultimate strength of bone tissue is accounted for by bone mineral density and the other contributors to fragility cannot yet be assessed non-invasively. Knowledge of risk factors is growing, but they cannot be used in lieu of bone mineral measurements to identify specific individuals with osteoporosis.

EPIDEMIOLOGY OF FRACTURES

Hip fractures have been recognized as a manifestation of osteoporosis for over a century (Cooper, 1842) and vertebral fractures have been virtually synonymous with post-menopausal osteoporosis since the time of Albright (Albright *et al.*, 1941). Only in the last decade, however, has it become obvious that osteoporosis represents an enormous public health problem. Literally millions of fractures each year can be attributed in part to osteoporosis and they exact a staggering toll of disability and expense. New knowledge is providing a better understanding of fracture epidemiology, especially with regard to the relative contributions to fracture pathogenesis of low bone mass and falls. It may be possible in the future to exploit these insights for fracture prevention.

HOW MANY PEOPLE HAVE FRACTURES?

Fractures are common, especially among the young and the elderly, so that the incidence of limb fractures as a function of age is bimodal (Melton, 1995a). While most fractures among the elderly are due in part to low bone mass (Seeley *et al.*, 1991), those that have been most closely linked to advanced age, and by extension to osteoporosis, share three distinctive features: incidence rates that are greater among women than men, rates that increase dramatically with aging, and occurrence at sites that contain a large proportion of cancellous bone. Fractures of the proximal femur, distal forearm and spine display these characteristics and have received the most attention. Their frequency can be assessed in terms of both annual incidence rates and cumulative incidence over a lifetime.

Incidence patterns

The classic example of an age-related injury is fracture of the proximal femur (Figure 4.4). Incidence rates rise expoentially with aging, reaching about 3% per year among white women aged 85 years and over in the United States and Northern Europe (Melton, 1995a). Rates for white men are about half as much at any age, but, because women live longer, 80% of all hip fractures are in women. The same pattern is seen in the United Kingdom, except that age-adjusted rates are around 35% lower (Donaldson *et al.*, 1990). Hip fractures are considerably less frequent in black populations (Jacobsen *et al.*, 1990a) and incidence rates in black men and women at any given age are closer than those in whites. Hip fracture incidence rates among Asians lie between those of whites and blacks, but a sharp increase in hip fracture incidence in some parts of the Far East in recent decades has brought rates closer to those observed in northern Europe (Lau *et al.*, 1990). Indeed, when projected population growth is taken

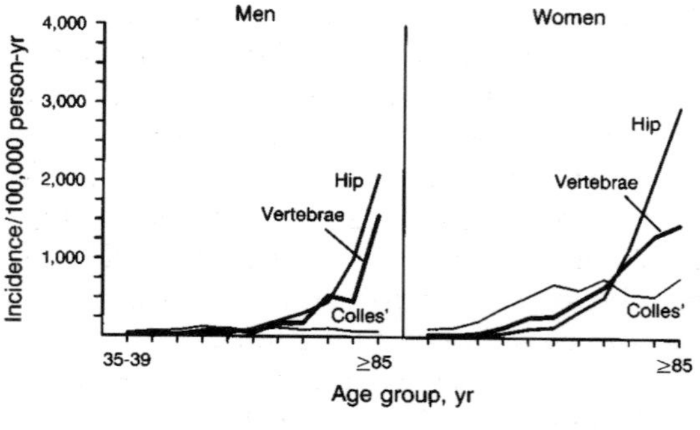

Figure 4.4 Age-specific incidence rates of hip, vertebral, and Colles' fracture in Rochester, Minnesota, men and women. From Cooper, C. and Melton III, L.J. (1992) Epidemiology of osteoporosis. *Trends Endocrinol Metab* **3**(6): 224–9.

into account, it is estimated that about half of the expected 6.3 million hip fractures world-wide in 2050 will occur in Asia (Cooper *et al.*, 1992b).

The incidence of vertebral fractures in white women and men has a similar pattern (Figure 4.4), but the number of affected individuals depends on who is counted. It has been estimated, for example, that 148 000 British women aged 50 and over might develop vertebral fractures each year if rates were the same as those in the United States (Cooper and Melton, 1992). Of these women, an estimated 50 000 would come to clinical attention and 12 000 would require hospitalization. Up to 17 000 British men might also be diagnosed annually if these rates applied. However, data on the actual frequency of vertebral fractures in the United Kingdom are inconsistent. Some investigators have reported a markedly lower prevalence of vertebral deformity than seen in the United States, while others have derived estimates that are much closer (Kanis and McCloskey, 1992). Such inconsistencies arise, at least in part, from variations in the method used to assess the prevalence of vertebral deformity. Thus, based on a new approach, only 2% of middle-aged women from Chingford, England, had severe vertebral fractures of the sort linked to chronic symptoms, but the prevalence was 10% using the methods employed in one of the studies in the United States (Spector *et al.*, 1993). The expected prevalence, based on the American rates, was 9%. Curiously, the prevalence of vertebral fractures among Asians seems to be as high as that in whites (Ross *et al.*, 1995), despite their lower hip fracture rates. Few data are available for other ethnic groups.

There is also a substantial female excess of distal forearm fractures, but the steep rise in incidence begins earlier in life and levels off at about age 60 (Figure 4.4). Incidence rates among men do not rise much after age 50. Consequently, rates in the elderly are only a fraction of those of hip fractures. Because the incidence is greater in midlife, however, where the population is larger, forearm fractures are as numerous as hip fractures and about 85% occur in women (Melton, 1995a). As with hip fractures, forearm fracture rates in the United Kingdom are around 30% lower than those in the United States but display the same pattern of age-specific increase in women (Donaldson *et al.*, 1990). Forearm fractures seem to be less frequent in black and Asian populations (Hagino *et al.*, 1989; Griffin *et al.*, 1992), but the epidemiological picture is generally the same.

Cumulative incidence

While the yearly risk of various fractures may seem relatively modest, annual rates accumulate quickly over a lifetime that, in the United States for example, averages 78.9 years for white women and 72.3 years for white men. Thus, the lifetime risk of a hip fracture has been estimated at 17.5% in white women and 6.0% in white men (Table 4.3). Some perspective is provided by the observation that these figures are approximately equivalent, respectively, to the lifetime risk in women of developing breast, ovarian and endometrial cancer and the lifetime risk in men of developing prostate cancer (Seidman *et al.*, 1978). The lifetime risk of hip fracture has been estimated at 5.6% for black women and 2.8% for black men from age 50 years onward (Cummings *et al.*, 1989). The lifetime risk of a clinically detected vertebral fracture is 15.6% in white women and 5.0% in white men (Table 4.3). Because a substantial proportion of vertebral fractures are asymptomatic and never diagnosed, these are probably low estimates. The lifetime risk of a distal forearm fracture is 16.0% in white women and 2.5% in white men (Table 4.3) on the basis of 1945–74 data (Owen *et al.*, 1982). More recent data are unavailable for the United States, but studies elsewhere suggest that forearm fracture rates may be rising (Obrant *et al.*, 1989) so this estimate could be outdated. Despite the fact that two of the

Table 4.3 Estimated lifetime fracture risk in 50-year-old white women and men. From Melton *et al.* (1992)

	Women % (95% CI)	*Men* % (95% CI)
Proximal femur fracture	17.5 (16.8–18.2)	6.0 (5.6–6.5)
Vertebral fracture¶	15.6 (14.8–16.3)	5.0 (4.6–5.4)
Distal forearm fracture	16.0 (15.2–16.7)	2.5 (2.2–3.1)
Any of the three	39.7 (38.7–40.6)	13.1 (12.4–13.7)

¶Using incidence of clinically diagnosed fractures only.

three fracture-specific estimates may be conservative, the lifetime risk of any one of the three fractures is 39.7% for white women from age 50 years onward and 13.1% for white men (Melton *et al.*, 1992). Moreover, hip, forearm and vertebral fractures are not the only ones associated with osteoporosis.

WHO IS AT RISK OF FRACTURE?

The exponential increase in hip fracture incidence with aging resembles that of other 'Gompertzian' (after the British actuary, Benjamin Gompertz, who first described the exponential nature of mortality) diseases like osteoarthritis, adenocarcinoma, atherosclerosis and stroke (Melton, 1990). These disorders have certain features in common including the onset of a pathophysiologic process early in life, with insidious progression until a symptomatic threshold is reached after a long latent period. Most common chronic degenerative diseases are of this type and the majority of the population is at risk to some degree. These diseases do not have a single 'cause'; instead, individual risk results from the interplay of multiple factors. In the case of hip fractures, these include the risk factors related to low bone mass (previously reviewed) and others that are associated with an increased likelihood of falling. Based on the preceding observations, however, no single factor would be expected to account for the majority of fractures.

Such interrelationships also lead to uncertainty about the mechanisms through which prominent risk factors like gender, race and age exert their effects. For example, the greater hip fracture incidence in men than women of all races and whites than nonwhites (Figure 4.5) has been attributed to differences in bone mass, with American blacks said to have substantially greater bone mineral density than whites of the same age and sex (Cauley *et al.*, 1994). The African Bantu, however, who have the lowest hip fracture incidence rates of any population, have values for metacarpal bone density that are lower than those of Johannesburg whites, who display the usual Western pattern of hip fracture incidence (Solomon, 1979). The Bantu do have better skeletal preservation during midlife, presumably as a result of physically demanding labor. Greater strength and fitness may also account for the lower risk of falling in black than white women (Nevitt *et al.*, 1989) and for the lower hip fracture risk that Japanese women enjoy (Ross *et al.*, 1991b). It remains uncertain whether exercise, diet and other such factors can account for the surprising variation in fracture incidence observed within populations (Jacobsen *et al.*, 1990b; Johnell *et al.*, 1992).

Similar observations can be made with respect to gender. A substantial proportion of elderly women are susceptible to fractures because of their fragile skeletons. However,

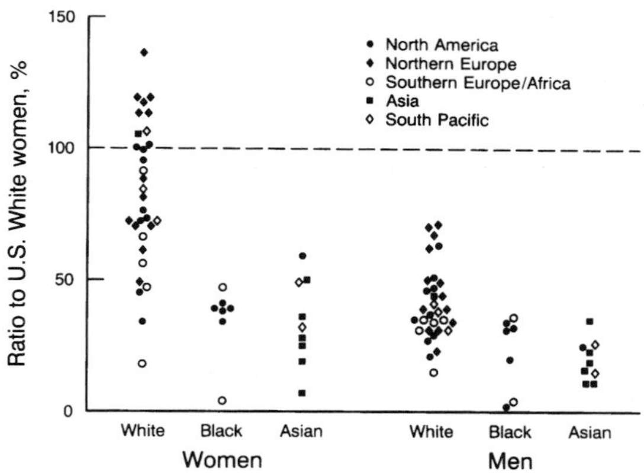

Figure 4.5 Hip fracture incidence around the world as a ratio of the rates observed to those expected for United States white women of the same age. From Melton (1991).

their likelihood of falling is also great, rising annually from about one in five women at 45–49 years old to nearly half of those aged 85 years and over (Winner *et al.*, 1989). The risk of falling is generally much less in men. Based on the data of Winner and colleagues (1989), women aged 65 years and over were 50% more likely to report a fall in the previous year than were elderly men. The pathophysiology of these falls is poorly understood and, in a specific patient, usually results from a complex interaction of several factors. While environmental factors play a role, half or more of the falls among elderly persons are associated with organic dysfunction such as diminished postural control, gait changes, muscular weakness, decreased reflexes or poor vision (Table 4.4). The proportion of persons with one or more of these problems increases with age and the risk of falling is directly correlated with the number of conditions present (Tinetti *et al.*, 1988).

It is important to point out, however, that most falls to not result in an injury, even among the elderly. Only about 5% of falls lead to a fracture and only one in 100 ends in a hip fracture (Gibson, 1987). Therefore, additional risk factors are needed to account for the full spectrum of fall outcomes. These likely relate to the mechanics of falling (Melton and Riggs, 1985). Recent data indicate, for example, that the likelihood of hip fracture among community fallers is influenced by the orientation of the fall, the potential energy of the faller and the amount of soft tissue padding over the hip, as well as by the bone density of the proximal femur

Table 4.4 Risk factors for falling. Modified from Tinetti, M.E. and Speechley, M. (1989) Prevention of falls among the elderly. *N Engl J Med* **320**(16): 1055–9.

Reduced visual acuity, dark adaptation and perception
Reduced hearing
Vestibular dysfunction
Proprioceptive dysfunction, cervical degenerative disorders and peripheral neuropathy
Dementia
Musculoskeletal disorders
Foot disorders (calluses, bunions, deformities)
Postural hypotension
Use of medications (benzodiazepines, phenothiazines, antidepressants, antihypertensives, antiarrhythmics, anticonvulsants, diuretics, alcohol, etc.)

(Greenspan *et al.*, 1994). However, most elderly individuals have bone density levels low enough to put them at increased risk. Consequently, prevention of the clinical manifestations of osteoporosis will depend, in part, on reducing the frequency and severity of falls. Unfortunately, fall prevention programs are of uncertain effectiveness (Report of the US Preventive Services Task Force, 1989), but preliminary data indicate that energy-absorbing protective devices worn externally may be able to lower the risk of hip fractures among frequent fallers (Lauritzen *et al.*, 1992).

Given the complex pathophysiology involved, it is not surprising that efforts to predict fractures directly from risk factor data have met with limited success. For example, a risk factor score was able to discriminate among 1014 Dutch women aged 45–64 years who did and did not have subsequent fractures over nine years of follow-up, but sensitivity was low and specificity was modest (Van Hemert *et al.*, 1990). Various risk factors were also unable to predict vertebral fractures among a group of 704 Japanese-American women (Table 4.5). The lack of specificity was emphasized by the fact that all of the women had at least two of the risk factors and 91% had four or more of them (Wasnich *et al.*, 1987). Likewise, the positive predictive value of an elevated risk factor score was only 9–17%, depending on the cut-off value used, in identifying vertebral fractures among 1012 women in the United Kingdom (Cooper *et al.*, 1991). Most of that very modest predictive power was contributed by a history of vertebral fracture per se. In the most recent report, an exhaustive set of potential risk factors was evaluated in a prospective study of 9516 white and Asian-American women (Cummings *et al.*, 1995). Hip fracture incidence was 17 times greater among 15% of the women who had five or more risk factors, exclusive of bone density, compared to 47% of the women who had two risk factors or less. However, women with five risk factors or more had an even higher risk of hip fracture if their bone density Z-score was in the lowest tertile. While these data suggest that risk factors can be used in combination with bone density measurements to sharpen the prediction of future fracture risk, no consistent set of risk factors has emerged from the different studies.

WHAT ARE THE ADVERSE OUTCOMES OF FRACTURES?

Adverse fracture outcomes fall into three broad categories: mortality, morbidity and

Table 4.5 Risk factor prevalence and relative risk of spine fracture. Modified from Wasnich *et al.* (1987)

	Prevalence	*Relative risk*	*P value*
Premature menopause (≤ age 40)	4.7%	1.6	NS
Family history (+ or -)	1.7%	2.7	NS
Short stature (ht ≤ 62 in)	87.2%	1.6	NS
Leanness (BMI ≤ 19.7)	14.7%	1.7	NS
Calcium deficiency (≤ 500 mg)	83.9%	1.2	NS
Physical activity (PAI ≤ 26.9)	7.8%	2.5	NS
Nulliparity (+ or -)	5.7%	1.6	NS
Smoking (+ or -)	16.8%	1.2	NS
Alcohol (≥ 2 g/day)	4.8%	1.7	NS
Asian ancestry (+ or -)	100.0%	–	–
Caffeine (≥ 300 mg/day)	29.6%	2.1	NS
Chronic gastrointestinal disease (+ or -)	4.1%	1.0	NS

cost. From the social perspective, hip fractures dominate each category but vertebral and forearm fractures contribute significantly. Almost no data are available with regard to the mortality, morbidity or social cost of any of the other kinds of osteoporosis-related fractures. This is a noteworthy deficiency because it means that any intervention for osteoporosis will be undervalued relative to its cost and therefore handicapped in competition for scarce health-care resources.

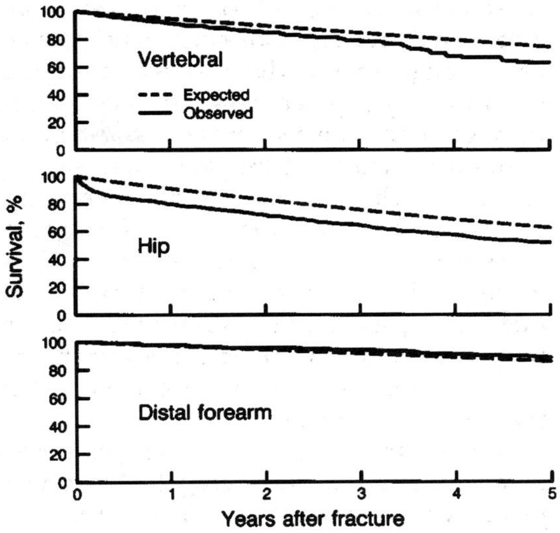

Figure 4.6 Survival following the diagnosis of vertebral, hip and distal forearm fracture among Rochester, Minnesota, residents. Figures show observed survival and that expected using death rates of West North Central United States residents in 1980. From Cooper *et al.* (1993).

Mortality

The influence of osteoporotic fractures on survival varies with the type of fracture for reasons that are not well understood. Hip fractures are the most serious, leading to an overall 5–20% reduction from expected survival (Melton, 1995a). The excess deaths occur soon after the fracture and diminish with time so that, after six months or so, subsequent survival is comparable to that of similar-aged men and women in the general population (Figure 4.6). While some of these early deaths are related to surgical misadventures and acute complications, the majority appear to be due to serious coexisting illnesses (Poór *et al.*, 1995). The deaths seem unrelated to falling per se, since distal forearm fractures are all due to falls but impose no excess risk of death. Likewise, a third of clinically diagnosed vertebral fractures have been attributed to falling (Cooper *et al.*, 1992a), but there is no early excess of vertebral fracture deaths like that seen for hip fractures. Instead, survival appears to worsen with the passage of time (Figure 4.6), probably the result of a variety of comorbid conditions (Cooper *et al.*, 1993). Comorbidity is also the most likely explanation for the higher death rates seen among women with low bone mass (Browner *et al.*, 1991).

Morbidity

Chrischilles and colleagues (1991) have estimated that osteoporotic fractures of the hip, spine and forearm would cause an extra 6.7% of white women to become dependent in the activities of daily living, over and above background levels of dependency in the community, and precipitate admission of an additional 7.8% of women into nursing homes for long-term care (Chrischilles *et al.*, 1991). Hip fractures contribute the most to these problems. Almost all hip fractures require hospitalization, leading to over 7 million restricted activity days (62.5 days per episode) among non-institutionalized individuals in the United States each year (Holbrook *et al.*, 1984). Patients may also develop complications, such as pressure sores, pneumonia and urinary tract infections, and they may become severely depresed (Anon., 1990). The most important problem, however, is impaired ambulation. Many patients are non-ambulatory prior to fracture but, of those able to walk before, half cannot walk independently afterward (Koval *et al.*,

1995). Poor ambulation is an important predictor of nursing home admission (Bonar *et al.*, 1990) and 60 000 nursing home admissions are attributed to hip fractures in the United States each year (Phillips *et al.*, 1988). There is a possibility, however, that disability related to hip fractures could be reduced through more aggressive rehabilitation (Bourgquist *et al.*, 1991).

Vertebral fractures may result in acute pain which usually resolves after several weeks of bed rest (Cooper and Melton, 1992), but the majority are not medically attended and the fracture is often found incidentally on a radiograph taken for some other purpose (Cooper *et al.*, 1992a). Nonetheless, vertebral fractures in patients aged 65 years or older account for 150 000 hospital admissions each year (Jacobsen *et al.*, 1992), along with 161 000 physician office visits and over 5 million restricted activity days for those aged 45 years and over (Holbrook *et al.*, 1984). There are few data on long-term outcomes, but such fractures may lead to progressive loss of height, kyphosis, postural changes and persistent pain that interferes with the activities of daily living (Sinaki, 1995). In the control arm of one treatment study (Ringe, 1987), for example, most patients were noted to have persistent pain for six months following the fracture. However, physical function, self-esteem, body image and mood are adversely affected mainly in those with the more severe vertebral deformities (Ross *et al.*, 1991a) and only an estimated 4.2% of patients with a vertebral fracture became dependent because of the fracture, though nearly half of them needed nursing home placement (Chrischilles *et al.*, 1991). In the best study to date, Ettinger and colleagues (1992) found that elderly women with a mild or moderate vertebral deformity were only slightly more likely to have constant or severe back pain, back disability or substantial height loss than were those with no evidence of vertebral fracture (Table 4.6). Ten percent of elderly women had a severe (four standard deviations) deformity and only in this latter group was there a statistically significantly increased risk of these problems.

Despite the fact that only about one-fifth of the patients with wrist fractures are hospitalized (Garraway *et al.*, 1979), they account for nearly 50 000 hospital admissions and over 400 000 physician office visits by persons 45 years of age or older in the United States each year (Holbrook *et al.*, 1984). Distal forearm fractures also lead to over 6 million restricted activity days annually but they have traditionally been considered free of long-term disability. However, more recent reviews show that persistent pain, loss of function, neuropathies and post-traumatic arthritis are quite common (de Bruijn, 1987; Kanis and Pitt, 1992). While it has been estimated that less than 1% of forearm fracture patients become dependent as a result of the fracture (Chrischilles *et al.*, 1991), nearly half report only fair or poor functional outcomes at six months (Kaukonen *et al.*, 1988). The

Table 4.6 Prevalence (%) of chronic problems by grade of worst vertebral deformity. Modified from Ettinger *et al.* (1992)

Deformity grade	*Back pain most or all of the time*	*Back pain moderate or severe*	*Back disability score ≥ 6*	*Height loss > 4 cm*
None	13.8	42.0	3.8	23.0
2 SD	15.4	45.1	4.3	27.0
3 SD	16.3	44.0	5.0	32.1
4 SD	24.3†	57.7†	10.2	50.2†

† $P < 0.001$.

proportion with good or excellent outcomes decreases with age and is lower in women.

Cost

The total cost of fractures may be as much as $20 billion per year in the United States (Praemer *et al.*, 1992) and osteoporosis accounts for at least a third of this (Holbrook *et al.*, 1984). Because most of these fractures are in elderly individuals, wages foregone and years of life lost are not the important determinants of cost (Eiskjaer *et al.*, 1992). Costs relate instead to inpatient and outpatient medical services and nursing home care. These included an estimated 322 000 hospitalizations and almost 4 million hospital days for women 45 years old and over in the United States in 1986, where osteoporosis-related conditions were the primary cause of admission; more than half of the total was for hip fractures (Phillips *et al.*, 1988). Osteoporosis was a contributing cause for another 170 000 hospitalizations and 290 000 more hospital days. Additionally, there were 2.3 million physician visits for osteoporosis in 1986; at each visit, a third of the women needed an X-ray, a quarter required physiotherapy and most received a prescribed medication. There were also an estimated 83 000 nursing home stays for osteoporosis-related causes in the United States in 1986, with an average duration of stay of one year. Altogether, these direct costs of osteoporosis totaled $5.2 billion for postmenopausal women alone (Phillips *et al.*, 1988). Hip fracture patients occupied one-fifth of all orthopedic beds in England and Wales in 1988, at a direct cost of £160 million (Hoffenberg *et al.*, 1989). In France, an estimated 40 000–65 000 vertebral fractures, 56 000 hip fractures and 35 000 distal forearm fractures together cost FF3.7 billion each year (Levy, 1989). Such figures are a source of great concern to government officials in almost every country.

Unless some dramatic change occurs, these costs can only rise in the future. Because hip fracture incidence rates rise exponentially with aging, continuation of the demographic trends described earlier could increase the number of hip fractures from an estimated 1.7 million in 1990 to a projected 6.3 million in 2050 (Cooper *et al.*, 1992b). In the United States, the number of hip fractures and their associated costs could triple by 2040 (Schneider and Guralnik, 1990) and other estimates are comparable. Hip fractures might increase in the United Kingdom from 46 000 in 1985 to 60 000 in 2016 (Hoffenberg *et al.*, 1989) and in Australia from 10 150 in 1986 to 18 550 in 2011 (Lord and Sinnett, 1986). Health authorities in Finland expect a 38% increase in the number of hip fractures between 1983 and 2010 and a 71% increase in resulting hospital bed-days (Simonen, 1988). Any rise in fracture incidence, over and above that due to population aging, will increase the number of future fractures still further. Indeed, dramatic increases in incidence have been seen in all areas of the world (Figure 4.7), although age-adjusted rates appear to have leveled off in the United States (Melton *et al.*, 1987), Sweden (Naessén *et al.*, 1989) and Great Britain (Spector *et al.*, 1990). Additionally, there is evidence that the incidence of distal forearm fractures, ankle fractures, proximal humerus fractures, proximal tibia fractures and possibly vertebral fractures is increasing (Obrant *et al.*, 1989). No convincing explanation for these secular trends has been forthcoming.

WHAT ARE THE IMPLICATIONS FOR PATIENT MANAGEMENT?

As noted previously, the therapies for osteoporosis that are now available cannot restore skeletal strength to normal. Even if they could, fractures would continue to occur as a result of traumatic events, especially falls. These falls are extremely common and their pathophysiology is poorly understood. In a specific patient, falls usually result from a complex interaction of factors that are

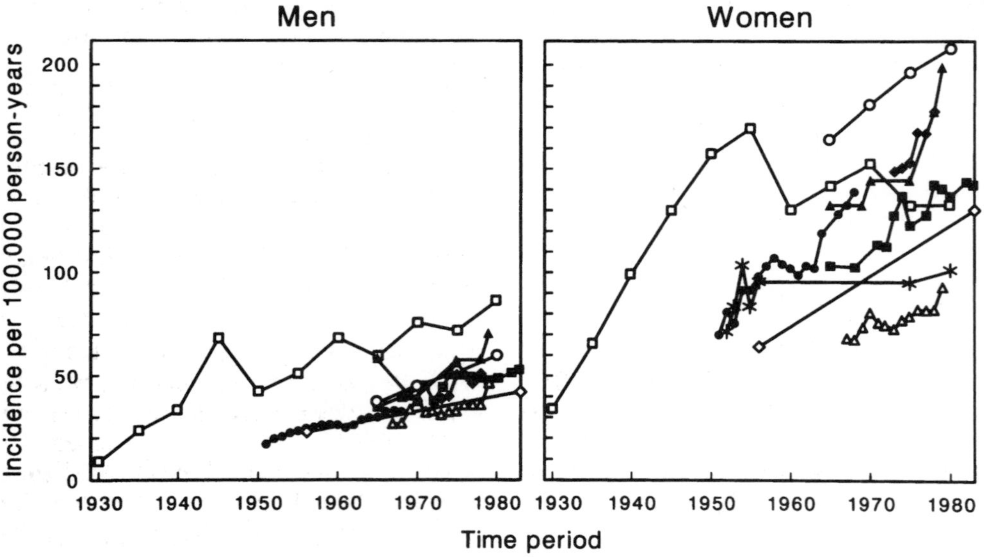

Figure 4.7 Incidence of hip fractures over time as reported from various studies: ❑ – ❑ Rochester, Minnesota; ■ – ■ United States; ◊ – ◊ Oxford, England; ◆ – ◆ Funen County, Denmark; Δ – Δ Holland; ▲ – ▲ Göteborg, Sweden; ❍ – ❍ Uppsala, Sweden; , ● – ●, New Zealand; * – * Dundee, Scotland. From Melton *et al.* (1987).

unlikely to be affected by treatment of bone mass. While only a small percentage of falls lead to fracture, prevention of the clinical manifestations of osteoporosis will depend in large part on ultimately reducing the frequency and severity of falls. However, the only action that can be taken now to prevent fractures in the future is to preserve bone mass. This is crucial because demographic changes alone can be expected to cause the number of fractures to increase dramatically. Any hope for limiting the rising disability and social costs depends on preventing these fractures.

CONCLUSION

A variety of pathophysiologic mechanisms contribute to the decline in bone mineral density (a pathogenic trait), which causes a disproportionate decrease in bone strength (asymptomatic disease) and leads to an increase in fractures (symptomatic disease), which are the sole clinical manifestation of osteoporosis. While osteoporosis is widely viewed as a major public health concern, the exact magnitude of the problem depends on how the condition is defined. Whether assessed on the basis of low bone mass or the occurrence of specific fractures, however, osteoporosis is a very common condition. Because there are no symptoms of osteoporosis until fractures occur, relatively few people are diagnosed in time for effective therapy to be administered. Consequently, a large number of individuals experience the pain, expense, disability and decreased quality of life caused by these age-related fractures. This important public health problem will worsen in the future as the population ages and, if the enormous costs associated with these fractures are to be reduced, increased attention must be given to the design and implementation of effective control programs. Because so many people are and will be affected, public health approaches will be crucial. However, research is also needed to improve interventions for high-risk individuals. The following chapters describe clinical strategies for identifying and treating those believed to be at greatest risk. Such efforts may be expensive, but the potential benefits are great as well.

ACKNOWLEDGEMENTS

The authors would like to thank Mrs Mary Roberts for help in preparing the manuscript.

This study was supported by grants AR 27065 and AG 04875 from the National Institutes of Health, US Public Health Service.

REFERENCES

Albright, F., Smith, P.N. and Richardson, A.M. (1941) Postmenopausal osteoporosis. *J Am Med Assoc* **116**(22): 2465–74.

Anon. (1990) Osteoporosis. In: *The Second Fifty Years: Promoting Health and Preventing Disability*, (eds Berg, R.L. and Cassells, J.S.), National Academy Press, Washington, DC, pp. 76–100.

Bauer, D.C., Browner, W.S., Cauley, J.A. *et al.* for the Study of Osteoporotic Fractures Research Group (1993) Factors associated with appendicular bone mass in older women. *Ann Intern Med* **118**(9): 741–2.

Bonar, S.K., Tinetti, M.E., Speechley, M. *et al.* (1990) Factors associated with short- versus long-term skilled nursing facility placement among community-living hip fracture patients. *J Am Geriatr Soc* **38**(10): 1139–44.

Borgquist, L., Lindelöw, G. and Thorngren, K.-G. (1991) Costs of hip fracture. Rehabilitation of 180 patients in primary health care. *Acta Orthop Scand* **62**(1): 39–48.

Browner, W.S., Seeley, D.G., Vogt, T.M. *et al.* for the Study of Osteoporotic Fractures Research Group (1991) Non-trauma mortality in elderly women with low bone mineral density. *Lancet* **338**(8763): 355–8.

Cauley, J.A., Gutai, J.P., Kuller, L.H., Scott, J. and Nevitt, M.C. (1994) Black-white differences in serum sex hormones and bone mineral density. *Am J Epidemiol* **139**(10), 1035–46.

Chrischilles, E.A., Butler, C.D., Davis, C.S. and Wallace, R.B. (1991) A model of lifetime osteoporosis impact. *Arch Intern Med* **151**(10): 2026–32.

Cooper, A. (1842) *A Treatise on Dislocations and Fractures of the Joints*, (ed. Cooper, B.B.), John Churchill, London.

Cooper, C. and Eastell, R. (1993) Bone gain and loss in premenopausal women. *Br Med J* **306**(6889): 1357–8.

Cooper, C and Melton III, L.J. (1992) Vertebral fractures: how large is the silent epidemic? *Br Med J* **304**(6830): 793–4.

Cooper, C., Shah, S., Hand, D.J. *et al.* (The Multicentre Vertebral Fracture Study Group) (1991) Screening for vertebral osteoporosis using individual risk factors. *Osteoporosis Int* **2**(1): 48–53.

Cooper, C., Atkinson, E.J., O'Fallon, W.M. *et al.* (1992a) Incidence of clinically diagnosed vertebral fractures: a population-based study in Rochester, Minnesota, 1985–1989. *J Bone Miner Res* **7**(2): 221–7.

Cooper, C., Campion, G. and Melton III, L.J. (1992b) Hip fractures in the elderly: a world-wide projection. *Osteoporosis Int* **2**(6): 285–9.

Cooper, C., Atkinson, E.J., Jacobsen, S.J. *et al.* (1993) Population-based study of survival following osteoporotic fractures. *Am J Epidemiol* **137**(9), 1001–5.

Courtney, A.C., Wachtel, E.F, Myers, E.R. and Hayes, W.C. (1995) Age-related reductions in the strength of the femur tested in a fall-loading configuration. *J Bone Joint Surg* **77**A: 387–95.

Cummings, S.R., Black, D.M. and Rubin, S.M. (1989) Lifetime risks of hip, Colles', or vertebral fracture and coronary heart disease among white postmenopausal women. *Arch Intern Med* **149**(11): 2445–8.

Cummings, S.R., Black, D.M., Nevitt, M.C. *et al.* (1993) Bone density at various sites for prediction of hip fractures. *Lancet* **341**(8837): 72–5.

Cummings, S.R., Nevitt, M.C., Browner, W.S. *et al.* for the Study of Osteoporotic Fractures Research Group (1995) Risk factors for hip fracture in white women. *N Engl J Med* **332**(12): 767–73.

De Bruijn, H.P. (1987) The Colles fracture, review of literature. *Acta Orthop Scand* **58** (Suppl 223): 7–25.

Donaldson, L.J., Cook, A. and Thomson, R.G. (1990) Incidence of fractures in a geographically defined population. *J Epidemiol Community Health* **44**(3): 241–5.

Eiskjaer, S., Østgård, S.E., Jakobsen, B.W. *et al.* (1992) Years of potential life lost after hip fracture among postmenopausal women. *Acta Orthop Scand* **63**(3): 293–6.

Eisman, J.A., Kelly, P.J., Morrison, N.A. *et al.* (1993) Peak bone mass and osteoporosis prevention. *Osteoporosis Int* **3** (Suppl 1): S56–60.

Ettinger, B., Black, D.M., Nevitt, M.C. *et al.* (1992) Contribution of vertebral deformities to chronic back pain and disability. *J Bone Miner Res* **7**(4): 449–56.

Gallagher, J.C., Goldar, D. and Moy, A. (1987) Total bone calcium in normal women: effect of age and menopause status. *J Bone Miner Res* **2**(6): 491–6.

Garraway, W.M., Stauffer, R.N., Kurland, L.T. *et al.* (1979) Limb fractures in a defined population. I. Frequency and distribution. *Mayo Clin Proc* **54**(11): 701–7.

Gibson, M.J. (1987) The prevention of falls in later life. *Danish Med Bull* **34** (Suppl 4): 1–24.

Greenspan, S.L., Myers, E.R., Maitland, L.A., Resnick, N.M. and Hayes, W.C. (1994) Fall severity and bone mineral density as risk factors for hip fracture in ambulatory elderly. *J Am Med Assoc* **271**(2): 128–33.

Griffin, M.R., Ray, W.A., Fought, R.L. *et al.* (1992) Black-white differences in fracture rates. *Am J Epidemiol* **136**(11): 1378–85.

Hagino, H., Yamamoto, K., Teshima, R. *et al.* (1989) The incidence of fractures of the proximal femur and the distal radius in Tottori prefecture, Japan. *Arch Orthop Trauma Surg* **109**(1): 43–4.

Hoffenberg, R., James, O.F.W., Brocklehurst, J.C. *et al.* (1989) Fractured neck of femur: prevention and management. Summary and recommendations of a report of the Royal College of Physicians. *J R Coll Physicians London* **23**(1): 8–12.

Holbrook, T.L., Grazier, K., Kelsey, J.L. *et al.* (1984) *The Frequency of Occurrence, Impact and Cost of Selected Musculoskeletal Conditions in the United States*, American Academy of Orthopedic Surgeons, Chicago.

Hui, S.L., Slemenda, C.W. and Johnston Jr, C.C. (1988) Age and bone mass as predictors of fracture in a prospective study. *J Clin Invest* **81**(6): 1804–9.

Hui, S.L., Slemenda, C.W. and Johnston Jr, C.C. (1990) The contribution of bone loss to postmenopausal osteoporosis. *Osteoporosis Int* **1**(1), 30–4.

Jacobsen, S.J., Goldberg, J., Miles, T.P. *et al.* (1990a) Hip fracture incidence among the old and very old: a population-based study of 745,435 cases. *Am J Public Health* **80**(7): 871–3.

Jacobsen, S.J., Goldberg, J., Miles, T.P. *et al.* (1990b) Regional variation in the incidence of hip fracture: US white women aged 65 years and older. *J Am Med Assoc* **264**(4): 500–2.

Jacobsen, S.J., Cooper, C., Gottlieb, M.S. *et al.* (1992) Hospitalization with vertebral fracture among the aged: a national population-based study, 1986–1989. *Epidemiology* **3**(6): 515–18.

Johnell, O., Gullberg, B., Allander, E. *et al.* and the MEDOS Study Group (1992) The apparent incidence of hip fracture in Europe: a study of national register sources. *Osteoporosis Int* **2**(6): 298–302.

Johnston Jr, C.C. and Melton III, L.J. (1995) Bone densitometry. In: *Osteoporosis: Etiology, Diagnosis and Management*, 2nd edn, (eds Riggs, B.L., Melton III, L.J.), Lippincott-Raven Press, Philadelphia, pp. 275–97.

Johnston Jr, C.C., Melton III, L.J., Lindsay, R. *et al.* (1989) Clinical indications for bone mass measurements: a report from the Scientific Advisory Board of the National Osteoporosis Foundation. *J Bone Miner Res* **4** (Suppl 2): 1–28.

Johnston, C.C., Miller, J.Z., Slemenda, C.W. *et al.* (1992) Calcium supplementation and increases in bone mineral density in children. *N Engl J Med* **327**(2): 82–7.

Kanis, J.A. and McCloskey, E.V. (1992) Epidemiology of vertebral osteoporosis. *Bone* **13** (Suppl 1): S1–10.

Kanis, J.A. and Pitt, F.A. (1992) Epidemiology of osteoporosis. *Bone* **13** (Suppl 1): S7–15.

Kanis, J.A., Melton III, L.J., Christiansen, C., Johnston Jr, C.C. and Khaltaev, N. (1994) Perspective: the diagnosis of osteoporosis. *J Bone Miner Res* **9**(8): 1137–41.

Kaukonen, J.-P., Karaharju, E.O., Porras, M. *et al.* (1988) Functional recovery after fractures of the distal forearm: analysis of radiographic and other factors affecting the outcome. *Ann Chir Gynaecol* **77**(1): 27–31.

Khosla, S. and Melton III, L.J. (1995) Secondary osteoporosis. In: *Osteoporosis: Etiology, Diagnosis and Management*, 2nd edn, (eds Riggs, B.L. and Melton III, L.J.), Lippincott-Raven Press, Philadelphia, pp. 183–204.

Koval, K.J., Skovron, M.L., Aharonoff, G.B., Meadows, S.E. and Zuckerman, J.D. (1995) Ambulatory ability after hip fracture: a prospective study in geriatric patients. *Clin Orthop Rel Res* **310**: 150–9.

Lau, E.M.C., Cooper, C., Wickham, C. *et al.* (1990) Hip fracture in Hong Kong and Britain. *Int J Epidemiol* **19**(4): 1119–21.

Lauritzen, J.B., Petersen, M.M. and Lund, B. (1992) Hip fractures prevented by external hip protectors. A randomized nursing home study. *Acta Orthop Scand* **63** (Suppl 248): (abstract) 84.

Levy, E. (1989) Cost analysis of osteoporosis related to untreated menopause. *Clin Rheumatol* **8** (Suppl 2): 76–82.

Looker, A.C., Johnston Jr, C.C., Wahner H.W. *et al.* (1995) Prevalence of low femoral bone density in older U.S. women from NHANES III. *J Bone Miner Res* **10**(5): 797–802.

Lord, S.R. and Sinnett, P.F. (1986) Femoral neck fractures: admissions, bed use, outcome and projections. *Med J Aust* **145**(10): 493–6.

Madhok, R., Melton III, L.J., Atkinson, E.J. *et al.* (1993) Urban vs rural increase in hip fracture incidence: age and sex of 901 cases 1980–89 in Olmsted County, U.S.A. *Acta Orthop Scand* **64**(5): 543–8.

Mazess, R.B. (1987) Bone density in diagnosis of osteoporosis: thresholds and breakpoints. *Calcif Tissue Int* **41**(3): 117–18.

Melton III, L.J. (1990) A 'Gompertzian' view of osteoporosis. *Calcif Tissue Int* **46**(5): 285–6.

Melton III, L.J. (1991) Differing patterns of osteoporosis across the world. *Proceedings of the Second Asian Symposium on Osteoporosis, New Dimensions in Osteoporosis in the 1990s*, (ed. Chesnut, C.H.), Excerpta Medica Asian, Hong Kong, pp. 13–18.

Melton III, L.J. (1995a) Epidemiology of fractures. In: *Osteoporosis: Etiology, Diagnosis and Management*, 2nd edn, (eds B.L. Riggs and L.J. Melton III), Lippincott-Raven Press, Philadelphia, pp. 225–47.

Melton III, L.J. (1995b) Perspectives: How many women have osteoporosis now? *J Bone Miner Res* **10**(2): 175–7.

Melton III, L.J. and Riggs, B.L. (1985) Risk factors for injury after a fall. *Clin Geriatr Med* **1**(3), 525–39.

Melton III, L.J. and Wahner, H.W. (1989) Defining osteoporosis. *Calcif Tissue Int* **45**(5): 263–4.

Melton III, L.J., O'Fallon, W.M. and Riggs, B.L. (1987) Secular trends in the incidence of hip fractures. *Calcif Tissue Int* **41**(2): 57–64.

Melton III, L.J., Chao, E.Y.S. and Lane, J. (1988) Biomechanical aspects of fractures. In: *Osteoporosis: Etiology, Diagnosis, and Management*, (eds Riggs, B.L. and Melton III, L.J.), Raven Press, New York, pp. 111–31.

Melton III, L.J., Chrischille, E.A., Cooper, C. *et al.* (1992) How many women have osteoporosis? *J Bone Miner Res* **7**(9): 1005–10.

Melton III, L.J., Bryant, S.C., Wahner, H.W. *et al.* (1993a) Influence of breastfeeding and other reproductive factors on bone mass later in life. *Osteoporosis Int* **3**(2): 76–83.

Melton III, L.J., Atkinson, E.J., O'Fallon, W.M. *et al.* (1993b) Long-term fracture prediction by bone mineral assessed at different skeletal sites. *J Bone Miner Res* **8**(10): 1227–33.

Naessén, T., Parker, R., Persson, I. *et al.* (1989) Time trends in incidence rates of first hip fracture in the Uppsala Health Care Region, Sweden, 1965–1983. *Am J Epidemiol* **130**(2): 289–99.

Nevitt, M.C., Cummings, S.R., Kidd, S. *et al.* (1989) Risk factors for recurrent nonsyncopal falls. A prospective study. *J Am Med Assoc* **261**(18): 2663–8.

Nordin, B.E.C. (1987) The definition and diagnosis of osteoporosis. *Calcif Tissue Int* **40**(2): 57–8.

Obrant, K.J., Bengnér, U., Johnell, O. *et al.* (1989) Increasing age-adjusted risk of fragility fractures: a sign of increasing osteoporosis in successive generations? *Calcif Tissue Int* **44**(3): 157–67.

Owen, R.A., Melton III, L.J., Johnson, K.A. *et al.* (1982) Incidence of Colles' fracture in a North American community. *Am J Public Health* **72**(6): 605–7.

Peck, W.A., Riggs, B.L., Bell, N.H. *et al.* (1988) Research directions in osteoporosis. *Am J Med* **84**(2): 275–82.

Phillips, S., Fox, N., Jacobs, J. *et al.* (1988) The direct medical costs of osteoporosis for American women aged 45 and older, 1986. *Bone* **9**(5): 271–9.

Pocock, N., Eisman, J., Gwinn, T. *et al.* (1989) Muscle strength, physical fitness, and weight but not age predict femoral neck bone mass. *J Bone Miner Res* **4**(3): 441–8.

Poór, G., Atkinson, E.J., O'Fallon, W.M. and Melton III, L.J. (1995) Determinants of reduced survival following hip fracture in men. *Clin Orthop Rel Res* **319**: 260–5.

Praemer, A., Furner, S. and Rice, D.P. (1992) *Musculoskeletal Conditions in the United States*, American Academy of Orthopaedic Surgeons, Park Ridge, Illinois.

Report of the US Preventive Services Task Force (1989) Counseling to prevent household and environmental injuries. *Guide to Clinical Preventive Services*, Williams and Wilkins, Baltimore, pp. 321–9.

Riggs, B.L. and Melton III, L.J. (1986) Medical progress: involutional osteoporosis. *N Engl J Med* **314**(26): 1676–86.

Riggs, B.L. and Melton III, L.J. (1992) The prevention and treatment of osteoporosis. *N Engl J Med* **327**(9): 620–7.

Ringe, J.D. (1987) Clinical evaluation of salmon calcitonin in bone pain. In: *Osteoporosis 1987, Volume 2. Proceedings of the International Symposium on Osteoporosis*, (eds Christiansen, C., Johansen, J.S. and Riis, B.J.), Osteopress ApS, Copenhagen, pp. 1262–4.

Ross, P.D., Davis, J.W., Vogel, J.M. *et al.* (1990) A critical review of bone mass and the risk of fractures in osteoporosis. *Calcif Tissue Int* **46**(3), 149–61.

Ross, P.D., Ettinger, B., Davis, J.W. *et al.* (1991a) Evaluation of adverse health outcomes associated with vertebral fractures. *Osteoporosis Int* **1**(3): 134–40.

Ross, P.D., Norimatsu, H., Davis, J.W. *et al.* (1991b) A comparison of hip fracture incidence among native Japanese, Japanese Americans, and American Caucasians. *Am J Epidemiol* **133**(8): 801–9.

Ross, P.D., Fujiwara, S. Huang, C. *et al.* (1995) Vertebral fracture prevalence in women in Hiroshima compared to Caucasians or Japanese in the US. *Int J Epidemiol* **24**: 1171–7.

Schapira, D. and Schapira, C. (1992) Osteoporosis: the evolution of a scientific term. *Osteoporosis Int* **2**(4): 164–7.

Schneider, E.L. and Guralnik, J.M. (1990) The aging of America: impact on health care costs. *J Am Med Assoc* **263**(17): 2335–40.

Seeley, D.G., Browner, W.S., Nevitt, M.C. *et al.* for the Study of Osteoporotic Fractures Research Group (1991) Which fractures are associated with low appendicular bone mass in elderly women? *Ann Intern Med* **115**(11): 837–42.

Seidman, H., Silverberg, E. and Bodden, A. (1978) Probabilities of eventually developing and of dying of cancer (risk among persons previously undiagnosed with the cancer). CA: *Cancer J for Clinicians* **28**(1): 33–46.

Simonen, O. (1988) Epidemiology and socioeconomic aspects of osteoporosis in Finland. *Ann Chir Gynaecol* **77**(5–6): 173–5.

Sinaki, M. (1995) Musculoskeletal rehabilitation. In: *Osteoporosis: Etiology, Diagnosis and Management*, 2nd edn, (eds Riggs, B.L. and Melton III, L.J.), Lippincott-Raven Press, Philadelphia, pp. 435–73.

Slemenda, C.W., Hui, S.L., Longcope, C. *et al.* (1990) Predictors of bone mass in perimenopausal women: a prospective study of clinical data using photon absorptiometry. *Ann Intern Med* **112**(2): 96–101.

Slemenda, C.W., Miller, J.Z., Hui, S.L. *et al.* (1991) Role of physical activity in the development of skeletal mass in children. *J Bone Miner Res* **6**(11): 1227–33.

Solomon, L. (1979) Bone density in ageing Caucasian and African populations. *Lancet* **2**(8156–8157): 1326–30.

Spector, T.D., Cooper, C. and Lewis, A.F. (1990) Trends in admissions for hip fractures in England and Wales, 1969–85. *Br Med J* **300**(6733): 1173–4.

Spector, T.D., McCloskey, E.V., Doyle, D.V. *et al.* (1993) Prevalence of vertebral fracture in women and the relationship with bone density and symptoms: the Chingford Study. *J Bone Miner Res* **8**(7): 817–22.

Tinetti, M.E., Speechley, M. and Ginter, S.F. (1988) Risk factors for falls among elderly persons living in the community. *N Engl J Med* **319**(26): 1701–7.

Van Hemert, A.M., Vandenbroucke, J.P. and Birkenhäger, J.C. (1990) Prediction of osteoporotic fractures in the general population by a fracture risk score: a 9-year follow-up among middle-aged women. *Am J Epidemiol* **132**(1): 123–35.

Wasnich, R.D., Ross, P.D., MacLean, C.J. *et al.* (1987) The relative strengths of osteoporotic risk factors in a prospective study of postmenopausal osteoporosis. In: *Osteoporosis 1987, Volume 1. Proceedings of the International Symposium on Osteoporosis*, (eds Christiansen, C., Johansen, J.S., Riis, B.J.), Osteopress ApS, Copenhagen, pp. 394–5.

Winner, S.J., Morgan, C.A. and Evans, J.G. (1989) Perimenopausal risk of falling and incidence of distal forearm fracture. *Br Med J* **298**(6686): 1486–8.

BONE HISTOMORPHOMETRY 5

J. Compston

INTRODUCTION

Histopathological examination of tissue is fundamental to the understanding of disease states. An increasingly ingenious array of imaging, densitometric and biochemical tests facilitate diagnosis and management for the clinician but the secrets of disease aetiology and pathophysiology can only be unravelled by detailed analysis of the affected tissue. The development of techniques for preparation of undecalcified sections and the discovery that tetracycline could be used as a marker of current bone formation provided a base from which fundamental concepts about bone physiology were developed and subsequently applied to disease states. Whilst qualititative assessment of bone tissues enabled some important observations to be made, detection of more subtle alterations required a quantitative approach; techniques for bone histomorphometry were developed, initially using grids, graticules and direct measurement and later utilizing interactive computerized methods.

Over recent years there have been considerable advances in bone histomorphometry, yet its potential as a research tool in the study of osteoporosis is underrealized. Perceived problems associated with obtaining biopsy material *in vivo* and the labour intensiveness of section preparation and analysis have been major contributory factors; obscure and sometimes unintelligible terminology has not enhanced its general appeal. There is, however, a growing realization that the cellular pathophysiology of different forms of osteoporosis and the mechanism by which drugs act on bone can only be established by histomorphometric assessment of bone remodelling and structure.

BONE BIOPSY

The iliac crest is the site from which bone biopsies are obtained *in vivo* in patients with metabolic bone disease. A transverse approach is now generally preferred although a few still use vertical sampling. The advantage of the transverse approach is that two cortices are obtained with intervening trabecular bone, whereas a vertical biopsy has only one cortical plate with variable amounts of trabecular bone. Several biopsy trephines are commercially available, most of which have an internal diameter of 5–8 mm.

The biopsy can be carried out as an outpatient procedure and takes approximately 30 minutes. Transiliac biopsies are taken one inch below and behind the anterior superior spine. The patient lies in the supine position and a mild sedative, such as midazolam 5–7.5 mg, is injected intravenously; the dose required to produce adequate sedation varies between individuals and care must be taken to avoid respiratory depression, especially in the elderly.

Osteoporosis. Edited by John C. Stevenson and Robert Lindsay. Published in 1998 by Chapman & Hall, London.
ISBN 0 412 48870 1

The area around the anterior superior iliac spine is cleaned and draped under sterile conditions. 1% lignocaine (10 ml) is then infiltrated under the skin and into the subcutaneous tissue down to the outer cortex of the iliac crest. The author then uses a thin trocar and stilette to administer local anaesthetic to the periosteum covering both cortices. This is achieved by driving the trocar and stilette a short distance with the weighted head of the introducer (Figure 5.1) until it lies just underneath the outer cortex; 5 ml of 1% lignocaine is then infiltrated (slowly, since stretching the periosteum may cause discomfort) and the trocar and stilette are then advanced further, through trabecular bone until the inner cortex is reached, when another 5 ml of 1% lignocaine is injected. No more than 20 ml of 1% lignocaine in total should be given during a single biopsy procedure. In most cases cortical and trabecular bone can be clearly differentiated by the ease with which the trocar and stilette can be advanced; when the cortices are thin or there is loss of corticomedullary differentiation the point at which local anaesthetic should be infiltrated is judged empirically on the average thickness of the iliac crest at the biopsy site (approximately 1 cm). Adequate local anaesthesia of both the outer and inner periosteum is essential to minimize discomfort associated with the biopsy procedure.

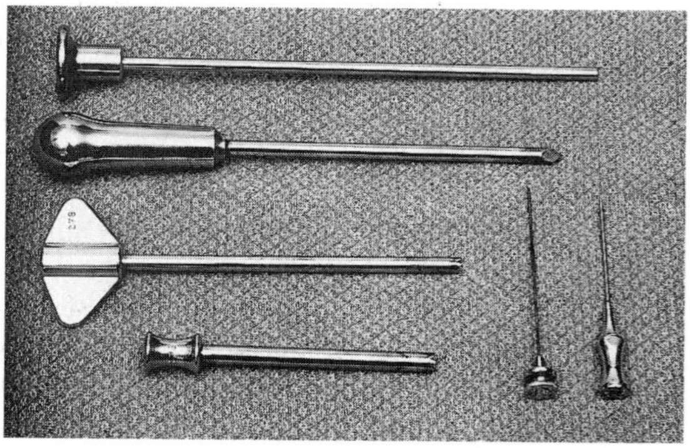

Figure 5.1 Bone biopsy trephine. From top to bottom: 1) outer cannula; 2) inner cannula; 3) rod for removal of biopsy from inner cannula; 4) introducer. On right: 5) trocar and stillette for administration of local anaesthetic.

The trocar and stilette are then withdrawn and a skin incision, approximately 1 cm long, is made. Using the introducer, the wider diameter, shorter cannula is inserted so that its serrated edge lies in contact with the outer periosteum; it should be perpendicular to the plane of the iliac crest and aimed along a line between the iliac crest and the umbilicus. The introducer is then withdrawn, keeping the cannula firmly in contact with the outer periosteum, and the longer, smaller diameter cannula is then inserted through the outer one. Using the latter as an anchor, the inner cannula is then steadily advanced through the iliac crest by rotating the instrument with alternating clockwise and anticlockwise movements. If the serrated edges of the inner cannula are sharp, this requires only relatively gentle pressure. When the inner cannula has been advanced through the entire thickness of iliac crest, the handle is then rotated through 360° to ensure that the biopsy is completely freed from the adjoining tissue and the two cannulas are withdrawn. The biopsy is removed from the end of the inner cannula using the metal rod (Figure 5.1). Finally, the skin incision is repaired with subcutaneous, absorbable sutures and a pressure dressing placed over the biopsy site. The patient is then instructed to lie on the side of the biopsy for at least one hour, in order to reduce the risk of haematoma formation. They should be advised to rest for the remainder of the day.

Bone biopsy is safe and generally well tolerated. No mortality from the procedure has been reported; the morbidity is low and due mainly to haematoma formation. Varying degrees of discomfort may be experienced after biopsy, generally lasting only 24–48 hours, although occasionally pain may be more severe and prolonged. Haematoma following biopsy is more common in obese subjects and in those with bleeding diatheses, for example patients on haemodialysis or with chronic liver disease; severe coagulopathies and current anticoagulant therapy are contraindications to bone biopsy. Rarely, infection may occur (less than 0.1% incidence in the author's experience); other reported rare complications include avulsion of the superior ramus of the iliac crest, fracture of the iliac crest, osteomyelitis and femoral nerve palsy, probably due to internal haematoma. The incidence of all complications from 9131 transiliac biopsies in a series compiled from the literature and from a multicentre survey was 0.7% (Rao, 1983).

BONE BIOPSY IN OSTEOPOROSIS

Bone biopsy is not a useful diagnostic test for osteoporosis because of the heterogeneity of bone loss associated with the disease and the non-relevance of the iliac crest as a site of clinical involvement. Thus, although correlations have been demonstrated between bone mass in iliac crest biopsies and other sites assessed by bone densitometry, these relationships are far from predictive and bone mass in iliac crest biopsies may be normal in patients with multiple osteoporotic vertebral fractures (Compston *et al.*, 1980a). However, bone biopsy provides a valuable research tool for the investigation of pathophysiological changes in untreated and treated osteoporosis and in certain cases should be performed to exclude other forms of bone disease, particularly osteomalacia, which may cause similar radiological and densitometric abnormalities to those encountered in osteoporosis. Bone biopsy should thus be considered as a part of the routine clinical investigation of osteoporosis in patients at increased risk of osteomalacia, for example those with malabsorption and elderly housebound or institutionalized subjects.

MEASUREMENT TECHNIQUES IN BONE HISTOMORPHOMETRY

The conventional histological sections on which bone histomorphometry is usually performed are viewed as a two-dimensional image in which profiles of three-dimensional structures are seen. Extrapolation of two-dimensional data to three-dimensional quantities necessitates the application of stereological formulae, which are based on the assumption that sampling is unbiased and random and, for most applications, that the structure is isotropic, i.e. evenly dispersed and randomly orientated in space (Parfitt, 1983). None of these conditions can be totally fulfilled in the case of bone and the expression of histomorphometric indices as three-dimensional quantities is thus subject to some error. Some histomorphometrists prefer to express their data as two-dimensional values whereas others apply stereological formulae to convert these to three-dimensional quantities. The format chosen will affect absolute values and hence accuracy, but should not influence comparisons between patient groups or the diagnostic value of histomorphometry, provided that the approach adopted is consistent.

The use of vertical sections to obtain unbiased stereological estimates from histological sections was first described by Baddeley *et al.* (1986) and subsequently applied to bone by Vesterby *et al.* (1987). The cycloid test system employed has the same axis as the sections and the test lines are defined in relation to the axis (sine weighted). The bone biopsy is randomly rotated around its long axis before embedding and all sections are cut parallel to this axis (the latter also being the case for conventionally prepared sections); the vertical axis of the sections must be kept parallel to the vertical axis of the test system. This procedure has clear theoretical advantages over the non-random sampling and biased measurement methods used by the majority of histomorphometrists, although the practical significance of these has not been established. Because of the need for random rotation before embedding, vertical sections as described above cannot be prepared from archival material.

GRIDS

These are composed of arrangements of lines and points which are either inserted into the eyepiece of the microscope or outlined on a flat surface on to which the microscope image can be projected. A number of different systems have been described. Some of these contain horizontal and/or vertical lines with points, for example the Zeiss Integrationsplatte 1 and 11; random test line orientation, which is theoretically superior, can be achieved using alternating hemispherical lines or, for vertical sections, a cycloid test grid. Alternatively, random orientation of the test lines may be achieved by random rotation of the graticule between each field of measurement (Kragstrup *et al.*, 1982a). Areas are measured by counting the grid points which fall on a profile and perimeters using intersection by test lines. Distances such as osteoid seam and wall width are measured using an eyepiece micrometer; in order to avoid systematic sampling errors in width measurements, Kragstrup *et al.* (1982b) have described a method in which a measuring grid is moved over the section in equidistant steps and orthogonal intercepts on the structures undergoing width measurements are sampled. This method provides a systematic sampling procedure which takes into account the surface extent of the structure.

COMPUTERIZED IMAGE ANALYSIS

The advent of interactive computerized systems for bone histomorphometry has superseded the use of grids and micrometers. These systems are much less labour intensive and tedious for the operator and possess the ability to perform complex measurements such as cancellous bone structural analysis, which cannot easily be achieved using non-computerized techniques. Several purpose-built systems are now commercially available; alternatively, in-house systems can be designed using relatively simple hardware, providing that programming expertise is available.

An example of such a system is illustrated in Figure 5.2. The system is developed around a PC386 computer (Elonex UK Ltd). Direct measurements are made using a digitizing tablet and cursor with an LED point light source and a binocular transmitted light microscope with a drawing attachment. Sections are viewed directly through the microscope, the cursor light being superimposed on the section. The field of measurement is defined by a square etched on the eyepiece graticule; the square is mapped to correspond with an active area on the tablet and an active drawing area on a video monitor. The system is calibrated for each magnification used. Perimeter measurements are made by tracing with the cursor LED and distance measurements are made either by dotting with the cursor on either side of the structure at appropriately spaced points or by tracing the outline of the structure (for example, a bone structural unit), distances between the outer and inner boundaries then being made automatically at four equidistant points. For cancellous bone structural analysis (Garrahan *et al.*, 1986), the system used incorporates a frame-store board to capture images

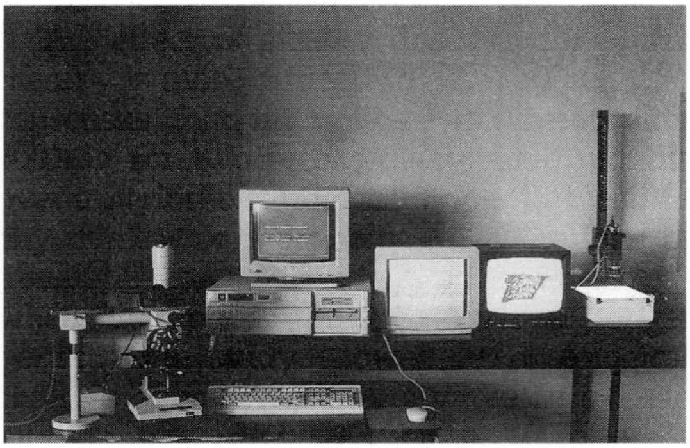

Figure 5.2 Image analysis system used for cancellous bone structural analysis. The image of the biopsy section is captured by a CCD television camera on to a video monitor.

from a CCD television camera on a video monitor.

HISTOMORPHOMETRIC INDICES – NOMENCLATURE AND UNITS

In 1987 the American Society of Bone and Mineral Research Histomorphometry Nomenclature Committee proposed a standardized system for the description of histomorphometric indices derived from two-dimensional histological sections (Parfitt *et al.*, 1987). The proposed nomenclature has become widely accepted and has provided a much needed clarification of the sometimes arbitrary and often unintelligible formats used previously. The revised system set out to simplify existing terminology and to separate clearly primary measurements from derived indices; all data are expressed in the format of source (the structure on which the measurement is made, for example bone tissue or surface), the measurement (primary or derived) and the referent (area or perimeter in two-dimensional and volume or surface in three-dimensional terminology) (Table 5.1). The recommended order and format to be used (including punctuation) is source – measurement/referent. In practice, because only one source is often used in any one study, it is unnecessary to specify this once it has been defined. The most commonly used source in bone histomorphometry is cancellous bone tissue (Cn); other possible sources include cortical bone tissue (Ct), endocortical surface (Ec), periosteal surface (Ps) and transitional zone (Tr.Z). It should be noted that although the term 'cancellous' is preferred to 'trabecular' when referring to the source, 'trabecular' rather than 'cancellous' is used in descriptions of some structural indices. Abbreviations or symbols are constructed from the first letters in the order of the words of the descriptive term, a single capital letter generally being used for the more commonly used terms and an additional lower case letter being used for less frequently used terms. The use of a single lower case letter denotes terms related to time; here the system is somewhat inconsistent, since words such as 'hit, single, double and active' are included in this category.

The primary measurements are referred to as area, perimeter and width when expressed in two dimensions and volume, surface and thickness in three dimensions. The fourth type of primary measurement, number, cannot be extrapolated to a three-dimensional value unless serial sections are examined. Absolute area and perimeter measured in two dimensions have no three-dimensional equivalent but if three-dimensional nomenclature is adopted these quantities are referred to as volume and surface although the absolute values are identical. Values for width can be converted to thickness by dividing width by

Table 5.1 Referents commonly used in bone histomorphometry. From Parfitt *et al.* (1987)

Referent (3D/2D)	*Abbreviation (3D/2D)*
Bone surface/perimeter	BS/B.Pm
Bone volume/area	BV/B.Ar
Tissue volume/area	TV/T.Ar
Core volume/area	CV/C.Ar
Osteoid surface/perimeter	OS/O.Pm
Eroded surface/perimeter	ES/E.Pm
Mineralized surface/perimeter	Md.S/Md.Pm
Osteoblast surface/perimeter	Ob.S/Ob.Pm
Osteoclast surface/perimeter	Oc.S/Oc.Pm

$4/\pi$ (1.273) for isotropic structures or 1.2 for human iliac cancellous bone (Schwartz and Recker, 1981; Parfitt, 1983); the one exception to this rule is cortical width and thickness, which are numerically equal. Measurements of width may be obtained directly or indirectly by calculation from area and perimeter; the former method has the advantage of providing a frequency distribution of widths within a biopsy. Commonly used primary histomorphometric indices are shown in Table 5.2.

Area, perimeter and number have meaning only if expressed in terms of a referent, whereas distance measurements do not require any referent. Areas and perimeters (two-dimensional) or volumes and surfaces (three-dimensional) are used as referents for most measurements. When measurements with a surface referent (three-dimensional nomenclature) are expressed as a percentage, the referent is termed bone surface (or a subdivision of it) and equivalent to two-dimensional perimeter values; however, in the new nomenclature, the term 'bone surface' is also used specifically to denote bone surface to tissue volume ratio or surface density, a three-dimensional quantity expressed in units of mm^2/mm^3. This and the other surface/volume and volume/volume ratios are derived from the corresponding two-dimensional perimeter/area ratios using a multiplication factor of $4/\pi$ or 1.2 (see above). The main surface and volume referents BS, BV and TV can be interconverted using the ratios BS/BV and BS/TV.

Bone histomorphometry is most commonly applied to cancellous bone. This has a considerably higher turnover than cortical bone and hence a potentially greater capacity to exhibit alterations in bone remodelling. Cancellous bone may be subdivided into corticoendosteal and midcancellous regions; changes at the corticoendosteal region are particularly important as they may affect both cortical and cancellous bone mass and structure (Brown *et al.*, 1987). Cortical bone is largely ignored by most histomorphometrists in spite of its predominance in the skeleton and its importance as a determinant of fracture risk. Frost (1969) pioneered the application of histomorphometric techniques to cortical bone and more recently detailed analysis of the bone remodelling cycle in iliac crest cortical bone

Table 5.2 Primary histomorphometric indices of bone remodelling

Name	*Abbreviation*	*Units*
Bone area	B.Ar/T.Ar	%
Osteoid area	O.Ar/T.Ar or O.Ar/B.Ar	%
Osteoid perimeter	O.Pm/B.Pm	%
Osteoblast perimeter	Ob.Pm/B.Pm	%
Osteoid width	O.Wi	μm
Interstitial width	It.Wi	μm
Trabecular width	Tb.Wi	μm
Eroded perimeter	E.Pm/B.Pm	%
Osteoclast perimeter	Oc.Pm/B.Pm	%
Mineralizing surface	Md.Pm/B.Pm	%
Mineral apposition rate	MAR	μm/d
Wall width	W.Wi	μm
Erosion depth	E.De	μm
Erosion length	E.Le	μm
Erosion area	E.Ar	μm^2
Cavity number	N.Cv./B.Pm or /TA	No./mm or /mm^2

has been reported (Agerbaek *et al.*, 1991). However, nearly all histomorphometric data derived from patients with osteoporosis relate to cancellous bone and the discussion of bone histomorphometry in this chapter will be largely confined to this. Two-dimensional nomenclature is used throughout.

UNITS AND DIMENSIONS

The units recommended for the new nomenclature are micrometre and millimetre for length and day and year for time. Surface/surface and volume/volume ratios are expressed as percentages rather than decimal fractions whilst surface to volume ratios are expressed in mm^2/mm^3. Formation rates with volume referents are expressed as %/year. Table 5.3 shows some commonly used derived histomorphometric indices, with their abbreviations and units.

ASSESSMENT OF BONE AREA

Assessment of bone area is a relatively simple procedure in bone histomorphometry although it is subject to a large sampling error and this, together with the heterogeneity of bone loss in osteoporosis, makes it unreliable as a diagnostic index. Accurate measurement of cancellous bone area in a biopsy requires good quality sections with minimal bone dust and trabecular shattering; agreement between observers depends critically upon the criteria used for corticomedullary demarcation. In practice, decisions about corticomedullary delineation are often subjective and arbitrary and rarely specified in publications. Because of the variable angle at which the biopsy is obtained relative to the perpendicular axis of the iliac crest and the varying structure of the corticoendosteal region, it is difficult to establish absolute criteria. One approach has been to use twice the thickness of the largest trabecula attached to either cortex as a starting point for measurement (Brown *et al.*, 1987); in the author's laboratory the first 1100 μm (one field at ×62.5 magnification) immediately inside each inner cortical boundary is omitted from the measurement (Wright *et al.*, 1992). Because bone area is used as a referent for other measurements, it is essential that for

Table 5.3 Derived histomorphometric indices of bone remodelling

Name	*Abbreviation*	*Units*
Adjusted apposition rate	Aj.AR	μm/d
Bone formation rate	BFR/B.Pm	$\mu m^2/\mu m/d$
	BFR/B.Ar	%/y
Erosion rate	ER	μm/d
Mineralization lag time	Mlt	d
Osteoid maturation period	Omt	d
Formation period	FP	d
Active formation period	FP(a+)	d
Erosion period	EP	d
Reversal period	Rv.P	d
Quiescent period	QP	d
Remodelling period	Rm.P	d
Total period	Tt.P	d
Activation frequency	Ac.f	/y
Trabecular separation*	Tb.Sp.	μm or mm
Trabecular number*	Tb.N.	/mm

* May also be measured directly. d = day; y = year

any one set of measurements the same criteria are applied for corticomedullary delineation.

Cortical width is also subject to considerable sampling error and is rarely assessed in iliac crest biopsies. Cortical bone area can also be measured and the number and area of individual Haversian systems characterized.

ASSESSMENT OF MINERALIZATION

On undecalcified bone sections mineralized bone can be easily differentiated from unmineralized bone or osteoid, using a number of stains including von Kossa (Plate 1), Goldner's and toluidine blue; the latter may also be used to demonstrate calcification fronts (Plate 2). The most important primary measurement in the assessment of mineralization is osteoid width, an increase in which indicates defective mineralization. Osteoid width in turn is determined by two variables, namely the mineral apposition rate and the mineralization lag time or, when averaged over the entire osteoid surface, osteoid apposition rate and osteoid maturation period. Since mineralization defects may sometimes be focal as, for example, in bisphosphonate-induced osteomalacia (Boyce *et al.*, 1984), osteoid width values averaged over the entire osteoid surface may be misleading.

OSTEOID WIDTH

Osteoid width should be measured directly since calculation from osteoid area and perimeter (expressed as percentages rather than absolute values) may give inaccurate results, especially when amounts of osteoid are small (Vedi and Compston, 1984). Width may be measured using a graticule or cursor; the latter method is quicker and gives comparable results.

MINERAL APPOSITIONAL RATE

This is calculated as the distance between two time-spaced tetracycline labels (Plate 3) divided by the time interval between administration of those labels. The point of measurement is usually taken as the midpoint of each label, measured at approximately equidistant points along the site of measurement and the interlabel period as the number of days between the midpoints of the two labelling periods (Frost, 1983a). When three-dimensional nomenclature is used, the value obtained should be multiplied by $\pi/4$ or 1.2 (Parfitt *et al.*, 1987). The regimen used for tetracycline labelling is described in the section on assessment of bone turnover, below.

Mineral apposition rate is used in the calculation of many derived indices of bone remodelling and hence accurate measurement is of key importance. The mean value obtained for a biopsy is used in these calculations; however, it should be noted that in focal osteomalacia, this may be misleading. In the absence of tetracycline uptake, mineral apposition rate and indices derived from it should be treated as missing data. Since mineral apposition rate has a finite lower limit of 0.3 μm/day, this value should be used for the calculation of derived indices in biopsies in which single labels only can be detected (Foldes *et al.*, 1990).

ADJUSTED APPOSITION RATE

This represents the mineral apposition rate or the bone formation rate averaged over the osteoid surface. In the absence of a mineralization defect, the formation of matrix and mineral, although not synchronous, can be assumed to occur at the same rate and under these circumstances the adjusted apposition rate is equivalent to the osteoid apposition rate. It is calculated as follows:

$$\text{Aj.AR or OAR} = \text{MAR} \times \text{Md.Pm/O.Pm}.$$

It is clear from the above formula that Aj.AR is usually less than and can never exceed MAR.

MINERALIZATION LAG TIME

This is the time interval between the deposition and mineralization of a given amount of osteoid, averaged over the lifespan of the osteoid seam. It is calculated as follows:

Mlt = O.Wi/Aj.AR.

OSTEOID MATURATION PERIOD

This represents the time interval between the onset of deposition and the onset of mineralization of a given amount of osteoid and results from processes such as collagen crosslinking which are required before mineralization can proceed (Parfitt, 1983). In humans it is generally shorter than the Mlt and never exceeds it. It is calculated as follows:

Omt = O.Wi/MAR.

ASSESSMENT OF BONE TURNOVER

IN VIVO TETRACYCLINE LABELLING

The administration of two time-spaced tetracycline labels prior to biopsy enables measurement of the surface extent of mineralization, from which a number of dynamic indices of bone formation and resorption can be calculated (Frost, 1983a) (Figure 5.6). The regimen and preparation used vary between centres, but the author uses demeclocycline hydrochloride (Ledermycin, Lederle) in the following regimen:

- day 1 and 2 – 150 mg twice daily
- 10 days – no demeclocycline
- day 13 and 14 – 150 mg twice daily.

The bone biopsy is performed 4–5 days after the last dose of demeclocycline.

Adverse reactions to demeclocycline are rare but include gastrointestinal symptoms, particularly diarrhoea, and, rarely, skin rashes which may be severe and exhibit photosensitivity. Patients should be questioned about prior sensitivity to tetracyclines before the labels are administered and should be warned to stop taking the tablets and to avoid sunlight if a rash appears after ingestion of the drug.

The two tetracyclines most commonly used as bone labels in humans are oxytetracycline and demeclocycline which fluoresce green and yellow respectively when viewed on unstained sections under ultraviolet light. There is evidence that these two compounds differ with respect to their uptake on mineralizing surfaces, demeclocycline producing a greater surface extent of fluorescence than oxytetracycline (Parfitt *et al.*, 1991). This may significantly affect values obtained for mineralizing perimeter and derived indices such as bone formation rate and adjusted appositional rate.

MINERALIZING PERIMETER

The mineralizing perimeter is assessed from the extent of the bone perimeter which exhibits tetracycline fluorescence after an appropriate time-spaced label. Because of the labelling escape error, which occurs because of initiation of mineralization before the first label or termination of mineralization between the two markers, a proportion of the perimeter exhibits a single label only and use of the double-labelled perimeter only would considerably underestimate the true mineralizing surface (Frost, 1983b). In addition, a small proportion of single label may be due to the 'on–off' phenomenon, a state in which osteoid seams become inactive or resting. In order to correct for these sources of inaccuracy, the double plus half the single-labelled perimeter is used to assess mineralizing perimeter. Since both mineral apposition rate and mineralized perimeter are significantly underestimated in sections of 20 μm thickness, the sections used for fluorescence microscopy should be as thin as possible; in practice, between 5 and 10 μm (Birkenhäger-Frenkel and Birkenhäger-Frenkel, 1987).

A zero value for mineralizing perimeter is

possible and, if obtained, should be used for derived indices if mineralizing perimeter is in the numerator. However, if zero values for mineralizing perimeter are used in the denominator, as for example in mineralization lag time and formation period, an infinite value would be obtained; the suggested solution is to use the reciprocals of these indices, thus restoring mineralizing perimeter to the numerator. These reciprocal indices are referred to as osteoid mineralization rate and osteoblast vigour respectively. Finally, where only single labels can be detected, the mineralizing perimeter may be expressed as half the single-labelled perimeter (Foldes *et al.*, 1990).

BONE FORMATION RATES

Bone formation rate may be defined in relation to a number of different referents but the two most commonly used are /bone perimeter and /bone area. When osteoid perimeter is used as a referent, bone formation rate is equivalent to the adjusted apposition rate. Bone formation rate/bone perimeter indicates the tissue-based formation rate and is calculated as follows:

$$\text{BFR/B.Pm} = \text{MAR} \times \text{Md.Pm/B.Pm}$$

Bone formation rate/bone area indicates bone turnover rate which is an important determinant of bone age. It is calculated as follows:

$$\text{BFR/B.Ar} = \text{MAR} \times \text{Md.Pm} \times (\text{B.Pm/B.Ar}) \times 100.$$

BONE RESORPTION RATES

At present resorption rates cannot be measured directly by histomorphometric techniques; calculation is based on the assumptions that bone resorption and formation are coupled both in time and space and that bone remodelling is in a steady state. Neither of these assumptions may be tenable in untreated or treated disease states and accurate estimation of resorption rates must await the development of techniques which reliably assess current resorption, analogous to the use of tetracycline markers for bone formation.

Using the above assumptions, erosion rate can be calculated as follows:

$$\text{ER} = \text{E.De/EP}$$

where the erosion period (EP) is calculated as shown below. It should be noted that, in contrast to bone formation rate, erosion rate is not related to a perimeter or area referent but is expressed in μm/day and defines the movement of the erosion front perpendicular to the surface, averaged throughout the erosion period.

REMODELLING PERIODS

The formation period is the time taken to form a new bone structural unit and is calculated as follows:

$$\text{FP} = \text{W.Wi/Aj.AR}.$$

Formation period can be subdivided into the active formation period (FP(a+)) and the inactive formation period (FP(a-)). These are calculated as follows:

$$\text{FP(a+)} = \text{W.Wi/MAR}$$
$$\text{FP(a-)} = \text{FP-FP(a+)}.$$

The inactive formation period is a measure of 'off-time', the phenomenon responsible for the discrepancy between osteoid and mineralizing perimeter after correction for label escape (Frost, 1983b).

On the basis of the principle that, in a steady state, fractions of space are equivalent to fractions of time the erosion, reversal and quiescent remodelling periods can be calculated as follows (Parfitt, 1983):

$$\text{EP} = \text{E.Pm/B.Pm} \times \text{FP}$$
$$\text{Rv.P} = \text{Rv.Pm/B.Pm} \times \text{FP}$$
$$\text{QP} = \text{Q.Pm/B.Pm} \times \text{FP}.$$

The average duration of a single remodelling cycle is referred to as the remodelling period and is calculated as follows:

$$\text{Rm.P} = \text{EP} + \text{Rv.P} + \text{FP}.$$

The average time between the initiation of two successive remodelling cycles at the same site on the trabecular surface is referred to as the total period and is calculated as follows:

Tt.P = Rm.P + QP.

ACTIVATION FREQUENCY

Increased bone turnover is quantitatively the most important mechanism of bone loss in osteoporosis (Frost, 1985) and assessment of activation frequency is therefore of key importance. However, the process of activation cannot be detected by histomorphometric techniques and assessment of activation frequency is at present limited to calculation of the frequency with which a given site on the bone surface undergoes new remodelling, represented by the reciprocal of the total remodelling period (Parfitt, 1983; Eriksen, 1986):

Ac.f = 1/Tt.P.

Using the original primary data, this formula can be reduced to a simpler equation, as follows (Parfitt *et al.*, 1987):

Ac.f = (BFR/B.Pm)/W.Wi.

It should be noted that these formulae define activation frequency as the reciprocal of the time taken from initiation of one remodelling cycle to initiation of a new remodelling cycle at the same site, thus implying its dependence on the lifespan of previously activated units. Conceptually, however, activation frequency describes the number of new remodelling units activated anywhere on the bone surface within a given time; in view of the relatively small proportion of the surface normally undergoing remodelling at any one time it seems unlikely that it would be related to the lifespan of previously activated bone remodelling units. Furthermore, calculation of activation frequency from indices of bone formation is unlikely to be accurate unless bone is in a steady state with regard to remodelling, an untenable assumption in osteoporosis, untreated or treated. Accurate estimation frequency requires the development of markers of activation or active resorption in undecalcified bone sections.

ASSESSMENT OF REMODELLING BALANCE

BONE FORMATION

Accurate assessment of remodelling balance requires measurement of both components, namely formation and resorption. The average amount of bone formed in individual remodelling units is referred to as the wall width (Frost, 1963; Lips *et al.*, 1978); the mean width of completed trabecular bone packets without resorption lacunae or osteoid is measured. The bone structural units may be identified under polarized light or by identification of cement lines using toluidine blue or gallocyanine staining (Plate 4). The latter method gives lower values than the former; in addition, the sampling technique used for measurement may affect the result obtained (Compston and Croucher, 1991).

One problem associated with the measurement of wall width in non-steady state conditions is the difficulty in differentiating those units which were present before the onset of disease or its treatment from those formed subsequently. Uncompleted bone structural units can be identified by their covering of osteoid and represent current remodelling activity. Reconstruction of these forming sites can be made using paired values for osteoid width and uncompleted wall width, growth curves for matrix and bone mineral being obtained. The mean growth curves for mineralized bone and for mineralized bone plus osteoid are then constructed and the completed wall width is obtained from the convergent endpoints of these curves (Steiniche *et al.*, 1992).

BONE RESORPTION

Assessment of the amount of bone resorbed in individual remodelling units presents a number of problems. The identification of resorption cavities can be difficult and has a considerable subjective element; moreover, some methods for measuring cavity depth involve reconstruction of the eroded surface. The use of polarized light microscopy to demonstrate cut-off lamellae at the edges of the cavity assists recognition (Vedi *et al.*, 1984) and may be used as a criterion for inclusion. The presence of osteoclast, mononuclear or preosteoblast-like cells within the cavity also helps to identify resorption cavities (Eriksen *et al.*, 1984), although such cells are morphologically heterogeneous and their presence and appearance depend to some extent on the level and plane of sectioning. At present these cells are generally identified on purely morphological grounds; tartrate-resistant acid phosphatase can be demonstrated in osteoclasts by histochemical techniques, but is not specific to these cells (Burstone, 1959; Evans *et al.*, 1979). Finally, it is not usually possible to identify those cavities which have resulted in trabecular penetration.

For the assessment of remodelling balance, measurement of completed or final resorption depth is required. The presence of a thin layer of osteoid at the base of a resorption cavity ensures that resorption has been completed within that unit (Cohen-Solal *et al.*, 1991) although other completed cavities in the reversal phase of remodelling will be omitted from analysis if this is the sole criterion used and the number available for measurement will be very small in most biopsies. The presence of preosteoblast-like cells in the cavity may indicate that resorption has been completed (Eriksen *et al.*, 1984) but these cells can be difficult to identify. Finally, some cavities may persist in a state of arrested resorption; this phenomenon produces small cavities in which subsequent formation does not occur (Parfitt, 1983).

Measurement or calculation of interstitial width has been used to assess resorption depth, based on the postulate that the distance between two bone structural units on opposite sides of a trabecula is inversely proportional to resorption depth (Courpron *et al.*, 1980). Thus interstitial width is calculated as follows:

$$\text{It.Wi} = \text{Tb.Wi} - (2 \times \text{W.Wi}).$$

However, the relationship between interstitial width and resorption depth is not a simple inverse one since, depending on the concomitant changes in wall width and trabecular width, decreasing interstitial width may be associated with decreased, constant or increased resorption depth and a constant interstitial width may occur with decreasing or constant resorption depth (Croucher *et al.*, 1989; Parfitt and Foldes, 1991).

Direct assessment of resorption depth in cancellous bone was first described by Eriksen *et al.* (1984), using a technique in which the number of lamellae eroded beneath the bone surface was counted in cavities containing osteoclasts, mononuclear cells and preosteoblast-like cells; it was proposed that these cells were specifically associated with increasing stages of completion of the resorptive phase. Accurate identification of these cell types within the cavities undergoing measurement is a central prerequisite of this method and even in the authors' hands 24% of resorption cavities were excluded from measurement because of failure to subdivide by cell type or inability to define and count the eroded lamellae. This technique, although ingenious, is technically difficult and laborious and has not been widely adopted. Moreover, the values reported using this method for final resorption depth in normal biopsies are considerably in excess of reported values for wall width (Compston and Croucher, 1991), indicating a remodelling imbalance greater than is consistent with documented changes in trabecular width (Parfitt, 1991). Factors contributing to this overestimation of resorption depth include the sampling technique used, which favours the selection of larger cavities, and the assumption that the eroded lamellae are parallel to the bone surface and hence have a constant width. A simplified version of the method, in which the eroded lamellae are counted without subdivision of cavities by cell type, has been practised (Palle *et al.*, 1989); this approach provides an estimate of the mean depth of cavities in all stages of completion and hence considerably underestimates final resorption depth.

The computerized technique developed by Garrahan *et al.* (1990) involves reconstruction of the eroded mineralized surface by a curve-fitting technique (cubic spline) and enables measurement of a number of resorption cavity characteristics including mean and maximum depth, area, surface extent and cavity number. The technique is simple to perform and can be adapted for use in most image analysis systems used for bone histomorphometry; since all identified cavities >3 μm depth are included in the analysis, the mean value obtained for depth (mean or maximum) considerably underestimates final resorption depth. Cohen-Solal *et al.* (1991) have described a modification of this technique in which the eroded bone surface is reconstructed interactively; only those cavities with a layer of osteoid are included for measurement, ensuring that resorption is complete, although some completed cavities are likely to be omitted. Application of this method to normal human biopsies resulted in mean values approximately 17% lower than those obtained in the same biopsies by the technique of counting eroded lamellae and were more consistent with reported age-related changes in trabecular width (Weinstein and Hutson, 1987; Mellish *et al.*, 1989).

Further work is thus needed to improve existing techniques for the assessment of resorption cavity depth and other characteristics. The technique described by Eriksen *et al.* (1984) almost certainly overestimates true erosion depth; values generated using the method reported by Cohen-Solal *et al.* (1991) are probably more accurate. Inclusion of all resorption cavities for measurement will inevitably underestimate final erosion depth but can yield valuable information about the frequency distribution of cavity size in bone (Compston and Croucher, 1991). Accurate identification of the different stages of resorption and associated cell types is required before significant methodological advances can occur.

ASSESSMENT OF BONE STRUCTURE

The importance of bone structure as a determinant of bone strength has received increasing recognition and a number of histomorphometric techniques have been developed to assess cancellous bone structure and, in particular, its connectivity. Cancellous bone loss may be associated with trabecular thinning and/or penetration through and erosion of trabecular plates; these two processes are likely to be interdependent and are determined by the underlying changes in bone remodelling associated with bone loss (Compston *et al.*, 1989a). Trabecular thinning is favoured by low turnover states and is associated with relative preservation of architecture, whilst trabecular erosion and penetration occur in high turnover states and situations in which a negative remodelling balance is due to increased resorption depth. Disruption of cancellous bone structure is an inevitable consequence of bone loss and contributes to the resulting decrease in bone strength; the most important consquences of structural changes, however, lie in their therapeutic implications and, in particular, whether cancellous structure can be restored.

With the exception of high resolution microcomputed tomography (see below), all histomorphometric techniques presently available are performed on two-dimensional histological sections; although three-dimensional images can now be produced using a variety of techniques, quantitative assessment of such images is problematic, not least because of superimposition of structures. The extrapolation of two-dimensional data to three-dimensional structure requires further study but there are several lines of evidence to support the contention that structural indices obtained from two-dimensional sections do reflect changes in three-dimensional structure.

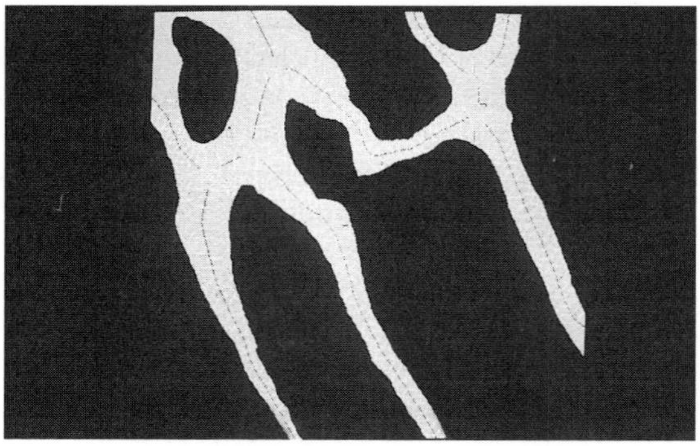

Figure 5.3 Measurement of trabecular width. The binary image is skeletonized and circles are generated around the symmetric axis; the circles are automatically adjusted until they are simultaneously tangential to the two opposing boundaries and the diameter of each circle represents the trabecular width at that point

TRABECULAR WIDTH, SEPARATION AND NUMBER

These indices of cancellous bone structure may either be measured directly or calculated. In spite of the sometimes questionable assumptions upon which some of these calculations are based, much valuable information has been obtained about cancellous bone structure using this approach, although it can only provide indirect evidence about connectivity.

Direct measurements of trabecular width can be made using an eyepiece graticule or grid; however, these are time consuming, provide values for width only at relatively widespread points along the trabeculae and usually omit measurements at nodes (Wakamatsu and Sissons, 1969; Whitehouse, 1974; Aaron *et al.*, 1987). More recently, computerized techniques have been described (Clermonts and Birkenhäger-Frenkel, 1985; Garrahan *et al.*, 1987); these enable rapid measurements of width to be made at intervals of the operator's choice and include width measurements at the nodes. One such technique involves skeletonization of the cancellous bone and subsequent generation of circles around the symmetric axis which are simultaneously tangential to the two opposing boundaries (Figure 5.3). Measurements are performed automatically on stored, edited binary images (Garrahan *et al.*, 1987).

Alternatively, trabecular width can be calculated from area and perimeter measurements (Parfitt *et al.*, 1983); the validity of this approach depends on the assumption that the width of the measured structures is small relative to length and this is generally, although not always, true of cancellous bone in the iliac crest. Assessment of trabecular width calculated in this way shows a good correlation with directly measured width; however, only direct techniques provide information about intraindividual variations in trabecular width.

Trabecular separation may also be measured directly using an eyepiece graticule or grid (Wakamatsu and Sissons, 1969; Aaron *et al.*, 1987); these measurements are made between the midpoints of the trabeculae and hence are unaffected by trabecular thinning. Trabecular spacing, also defined as the distance between midpoints, can be calculated as the reciprocal of trabecular number (Parfitt *et al.*, 1987). More commonly, trabecular separation is calculated as follows (Parfitt *et al.*, 1983):

$$\text{Trabecular separation} = \text{trabecular width} \times [100/(\text{BV}/\text{TV}) - 1]$$

This method of calculation is based on the assumption that bone consists of parallel trabecular plates and defines the distance between the edges of the trabeculae; the values obtained are thus influenced by changes in trabecular width.

Trabecular number or density can be assessed directly by counting but is usually calculated according to the parallel plate model as follows (Parfitt *et al.*, 1983):

$$\text{Trabecular number} = (\text{BV/TV}\ \% \times 10)/\text{Trabecular width.}$$

STRUT ANALYSIS

In 1986 Garrahan *et al.* described a new technique for the quantitative analysis of cancellous bone structure, based on the topological classification of trabeculae or struts and on the definition of free ends (termini) and nodes (junctions). Using a computerized image analysis system, the number of free ends and nodes are counted automatically and a node/free end ratio derived. The different strut types are classified as shown in Figure 5.4; node to loop and node to node strut types are positively related to connectivity whereas struts with free ends are inversely related. The total length of each individual strut type within a section is measured automatically and expressed as a percentage of the total

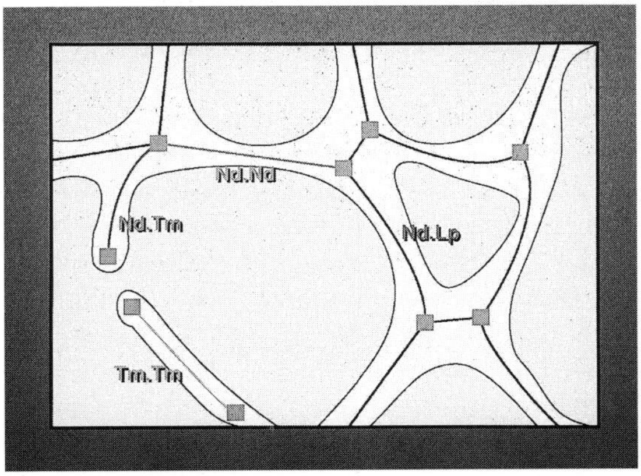

Figure 5.4 Trabecular strut analysis. Diagrammatic representation of the different strut types.

strut length within the section. Whilst free ends may clearly be created artefactually by the process of sectioning, nodes, node to node and node to loop struts are true indices of connectivity although their number may be underestimated.

This technique was originally based on expensive hardware (Ibas 11 image analyser) but has now been adapted for use on simpler and more widely used systems. Indices such as nodes, free ends and different strut types may also be counted manually (Mellish *et al.*, 1991), although this approach is relatively labour intensive.

STAR VOLUME

The star volume is defined as the mean volume of solid material or empty space that can be seen unobscured from a point of measurement chosen at random inside the material (Serra, 1982). The application of this parameter to bone was described by Vesterby (1990) using the vertical section technique (Baddeley *et al.*, 1986) and a cycloid test system (Figure 5.5). The method provides an unbiased stereological estimate of the mean size of the trabeculae and of the marrow space and can be used both for measurements of trabecular width (trabecular star volume) and trabecular separation or connectivity (marrow star volume); it was initially applied to assessment of vertebral bone structure but, with some modifications, can also be used in iliac crest bone. The technique is conceptually ingenious and theoretically superior to other approaches currently used, although practical evidence for its superiority is lacking. The requirement for randomly orientated 'vertical sections' is probably not absolute, since random rotation of the biopsy core is likely to occur during the normal embedding process. Hence the technique may be applicable to archival material, provided that the cycloid test system is used.

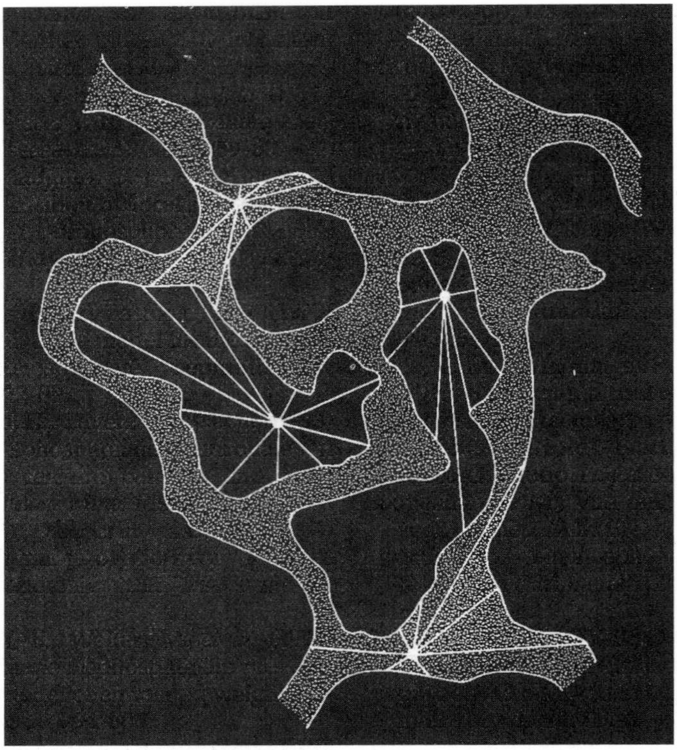

Figure 5.5 The marrow star volume.

EULER NUMBER AND THE CONNEULER

The Euler number is a topological property based on the number of holes and connected components in an object and provides a direct measure of connectivity. The ConnEuler, described by Gundersen *et al.* (1993), is a method in which the Euler number is calculated on projections through parallel thin section pairs, or disectors, spaced 10–40 μm apart. The Euler number is calculated from the numbers of islands, holes and bridges identified in the disectors. Further modifications may now enable correct, direct connectivity density measurements (Thomsen *et al.*, 1996).

TRABECULAR BONE PATTERN FACTOR

This index is related to trabecular connectivity and is based on the concept that patterns or structures can be defined by the relationship between convex and concave surfaces (Hahn *et al.*, 1992), convexity indicating poor connectivity and concavity being associated with structural integrity. Convexity and concavity are assessed by the measurement of bone perimeter and area before and after dilatation of a structure; thickening of convex structures increases the perimeter whilst the reverse applies to concave structures. The change in bone perimeter after dilatation thus depends on the ratio of convex to concave structures. Computer-based dilatation is carried out on binary images and the trabecular bone pattern factor (TBFf) is calculated as follows:

TBPf = (P1–P2)/(A1–A2)

where P1 = first perimeter measurement

P2 = second perimeter measurement
A1 = first area measurement
A2 = second area measurement.

HIGH-RESOLUTION MICROCOMPUTED TOMOGRAPHY

This technique generates a three-dimensional reconstruction array from which bone area, bone perimeter, trabecular width, separation and density can be determined and structural anisotropy examined (Feldkamp *et al.*, 1989). Connectivity is assessed using the Euler number, which in turn is calculated from the number of nodes and the number of branches. Breaking a single connection increases the Euler number by 1, whilst the creation of a connection decreases it by the same amount. An alternative approach to the production of three-dimensional images is reconstruction of serial sections, for which automated techniques have recently been described (Odgäard *et al.*, 1990).

Connectivity is independent of trabecular shape, size or orientation and its ability to predict the mechanical strength of bone is thus limited; Goldstein *et al.* (1993) reported that bone volume and anisotropy accounted for 90% of the variance in elastic modulus and ultimate strength in human metaphyseal bone. Correlations have been demonstrated between a number of two-dimensional structural indices and mechanical strength. Thus Dempster *et al.* (1993) reported a significant relationship between trabecular thickness and ultimate compressive strength in the second lumbar vertebra and structural indices obtained by strut analysis have also been shown to correlate with mechanical strength at this site (Mellish *et al.*, 1991). The marrow star volume of vertebral bone is also correlated with compressive strength (Vesterby *et al.*, 1991a); however, in all these studies, bone volume overshadowed structure as a predictor of strength.

FRACTAL ANALYSIS

Fractal objects are characterized by scale invariance or self-similarity over a wide range of magnification (Mandelbrot, 1977). The fractal dimension, D, describes how the object occupies space and is related to the complexity of the structure.

Some preliminary data indicate that fractal analysis can be applied to cancellous bone and may provide information about trabecular number and connectivity (Weinstein *et al.*, 1992). Clear differences in the fractal dimension (D) were demonstrated in iliac crest bone from osteoporotic patients when compared to normal subjects; however, the numbers examined were small and further studies are required. In contrast, Cross *et al.* (1993) were unable to define fractal geometry in iliac crest cancellous bone.

BONE REMODELLING IN OSTEOPOROSIS

MECHANISMS OF BONE LOSS

At the cellular level, bone loss may occur by two mechanisms (Figure 5.6). First, within individual remodelling units a negative balance results if bone formation is reduced relative to bone resorption; this is termed 'remodelling imbalance' and may reflect an increase in the amount of bone resorbed, a

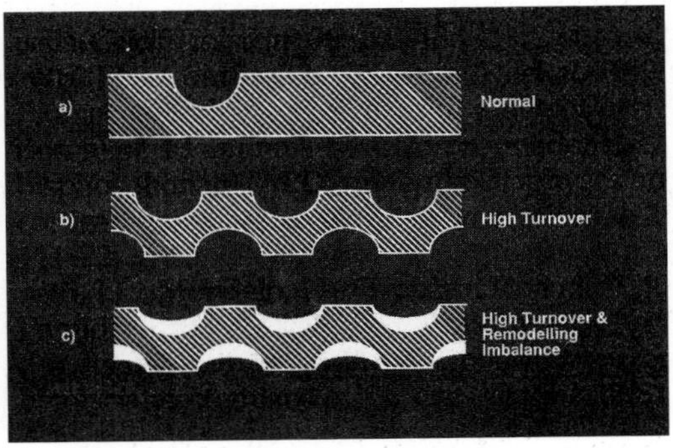

Figure 5.6 Diagrammatic representation of the cellular mechanisms of bone loss in osteoporosis.

decrease in the amount formed or both. Once the remodelling sequence has been completed within that unit, this form of bone loss is irreversible. Secondly, bone loss occurs when the number of remodelling units undergoing resorption is increased, due to an increase in activation frequency. This is described as high bone turnover and represents quantitatively the most important mechanism of bone loss in osteoporosis; provided that remodelling balance is maintained, this form of bone loss is potentially reversible.

The structural changes which occur, both in cortical and cancellous bone, are a consequence of the underlying alterations in bone remodelling. High bone turnover states, with or without an increase in erosion depth, favour trabecular penetration and disruption of cancellous architecture whereas low bone turnover and reduced bone formation within individual remodelling units result in trabecular thinning with relative preservation of connectivity. In reality, since trabecular thinning and penetration are to some extent interdependent (Compston *et al.*, 1989a), varying combinations of the two are generally encountered in osteoporosis although an increase in mean trabecular width, presumably due to the disappearance of thinner trabeculae, has been reported in some studies of postmenopausal osteoporosis.

LIMITATIONS OF BONE HISTOMORPHOMETRY

Bone histomorphometry enables unique information to be obtained *in vivo* about disease processes and their response to treatment but, like many techniques, it has limitations and is subject to error from a variety of causes (de Vernejoul *et al.*, 1981; Chavassieux *et al.*, 1985; Wright *et al.*, 1992). Measurement variance in bone histomorphometry is considerable and has many components including intra- and interobserver variation, intersection variation, intermethod variation (which includes factors such as magnification, corticomedullary differentiation and staining techniques as well as the method used for quantitation) and sampling variation. The latter applies not only to variation within the iliac crest but also throughout the skeleton; this is particularly important for osteoporosis, in which skeletal heterogeneity is well documented and the interactions between haematopoietic bone marrow and bone remodelling underline the probability of regional differences in bone turnover throughout the skeleton. The critical question of whether changes in iliac crest bone remodelling reflect those at sites of greater clinical relevance such as the spine and femur requires further study; differences in bone remodelling at different skeletal sites are well documented (Eventov *et al.*, 1991) but the contribution of measurement variance to these is unclear. The clear demonstration in iliac crest bone of significant deviations from the norm in osteoporosis, both primary and secondary, and of corresponding changes in response to treatment indicates that the observed changes reflect those occurring elsewhere qualitatively if not quantitatively.

In the case of bone structure, there are clear variations in cancellous architecture throughout the skeleton and extrapolation between sites is even more problematic. However, whilst differences in absolute values for structural indices may vary considerably, significant correlations have been demonstrated between indices of connectivity in the iliac crest and lumbar vertebrae (Mellish *et al.*, 1991). Thus iliac crest biopsy data can provide relevant information about structural changes occurring elsewhere in the skeleton; nevertheless, because of the unique structural composition of bone at sites such as the spine and femur, detailed analysis of changes associated with ageing or disease requires direct examination of the site in question.

BONE HISTOMORPHOMETRY IN OSTEOPOROSIS

POSTMENOPAUSAL OSTEOPOROSIS

Histomorphometric data in postmenopausal osteoporosis are relatively sparse and almost exclusively cross-sectional. The main finding has been that of striking heterogeneity in indices of bone turnover (Meunier *et al.*, 1981; Whyte *et al.*, 1982; de Vernejoul *et al.*, 1988; Eriksen *et al.*, 1990; Kimmel *et al.*, 1990); increased, normal and reduced tissue-based bone formation rates have been reported within patient groups, similar variability being documented in osteoclast count and in osteoclastic and osteoblastic surfaces. These changes may indicate disease subgroups with high or low bone turnover or may reflect intermittent changes in bone turnover, skeletal heterogeneity or measurement variance. Another possible explanation, for which there is some evidence, is that changes in bone turnover are sequential, high bone turnover in the immediate postmenopausal phase being followed by low turnover in later years (Heaney *et al.*, 1978; Eastell *et al.*, 1988). However, in spite of the heterogeneity in indices of bone turnover, one relatively consistent finding has been a reduction in wall width relative to that found in age-matched controls (Darby and Meunier, 1981; Carasco *et al.*, 1989; Arlot *et al.*, 1990; Eriksen *et al.*, 1990; Kimmel *et al.*, 1990). This may indicate a specific osteoblast defect in women with postmenopausal osteoporosis (Arlot *et al.*, 1984); alternatively, postmenopausal osteoporosis may result from normal age-related bone loss in women with low peak bone mass and, perhaps, smaller bone structural bone units. Measurement of the formation period in patients with primary osteoporosis has generally demonstrated no significant difference from control values (Carasco *et al.*, 1989; Eriksen *et al.*, 1990; Kimmel *et al.*, 1990) although in one study (Arlot *et al.*, 1990), a significant reduction in the active formation period was shown in women with postmenopausal osteoporosis. Normal values for mineral apposition rate and mineralization lag time have been reported in most studies (Carasco *et al.*, 1989; Arlot *et al.*, 1990; Kimmel *et al.*, 1990); however, a significanat reduction in mineral apposition rate was reported by Eriksen *et al.* (1990).

Measurements of resorption cavity depth in women with postmenopausal osteoporosis have not demonstrated any significant increase (Eriksen *et al.*, 1990; Cohen-Solal *et al.*, 1991; Croucher *et al.*, 1992), although in the study by Eriksen *et al.* (1990), a non-significant increase was reported which, together with a reduction in wall width, resulted in a substantial negative remodelling balance. Cohen-Solal *et al.* (1991) were unable to show any difference in completed resorption depth between normal and osteoporotic subjects, whilst Croucher *et al.* (1992) reported that the mean depth of all cavities was similar in patients and control groups.

The magnitude of the remodelling imbalance observed in women with postmenopausal osteoporosis is disputed. Eriksen *et al.* (1990) reported a median value of -16.1 μm whereas in the study of Cohen-Solal *et al.* (1991), the mean deficit of -6.11 μm was considerably smaller. This discrepancy between studies is likely to be due to the different techniques used to assess completed resorption depth; as Parfitt (1991) has pointed out, the remodelling imbalance reported by Eriksen *et al.* (1990) is almost certainly an overestimate, since in conjunction with the calculated activation frequency, this degree of imbalance would lead to complete disappearance of all trabeculae by the age of 66 years. Most existing data would support the contention that erosion depth is normal or reduced in patients with postmenopausal osteoporosis and that the trabecular thinning demonstrated in most studies is due to a reduction in wall width.

Changes in bone remodelling at cortico-endosteal surfaces also contribute to bone loss in postmenopausal osteoporosis. Brown *et al.* (1987) reported that women with postmenopausal osteoporosis exhibited a significant increase in bone turnover at corticoendosteal surfaces when compared to midcancellous bone; these changes are likely to contribute to the reduction in cortical width which occurs in such patients (Arlot *et al.*, 1990; Kimmel *et al.*, 1990).

The cellular pathophysiology of postmenopausal osteoporosis thus remains only partially defined. The heterogeneity observed both between patients (Meunier *et al.*, 1981; Whyte *et al.*, 1982; Eriksen *et al.*, 1990; Kimmel *et al.*, 1990) and within patients over relatively short periods of time (de Vernejoul *et al.*, 1988) probably reflects a number of factors, not least the large measurement variance associated with bone histomorphometry. Nevertheless, there is strong biochemical evidence, backed by some histomorphometric data (Vedi *et al.*, 1983; Eastell *et al.*, 1988) that increased activation frequency contributes to bone loss (Christiansen *et al.*, 1984; Stepán *et al.*, 1987), although this may be transient, and that bone formation rate at the cellular level is reduced. The fundamental question of whether postmenopausal osteoporosis represents a distinct pathogenetic entity or results from physiological bone loss in women with low peak bone mass remains unresolved. The demonstration in some, but not all, studies that a minority of women have significantly increased rates of bone loss during the menopause (Christiansen *et al.*, 1987) would suggest that postmenopausal osteoporosis results from bone loss which differs qualitatively or quantitatively from that which occurs in the majority of women; alternatively, the marked heterogeneity in rates of bone loss may be attributable to its phasic nature, the magnitude of bone loss over longer periods of time being similar in all women (Hui *et al.*, 1990).

FEMORAL NECK FRACTURES IN THE ELDERLY

Because of the inability to perform double tetracycline labelling prior to femoral neck fracture, information about bone remodelling in such patients is limited. Some early reports from the UK indicated that the prevalence of osteomalacia was considerably increased in hip fracture patients (Jenkins *et al.*, 1973; Aaron *et al.*, 1974; Faccini *et al.*, 1976); the diagnostic criteria used were, however, inadequate and based primarily on increased osteoid perimeter, which reflects increased bone turnover rather than defective mineralization. Subsequent studies, using stricter criteria, have generally demonstrated that the prevalence of histological osteomalacia is low in patients with hip fracture and similar to that encountered in the non-fracture elderly UK and other western European populations (Evans *et al.*, 1981; Lips *et al.*, 1982; Compston *et al.*, 1991). However, in a recent study from Leeds, UK, the prevalence of histological osteomalacia in 78 hip fracture patients was 12% (Hordon and Peacock, 1990a); this may indicate geographical variations in vitamin D status and osteomalacia within the UK.

The increased extent of osteoid perimeter noted in some patients with hip fracture indicates increased bone turnover and there is now evidence to support this contention. The concept of 'subclinical vitamin D deficiency', in which vitamin D status is insufficiently low to result in osteomalacia but sufficient to stimulate parathyroid hormone secretion (Parfitt *et al.*, 1982), has gained increasing acceptance and is backed by biochemical and clinical evidence (Compston *et al.*, 1989b; Chapuy *et al.*, 1992). Most of these studies have been conducted in western Europe, where low serum 25-hydroxyvitamin D levels are relatively common in the elderly. In the largest histomorphometric study to date, Lips *et al.* (1982) reported that a subgroup (21%) of patients with hip fracture had evidence of increased bone turnover (increased osteoid perimeter and eroded surface), increased osteoid perimeter being associated with low serum 25-hydroxyvitamin D and positively correlated with serum parathyroid hormone levels. Furthermore, osteoid perimeter has

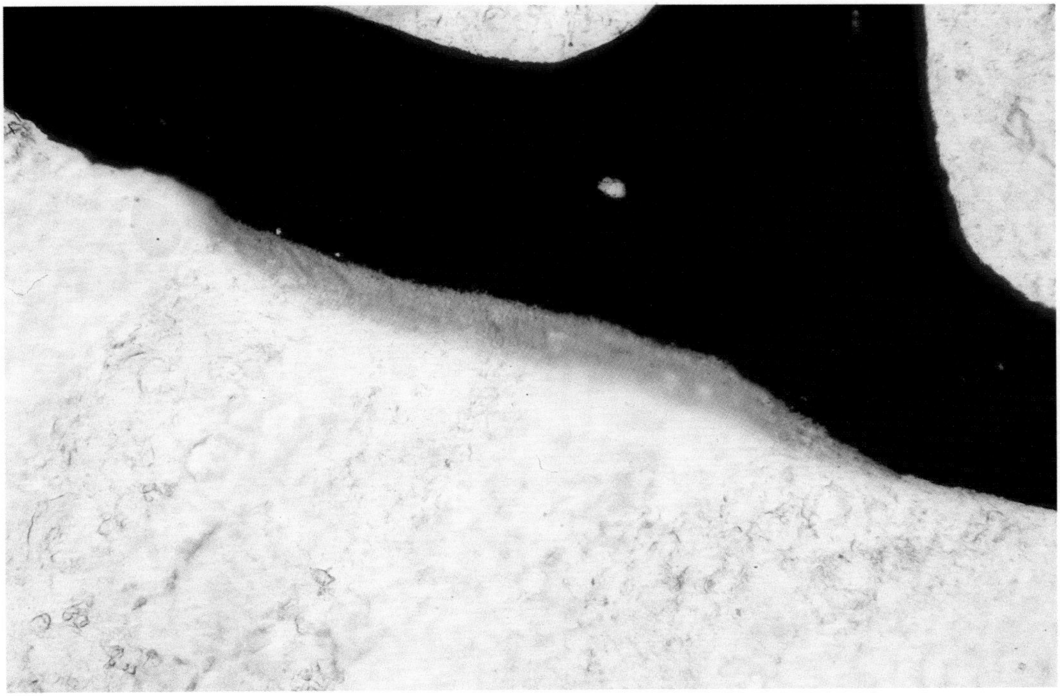

Plate 1 Iliac crest trabecular bone stained with the von Kossa stain and van Giesen counterstain to show mineralized bone (stained black) and osteoid (stained pink).

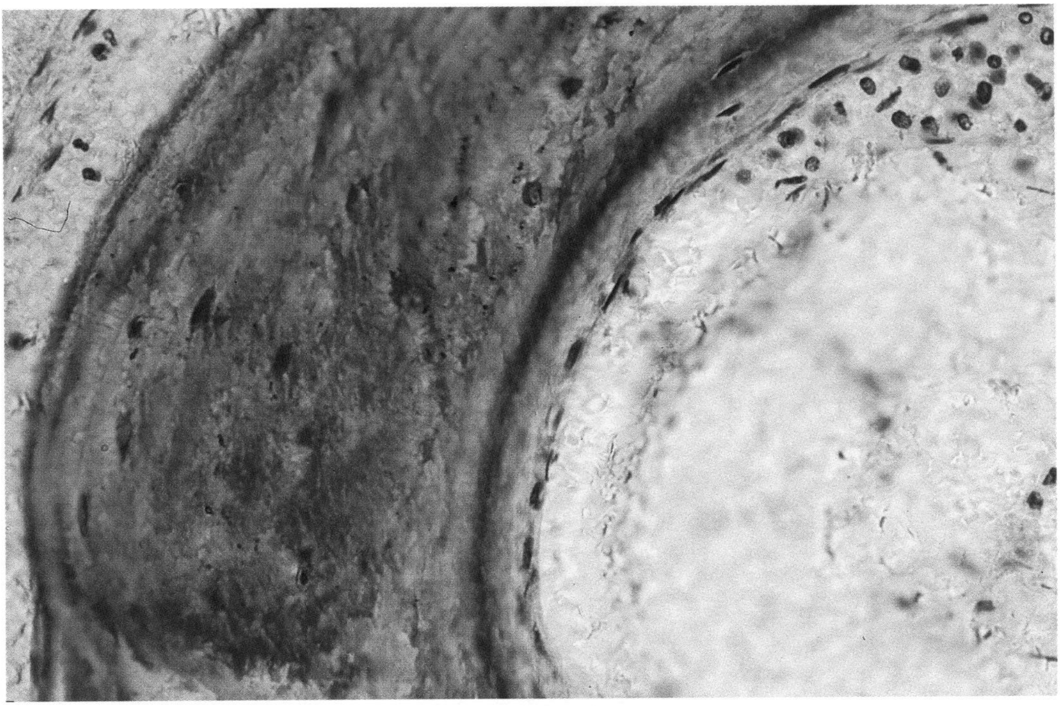

Plate 2 Iliac crest trabecular bone stained with toluidine blue to show mineralized bone (purple/blue) and osteoid (pale blue). The calcification front can be seen as a dark blue line at the interface of the osteoid and mineralized bone.

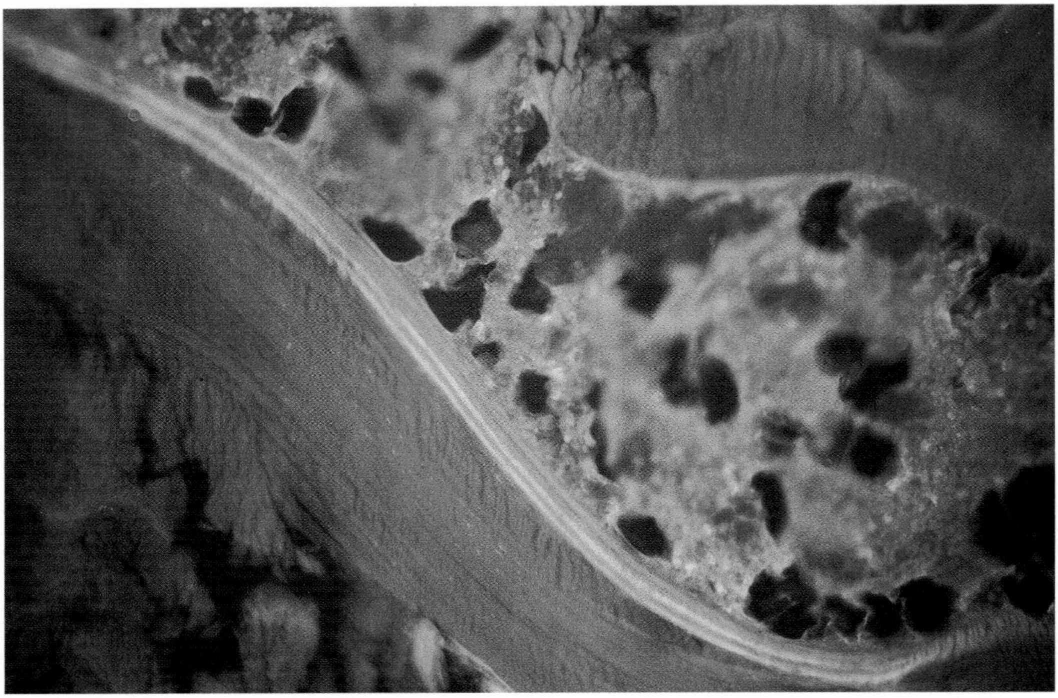

Plate 3 Unstained iliac crest biopsy section viewed by fluorescence microscopy. Two sets of double tetracycline labels can be seen as yellow fluorescent lines.

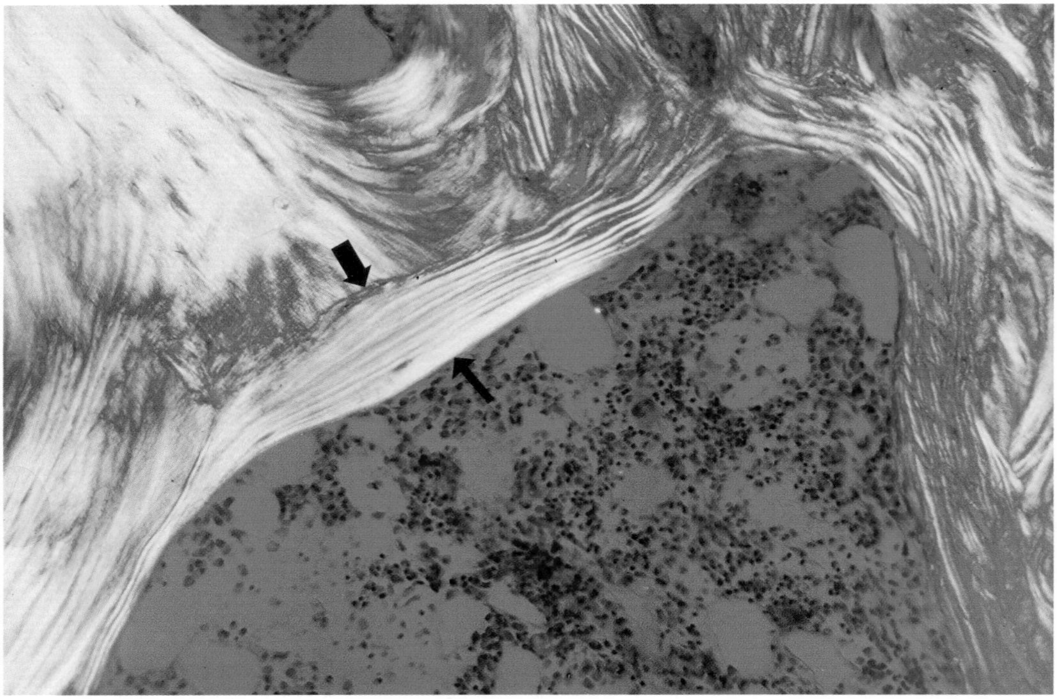

Plate 4 Iliac crest trabecular bone viewed under polarized light to show a completed bone structural unit, bounded by the cement line (thick arrow) and the mineralized bone surface (thin arrow).

been shown to correlate negatively with cortical bone mineral density in the forearm, implicating increased endosteal bone turnover in the pathogenesis of cortical thinning (Lips *et al.*, 1990). However, most histomorphometric studies of hip fracture patients show marked heterogeneity in most indices and only a minority show increased bone turnover.

When compared to control subjects, reduced iliac crest cancellous bone area and cortical width have been reported in hip fracture patients and in one study (Lips *et al.*, 1982), cancellous bone area was significantly lower in patients with trochanteric than with cervical fractures, although similar values for bone area in the two fracture groups have also been reported (Hordon and Peacock, 1990a). A significant reduction in wall width and trabecular width was reported in patients with trochanteric but not cervical fractures (Uitewaal *et al.*, 1987) whilst in another study (Hordon and Peacock, 1990b) cortical width was lower in patients with trochanteric fractures; these patients were, however, significantly older than the group with cervical fracture. The viability of osteocytes, demonstrated histochemically using lactate dehydrogenase, decreases with age, suggesting that 'bone death' may contribute to hip fracture; in one study, extensive osteocyte death was noted in femoral head bone from some hip fracture cases, although in others the bone appeared viable (Dunstan *et al.*, 1990). The positive, although weak, relationship between osteocyte viability and microfracture callus indicates that failure to repair microfractures may contribute to reduced bone strength.

To date, histomorphometric studies in hip fracture patients have been restricted to iliac crest bone; the observed changes at that site, particularly with respect to cortical bone, are unlikely to reflect accurately changes affecting the femoral neck with its unique cortical and cancellous bone structure. Moreover, appropriate control biopsy data in the very elderly age groups are difficult if not impossible to obtain and the use of autopsy data is known to be unreliable. It is thus uncertain whether hip fracture patients have specific abnormalities in cortical and/or cancellous bone remodelling and structure or whether they simply represent one end of the spectrum of 'physiological' bone loss; low bone mass is almost universal in many elderly populations and in these circumstances trauma becomes the major determinant of fracture risk.

BONE STRUCTURE IN PRIMARY OSTEOPOROSIS

Cancellous bone structure varies throughout the skeleton, as would be predicted from the different load-bearing functions at different sites. Iliac crest bone consists mainly of curved plates which are interconnected by thick bars (Whitehouse, 1974; Dempster *et al.*, 1986); vertebral bone shows much more marked anisotropy with its arrangement of vertical and horizontal plates and bars (Arnold and Wei, 1972). Both trabecular thinning and erosion occur during age-related bone loss, leading to progressive thinning and perforation of plates and, eventually, disappearance of whole trabecular elements. Measurement of trabecular width by a variety of different methods has shown an age-related reduction in both sexes, generally more marked in men (Wakamatsu and Sissons, 1969; Parfitt *et al.*, 1983; Weinstein and Hutson, 1987; Mellish *et al.*, 1989), although this finding has not been universal (Aaron *et al.*, 1987; Birkenhäger-Frenkel *et al.*, 1988; Vesterby *et al.*, 1989b). There is general agreement that in women, trabecular erosion with consequent disruption of structure is the predominant mechanism of bone loss (Compston *et al.*, 1987; Weinstein and Hutson, 1987; Vesterby *et al.*, 1989a; Hahn *et al.*, 1992), although whether this is attributable solely to increased bone turnover and trabecular thinning or whether increased osteoclastic activity and resorption depth also contribute is controversial. Statistical models of menopausal bone loss indicate that the observed loss of bone structure results from a combination of the two mechanisms (Reeve, 1986); however, the assumption made in these analyses that activation is randomly located on the cancellous surface is unlikely to be correct (Compston *et al.*, 1989a). In vertebral bone, age-related bone loss is associated with preferential thinning and loss of horizontal trabeculae, the vertical trabeculae remaining well preserved (Mosekilde, 1988).

The contribution of bone structure to mechanical strength is well established; however, whilst there is no doubt that bone mass is a major determinant of fracture risk, it is less clear whether changes in cancellous structure in osteoporosis contribute independently (Parfitt, 1992). Cortical bone, both in the vertebrae and elsewhere, has a major influence on bone strength and indices of trabecular connectivity do not predict mechanical strength better than does cancellous bone area (Mellish *et al.*, 1991; Versterby *et al.*, 1991a). However, two clinical studies provide some support for an independent contribution of cancellous bone structure to fracture risk (Kleerekoper *et al.*, 1985; Recker and Kimmel, 1991). When patients with postmenopausal osteoporosis and vertebral fracture were matched for cancellous bone area with non-fracture control subjects, indices of connectivity were found to be significantly reduced in the patient group; these changes were accompanied by a greater trabecular width. In contrast, Croucher *et al.* (1994) reported that although indices of connectivity showed highly significant reductions in patients with primary osteoporosis when compared to controls, these differences disappeared when patients and controls were matched for trabecular bone area (Figure 5.7). In this study, cancellous width was reduced in the osteoporotic group, a finding consistent with most other studies which indicate that bone loss in postmenopausal osteoporosis is associated both with trabecular thinning and loss of trabecular elements, the latter mechanism predominating (Parfitt *et al.*, 1983; Podenphant *et al.*, 1987; Kimmel *et al.*, 1990). The finding of a higher trabecular width in biopsies from fracture patients than controls in the studies of Kleerekoper *et al.* (1985) and Recker and Kimmel (1991) is thus atypical and may reflect factors related to the selection of patients and/or controls. The results of Croucher *et al.* (1994) suggest that changes in cancellous bone structure in primary osteoporosis do not differ qualitatively from those occurring during age-related bone loss, but that subjects with osteoporosis may simply have 'older bones' than their age-matched, non-osteoporotic equivalent. The observation that low bone mass is associated with greater non-trauma mortality and may thus be a manifestation of biological ageing (Aitken, 1987; Browner *et al.*, 1991) would support this contention.

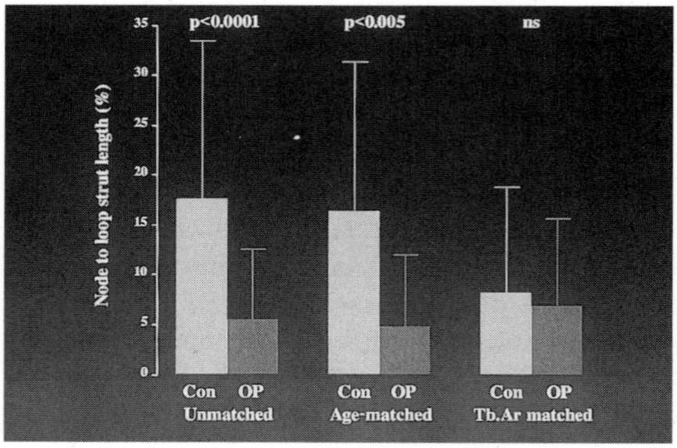

Figure 5.7 Node to loop strut length (% total strut length) in iliac crest cancellous bone from patients with primary osteoporosis. Results are expressed as the geometric mean value and 95% range. On the left, values in 39 patients have been compared with those obtained from 41 controls; in the middle column, a subgroup of patients were age-matched with controls and in the right column, a subgroup has been matched for cancellous bone area.

THE EFFECTS OF DRUGS ON BONE REMODELLING

GENERAL CONSIDERATIONS

If current concepts of bone remodelling are correct and apply both in health and disease, the capacity to respond to treatment should be critically dependent on bone turnover. If this is high, a reduction in activation frequency will be followed by an initial gain in bone mass and prevention of further bone loss; the magnitude of the transient increase in bone mass will be proportional to initial bone turnover and if remodelling balance is also improved, the increase in bone mass for any given bone turnover will be proportionately greater. Low bone turnover states per se do not result in bone loss unless combined with a negative remodelling balance; this combination will lead to relatively slow bone loss and the capacity to increase bone mass in response to treatment will be limited by the small proportion of the trabecular surface occupied by remodelling units, unless activation frequency is first increased.

In the light of these considerations, it would be expected that the response to treatment with drugs such as oestrogens and bisphosphonates, which act predominantly by reducing activation frequency, should be greatest in high turnover disease, whilst those with low or normal bone turnover (the majority of patients with postmenopausal osteoporosis) would be expected to show a smaller or even zero response. At present, however, there is no evidence that this is the case and, with the exception of sodium fluoride therapy, the issue of whether there are true nonresponders has not been specifically addressed. In densitometric studies, the effect of a drug is usually assessed by comparison of rates of bone loss in treated and placebo groups; rates of bone loss prior to treatment are seldom measured and maintenance of bone mass in postmenopausal women is often taken as an indication of drug responsiveness. However, low bone turnover prior to treatment in some subjects may be responsible for low or zero rates of bone loss during treatment; this phenomenon would explain the surprisingly low rates of bone loss in some placebo groups and could also misclassify some treated patients as responders.

The question of whether anabolic effects occur at the level of the individual remodelling unit is unresolved. Whilst some drugs may have the ability to restore a previously negative remodelling balance to normal, it seems less likely that osteoblasts will continue to form bone after the original resorption cavity has been filled, leading to a positive remodelling balance. If this assumption is correct, decreases in resorption depth would be associated with proportional reductions in wall width and would not result in any overall improvement in remodelling balance. Clarification of this issue requires improved techniques for the assessment of remodelling balance; at present, the mechanisms by which drugs produce anabolic effects in bone are unclear.

HORMONE REPLACEMENT THERAPY

Densitometric studies have shown that hormone replacement therapy is associated with prevention of bone loss, often with small increases in bone mass which are presumed to be due to filling in of the remodelling space. Histomorphometric data in women treated with hormone replacement are sparse and only two longitudinal studies have been reported (Steiniche *et al.*, 1989; Lufkin *et al.*, 1992); in both of these a significant reduction in activation frequency and tissue-based bone formation rate was demonstrated after one year's treatment but no effect on wall width was shown (Steiniche *et al.*, 1989). Longer term, longitudinal studies in which both resorption depth and wall width are assessed are required to demonstrate the effects of oestrogens on remodelling balance; in rats there is evidence that high doses of oestrogens stimulate *de novo* bone formation (Tobias *et al.*, 1991; Lean *et al.*, 1992) but there is no evidence for an anabolic effect in humans.

BISPHOSPHONATES

A significant reduction in activation frequency and tissue-based bone formation rate has also been shown in women treated with the bisphosphonate etidronate in a cyclic, intermittent regime (Steiniche *et al.*, 1991); the final resorption depth decreased significantly but no change was observed in wall width and although remodelling balance improved from a median value of –1.7 to +5.0 μm after treatment, this change was not statistically significant. The beneficial effects on activation frequency and correction of remodelling imbalance are consistent with the reported increase of around 5% in spinal bone mineral density after 2–3 years' treatment (Storm *et al.*, 1993; Ott *et al.*, 1994). Reduced activation frequency and resorption depth would also be expected to protect cancellous bone against adverse structural and hence biomechanical changes; however, suppression of activation frequency to abnormally low levels may lead to an increase in bone age and a reduction in the ability to repair fatigue microdamage, resulting in reduced bone strength.

The ability of bisphosphonates to inhibit mineralization varies between compounds and is unrelated to antiresorptive potency. Defective mineralization has been reported in patients with Paget's disease after treatment with etidronate (Boyce *et al.*, 1984) and pamidronate (Adamson *et al.*, 1993); as yet no evidence of similar changes has been reported in patients undergoing treatment for osteoporosis but further studies are needed.

ANABOLIC AGENTS – PARATHYROID HORMONE AND SODIUM FLUORIDE

The mechanisms by which agents such as sodium fluoride and parathyroid hormone produce anabolic effects on bone are of considerable interest and cannot easily be explained on the basis of current concepts of bone remodelling. Both agents produce large increases in cancellous bone volume; after four years, a mean increase in lumbar bone mineral density of 35% was observed in women with postmenopausal osteoporosis treated with a mean daily dose of 75 mg sodium fluoride (Riggs *et al.*, 1990) and large increases in spinal bone density have also been reported after treatment with 1–34 or 1–38 human parathyroid hormone (Slovik *et al.*, 1986; Hesch *et al.*, 1989; Reeve *et al.*, 1990; Hodsman *et al.*, 1991). The effects on cortical bone mass are considerably smaller and, in some studies, negative changes have been reported (Riggs *et al.*, 1990; Reeve *et al.*, 1990). An increase in activation frequency was reported after 200 days in which two 14-day cycles of 1–38 human parathyroid hormone were administered (Hodsman *et al.*, 1991); in an earlier study of the effects of 1–34 human parathyroid hormone given daily for 6–24 months to patients with osteoporosis, significant increases in osteoid and eroded perimeter were seen, although activation frequency was not assessed (Reeve *et al.*, 1980). A recent study, however, suggests that parathyroid hormone may stimulate *de novo* bone formation rather than increasing bone turnover via the expected sequence of resorption followed by formation. Thus biopsies obtained before and immediately after 28 days of parathyroid hormone fragment exhibited an increase in bone-forming surfaces and bone formation rates (Hodsman and Steer, 1992); the time course of the study makes it unlikely that the resorption/reversal phases of the normal remodelling cycle could have been completed before the observed increase in bone formation. Increases in wall width have also been reported after treatment with parathyroid hormone (Reeve *et al.*, 1991) and may contribute to the anabolic effect, although there are no data on resorption depth in these patients.

The effects of sodium floride on activation

frequency are less well documented. Increases in osteoid perimeter, eroded perimeter and mineralizing perimeter after 1–3 years of therapy have been reported and are compatible with increased bone turnover (Baylink and Bernstein, 1967; Jowsey *et al.*, 1972; Briancon and Meunier, 1981; Pak *et al.*, 1989; Aaron *et al.*, 1991) but there are no data on short-term changes in activation frequency in cancellous bone, although Kragstrup *et al.* (1989) demonstrated increased activation frequency in cortical bone after six months' treatment with fluoride, calcium and vitamin D. In a comprehensive study of the effects of five years of combined therapy with sodium fluoride, calcium, phosphate and vitamin D_2 in patients with postmenopausal osteoporosis (Eriksen *et al.*, 1985), a significant increase in remodelling balance was observed, from –7.7 to +9.1 μm; this was due to an increase in wall width, with no significant change in the completed resorption depth. Although large amounts of woven bone are seen in fluoride-treated patients after 1–2 years (Melsen *et al.*, 1977), predominantly lamellar bone was present after five years. An increase in osteoid seam width and mineralization lag time was also observed, indicating a mineralization defect; similar findings have been reported by several other groups (Compston *et al.*, 1980b; Boivin *et al.*, 1988; Kragstrup *et al.*, 1989). The effects of sodium fluoride on cortical bone are of particular interest in view of the small positive, neutral or negative effects on cortical bone mass reported in densitometric studies. Kragstrup *et al.* (1989) were unable to demonstrate any effects on remodelling balance or on cortical thickness after five years' treatment; in this study, like most others, sodium fluoride was given in conjuction with vitamin D and calcium supplements.

Thus sodium fluoride and parathyroid hormone appear to increase cancellous bone mass by both increasing activation frequency and improving remodelling balance; *de novo* bone formation may also occur, at least in response to parathyroid hormone, although further evidence is required. In some studies activators of bone remodelling have been used with drugs which depress osteoclastic resorption (ADFR regime; Frost, 1981), but no additional benefits on remodelling balance have been observed (Hodsman *et al.*, 1991; Steiniche *et al.*, 1991).

THE EFFECTS OF DRUGS ON BONE STRUCTURE

In view of the likely irreversibility of cancellous bone structural changes in osteoporosis, the effects of drugs on bone architecture are of particular interest. Trabecular thickening after sodium fluoride or parathyroid hormone therapy is well documented but the effects of these and other drugs on connectivity are less clear. Vesterby *et al.* (1991a) reported a significant reduction in marrow space star volume after five years' treatment with sodium fluoride in 11 patients with osteoporosis, indicating an increase in cancellous bone connectivity; however in contrast to previous reports, no significant change in cancellous bone volume was observed with treatment and the mean trabecular width decreased. In the study of Aaron *et al.* (1991), the expected increases in cancellous bone area and trabecular width were demonstrated in 15 patients after two years' treatment, but no change occurred in either trabecular number or the free end count, indicating that connectivity was unaffected. The demonstration by Quarles *et al.* (1988) that high doses of aluminium stimulate *de novo* bone formation in dogs indicates the potential for restoration of trabecular connectivity in humans. Alternatively, trabecular connectivity may be improved in the absence of *de novo* bone formation if trabecular thickening is followed by intratrabecular resorption, as occurs in Paget's disease; this may occur in response to parathyroid hormone therapy but is not seen in patients treated with sodium fluoride (Aaron *et al.*, 1992). However, with either mechanism it is unlikely that the original structure would be restored.

Much remains to be learnt about the effects of drugs on bone remodelling and structure. There are, for example, very few histomorphometric data on the effects of calcium on bone although it is widely used as an adjunct to the treatment of osteoporosis and its demonstrated effects on biochemical indices of bone remodelling; likewise the mechanisms by which vitamin D and its metabolites preserve bone mass in postmenopausal women and in the elderly have been little studied. In spite of the known adverse effects of oestrogen deficiency on cancellous bone mass and structure, the actions of oestrogens on bone remodelling are only partially understood and no study has yet addressed the effects of oestrogens on cancellous bone architecture in humans. Information of this kind can only be obtained by incorporation of bone histomorphometry into trial protocols; new techniques such as *in situ* hybridization and immunohistochemistry should expand the already considerable potential of bone histomorphometry to provide further insights into bone physiology and the effects upon it of disease and its treatment.

REFERENCES

Aaron, J.E., Gallagher, J.C., Anderson, J. *et al.* (1974) Frequency of osteomalacia and osteoporosis in fractures of the proximal femur. *Lancet* **i**: 229–33.

Aaron, J.E., Makins, N.B. and Sagreiya, K. (1987) The microanatomy of trabecular bone loss in normal aging men and women. *Clin Orthop Rel Res* **215**: 260–71.

Aaron, J.E., de Vernejoul, M.-C. and Kanis, J.A. (1991) The effect of sodium fluoride on trabecular architecture. *Bone* **12**: 307–10.

Aaron, J.E., de Vernejoul, M.-C. and Kanis J.A. (1992) Bone hypertrophy and trabecular generation in Paget's disease and in fluoride-treated osteoporosis. *Bone Mineral* **17**: 399–413.

Adamson, B.B., Gallacher, S.J., Byars, J. *et al.* (1993) Mineralisation defects with pamidronate therapy for Paget's disease. *Lancet* **342**: 1459–60.

Agerbaek, M.O., Eriksen, E.F, Kragstrup, J., Mosekilde L. and Melsen, F. (1991) A reconstruction of the remodelling cycle in normal cortical iliac bone. *Bone Mineral* **12**: 101–12.

Aitken, J.M. (1987) Relationship between mortality after femoral neck fracture and osteoporosis. In: *Osteoporosis 1987* (eds Christiansen, C., Johansen, J.S. and Riis, B.J.), Osteopress ApS, Copenhagen, pp. 45–8.

Arlot, M.E., Delmas, P.D., Chappard, D. and Meunier, P. (1990) Trabecular and endocortical bone remodelling in postmenopausal osteoporosis: comparison with normal postmenopausal women. *Osteoporosis Int* **1**: 41–9.

Arlot, M., Edouard, C., Meunier, P.J., Neer, R.M. and Reeve, J. (1984) Impaired osteoblast function in osteoporosis: comparison between calcium balance and dynamic histomorphometry. *Br Med J* **289**: 517–20.

Arnold, J.S. and Wei, L.T. (1972) Quantitative morphology of vertebral trabecular bone. In: *Radiobiology of Plutonium*, (eds Stover, B. and Jee, W.S.S.), JW Press, Salt Lake City, pp. 333–54.

Baddeley, A.J., Gundersen, H.J.G. and Cruz Orive, L.M. (1986) Estimation of surface area from vertical sections. *J. Microsc* **142**: 259–76.

Baylink, D.J. and Bernstein, D.S. (1967) The effect of fluoride therapy on metabolic bone disease: a histologic study. *Clin Orthop* **55**: 51–85.

Birkenhäger-Frenkel, D.H. and Birkenhäger-Frenkel, J.C. (1987) Bone appositional rate and percentage of doubly and singly labelled surfaces: comparison of data from 5 and 20 μm sections. *Bone* **8**: 7–12.

Birkenhäger-Frenkel, D.H., Courpron, P. Hüpscher, E.A. *et al.* (1988) Age-related changes in cancellous bone structure. A two-dimensional study in the transiliac and iliac crest biopsy sites. *Bone Mineral* **4**: 197–216.

Boivin, G., Chapuy, M.C., Baud, C.A. and Meunier, P.J. (1988) Fluoride content in human iliac bone; results in controls, patients with fluorosis, and osteoporotic patients treated with fluoride. *J Bone Miner Res* **3**: 497–501.

Boyce, B.F., Fogelman, I., Ralston, S. *et al.* (1984) Focal osteomalacia due to low-dose diphosphonate therapy in Paget's disease. *Lancet* **i**: 821–4.

Briancon, D. and Meunier, P.J. (1981) Treatment of osteoporosis with fluoride, calcium and vitamin D. *Orthop Clin North Am* **12**: 629–48.

Brown, J.P., Delmas, P.D., Arlot, M. and Meunier, P.J. (1987) Active bone turnover of the cortico-endosteal envelope in postmenopausal osteoporosis. *J Clin Endocrinol Metab* **64**: 954–9.

Browner, W.S., Seeley, D.G., Vogt T.M. and Cummings, S.R. (1991) Non-trauma mortality in elderly women with low bone mineral density. *Lancet* **338**: 355–8.

Burstone, M.S. (1959) Histochemical demonstration of acid phosphatase activity in osteoclasts. *J Histochem Cytochem* **7**: 39–41.

Carasco, M.G., de Vernejoul, M.C., Sterkers, Y. *et al.* (1989) Decreased bone formation in osteoporotic patients compared with age-matched controls. *Calcif Tissue Int* **44**: 173–5.

Chapuy, M.C., Arlot, M.E., DuBoeuf, F. *et al.* (1992) Vitamin D3 and calcium to prevent hip fractures in elderly women. *N Engl J Med* **327**: 1637–42.

Chavassieux, P.M., Arlot, M.E. and Meunier, P.J. (1985) Intermethod variation in bone histomorphometry: comparison between manual and computerised methods applied to iliac bone biopsies. *Bone* **6**: 211–19.

Christiansen, C, Riis, B.J. and Rodbro, P. (1987) Prediction of rapid bone loss in postmenopausl women. *Lancet* **i**: 1105–8.

Christiansen, C., Rodbro, P. and Tjellesen, L. (1984) Serum alkaline phosphatase during hormone treatment in early postmenopausal women. *Acta Med Scand* **216**: 11–17.

Clermonts, E.C.G.M. and Birkenhäger-Frenkel, D.H. (1985) Software for bone histomorphometry by means of a digitizer. *Comput Math Prog Biomed* **21**: 185–94.

Cohen-Solal, M.E., Shih, M.-S., Lundy, M.W. and Parfitt, A.M. (1991) A new method for measuring cancellous bone erosion depth: application to the cellular mechanisms of bone loss in postmenopausal osteoporosis. *J Bone Miner Res* **6**: 1331–8.

Compston, J.E. and Croucher, P.I. (1991) Histomorphometric assessment of trabecular bone remodellng in osteoporosis. *Bone Mineral* **14**: 91–102.

Compston, J.E., Crowe, J.P., Wells, I.P. *et al.* (1980a) Vitamin D prophylaxis and osteomalacia in chronic cholestatic liver disease. *Dig Dis* **25**: 28–32.

Compston, J.E., Chadha, S. and Merrett A.L. (1980b) Osteomalacia developing during treatment of osteoporosis with sodium fluoride and vitamin D. *Br Med J* **281**: 910–1.

Compston, J.E., Mellish, R.W.E. and Garrahan, N.J. (1987) Age-related changes in the iliac crest trabecular microanatomic bone structure in man. *Bone* **8**: 289–92.

Compston, J.E., Mellish, R.W.E., Croucher, P.I. Newcombe, R. and Garrahan, N.J. (1989a) Structural mechanisms of trabecular bone loss in man. *Bone Mineral* **6**: 339–50.

Compston, J.E., Silver, A.C., Croucher, P.I., Brown, R.C. and Woodhead, J.S. (1989b) Elevated serum intact parathyroid hormone levels in elderly patients with hip fracture. *Clin Endocrinol* **31**: 667–72.

Compston, J.E., Vedi, S. and Croucher, P.I. (1991) Low prevalence of osteomalacia in elderly patients with hip fracture. *Age Ageing* **20**: 132–4.

Courpron, P., Lepine, P., Arlot, M., Lips, P. and Meunier, P.J. (1980) Mechanisms underlying the reduction with age of the mean wall thickness of trabecular basic structure unit (BSU) in human iliac bone. *Bone Histomorphometry. Third International Workshop*, (eds Jee, W.S.S. and Parfitt, A.M.), Armour Montagu, Paris, pp. 323–9.

Cross, S.S., Rogers, S., Silcocks, P.B. and Cotton, D.W.K. (1993) Trabecular bone does not have a fractal structure on light microscopy. *J Pathol* **170**: 311–13.

Croucher, P.I., Mellish, R.W.E., Vedi, S., Garrahan, N.J. and Compston, J.E. (1989) The relationship between resorption depth and mean interstitial bone thickness: age-related changes in man. *Calcif Tissue Int* **45**: 15–19.

Croucher, P.I., Garrahan, N.J. and Compston, J.E. (1992) Assessment of resorption cavity characteristics in trabecular bone: changes in primary and secondary osteoporosis. *Bone* **13**: A9.

Croucher, P.I., Garrahan, N.J. and Compston, J.E. (1994) Structural mechanisms of trabecular bone loss in primary osteoporosis: specific disease mechanism or early ageing? *Bone Mineral* **25**: 111–21.

Darby, A.J. and Meunier, P.J. (1981) Mean wall thickness and formation periods of trabecular bone packets in idiopathic osteoporosis. *Calcif Tissue Int* **33**: 199–204.

Dempster, D.W., Shane, E., Horbert, W. and Lindsay, R. (1986) A simple method for correlative light and scanning electron microscopy of human iliac crest bone biopsies: qualitative observations in normal and osteoporotic subjects. *J Bone Miner Res* **1**: 15–21.

Dempster, D.W, Ferguson-Pell, M.W., Mellish, R.W.E. *et al.* (1993) Relationship between bone structure in the iliac crest and bone structure and strength in the lumbar spine. *Osteoporosis Int* **3**: 90–6.

De Vernejoul, M.C., Kuntz, D., Miravet, L., Goutalier, D. and Ryckewaert, A. (1981) Histomorphometric reproducibility in normal patients. *Calcif Tissue Int* **33**: 369–74.

De Vernejoul, M.C., Belenguer-Prieto, R., Kuntz, D. *et al.* (1988) Bone histological heterogeneity in postmenopausal osteoporosis: a sequential histomorphometric study. *Bone* **8**, 339–42.

Dunstan, C.R., Evans, R.A., Hills, E., Wong, S.Y.P. and Higgs, R.J.E.D. (1990) Bone death in hip fracture in the elderly. *Calcif Tissue Int* **47**, 270–5.

Eastell, R., Delmas, P.D., Hodgson, S.F. *et al.* (1988) Bone formation rate in older normal women: concurrent assessment with bone histomorphometry, calcium kinetics, and biochemical markers. *J Clin Endocrinol Metab* **67**, 741–8.

Eriksen, E.F. (1986) Normal and pathological remodelling of human trabecular bone: three-dimensional reconstruction of the remodelling sequence in normals and in metabolic bone disease. *Endocr Rev* **7**: 379–408.

Eriksen, E.F., Gundersen, H.J.G., Melsen, F. and Mosekilde, L. (1984) Reconstruction of the resorptive site in iliac trabecular bone: a kinetic model for bone resorption in 20 normal individuals. *Metab Bone Dis Rel Res* **5**: 235–42.

Eriksen, E.F., Mosekilde, L. and Melsen, F. (1985) Effect of sodium fluoride, calcium phosphate and Vitamin D_2 on trabecular bone balance and remodelling. *Bone* **6**: 381–91.

Eriksen, E.F., Hodgson, S.F., Eastell, R. *et al.* (1990) Cancellous bone remodelling in Type 1 (postmenopausal) osteoporosis: quantitative assessment of rates of formation, resorption, and bone loss at tissue and cellular levels. *J Bone Miner Res* **5**: 311–19.

Evans, R.A., Dunstan, C.R. and Baylink, D.J. (1979) Histochemical identification of osteoclasts in undecalcified sections of human bone. *Miner Elect Metab* **2**: 179–85.

Evans, R.A., Ashwell, J.R. and Dunstan, C.R. (1981) Lack of metabolic bone disease in patients with fracture of the femoral neck. *Aust NZ J Med* **11**: 158–61.

Eventov, I., Frisch, B., Cohen, Z. and Hammel, I. (1991) Osteopenia, hematopoiesis, and bone remodelling in iliac crest and femoral biopsies: a prospective study of 102 cases of femoral neck fractures. *Bone* **12**, 1–6.

Faccini, J.M., Exton-Smith, A.N. and Boyde, A. (1976) Disorders of bone and fractures of the femoral neck. *Lancet* **i**, 1089–92.

Feldkamp, L.A., Goldstein, S.A., Parfitt, A.M., Jesion, G. and Kleerekoper, M. (1989) The direct examination of three-dimensional bone architecture in vitro by computed tomography. *J Bone Miner Res* **4**: 3–11.

Foldes, J., Shih, M.-S. and Parfitt, A.M. (1990) Frequency distributions of tetracycline-based measurements: implications for the interpretation of bone formation indices in the absence of double-labelled surfaces. *J Bone Miner Res* **5**: 1063–7.

Frost, H.M. (1963) Mean formation time of human osteons. *Can J Biochem Physiol* **41**: 1307–10.

Frost, H.M. (1969) Tetracycline-based histological analysis of bone remodelling. *Calcif Tissue Int* **3**: 211–37.

Frost, H.M. (1981) Coherence treatment of osteoporosis. *Orthop Clin North Am* **12**: 649–69.

Frost, H.M. (1983a) Bone histomorphometry: analysis of trabecular bone dynamics. In: *Bone Histomorphometry. Techniques and Interpretations*, (ed. Recker, R.), CRC Press, Boca Raton, pp. 109–31.

Frost, H.M. (1983b) Bone histomorphometry: choice of marking agent and labelling schedule. In: *Bone Histomorphometry. Techniques and Interpretations*, (ed. Recker, R.), CRC Press, Boca Raton, pp. 37–51.

Frost, H.M. (1985) The pathomechanics of osteoporosis. *Clin Orthop Rel Res* **200**: 198–225.

Garrahan, N.J., Mellish, R.W.E. and Compston, J.E. (1986) A new method for the analysis of two-dimensional trabecular bone structure in human iliac crest biopsies. *J Microsc* **142**: 341–9.

Garrahan, N.J., Mellish, R.W.E., Vedi, S. and Compston, J.E. (1987) Measurement of mean trabecular plate thickness by a new computerized method. *Bone* **8**: 227–30.

Garrahan, N.J., Croucher, P.I. and Compston, J.E. (1990) A computerised technique for the quantitative assessment of resorption cavities in trabecular bone. *Bone* **11**: 241–6.

Goldstein, S.A., Goulet, R. and McCubbrey (1993) Measurement and significance of three-dimensional architecture to the mechanical integrity of trabecular bone. *Calcif Tissue Int* **53** (Suppl 1): S127–33.

Gundersen, H.J.G., Boyce, R.W., Nyengaard, J.R. and Odgäard, A. (1993) The Conneulor: unbiased estimate of connectivity using physical disectors under projection. *Bone* **14**: 217–22.

Hahn, M., Vogel, M., Pompesius-Kempa, M. and Delling, G. (1992) Trabecular bone pattern factor – a new parameter for simple quantification of bone microarchitecture. *Bone* **13**: 327–30.

Heaney, R.P., Recker, R.R. and Saville, P.D. (1978) Menopausal changes in bone remodelling. *J Lab Clin Med* **92**: 964–70.

Hesch, R.-D., Busch, U., Prokop, M., Delling, G. and Rittinghaus, E.-F. (1989) Increase of vertebral density by combination therapy with pulsatile 1–38 PTH and sequential addition of calcitonin nasal spray in osteoporotic patients. *Calcif Tissue Int* **44**: 176–80.

Hodsman, A.B. and Steer, B.M. (1992) Early histomorphometric changes in response to parathyroid hormone therapy in osteoporosis: evidence for de novo bone formation on quiescent cancellous surfaces. *Bone* **13**: A13.

Hodsman, A.B., Steer, B.M., Fraher, L.J. and Drost, D.J. (1991) Bone densitometric and histomorphometric responses to sequential human parathyroid hormone (1–38) and salmon calcitonin in osteoporotic patients. *Bone Mineral* **14**: 67–83.

Hordon, L.D. and Peacock, M. (1990a) Osteomalacia and osteoporosis in femoral neck fracture. *Bone Mineral* **11**: 247–59.

Hordon, L.D. and Peacock, M. (1990b) The architecture of cancellous and cortical bone in femoral neck fracture. *Bone Mineral* **11**: 335–45.

Hui, S.L., Slemenda, C.W. and Johnston, C.C. (1990) The contribution of bone loss to postmenopausal osteoporosis. *Osteoporosis Int* **1**: 30–4.

Jenkins, D.H.R., Roberts, J.G., Webster, D. and Williams, E.O. (1973) Osteomalacia in elderly patients with fracture of the femoral neck. *J Bone Joint Surg* **55B**: 575–80.

Jowsey, J., Riggs, B.L., Kelly, P.J. and Hoffman, D.L. (1972) Effect of combined therapy with sodium fluoride, vitamin D and calcium in osteoporosis. *Am J Med* **53**: 43–9.

Kimmel, D.B., Recker, R.R., Gallagher, J.C., Vaswani, A.S. and Aloia, J.F. (1990) A comparison of iliac bone histomorphometric data in postmenopausal osteoporotic and normal subjects. *Bone Mineral* **11**: 217–35.

Kleerekoper, M., Villanueva, A.R., Stanciu, J., Rao, D.S. and Parfitt, A.M. (1985) The role of three-dimensional trabecular microstructure in the pathogenesis of vertebral compression fractures. *Calcif Tissue Int* **37**: 594–7.

Kragstrup, J., Gundersen, H.J.G., Mosekilde, L. and Melsen, F. (1982b) Estimation of the three dimensional wall thickness of completed remodelling sites in iliac trabecular bone. *Metab Bone Dis Rel Res* **4**: 113–19.

Kragstrup, J., Melsen, F. and Mosekilde, L. (1982a) Reduced wall thickness of completed remodelling sites in iliac trabecular bone following anticonvulsant therapy. *Metab Bone Dis Rel Res* **4**: 181–5.

Kragstrup, J., Shijie, Z., Mosekilde, L. and Melsen, F. (1989) Effects of sodium fluoride, vitamin D and calcium on cortical bone remodelling in osteoporotic patients. *Calcif Tissue Int* **45**: 337–41.

Lean, J.M., Chow, J.W.M. and Chambers, T.J. (1992) The increased bone formation induced by oestrogen in rats occurs on non-resorptive surfaces. *Bone* **13**: A20.

Lips, P., Courpron, P. and Meunier, P.J. (1978) Mean wall thickness of trabecular bone packets in the human iliac crest: changes with age. *Calcif Tissue Res* **26**: 13–17.

Lips, P., Netelenbos, J.C., Jongen, M.J.M. *et al.* (1982) Histomorphometric profile and vitamin D status in patients with femoral neck fracture. *Metab Bone Dis Rel Res* **4**: 85–93.

Lips, P., Hesp, R., Reeve, J. *et al.* (1990) High indices of remodelling in iliac trabecular bone predict reduced forearm cortical bone mass indices in patients with proximal femoral fractures. *Bone Mineral* **11**: 93–100.

Lufkin, E.G., Wahner, H., O'Fallon, W.M. *et al.* (1992) Treatment of postmenopausal osteoporosis with transdermal oestrogen. *Ann Intern Med* **117**: 1–9.

Mandelbrot, B.B. (1977) *Fractals: Form, Chance and Dimension*, W.H. Freeman, San Francisco.

Mellish, R.W.E., Garrahan, N.J. and Compston, J.E. (1989) Age-related changes in trabecular width and spacing in human iliac crest biopsies. *Bone Mineral* **6**: 331–8.

Mellish, R.W.E., Ferguson-Pell, M.W., Cochran, G.V.B., Lindsay, R. and Dempster, D. (1991) A new manual method for assessing two-dimensional cancellous bone structure: Comparison between iliac crest and lumbar vertebra. *J Bone Miner Res* **6**: 689–96.

Melsen, F., Mosekilde, L., Larsen, M.J., Christensen, M.S. and Melsen, B. (1977) Treatment of osteoporosis with sodium fluoride, calciferol and calcium phosphate. A two year study. *Calcif Tissue Res* **24** (Suppl): 17.

Meunier, P.J., Sellami, S., Briancon, D. and Edouard, C. (1981) Histological heterogeneity of apparently idiopathic osteoporosis. In: *Osteoporosis: Recent Advances in Pathogenesis and Treatment*, (eds DeLuca, H.F. *et al.*), University Park Press, Baltimore, pp. 293–301.

Mosekilde, L. (1988) Age-related changes in vertebral trabecular bone architecture – assessed by a new method. *Bone* **9**: 247–50.

Odgäard, A., Andersen, K., Melsen, F. and Gundersen, H.J.G. (1990) A direct method for fast three-dimensional serial reconstruction. *J Microsc* **159**: 335–42.

Ott, S.M., Woodson, G.C., Huffer, W.E., Miller, P.D. and Watts, N.B. (1994) Bone histomorphometric changes after cyclic therapy with phosphate and etidronate disodium in women with postmenopausal osteoporosis. *J Clin Endocrinol Metab* **78**: 968–72.

Pak, C.Y.C., Sakhaee, K., Zerwekh, J.E. *et al.* (1989) Safe and effective treatment of osteoporosis with intermittent slow release sodium fluoride: augmentation of vertebral bone mass and inhibition of fractures. *J Clin Endocrinol Metab* **68**: 150–8.

Palle, S., Chappard, D., Vico, L., Riffat, G. and Alexandre, C. (1989) Evaluation of the osteoclastic population in iliac crest biopsies from 36 normal subjects: a histoenzymologic and histomorphometric study. *J Bone Miner Res* **4**: 501–6.

Parfitt, A.M. (1983) The physiological and clinical significance of bone histomorphometric data. In: *Bone Histomorphometry. Techniques and Interpretations*, (ed. Recker, R.), CRC Press, Boca Raton, pp. 143–224.

Parfitt, A.M. (1991) Bone remodelling in Type 1 osteoporosis (letter). *J Bone Miner Res* **6**: 95–7.

Parfitt, A.M. (1992) Implications of architecture for the pathogenesis and prevention of vertebral fracture. *Bone* **13**: S41–7.

Parfitt, A.M. and Foldes, J. (1991) The ambiguity of interstitial bone thickness: a new approach to the mechanism of trabecular thinning. *Bone* **12**: 119–22.

Parfitt, A.M., Gallagher, J.C., Heaney, R.P. *et al.* (1982) Vitamin D and bone health in the elderly. *Am J Clin Nutr* **36**: 1014–37.

Parfitt, A.M., Mathews, C.H.E., Villanueva, A.R. *et al.* (1983) Relationship between surface, volume and thickness of iliac trabecular bone in aging and in osteoporosis: implications for the microanatomic and cellular mechanism of bone loss. *J Clin Invest* **72**: 1396–409.

Parfitt, A.M., Drezner, M.K., Glorieux, F.H. *et al.* (1987) Bone histomorphometry. Standardization of nomenclature, symbols and units. *J Bone Miner Res* **2**: 595–610.

Parfitt, A.M., Foldes, J., Villanueva, A.R. and Shih, M.S. (1991) Difference in length between demethylchlortetracycline and oxytetracycline: implications for the interpretation of bone histomorphometric data. *Calcif Tissue Int* **48**: 74–7.

Podenphant, J., Herss Nielsen, V.A., Riss, B.J., Gotfredsen, A. and Christiansen, C. (1987) Bone mass, bone structure and vertebral fractures in osteoporotic patients. *Bone* **8**: 127–30.

Quarles, L.D., Gitelman, J.J. and Drezner, M.K. (1988) Induction of de novo bone formation in the beagle: a novel effect of aluminium. *J Clin Invest* **81**: 1056–66.

Rao, D.S. (1983) Practical approach to bone biopsy. In: *Bone Histomorphometry: Techniques and Interpretation*, (ed. Recker, R.), CRC Press, Boca Raton, pp. 3–11.

Recker, R.R. and Kimmel, D.B. (1991) Changes in trabecular microstructure in osteoporosis occur with normal bone remodelling dynamics. *J Bone Miner Res* **6** (Suppl 1): S225.

Reeve, J. (1986) A stochastic analysis of iliac trabecular bone dynamics. *Clin Orthop Rel Res* **213**: 264–78.

Reeve, J., Meunier, P.J., Parsons, J.A. *et al.* (1980) Anabolic effect of human parathyroid hormone fragment on trabecular bone in involutional osteoporosis: a multicentre trial. *Br Med J* **280**: 1340–4.

Reeve, J., Davies, U.M., Hesp, R., McNally, E. and Katz, D. (1990) Treatment of osteoporosis with human parathyroid peptide and observations on the effect of sodium fluoride. *Br Med J* **301**: 314–18.

Reeve, J., Bradbeer, J.N., Arlot, M. *et al.* (1991) hPTH 1–34 treatment of osteoporosis with added hormone replacement therapy: biochemical, kinetic and histological responses. *Osteoporosis Int* **1**: 162–70.

Riggs, B.L., Hodgson, S.F., O'Fallon, W.M. *et al.* (1990) Effect of fluoride treatment on the fracture rate in postmenopausal women with osteoporosis. *N Engl J Med* **322**: 802–9.

Schwartz, M.P. and Recker, R.R. (1981) Comparison of surface density and volume of human iliac trabecular bone measured directly and by applied sterology. *Calcif Tissue Int* **33**: 561–5.

Serra, J. (1982) *Image Analysis and Mathematical Morphology*, Academic Press, London.

Slovik, D.M., Rosenthal, D.I., Doppelt, S. *et al.* (1986) Restoration of spinal bone in osteoporotic men by treatment with human parathyroid hormone (1–34) and 1,25-dihydroxyvitamin D. *J Bone Miner Res* **1**: 377–81.

Steiniche, T., Hasling, C., Charles, P. *et al.* (1989) A randomised study on the effects of estrogen/gestagen or high dose oral calcium on trabecular bone remodelling in postmenopausal osteoporosis. *Bone* **10**: 313–20.

Steiniche, T., Halsing, C., Charles, P. *et al.* (1991) The effects of etidronate on trabecular bone remodelling in postmenopausal spinal osteoporosis; a randomised study comparing intermittent treatment and an ADFR regime. *Bone* **12**: 155–63.

Steiniche, T., Eriksen, E.F., Kudsk, H. Mosekilde, L. and Melsen, F. (1992) Reconstruction of the formative site in trabecular bone by a new, quick, and easy method. *Bone* **13**: 147–52.

Stepán, J.J., Postichal, J., Presl, J. and Pacovsky, V. (1987) Bone loss and biochemical indices of bone remodelling in surgically induced postmenopausal women. *Bone* **8**: 279–84.

Storm, T., Steiniche, T., Thamsborg, G. and Melsen, F. (1993) Changes in bone histomorphometry after long-term treatment with intermittent cyclic etidronate for postmenopausal osteoporosis. *J Bone Miner Res* **8**: 199–208.

Thomsen, J.S., Barlach, J. and Mosekilde, L. (1996) Determination of connectivity density in human iliac crest bone biopsies assessed by a computerized method. *Bone* **18**: 459–65.

Tobias, J.H., Chow, J., Colston, K.W. and Chambers, T.J. (1991) High concentrations of 17β-oestradiol stimulate trabecular bone formation in adult female rats. *Endocrinology* **128**: 408–12.

Uitewaal, P.J.M., Lips, P. and Netelenbos, J.C. (1987) An analysis of bone structure in patients with hip fracture. *Bone Mineral* **3**: 63–73.

Vedi, S. and Compston, J.E. (1984) Direct and indirect measurements of osteoid seam width in human iliac crest biopsies. *Metab Bone Dis Rel Res* **5**: 269–74.

Vedi, S. Compston, J.E., Webb, A. and Tighe, J.R. (1983) Histomorphometric analysis of dynamic parameters of trabecular bone formation in iliac crest of normal British subjects. *Metab Bone Dis Rel Res* **5**: 69–74.

Vedi, S., Tighe, J.R. and Compston, J.E. (1984) Measurement of total resorption surface in iliac crest trabecular bone in man. *Metab Bone Dis Rel Res* **5**: 275–80.

Vesterby, A. (1990) Star volume of marrow space and trabeculae in iliac crest: sampling procedure and correlation to star volume of first lumbar vertebra. *Bone* **11**: 149–55.

Vesterby, A., Kragstrup, J., Gundersen, H.J.G. and Melsen, F. (1987) Unbiased stereologic estimation of surface density in bone using vertical sections. *Bone* **8**: 13–17.

Vesterby, A., Gundersen, H.J.G. and Melsen, F. (1989a) Star volume of marrow space and trabeculae of the first lumbar vertebra: sampling efficiency and biological variation. *Bone* **10**: 7–13.

Vesterby, A., Gundersen, H.J.G., Melsen, F. and Mosekilde, L. (1989b) Normal postmenopausal women show iliac crest trabecular thickening on vertical sections. *Bone* **10**: 333–9.

Vesterby, A., Mosekilde, L., Gundersen, H.J.G. *et al.* (1991a) Biologically meaningful determinants of the in vitro strength of lumbar vertebrae. *Bone* **12**: 219–24.

Vesterby, A., Gundersen, H.J.G., Melsen, F. and Mosekilde, L. (1991b) Marrow space star volume in the iliac crest decreases in osteoporotic patients after continuous treatment with fluoride, calcium and vitamin D. *Bone* **12**: 33–7.

Wakamatsu, E. and Sissons, H.A. (1969) The cancellous bone of the iliac crest. *Calcif Tissue Res* **4**: 147–61.

Weinstein, R.S. and Hutson, M.S. (1987) Decreased trabecular width and increased trabecular spacing contribute to bone loss with ageing. *Bone* **8**: 137–42.

Weinstein, R.S., Majumdar, S. and Genant, H.K. (1992) Fractal geometry applied to the architecture of cancellous bone biopsy specimens. *Bone* **13**: A38.

Whitehouse, W.J. (1974) The quantitative morphology of anisotropic trabecular bone. *J Microsc* **101**: 153–68.

Whyte, P.M., Bergfeld, M.A., Murphy, W.A., Avioli, L.V. and Teitelbaum, S.L. (1982) Postmenopausal osteoporosis. A heterogeneous disorder as assessed by histomorphometric analysis of iliac crest bone from untreated patients. *Am J Med* **72**: 192–202.

Wright, C.D.P., Vedi, S., Garrahan, N.J. *et al.* (1992) Combined inter-observer and inter-method variation in bone histomorphometry. *Bone* **13**: 205–8.

BIOLOGICAL MARKERS OF BONE TURNOVER IN OSTEOPOROSIS

6

P.D. Delmas and P. Garnero

SUMMARY

The non-invasive assessment of bone turnover has received increasing attention over the past few years, because of the need for sensitive markers in the clinical investigation of osteoporosis. Markers of bone formation include serum total and bone-specific alkaline phosphatase, serum osteocalcin and measurement of serum type I collagen extension peptides. Assessment of bone resorption can be achieved with measurement of urinary hydroxyproline and hydroxylysine glycosides, urinary excretion of the pyridinium crosslinks (pyridinoline and deoxypyridinoline) and associated peptides and by measurement of plasma tartrate-resistant acid phosphatase activity. Osteocalcin, the pyridinium crosslinks and the immunoassay of bone alkaline phosphatase appear to be the most efficient markers to assess the level of bone turnover at the menopause but also in elderly patients with osteoporosis. Programs combining bone mass measurement and assessment of bone turnover in women at the time of menopause have been developed, in an attempt to improve the assessment of the risk for osteoporosis. Recent data suggest that some of the new immunoassays for pyridinoline crosslinks and related peptides could predict the subsequent risk of hip fracture in elderly women. Thus, bone markers might be used in combination with bone mass measurement to improve the prognostic assessment of postmenopausal women, i.e. their risk of developing osteoporosis and ultimately fractures. Treatment of postmenopausal women with antiresorptive drugs such as estrogens, bisphosphonates and calcitonin is followed by rapid decrease of the levels of bone markers correlated with the long-term increase of bone mass as assessed by dual energy X-ray absorptiometry measurement. Thus, bone markers should be useful in monitoring treatment efficacy in patients with osteoporosis. In the near future, the use of a battery of various specific markers is likely to improve the assessment of the complex aspects of bone metabolism, especially in osteoporosis.

INTRODUCTION

Bone metabolism is characterized by two opposite activities, the formation of new bone by osteoblasts and the degradation (resorption) of old bone by the osteoclasts. Both are tightly coupled in time and space in a sequence of events which define the same remodeling unit. Bone mass depends on the balance between resorption and formation within a remodeling unit and on the number

Osteoporosis. Edited by John C. Stevenson and Robert Lindsay. Published in 1998 by Chapman & Hall, London. ISBN 0 412 48870 1

of remodeling units which are activated within a given period of time in a defined area of bone. Needless to say, bone formation and bone resorption are altered in most metabolic bone diseases, including osteoporosis.

Invasive techniques for measuring bone turnover have provided useful information but all have limitations. Histomorphometry of the iliac crest provides unique information on the rate of formation at the cell and tissue level and allows measurement of the activation frequency of remodeling units but the assessment of bone resorption is less accurate. In addition, measurement of bone turnover is limited to a small area of the cancellous and corticoendosteal envelope which may not reflect bone turnover at other sites of the skeleton (Delmas, 1988). Calcium kinetic studies have allowed us to quantify the increase in bone turnover after the menopause but measurement of calcium accretion rate – an index of bone formation – may be inaccurate in elderly women (Eastell *et al.*, 1988). Finally the whole body retention (WBR) of labeled bisphosphonates, a marker of bone turnover and bone formation, has not proved to be very sensitive (Thomsen *et al.*, 1987). These limitations, in addition to the need for non-invasive techniques that can be applied more widely and repeated several times in a single patient, explain the development of markers of bone turnover to be measured in blood and urine.

In contrast to metabolic bone diseases such as Paget's disease of bone or renal osteodystrophy characterized by dramatic changes of bone turnover, osteoporosis is a condition where subtle modifications of the bone remodeling activity can lead to a substantial loss of bone mass after a long period of time. This explains why most conventional markers are normal in an individual woman recently post menopausal, such as in a patient with well-characterized vertebral osteoporosis. Consequently there have been efforts to develop more sensitive biochemical markers of bone turnover.

The rate of formation or degradation of the bone matrix can be assessed either by measuring a prominent enzymatic activity of the bone-forming or resorbing cells, such as alkaline and acid phosphatase activity, or by measuring bone matrix components released into the circulation during formation or resorption (Table 6.1). These have been separated into markers of formation and resorption but it should be borne in mind that in disease states where both events are coupled and in balance, either of these markers will reflect the overall rate of bone turnover. As

Table 6.1 Biochemical markers of bone turnover

Formation	*Resorption*
Serum	*Plasma*
Osteocalcin (bone gla-protein)	Tartrate-resistant acid phosphatase
Total and bone-specific alkaline phosphatase	Pyridinoline and pyridinoline-containing peptides
Procollagen I carboxy and N terminal extension peptides	
	Urine
	Urinary pyridinoline and deoxypyridinoline (collagen crosslinks) and related type I collagen peptides
	Fasting urinary calcium and hydroxyproline
	Urinary hydroxylysine glycosides

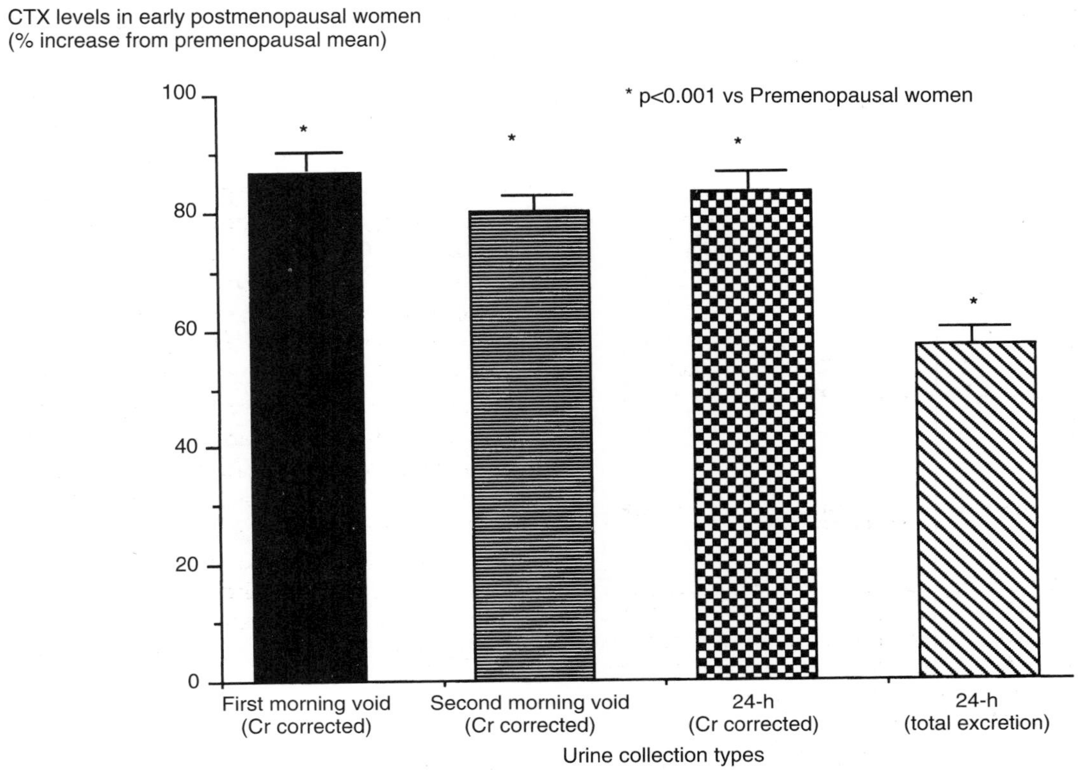

Figure 6.5 Increased levels of CTX excretion in postmenopausal women according to the type of urine collection. For each of the 170 early postmenopausal women, first morning void sample, second morning void sample and 24-h urine samples were collected for CTX and creatinine measurements. Bars represent mean CTX levels of postmenopausal women for each type of urine sample, expressed as a percentage increase and SEM over the mean of 134 premenopausal women. The increase of creatinine corrected CTX levels after the menopause was of similar amplitude in first, second and 24-h urine samples. The increase was less important for the total 24-h urinary collection.

postmenopausal increase in both bone formation and bone resorption is sustained long after the menopause, even in the elderly (Figure 6.6) (Garnero *et al.*, 1996). Thus the age-related bone loss which has been shown to persist at a significant rate at the hip until the ninth decade (Jones *et al.*, 1994) results primarily from the increased bone turnover, although the osteoblastic activity at the level of a remodeling unit declines with age as indicated by histomorphometric studies (Lips *et al.*, 1978; Parfitt *et al.*, 1983). Two independent studies have shown that in untreated postmenopausal women followed for 2–4 years, serum osteocalcin is correlated with the spontaneous rate of bone loss assessed by repeated measurements of the bone mineral content of the radius and the lumbar spine, i.e. the higher the bone turnover rate, the higher the rate of bone loss (Slemenda *et al.*, 1987; Johansen *et al.*, 1988). We have also shown that the combination of a single measurement of serum osteocalcin, urinary hydroxyproline and D-Pyr can predict the rate of bone loss over two years with an r value of 0.77 (Uebelhart *et al.*, 1991).

Whether slow and fast losers of bone do so for a prolonged period of time after the

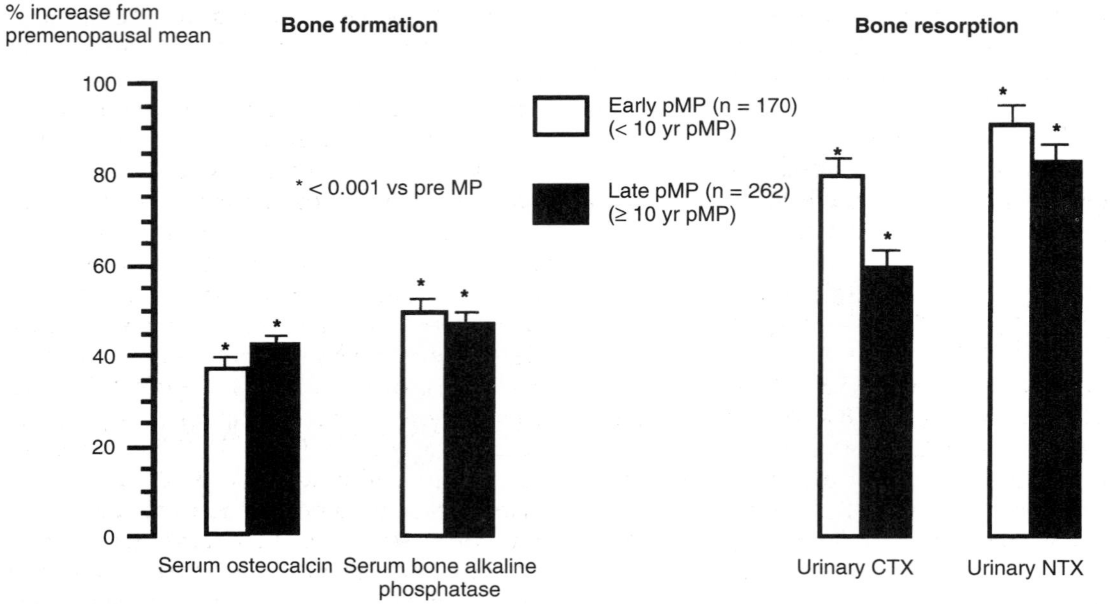

Figure 6.6 Increased levels of bone formation and bone resorption markers in early and late postmenopausal women. Postmenopausal women (n = 432) were divided in two groups: early postmenopausal women (Early pMP) within 10 years of the menopause (mean time postmenopause five years) and late postmenopausal women (late pMP), 10 years postmenopause and over (mean time postmenopause 20 years, 10–40 years pMP). For each marker in each group, mean levels are expressed as a percentage increase and SEM over the mean of 134 premenopausal women (31–57 years of age). Both bone formation and bone resorption markedly increased at the time of menopause and high bone turnover is maintained in late postmenopausal women and in elderly. NTX = type I crosslinked N telopeptides; CTX = type I C telopeptide breakdown products (see Fig. 6.2). Adapted from Garnero *et al.* (1996).

menopause is debated, but a recent long-term study suggests that the rate of bone loss measured over 12 years is increased in postmenopausal women classified as rapid losers from the initial bone marker measurements (Hansen *et al.*, 1991). Thus, despite identical bone mass at baseline, women who were diagnosed fast losers at the initial biochemical measurement had lost 50% more bone 12 years later than those diagnosed slow losers (total bone loss 26.6% versus 16.6%, $p<0.001$). The combination of bone mass measurement and assessment of bone turnover by a battery of specific markers is likely to be helpful in the future for the screening of patients at risk for osteoporosis who should be treated.

BONE TURNOVER IN POSTMENOPAUSAL WOMEN WITH VERTEBRAL OSTEOPOROSIS

In patients with untreated vertebral osteoporosis, there is a wide range of individual values of biochemical markers of bone turnover beyond normal which reflects the histological heterogeneity of the disease. Serum osteocalcin is in the lower range of normal in patients with a low osteoblastic activity and significantly increased in the one-third of patients having a high bone turnover. When serum osteocalcin is compared with the bone-remodeling activity measured on undecalcified iliac crest biopsy, there is a significant correlation with histological parameters reflecting bone formation but not with those reflecting resorption, both at the trabecular and the corticoendosteal envelope (Brown *et al.*, 1984, 1987; Podenphant *et al.*, 1987). In most studies, serum TRAP, urinary hydroxyproline and crosslink excretion tend to be higher and more scattered than in age-matched controls.

BONE TURNOVER IN THE ELDERLY AND IN PATIENTS WITH HIP FRACTURE

Despite the importance of hip fracture as a major health problem, few studies have been devoted to potential bone turnover abnormalities in these patients. Histological studies suggest an increased bone resorption as a consequence of secondary hyperparathyroidism. Increased serum alkaline phosphatase activity is thought to reflect the occurrence of osteomalacia which is not uncommon in Europe in the elderly. Serum osteocalcin and urinary hydroxyproline have been reported to be either low or normal (Thompson *et al.*, 1989; Delmi *et al.*, 1990) but the acute changes of body fluid – and perhaps of bone turnover – related to the trauma might obscure subtle changes of bone remodeling.

In a large group of patients studied immediately after hip fracture, we have found increased urinary crosslink excretion and decreased serum osteocalcin levels when comparing to age-matched healthy elderly, suggesting that increased bone resorption and decreased bone formation might be important determinants of the low bone mass which characterizes patients with hip fracture (Akesson *et al.*, 1993) (Figure 6.7). The cross-sectional data are supported by recent prospective studies. Riis *et al.* (1996) reported that women within three years of menopause classified as fast bone losers, i.e. with a high bone turnover rate, had a twofold higher risk of sustaining vertebral and peripheral fractures during a 15-year follow-up than women classified as normal or slow losers. In addition, women with both a low bone mass and a fast rate of bone loss just after the menopause had a higher risk of subsequently sustaining fractures than women with only one of the two risk factors.

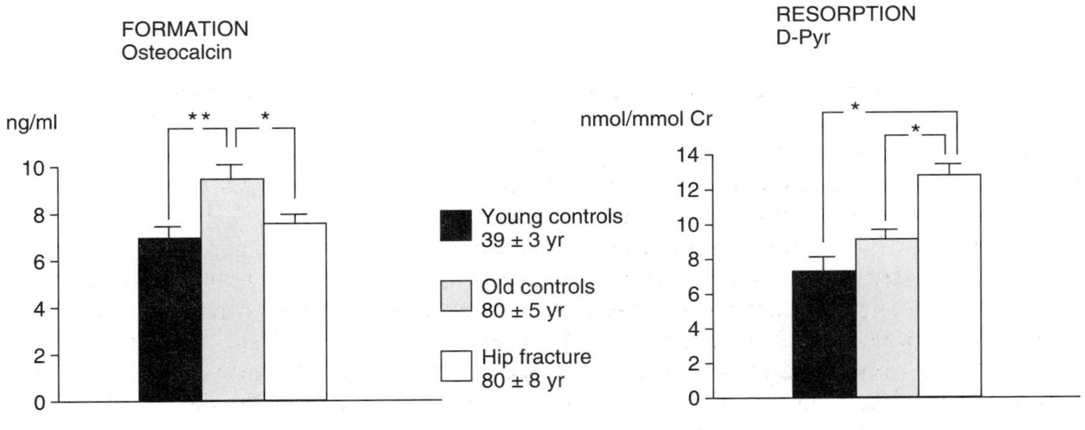

Figure 6.7 Serum osteocalcin and urinary deoxypyridinole (D-Pyr) in a large group of women who had sustained a hip fracture within the last 24 hours who were compared to age-matched women derived from the same community and to premenopausal healthy women. * $p < 0.01$–0.001; ** $p < 0.01$. Adapted from Akesson *et al.* (1993).

Concordant results have recently been obtained in a prospective study of risk factors for hip fractures conducted in a large cohort of elderly healthy women in France (Garnero *et al.*, 1996). In those women who had a hip fracture during a two-year follow-up, baseline measurements of urinary C-telopeptide breakdown products (CTX, CrossLaps™) and free D-Pyr (Pyrilink-D™) were higher than in non-fractured controls; increased CTX and free D-Pyr above the normal range of premenopausal women was associated with a 120% increase in the risk of hip fracture that was still significant after adjusting for hip bone mineral density (Table 6.3). Thus, the combination of bone mass and bone turnover measurements should be useful in improving the risk assessment of osteoporotic fractures.

As previously mentioned, osteocalcin contains three residues of γ carboxyglutamic acid, a vitamin K-dependent amino acid. The level of circulating undercarboxylated osteocalcin (that can be indirectly measured after incubation with hydroxyapatite) is significantly increased in elderly women and decreases with vitamin K treatment (Knapen *et al.*, 1989; Plantalech *et al.*, 1991). We have recently shown, in a prospective study in a cohort of elderly institutionalized women followed for three years, that serum undercarboxylated osteocalcin measured at baseline is significantly higher in those that subsequently sustained a hip fracture. In those women with an elevated level of circulating undercarboxylated osteocalcin, the relative risk of hip fracture was three times higher (Szulc *et al.*, 1993, 1996) (Table 6.4). Vitamin K deficiency is a common finding in the elderly, especially in those with hip fracture (Hodges *et al.*, 1991). In addition, serum undercarboxylated osteocalcin may reflect vitamin D status (Szulc *et al.*, 1993). Thus, the level of the γ

Table 6.3 Increased bone marker levels as predictors of hip fracture in elderly women. Adapted from Garnero *et al.* (1996) Elderly women in to the EPIDOS prospective study (7500 healthy female volunteers, 75 yrs of age and older). During an average 22-month follow-up, 109 women sustained a hip fracture. For each hip fracture patient there were 3 age-matched controls who did not sustain fracture during the same period. At baseline, 2 markers of bone formation (osteocalcin and bone alkaline phosphatase (BAP)) and 3 resorption markers (CTX, NTX and free D-Pyr) were assessed. The relative risk of hip fracture for an increased bone turnover, defined as bone marker levels either in the highest quartile of the values for the elderly controls or above the upper limit of the premenopausal range (mean + 2 SD of 134 premenopausal women 35–57 yrs), was estimated using odds ratio. Baseline increased levels of CTX and free D-Pyr were associated with an increased risk of sustaining hip fracture during the 2-yr follow-up, while markers of bone formation were not

	Odds ratio (95% CI)	
Bone markers (predictors)	*Highest quartile of elderly*	*Above upper limit of premenopausal range*
Osteocalcin	1.1 (0.7–1.9)	1.0 (0.6–1.6)
BAP	0.9 (0.6–1.4)	1.1 (0.7–1.7)
NTX	1.1 (0.7–1.9)	1.4 (0.9–2.2)
CTX	2.1 (1.3–3.3)	2.2 (1.3–3.6)
Free D-Pyr	1.5 (0.9–2.5)	1.9 (1.1–3.2)

Table 6.4 Serum undercarboxylated osteocalcin (ucOC) predicts hip fracture risk in elderly institutionalized women. 183 elderly institutionalized women (aged 70–95 yrs), in a randomized trial of the effect of calcium+vitamin D_3 supplementation, were prospectively followed for 3 yrs. During follow-up, 30 women sustained a hip fracture. We calculated the relative risk of hip fracture as a function of baseline ucOC levels assessed by the competitive hydroxyapatite-binding assay. Levels of ucOC in elderly women were categorized according to the number of SDs from the premenopausal mean (T score). The relative risk of hip fracture increased progressively with the increase of ucOC levels. Adapted from Szulc *et al.* (1996)

ucOC levels in T score	*Relative risk*	*95% CI*
T score ≤2	1.0	
2 <T score≤4	2.1	1.2–2.9
T score >4	2.9	2.2–3.7

carboxylation of osteocalcin appears to reflect the poor nutritional status of elderly patients with hip fracture and its significance deserves further investigation.

BONE MARKERS TO MONITOR TREATMENT OF OSTEOPOROSIS

In patients with osteoporosis, there is a wide range of individual values of biochemical markers of bone turnover beyond normal which reflects the histological heterogeneity of bone turnover in this disease. The subgroup of osteoporotic patients with high turnover, characterized by increased osteocalcin and hydroxyproline, showed a significant increase of spinal bone mineral density after one year of calcitonin therapy, whilst those with low turnover had no increase of bone mass despite the same therapy (Civitelli *et al.*, 1988). The authors suggested that patients with high turnover are more likely to benefit from calcitonin therapy. A larger effect on bone mass in high than in low turnover patients has not been well documented with other antiresorptive therapy, i.e. estrogen and bisphosphonates.

Antiresorptive therapies, such as estrogen and bisphosphonate, induce a significant decrease of resorption and formation markers that fall within the premenopausal range within 3–6 months, earlier for resorption than formation markers. Given the precision of bone mass measurement by dual energy X-ray absorptiometry of the lumbar spine and the expected change in bone mass induced by antiresorptive treatment, it is usually necessary to wait up to two years after initiating therapy to determine, in a single patient, if treatment is effective, i.e. it increases bone mass significantly. Conversely, repeating bone marker measurement within 3–6 months is likely to provide the same information on treatment effectiveness. As shown in Figure 6.8, a significant decrease of bone turnover after three months of bisphosphonate treatment in osteoporotic women was associated with an increase of BMD at the lumbar spine at three years with a low rate of false positives and false negatives (Garnero *et al.*, 1994c). Thus, repeating the measurement of a sensitive and specific marker of either bone formation or resorption 3–6 months after initiation of estrogen or bisphosphonate therapy is likely to be useful in the management of osteoporotic patients.

Finally, biochemical markers should also be useful to monitor patients on chronic corticosteroid therapy which inhibits osteoblastic activity, reflected by subnormal serum osteocalcin level (Reid *et al.*, 1986; Garrel *et al.*, 1988).

CONCLUSION

Currently there is no ideal marker of bone formation but circulating osteocalcin is the most satisfactory at the present time for the investigation of osteoporosis. Recent developments include the use of human osteocalcin and synthetic peptides as immunogens and of various monoclonal antibodies to measure specifically the intact molecule (sandwich assay) but also to identify fragments of osteo-

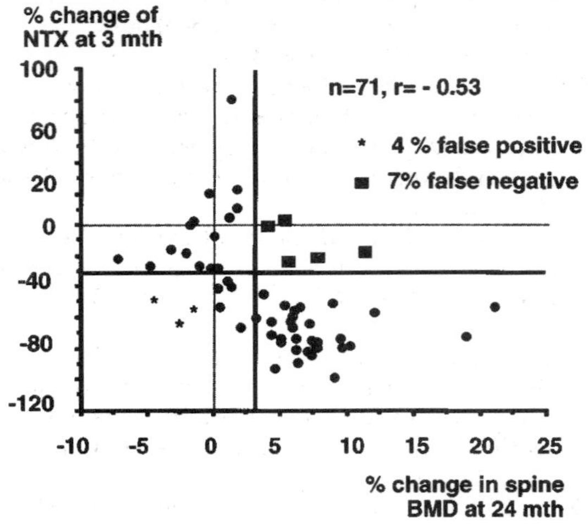

Figure 6.8 Use of bone markers to monitor the efficacy of antiresorptive therapy. The graph represents the correlation between the early percent change (from baseline to 3 months of treatment) of crosslinked N telopeptides (NTX) and the late percent change (from baseline to 24 months of therapy) of spinal BMD in patients treated orally with a bisphosphonate (alendronate) at different doses. Given a 1% precision error of spinal BMD measurements by dual-energy X ray absorptiometry, a 3% increase in BMD (bold vertical line) is needed to establish that the treatment is effective in a single patient. By setting the cut-off limit for the decrease in urinary NTX after 3 months of treatment (bold horizontal line) at –30%, the assessment of bone markers may allow identification as early as 3 months of most patients who will respond to treatment in terms of spinal BMD gain after 24 months, with only 7% false negatives (i.e. patients demonstrating a significant gain of bone mass after 24 months despite a lower than 30% decrease in urinary NTX after 3 months) and 4% false positives (patients in whom urinary NTX decreased by more than 30% after 3 months without increase in spinal BMD after 24 months). Adapted from Garnero *et al.* (1994c).

calcin. Unresolved questions include the volume of distribution of osteocalcin, its concentration in various compartments of bone (cortical versus trabecular) and the relative fraction of newly synthesized osteocalcin incorporated into the matrix and released into the circulation, which may vary in some diseases. The measurement of bone alkaline phosphatase with specific monoclonal antibodies and perhaps the assay of procollagen extension peptides and of other non-collagenous bone-related proteins will allow a more precise assessment of the complex osteoblastic dysfunction which is osteoporosis.

Finding a sensitive and specific marker of resorption is a challenge because most constituents of bone matrix are likely to be degraded into minute peptides during osteoclastic bone resorption. The measurement of pyridinium crosslinks and some of its related peptides is the most tangible improvement in this area. The use of well-characterized immunoassays will improve the assessment of the level of bone resorption in patients with osteoporosis. It should be remembered, however, that circulating markers reflect the activity of the whole skeleton, including cortical and trabecular bone, and depend on both the number and the activity of bone cells. Conversely, bone histomorphometry is limited to a small area of the trabecular envelope but allows detection of a specific defect at the cellular level. These differences should be kept in mind, as there is growing evidence that bone mass and bone turnover of osteoporotic patients before and during treatment vary in different appendicular/axial and cortical/trabecular compartments.

Therefore, biochemical markers, bone histomorphometry and bone densitometry should be seen as complementary techniques for the experimental investigation of osteoporosis. From a clinical point of view, bone densitometry and bone markers are likely to be widely used in the diagnosis and follow-up of osteoporotic patients.

NOTE IN PROOF

This chapter was written in May 1996 and reflects the state of research at that time.

REFERENCES

Akesson, K., Vergnaud, P., Gineyts, E., Delmas, P.D. and Obrant, K. (1993) Impairment of bone turnover in elderly women with hip fracture. *Calcif Tissue Int* **53**: 162–9.

Bataille, R., Delmas, P. and Sany, J. (1987) Serum bone gla-protein in multiple myeloma. *Cancer* **59**: 329–34.

Beardsworth, L.J., Eyer, D.R. and Dickson, I.R. (1990) Changes with age in the urinary excretion of lysyl- and hydroxylysylpyridinoline, two new markers of bone collagen turnover. *J Bone Miner Res* **5**: 671–6.

Black, D., Duncan, A. and Robins, S.P. (1988) Quantitative analysis of the pyridinium crosslinks of collagen in urine using ion-paired reversed-phase high-performance liquid chromatography. *Anal Biochem* **169**: 197–203.

Body, J.J. and Delmas, P.D. (1992) Urinary pyridinium cross-links as markers of bone resorption in tumor-associated hypercalcemia. *J Clin Endocrinol Metab* **74**(3): 471–5.

Bonde, H., Quist, P., Fidelins, C., Riss, B.J. and Christiansen, C. (1994) Immunoassay for quantifying type I collagen degradation products in urine evaluated. *Clin Chem* **40**: 2022–5.

Brown, J.P., Delmas, P.D., Malval, L. *et al.* (1984) Serum bone Gla-protein: a specific marker for bone formation in postmenopausal osteoporosis. *Lancet* **i**: 1091–3.

Brown, J.P., Delmas, P.D., Arlot, M. *et al.* (1987) Active bone turnover of the cortico-endosteal envelope in postmenopausal osteoporosis. *J Clin Endocrinol Metab* **64**: 954–9.

Charles, P., Poser, J.W., Mosekilde, L. and Jensen, F.T. (1985) Estimation of bone turnover evaluated by 47 calcium kinetics. Efficiency of serum bone gamma-carboxyglutamic acid containing protein, serum alkaline phosphatase and urinary hydroxyproline excretion. *J Clin Invest* **76**: 2254–8.

Cheung, C.K., Panesar, N.S., Haines, C., Masarei, J. and Swaminathan, R. (1995) Immunoassay of tartrate-resistant acid phosphatase in serum. *Clin Chem* **41**: 679–86.

Civitelli, R., Gonnelli, S., Zacchei, F. *et al.* (1988) Bone turnover in postmenopausal osteoporosis. Effect of calcitonin treatment. *J Clin Invest* **82**: 1268–74.

Colwell, A., Russell, R.G.G. and Eastell, R. (1993) Factors affecting the assay of urinary 3-hydroxy pyridinium crosslinks of collagen as markers of bone resorption. *Eur J Clin Invest* **23**: 341–9.

Crilly, R.G., Jones, M.M., Horsman, A. *et al.* (1980) Rise in plasma alkaline phosphatase at the menopause. *Clin Sci* **53**: 341–2.

Delmas, P.D. (1988) Biochemical markers of bone turnover in osteoporosis. In: *Osteoporosis: Etiology, Diagnosis and Management*, (eds Riggs, B.L. and Melton III, L.J.), Raven Press, New York, p. 297.

Delmas, P.D. (1990) Biochemical markers of bone turnover for the clinical assessment of metabolic disease. *Endocrinol Metab Clin North Am* **19**(1): 1–18.

Delmas, P.D., Stenner, D., Wahner, H.W. *et al.* (1983a) Serum bone gla-protein increases with aging in normal women: implications for the mechanism of age-related bone loss. *J Clin Invest* **71**: 1316–21.

Delmas, P.D., Wilson, D.M., Mann, K.G. *et al.* (1983b) Effect of renal function on plasma levels of bone gla-protein. *J Clin Endocrinol Metab* **57**: 1028–30.

Delmas, P.D., Malaval, L., Arlot, M.E. and Meunier, P.J. (1985) Serum bone gla-protein compared to bone histomorphometry in endocrine diseases. *Bone* **6**: 329–41.

Delmas, P.D., Demiaux, B., Malaval, L. *et al.* (1986) Serum bone gla-protein (osteocalcin) in primary hyperparathyroidism and in malignant hypercalcemia. Comparison with bone histomorphometry. *J Clin Invest* **77**: 985–91.

Delmas, P.D., Christiansen, C., Mann, K.G. and Price, P.A. (1990) Bone gla-protein (osteocalcin) assay standardization report. *J Bone Miner Res* **1**: 5–11.

Delmas, P.D., Schlemmer, A., Gineyts, E., Riis, B. and Christiansen, C. (1991) Urinary excretion of pyridinoline crosslinks correlates with bone turnover measured on iliac crest biopsy in patients with vertebral osteoporosis. *J Bone Miner Res* **6**: 639–44.

Delmi, M., Rapin, C.H., Bengoa, J.M. *et al.* (1990) Dietary supplementation in elderly patients with fractured neck of femur. *Lancet* **335**: 1013–16.

Duda, R.J., O'Brien, J.F., Katzmann, J.A. *et al.* (1988) Concurrent assays of circulating bone gla-protein and bone alkaline phosphatase: effects of sex, age, and metabolic bone disease. *J Clin Endocrinol Metab* **66**: 951–7.

Eastell, R., Delmas, P.D., Hodgson, S.F. *et al.* (1988) Bone formation rate in older normal women: concurrent assessment with bone histomorphometry, calcium kinetics and biochemical markers. *J Clin Endocrinol Metab* **67**: 741–8.

Eastell, R., Hampton, L. and Colwell, A. (1990) Urinary collagen crosslinks are highly correlated with radio isotopic measurements of bone resorption. Proceedings of the Third International Symposium on Osteoporosis, (eds Christiansen, C. and Overgaard, K.), Osteopress, Aalborg, pp. 469–70.

Eastell, R., Calvo, M.S., Burritt, M.F. *et al.* (1992) Abnormalities in circadian patterns of bone resorption and renal calcium conservation in type I osteoporosis. *J Clin Endocrinol Metab* **74**: 487–94.

Ebeling, P.R., Peterson, J.M. and Riggs, B.L. (1992) Utility of type I procollagen propeptide assays for assessing abnormalities in metabolic bone diseases. *J Bone Miner Res* **7**: 243–50.

Eyre, D.R. (1987) Collagen crosslinking aminoacids. *Methods Enzymol* **144**: 115–39.

Eyre, D.R., Koob, T.J. and Van Ness, K.P. (1984) Quantitation of hydroxypyridinium crosslinks in collagen by high-performance liquid chromatography. *Anal Biochem* **137**: 380–8.

Eyre, D.R., Dickson, I.R. and Van Ness, K.P. (1988) Collagen cross-linking in human bone and articular cartilage. Age-related changes in the content of mature hydroxypyridinium residues. *Biochem J* **252**: 495–500.

Farley, J.R., Chesnut, C.J. and Baylink, D.J. (1981) Improved method for quantitative determination in serum alkaline phosphatase of skeletal origin. *Clin Chem* **27**: 2002–7.

Fishman, W.H. and Green, S. (1967) Automated differential isoenzyme analysis. I. L-Phenylalanine-sensitive isoenzymes of human serum alkaline phosphatase. *Enzymologia* **33**: 88–99.

Garnero, P. and Delmas, P.D. (1993) Assessment of the serum levels of bone alkaline phosphatase with a new immunoradiometric assay in patients with metabolic bone disease. *J Clin Endocrinol Metab* **77**(4): 1046–53.

Garnero, P., Grimaux, M., Demiaux, B. *et al.* (1992) Measurement of serum osteocalcin with a human-specific two-site immunoradiometric assay. *J Bone Miner Res* **12**: 1389–98.

Garnero, P., Grimaux, M., Seguin, P. and Delmas, P.D. (1994a) Characterization of immunoreactive forms of human osteocalcin generated in vivo and in vitro. *J Bone Miner Res* **9**(2): 255–64.

Garnero, P., Gineyts, E., Riou, J.P. and Delmas, P.D. (1994b) Assessment of bone resorption with a new marker of collagen degradation in patients with metabolic bone disease. *J Clin Endocrinol Metab* **3**: 780–5.

Garnero, P., Shih, W.J., Gineyts, E., Karpf, D.B. and Delmas, P.D. (1994c) Comparison of new biochemical markers of bone turnover in late postmenopausal osteoporotic women in response to alendronate treatment. *J Clin Endocrinol Metab* **79**: 1693–700.

Garnero, P., Hausher, E., Chapuy, M.C. *et al.* (1996) Markers of bone resorption predict hip fracture risk in elderly women? The EPIDOS prospective study. *J Bone Miner Res* **11**: 1531–8.

Garnero, P., Sornay-Rendu, E., Chapuy, M.C. and Delmas, P.D. (1996) Increased bone turnover in late postmenopausal women is a major determinant of osteoporosis. *J Bone Miner Res* **11**: 337–49.

Garrel, D.R., Delmas, P.D., Welsh, C. *et al.* (1988) Effect of moderate physical training on prednisone-induced protein wasting: a study of whole bone and bone protein metabolism. *Metabolism* **37**: 257–62.

Gomez, B., Haugen, S., Ardakani, S. *et al.* (1995) Monoclonal antibody for measuring bone-specific alkaline phosphatase in serum. *Clin Chem* **41**: 1560–6.

Gundberg, C. and Weinstein, R.S. (1986) Multiple immunoreactive forms in uremic serum. *J Clin Invest* **77**: 1762–7.

Hansen, M.A., Kirsten, O. Riss, B.J. and Christiansen, C. (1991) Role of peak bone mass and bone loss in postmenopausal osteoporosis: 12 years study. *Br Med J* **303**: 961–4.

Hanson, D.A., Weiss, M.A.E., Bollen, A.M. *et al.* (1992) A specific immunoassay for monitoring human bone resorption: quantitation of type I collagen cross-linked N-telopeptides in urine. *J Bone Miner Res* **7**: 1251–8.

Harvey, R.D., McHardy, K.C. and Reid, I.W. (1991) Measurement of bone collagen degradation in hyperthyroidism and during thyroxine replacement therapy using pyridinium cross-links as specific urinary markers. *J Clin Endocrinol Metab* **72**(6): 1189–94.

Hassager, C., Ristelli, J., Ristelli, L., Jensen, S.B. and Christiansen, C. (1992) Diurnal variation in serum markers of type I collagen synthesis and degradation in healthy premenopausal women. *J Bone Miner Res* **7**: 1307–11.

Hassager, C., Fabbri-Mabelli, G. and Christiansen, C. (1993) The effect of the menopause and hormone replacement therapy on serum carboxyterminal propeptide of type I collagen. *Osteoporosis Int* **3**: 50–2.

Hassager, C., Jensen, L.T., Podenphant, J.,

Thomsen, K. and Christiansen, C. (1994) The carboxy-terminal pyridinoline cross-linked telopeptide of type I collagen in serum as a marker of bone resorption: the effect of nandrolone decanoate and hormone replacement therapy. *Calcif Tissue Int* **54**: 30–3.

Hassling, C., Eriksen, E.F., Melkko, J. *et al.* (1991) Effects of a combined estrogen-gestagen regimen on serum levels of the carboxy-terminal propeptide of human type I procollagen in osteoporosis. *J Bone Miner Res* **6**: 1295–300.

Hill, C.S. and Wolfert, R.L. (1990) The preparation of monoclonal antibodies which react preferentially with human bone alkaline phosphatase and not liver alkaline phosphatase. *Clin Chim Acta* **186**: 315–20.

Hodges, S.J., Pilkington, M.J., Stam, T.C.B. *et al.* (1991) Depressed levels of circulating menaquinones in patients with osteoporotic fractures of the spine and femoral neck. *Bone* **12**: 387–89.

Johansen, J.S., Riss, B.J., Delmas, P.D. *et al.* (1988) Plasma BGP: an indicator of spontaneous bone loss and effect of estrogen treatment in postmenopausal women. *Eur J Clin Invest* **18**: 191–5.

Jones, G., Nguyen, T., Kelly, P.J. and Eisman, J.A. (1994) Progressive loss of bone in the femoral neck in elderly people: longitudinal findings from the Dubbo osteoporosis epidemiology study. *Br Med J* **309**: 691–5.

Kivirikko, K.I. (1983) Excretion of urinary hydroxyproline peptide in the assessment of bone collagen deposition and resorption. In: *Clinical Disorders of Bone and Mineral Metabolism*, (eds Frame, B. and Potts, J.T. Jr), Excerpta Medica, Amsterdam, pp. 105–7.

Knapen, M.H.J., Hamulyak, K. and Vermeer, C. (1989) The effect of vitamin K supplemention on circulating osteocalcin (bone gla protein) and urinary calcium excretion. *Ann Intern Med* **111**: 1001–5.

Kraenzlin, M., Lau, K.H.W. and Liang, L. (1990) Development of an immunoassay for human serum osteoclastic tartrate-resistant acid phosphatase. *J Clin Endocrinol Metab* **71**: 442–51.

Krane, S.M. and Simon, L.S. (1987) Metabolic consequences of bone turnover in Paget's disease of bone. *Clin Orthop* **217**: 26–36.

Krane, S.M., Kantrowitz, F.G., Byrne, M., Pinnel, S.R. and Singer, F.R. (1977) Urinary excretion of hydroxylysine and its glycosides as an index of collagen degradation. *J Clin Invest* **59**: 819–27.

Li, C.Y., Chuda, R.A., Lam, W.K.W. *et al.* (1973) Acid phosphatase in human plasma. *J Lab Clin Med* **82**: 446–60.

Lian, J.B. and Gundberg, C.M. (1988) Osteocalcin. Biochemical considerations and clinical applications. *Clin Orthop Rel Res* **226**: 267–91.

Linkhart, S.G., Linkhart, T.A., Taylor, A.K. *et al.* (1993) Synthetic peptide-based immunoassay for amino-terminal propeptide of type I procollagen: application for evalation of bone formation. *Clin Chem* **39**: 2254–8.

Lips, P., Courpron, P. and Meunier, P.J. (1978) Mean wall thickness of trabecular bone packets in the human iliac crest: changes with age. *Calcif Tissue Res* **26**: 13–17.

Lowry, M., Hall, D.E. and Brosnan, J.J. (1985) Hydroxyproline metabolism by the rat kidney: distribution of renal enzymes of hydroxyproline catabolism and renal conversion of hydroxyproline to glycine and serine. *Metabolism* **39**: 955.

Minkin, C. (1982) Bone acid phosphatase: tartrate-resistant acid phosphatase as a marker of osteoclast function. *Calcif Tissue Int* **34**: 285–90.

Moro, L., Mucelli, R.S.P., Gazzarrini, C. *et al.* (1988) Urinary β-1-galactosyl-O-hydroxylysine (GH) as a marker of collagen turnover of bone. *Calcif Tissue Int* **42**: 87–90.

Moss, D.W. (1982) Alkaline phosphatase isoenzymes. *Clin Chem* **28**: 2007–16.

Parfitt, A.M., Mathews, C.H.E., Villanueva, A.R. *et al.* (1983) Relationship between surface, volume and thickness of iliac trabecular bone in aging and in osteoporosis. *J Clin Invest* **72**: 1396.

Parfitt, A.M., Simon, L.S., Vilanueva, A.R. *et al.* (1987) Procollagen type I carboxy-terminal extension peptide in serum as a marker of collagen biosynthesis in bone. Correlation with iliac bone formation rates and comparison with total alkaline phosphatase. *J Bone Miner Res* **2**: 427–36.

Piedra, C., Torres, R., Rapado, A. *et al.* (1989) Serum tartrate resistant acid phosphatase and bone mineral content in postmenopausal osteoporosis. *Calcif Tissue Int* **45**: 58–60.

Plantalech, L., Guillaumont, M., Leclerq, M. and Delmas, P.D. (1991) Impaired carboxylation of serum osteocalcin in elderly women. *J Bone Miner Res* **6**: 1211–16.

Podenphant, J., Johansen, J.S., Thomsen, K. *et al.* (1987) Bone turnover in spinal osteoporosis. *J Bone Miner Res* **2**: 497–503.

Price, P.A., Parthemore, J.G. and Deftos, L.J. (1980) New biochemical marker for bone metabolism. *J Clin Invest* **66**: 878–83.

Price, P.A., Williamson, M.K. and Lothringer, J.W. (1981) Origin of vitamin K-dependent bone protein found in plasma and its clearance by kidney and bone. *J Biol Chem* **256**: 12760–6.

Prockop, O.J. and Kivirikko, K.I. (1968) Hydroxyproline and the metabolism of collagen. In: *Treatise on Collagen*, (ed. Gould, B.S.), Academic Press, New York, pp. 215–46.

Prockop, O.J., Kivirikko, K.I., Tuderman, K. *et al.* (1979) The biosynthesis of collagen and its disorders. *N Engl J Med* **301**: 13–23.

Reid, I.R., Chapman, G.E., Fraser, T.R.C. *et al.* (1986) Low serum osteocalcin levels in glucocorticoid-treated asthmatics. *J Clin Endocrinol Metab* **2**: 379–83.

Riis, S.B.J., Hansen, A.M., Jensen, K. Overgaard, K. and Christiansen, C. (1996) Low bone mass and fast rate of bone loss at menopause-equal risk factors for future fracture. A 15 year follow-up study. *Bone* **19**: 9–12.

Ristelli, J., Elomaa, I., Niemi, S., Novamo, A. and Ristelli, L. (1993) Radioimmunoassay for the pyridinoline cross-linked carboxy-terminal telopeptide of type I collagen: a new serum marker of bone collagen degradation. *Clin Chem* **39**: 635–40.

Robins, S.P., Black, D., Paterson, C.R. *et al.* (1991) Evaluation of urinary hydroxypyridinium crosslink measurements as resorption markers in metabolic bone disease. *Eur J Clin Invest* **21**: 310–15.

Robins, S.P., Woitge, H., Hesley, R. *et al.* (1994) Direct, enzyme-linked immunoassay for urinary deoxypyridinoline as a specific marker for measuring bone resorption. *J Bone Miner Res* **9**: 1643–9.

Schlemmer, A., Hassager, C., Jensen, S.B. and Christiansen, C. (1992) Marked diurnal variation in urinary excretion of pyridinium crosslinks in premenopausal women. *J Clin Endocrinol Metab* **74**: 476–80.

Seibel, M.J., Gartenberg, F., Silverberg, S.J. *et al.* (1992) Urinary hydroxypyridinium crosslinks of collagen in primary hyperparathyroidism. *J Clin Endocrinol Metab* **74**(3): 481–6.

Seyedin, S., Zuk, R., Kung, V., Daniloff, Y. and Shepard, K. (1993) An immunoassay to urinary pyridinoline: the new marker of bone resorption. *J Bone Miner Res* **8**: 635–42.

Slemenda, C., Hui, S.L., Longcope, C. *et al.* (1987) Sex steroids and bone mass. A study of changes about the time of menopause. *J Clin Invest* **80**: 1261–9.

Smedsrod, B., Melkko, J., Ristelli, L. and Ristelli, J. (1990) Circulating C-terminal propeptide of type I procollagen is cleared mainly via the mannose receptor in liver endothelial cells. *Biochem J* **271**: 345–50.

Stepán, J.J., Silinkova-Malkova, E., Havrenek, T. *et al.* (1983) Relationship of plasma tartrate-resistant acid phosphatase to the bone isoenzyme of serum alkaline phosphatase in hyperparathyroidism. *Clin Chim Acta* **133**: 189–200.

Stepán, J.J., Pospichal, J., Presl, J. *et al.* (1987) Bone loss and biochemical indices of bone remodeling in surgically induced postmenopausal women. *Bone* **8**: 279–84.

Szulc, P., Chapuy, M.C., Meunier, P.J. and Delmas, P.D. (1993) Serum undercarboxylated osteocalcin is a marker of the risk of hip fracture in elderly women. *J Clin Invest* **91**: 1769–74.

Szulc, P., Chapuy, M.C., Meunier, P.J. and Delmas, P.D. (1996) Serum undercarboxylated osteocalcin is a marker of the risk of hip fracture: a three year follow-up study. *Bone* **5**: 487–8.

Taylor, A.K., Linkart, S., Mohan, S. *et al.* (1990) Multiple osteocalcin fragments in human urine and serum as detected by a midmolecule osteocalcin radioimmunoassay. *J Clin Endocrinol Metab* **70**: 467–72.

Thompson, S.P., White, D.A., Hosking, D.J., Wilton, T.J. and Pawley, E. (1989) Changes in osteocalcin after femoral neck fracture. *Ann Clin Biochem* **26**: 487–91.

Thomsen, K., Rodbro, P. and Christiansen, C. (1987) Bone turnover determined by urinary excretion of [99m TC] disphosphonate in the prediction of postmenopausal bone loss. *Bone Mineral* **2**: 125–31.

Tracy, R.P., Andrianorivo, A., Riggs, B.L. and Mann, K.G. (1990) Comparison of monoclonal and polyclonal antibody-based immunoassays for osteocalcin. A study of sources of variation in assay results. *J Bone Miner Res* **5**: 451–61.

Uebelhart, D., Gineyts, E., Chapuy, M.C. and Delmas, P.D. (1990) Urinary excretion of pyridinium crosslinks: a new marker of bone resorption in metabolic bone disease. *Bone Mineral* **8**: 87–96.

Uebelhart, D., Schlemmer, A., Johansen, J. *et al.* (1991) Effect of menopause and hormone replacement therapy on the urinary excretion of pyridinium crosslinks. *J Clin Endocrinol Metab* **72:** 367–73.

BONE MASS MEASUREMENTS 7

B. Lees, L.M. Banks and J.C. Stevenson

INTRODUCTION

Osteoporosis is generally defined as a disease characterized by low bone mass and microarchitectural deterioration of bone tissue leading to enhanced bone fragility and a consequent increase in fracture risk (Consensus Development Conference, 1991). The development of safe and non-invasive techniques for the measurement of bone mass has enabled clinicians to identify those individuals most at risk of developing osteoporosis before a fracture actually occurs.

This chapter describes the main techniques currently in use for the measurement of bone mass in both clinical and research settings. However, although bone mass is strongly correlated with compressive strength, there is a considerable overlap in bone density values between fracture and non-fracture cases, which indicates that other factors besides bone mass contribute to bone fragility. Trauma is obviously a major factor in determining fracture but other factors such as bone quality and architecture are also important and therefore the development of newer techniques which provide additional information on the structure and quality of bone may assist in improving the accuracy of fracture prediction in the future.

WHICH BONE SHOULD BE MEASURED?

The skeleton is composed of two types of bone, cortical and trabecular. Cortical bone forms the dense outer covering of all bones but is primarily found in the shafts of the long bones. It has well-defined periosteal and endosteal surfaces. Trabecular bone is contained within the cortical shell and has a branching lattice-like structure of small struts of bone separated by fatty or haematologenous marrow. This trabecular structure provides a large surface area to volume ratio and therefore increases the facility for bone turnover since this process occurs on the surface of bone. Although the total skeleton is composed of 80% cortical and 20% trabecular bone, the ratio of each type of bone varies throughout the skeleton and at different locations within the same bone (Table 7.1). Since trabecular bone has a potentially higher metabolic activity than cortical bone, techniques which measure trabecular bone alone or integral (cortical and trabecular) bone at locations where the trabecular/cortical ratio is high may be more sensitive to changes in bone mass than techniques that measure at more cortical sites. Additionally techniques that measure bone mass at sites which have a high fracture incidence, such as the distal forearm, spine and proximal femur, may provide the most clinically relevant information. For these reasons, techniques for measuring bone mass have been developed which measure at skeletal sites of high trabecular bone content, high fracture incidence or both.

Osteoporosis. Edited by John C. Stevenson and Robert Lindsay. Published in 1998 by Chapman & Hall, London.
ISBN 0 412 48870 1

Table 7.1 Percentage of cortical/trabecular bone at various skeletal sites using different techniques

Region	*Percentage of cortical/trabecular bone*
QCT	
Forearm	*0/100
Single-energy spine	*0/100
Dual-energy spine	*0/100
SPA/SXA	
Midradius	95/5
Distal third radius	75/25
Ultradistal radius	60/40
Os calcis	5/95
DPA/DXA	
Lumbar spine AP	50/50
Lumbar spine lateral	*10/90
Proximal femur	60/40
Total body	80/20
Ultrasound	
Os calcis	5/95
Photodensitometry	
Phalanx	60/40

*Depends on region of interest.

RADIOGRAPHS

Photodensitometry (PD) is the oldest quantitative technique for the evaluation of bone mass whereby the optical density of X-ray films of bone is measured. One of the first investigators to attempt to quantify bone on X-rays was Price in 1901 who used dental radiographs (Price, 1901). Current PD techniques tend to use X-rays of the phalanges. A standard step wedge, usually made of aluminium, is exposed alongside the bone to minimize errors due to variations in soft tissue thickness, voltage and film characteristics (Mack *et al.*, 1939; Omnell, 1957; Doyle, 1961; Vose *et al.*, 1964; Morgan *et al.*, 1967; Colbert *et al.*, 1970; Meema and Meema, 1972). However, PD suffers from poor accuracy and reproducibility and so has had limited use. Recently an improved method of PD has been described which utilizes a microdensitometer which scans the radiograph with a light beam and computes optical density and thus avoids the subjectivity of previous PD techniques, resulting in improvements in accuracy and precision error (Colbert and Bachtell, 1981). In one study this improved PD technique was able to predict low bone mass in the spine and femoral neck, as measured by dual photon absorptiometry, with a sensitivity of 90% and 82% respectively (Cosman *et al.*, 1991).

Semiquantitative measurements of bone mass can be obtained using the technique of radiogrammetry, which involves the measurement of the cortical thickness in the peripheral skeleton. The metacarpal shafts are a classic measurement site where the cortical thickness is measured from a hand X-ray using callipers (Barnett and Nordin, 1960). The proximal end of the radius (Meema and Meema, 1963) and shaft of the femur (Garn *et al.*, 1963) have also been used as measurement sites. One of the drawbacks of radiogrammetry is that it only gives information on the dimensions of bones and not on their intracortical porosity. Other drawbacks are that the reproducibility is poor and that the values obtained from the metacarpals, for example, may have little relevance to the hip and spine (Aitken, 1984; Sorenson and Cameron, 1987; Stevenson *et al.*, 1987), more clinically important sites of fracture. Despite its limitations, radiogrammetry was for many years the method of choice for assessing bone status and indeed, age-related bone loss in normal women has been demonstrated using this technique (Barnett and Nordin, 1960; Meema, 1962).

Singh (Singh *et al.*, 1970) developed a method which utilized the fact that trabeculae can be identified on X-rays of the spine and hip. The radioigraphic density (compared with a standard) was used to grade the change of the trabecular pattern of the upper end of the femur with increasing age and decreasing bone mass and thus produce an index of osteoporosis. The problem with this grading system is that it is highly subjective and any variations in radiographic technique may produce artefacts.

Plain radiographs are not sensitive enough to detect early osteoporosis because they only show recognizable bone loss when it is very advanced (Gordan and Vaughan, 1976), but they are often essential in the diagnosis of fracture.

Spinal radiographs can be used for the measurement of vertebral height and therefore to assess vertebral deformity. The interest in spinal morphometric measurements has increased with the suggestion from the American Food and Drug Administration (FDA) that fracture data as well as bone density measurements may be required for demonstrating efficacy of therapies for the prevention of osteoporosis. There is still some controversy regarding the definition of vertebral fracture (Eastell *et al.*, 1991; Adami *et al.*, 1992; NOFWP, 1995). Recent advances in morphometry measurements include the development of new computer software for measuring spinal deformity on digitized X-rays (Banks and Read, 1993). Digitization improves the quality of the X-rays, which not only enables more precise morphometric measurements to be made but also increases the number of vertebrae available for measurement. The dedicated software takes measurements of the anterior, middle and posterior height of each vertebral body and accuracy and precision are improved when compared with the traditional methods (Banks and Read, 1992). The high-resolution images provided by the new fan-beam dual energy X-ray absorptiometers allow the measurement of spinal deformities although as yet, the image quality is not good enough to replace film-based vertebral fracture determination (Gowin *et al.*, 1995; Lang *et al.*, 1995).

SINGLE-PHOTON ABSORPTIOMETRY (SPA)

Single photon absorptiometry (SPA) was introduced by Cameron and Sorenson in 1963 to measure bone mineral content of the appendicular skeleton. A narrow collimated beam of monoenergetic radiation (generally from a 200 mCi source of ^{125}I which provides 35 KeV γ rays) is passed through a limb and the transmitted photons are detected by a NaI scintillator. The number of photons transmitted is inversely proportional to the quantity of bone mineral in the path of the beam and is calculated by reference to a standard curve. Differences in the attenuation of the beam in bone and soft tissue and in soft tissue alone are proportional to bone mineral if the composition and thickness of soft tissue surrounding bone are of constant uniform thickness. This is achieved by submerging the limb (often the forearm) in a water bath or water bag or tissue-equivalent gel. The results are expressed as g of ashed bone in a cross-sectional piece of bone 1 cm in axial length (g/cm) and referred to as bone mineral content (BMC). BMC is normalized by dividing by the bone diameter of the scanning site to obtain an 'areal' density or bone mineral density (BMD) expressed in g/cm^2.

Because SPA requires the measurement site to be surrounded by a known thickness of tissue-equivalent material, measurement is limited to the peripheral skeleton. The radius is generally used but measurements of the calcaneus, femur, humerus, finger and whole hand and foot have been made. A single pass of source and detector is sufficient for measurement of the radial shaft which is homogeneous cortical bone but for more irregular anatomical trabecular areas such as the distal radius, a rectilinear scan is required. One of the disadvantages of SPA is that it is dependent on careful positioning of bone site during subsequent scanning and this is why the midshaft of the radius was originally used. It is almost entirely cortical and therefore, although BMC does not change rapidly with position, this also means it is not a very sensitive area for monitoring skeletal loss (Mazess, 1984). A more sensitive region is the distal third location where the proportion of trabecular bone is greater than in the midshaft (Lindsay, 1988). The distal third site is defined as the point one-third of the length of the ulna (measuring from the distal to the proximal end). The ultradistal site which corresponds to the point where the radius and ulna are separated by 5 mm has an even greater proportion of trabecular bone and therefore has enhanced sensitivity for detecting early and rapid bone loss (Lindsay, 1988).

Recently developed equipment uses an automatic search procedure to locate a fixed gap (8 mm) between the radius and the ulna. Several scans are then performed in a rectilinear fashion, both proximal (predominantly cortical bone) and distal to this site (higher proportion of trabecular bone), averaging the results at each site for the final measurements.

Measurements of appendicular bone mineral content by SPA have been shown to predict future forearm (Hui *et al.*, 1988), spine (Ross *et al.*, 1988), hip (Cummings *et al.*, 1990) and most appendicular (Seeley *et al.*, 1990) fractures. However, SPA has been criticized because although there is a correlation between bone density in the peripheral and central skeleton (Ott *et al.*, 1987; Stevenson *et al.*, 1987) the association is not strong enough to predict central bone mass from peripheral measurements in an individual (Grubb *et al.*, 1984; Stevenson *et al.*, 1987) and the spine and hip are more clinically important sites in terms of osteoporosis. A major disadvantage with SPA is that the source requires renewal every six months as the half-life of ^{125}I is approximately 60 days. However, the technique is well tolerated by patients, has good precision and accuracy (Cameron *et al.*, 1986), is rapid and has a low radiation dose (Table 7.2).

SINGLE-ENERGY X-RAY ABSOPTIOMETRY (SXA)

Recently single-energy X-ray absorptiometry (SXA) has been introduced for the assessment of bone density in the forearm. SXA utilizes an X-ray tube instead of a radionuclide source to provide the photon beam, thus eliminating the problem of source decay encountered with SPA. This should have advantages in terms of reduced running costs and improvement in the long-term precision of this technique. The region of interest is automatically determined from the point at which the radius and ulna are separated by 8 mm and the scanning proceeds in a distal to proximal direction. Scans of the distal and ultradistal forearm can be performed in under five minutes with a low radiation dose and low precision error (Kelly *et al.*, 1994). The recent development of peripheral dual-energy X-ray absorptiometry (p-DXA) for measurement of the forearm will eliminate the need for the water bath required by SPA and SXA to correct for soft tissue variations. Measurements can be performed at the ultradistal radius and ulna and at a more proximal site. However, as with SPA, measurements of bone density in the forearm by SXA and p-DXA may have a limited predictive value for BMD in the central skeleton.

DUAL-PHOTON ABSORPTIOMETRY (DPA)

The development of dual-photon absorptiometry (DPA) was a great step forwards in the measurement of bone mass as it allowed measurements to be performed in the clinically important sites of the lumbar spine and the proximal femur. However, DPA has now been largely superseded by dual-energy X-ray absorptiometry (DXA).

DPA is a modification of SPA and makes use of a radionuclide source that emits photons at two energy levels (Madsen *et al.*, 1976; Krolner and Nielsen, 1980). ^{153}Gd is a commonly used source because of its optimal energies at 44 and 100 KeV. The use of two energies eliminates the need to have a constant soft tissue thickness across the scanning path since the surrounding soft tissue is accounted for by calculating thickness of soft tissue and bone mineral separately from the attenuation of the two energies. This allows the measurement of deeper structures such as the spine and femur.

The patient lies on a purpose-built couch which houses the radiation source. The detector (in synchronization with the source) passes over the region of interest in a rectilinear fashion, picking up the transmitted energy point by point. The ratio of the attenuation of the two energies is used to calculate BMC values from calibration curves (originally derived from standards of ashed bone). The resulting series of transverse profiles are used to compile an image which is then used to select regions of interest. Usually L2–L4 of the lumbar spine is selected and the femoral neck, Ward's triangle and trochanteric regions of the proximal femur. The BMC is divided by the area measured and the result expressed as an 'areal' density (g/cm^2) and therefore, as with SPA, this is not a true volumetric density.

The accuracy of DPA and DXA BMD measurements may be influenced by an uneven fat distribution (Tothill *et al.*, 1989; Tothill and Pye, 1992) and the precision and accuracy may be affected by degenerative changes in the spine (e.g. osteophytes) and vascular calcification (Orwoll *et al.*, 1990; Reid *et al.*, 1991; Banks *et al.*, 1994). As a consequence some investigators have suggested that in elderly patients and those with lumbar fractures it is preferable to measure the hip or the calcaneum rather than the spine (Kotzski *et al.*, 1993). Difficulties may also arise in the accurate measurement of soft tissue baselines which can vary by as much as 10%, causing errors of up to 20% in BMD measurements. Artefacts that may affect baseline measurements include ribs, calcification of the aorta, transverse processes and iliac crest (Mazess, 1984). A major disadvantage of DPA is that source renewal is required every 12–18 months (the half-life of ^{153}Gd is 240 days). This is not only costly but may affect the long-term precision (Lindsay *et al.*, 1987). The examination time is fairly long (Table 7.2) and this may limit its use in elderly or osteoporotic patients and its suitability for broad screening programmes.

The advantages of DPA for measuring bone density are its low radiation dose (Table 7.2), good precision (Wilson and Matson, 1977; Tothill *et al.*, 1983; LeBlanc *et al.*, 1986; Stevenson *et al.*, 1989; Lees and Stevenson, 1992) and accuracy (Wilson and Matson, 1977) and the BMD values give a reasonable separation between normals and osteoporotics (Mazess, 1984). A good correlation is found between the incidence of hip and spine fractures and the density measurement at those sites (Riggs *et al.*, 1981; Wasnich *et al.*, 1985) and a recent study using DXA demonstrated that low bone density in the hip is a better predictor of hip fracture than low bone density at other sites such as the forearm or the spine (Cummings *et al.*, 1993).

Table 7.2 Comparison of techniques for measuring BMD

Method	*Precision (%)*	*Accuracy (%)*	*Effective dose equivalent (μSv)*	*Average scan time (min)*
QCT				
Forearm	1–2	2–8	≈1	10
Spine				
Single-energy	2–4	5–15	≈60	15
Dual-energy	4–6	3–6	≈90	20
SPA				
Radius	1–2	4–6	<1	10
Os calcis	1–2	4–6	<1	15
SXA				
Radius	1	4–6	<1	4
DPA				
Lumbar spine	2–4	5–10	≈5	30
Proximal femur	3–5	5–10	≈3	30
Total body	2–3	2	≈3	90
DXA				
AP spine	1–2	4–8	≈1	5
Lateral spine	1–5	5–10	≈5	15
Proximal femur	1–3	4–8	≈1	5
Total body	1	2	≈3	10
Ultrasound				
Os calcis	1–4	?	Nil	3
Photodensitometry				
Phalanx/metacarpal	2	6	≈5	5
NAA				
Total body	2–4	5–8	≈10 000	30

DUAL-ENERGY X-RAY ABSORPTIOMETRY (DXA)

Dual-energy X-ray absorptiometry (DXA), which has now generally replaced DPA, is exactly the same in principle but makes use of a X-ray tube instead of a radionuclide source (Figure 7.1). The necessary pairs of effective energies are obtained by k-edge filtering using cerium or samarium (Mazess *et al.*, 1989) or by rapidly switching the generator potential (Stein *et al.*, 1987). The X-ray tube produces a higher radiation flux than the radioisotope source which allows the use of a smaller radiation source collimator, resulting in increased scanning speed, reduced radiation dose and better image resolution. Scanning speed is reduced from about 20 minutes with DPA to about five minutes with DXA. For a typical spine scan radiation dose is reduced from about 5 μSv with DPA to <1 μSv with DXA. Pixel size is reduced from 4.5 mm × 4.5 mm for a typical spine scan using DPA to 1.2 mm × 1.2 mm with DXA. Precision is increased by the improved spatial resolution of DXA and the stable X-ray tube which does not decrease in source strength with time (Lees and Stevenson, 1992). These

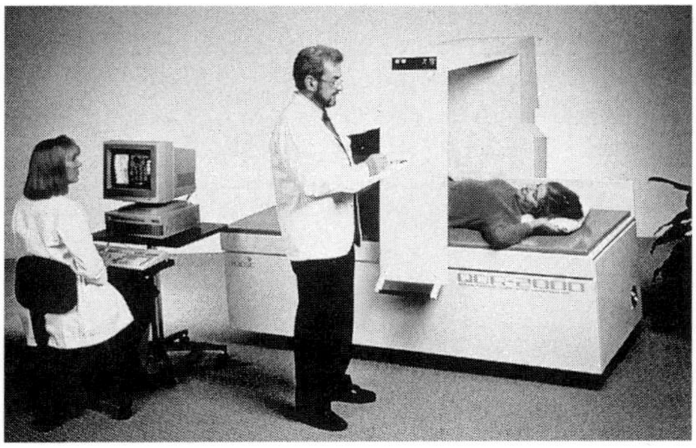

Figure 7.1 Dual-energy X-ray absorptiometer (DXA). This system (Hologic QDR-2000) uses a multiple fan-beam design with multiple channel detector array. The C arm design allows lateral scanning of the spine without patient repositioning. Courtesy of Hologic Inc.

improvements in precision have enhanced the ability to monitor BMD changes longitudinally in individual patients. As with DPA, DXA scans are usually performed on the lumbar spine and proximal femur (Figure 7.2).

For scans of the lumbar spine, the patient's legs are raised on a foam block 30 cm high to decrease the lumbar lordosis. This not only increases the ability to separate individual vertebrae on the image by optimizing the resolution of the disc spaces but it also decreases the variation in distance between the spine and the table top as the measured results are not completely independent of position in X-ray beam. With hip scanning, the foot is placed in a positioning brace with the leg abducted and rotated inwards. This procedure ensures that a reasonably constant position is achieved and that there is sufficient separation between the ischium and the femoral neck for analysis. The analysis software is highly automated, usually requiring minimal adjustment by the operator.

DXA BMD data are usually expressed as absolute BMD (g/cm^2) and these values may be expressed as a percentage compared to a sex-, age-, weight- and ethnic group-matched population. The BMD data may also be expressed as the number of standard deviations (SD) from the mean for young normals (T-score) and the number of SD from the mean of age-matched controls (Z-score). Recent World Health Organization guidelines suggest that a T-score of less than -1 be referred to as 'osteopenia' and a T-score of less than -2.5 be referred to as 'osteoporosis' (WHO Study Group, 1994).

Most DXA scanners have the ability to display and directly compare a patient's previous scan image with their current scan. This facility may help to reduce intra- and interoperator error and ensures that comparable regions of interest are selected for analysis.

There is a high correlation between DPA and DXA with correlations exceeding 0.95 in most cases, but differences in the absolute BMD (Wahner *et al.*, 1988; Lees and Stevenson, 1992). Similarly there is a high correlation in BMD values between different DXA instruments from different manufacturers but large differences in the absolute BMD values, resulting in variations of up to 20% (Reid *et al.*, 1990). The differences in BMD values between DXA instruments are due to differences in the bone mineral calibration, assumptions regarding marrow composition, bone edge detection algorithms and, particularly for proximal femur scans, differences in the definition of the regions of interest. The differences in absolute BMD values and the lack of standardization between instruments has led to the development of a geometrically defined, closely anthropomorphic spine phantom – the European Spine Phantom (ESP) (Kalender *et al.*, 1995) (Figure 7.3). This phantom is currently being evaluated for the calibration of DXA (Genant *et al.*, 1994) and quantitative computed tomography (QCT) instruments.

In addition to the standard spine and hip determinations, many DXA scanners have the capability of measuring BMD of the total body (Figure 7.4), rapidly (10–20 minutes versus 90 minutes with DPA) and with a

WYNN DIVISION OF
METABOLIC MEDICINE
National Heart and Lung Institute

PATIENT ID:	SCAN:	3.6z	22.09.94
NAME: S, F	ANALYSIS:	3.6z	22.09.94

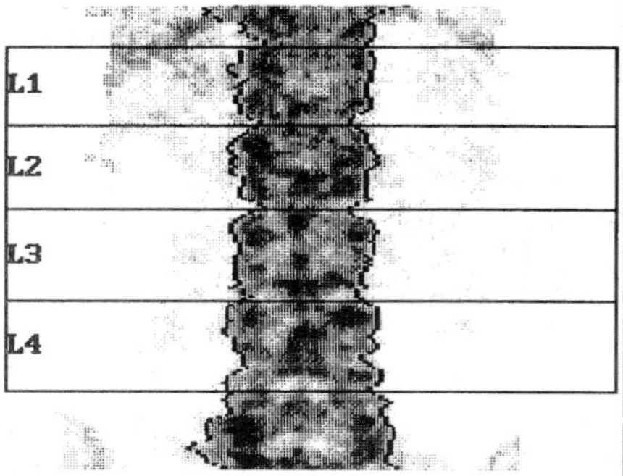

LUNAR®

IMAGE NOT FOR DIAGNOSIS

ID: **SCAN DATE: 22.09.94**

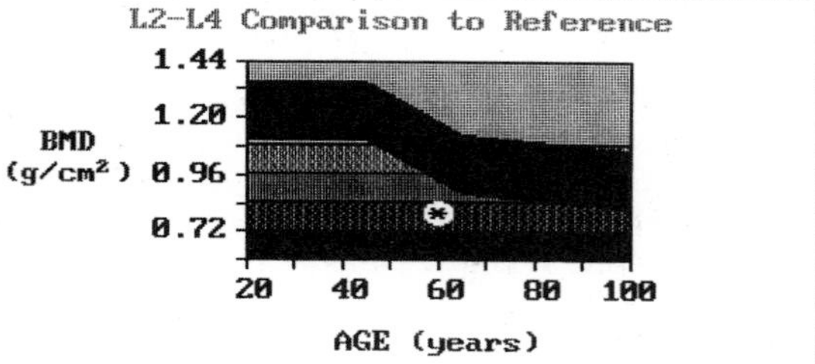

L2-L4 BMD (g/cm²)1	0.798 ± 0.01
L2-L4 % Young Adult2	66 ± 3
L2-L4 % Age Matched3	76 ± 3

Age (years).........	60	Large Standard......	272.43	Scan Mode.......	Medium
Sex.................	Female	Medium Standard.....	205.25	Scan Type...........	DPX
Weight (Kg).........	72.0	Small Standard......	144.28	Collimation (mm).....	1.68
Height (cm).........	169	Low keV Air (cps)...	667477	Sample Size (mm).....	1.2x 1.2
Ethnic..............	White	High keV Air (cps)..	441867	Current (uA).........	750
System..............	6254	Rvalue (%Fat).......	1.317(37.4)		

REGION	BMD[1] g/cm²	Young Adult[2] %	Young Adult[2] Z	Age Matched[3] %	Age Matched[3] Z
L1	0.743	66	-3.23	75	-2.02
L2	0.821	68	-3.16	78	-1.95
L3	0.804	67	-3.30	76	-2.09
L4	0.773	64	-3.56	73	-2.35
L1-L2	0.783	68	-3.06	78	-1.85
L1-L3	0.791	68	-3.16	77	-1.95
L1-L4	0.786	67	-3.29	76	-2.08
L2-L3	0.812	68	-3.23	77	-2.02
L2-L4	0.798	66	-3.35	76	-2.14
L3-L4	0.788	66	-3.44	75	-2.23

1 - See appendix E on precision and accuracy. Statistically 68% of repeat scans will fall within 1 SD.
2 - UK AP Spine Reference Population, Ages 20-45. See Appendices.
3 - Matched for Age, Weight (males 50-100kg; females 35-80kg), Ethnic.

Figure 7.2 (a) Printout of a DXA scan (Lunar DPX instrument) of the lumbar spine of a 60-year-old post-menopausal woman. Note that the BMD value for L2–L4 is more than 3SD below the young adult value.

WYNN DIVISION OF
METABOLIC MEDICINE
National Heart and Lung Institute

PATIENT ID:	SCAN:	3.6z	22.09.94
NAME: S, F	ANALYSIS:	3.6z	22.01.96

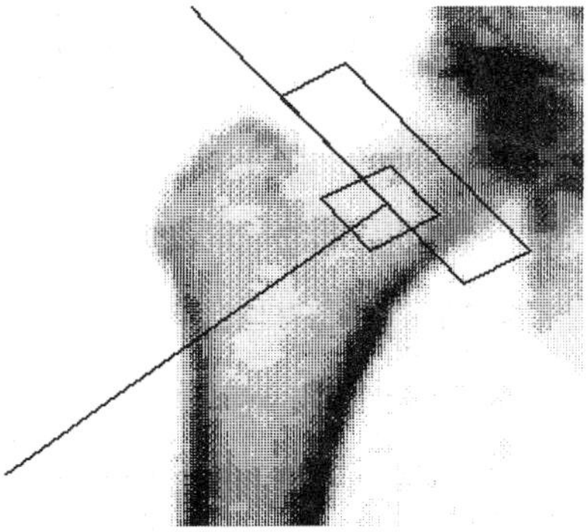

LUNAR®

IMAGE NOT FOR DIAGNOSIS

ID: SCAN DATE: 22.09.94

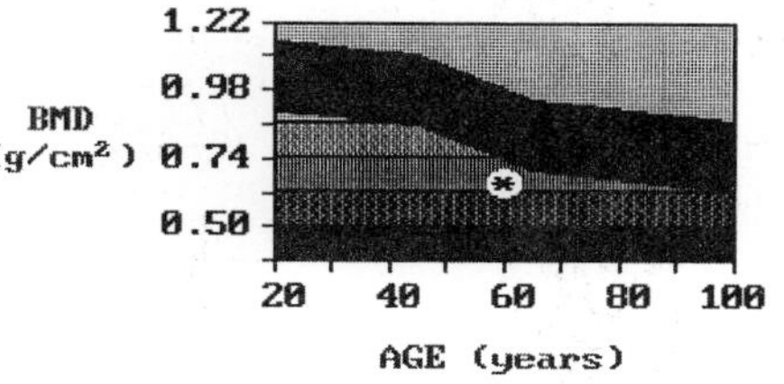

NECK BMD (g/cm²)1	0.657 ± 0.02
NECK % Young Adult2	67 ± 3
NECK % Age Matched3	77 ± 3

Age (years).........	60	Large Standard......	272.43	Scan Mode.......	Medium
Sex.................	Female	Medium Standard.....	205.25	Scan Type...........	DPX
Weight (Kg).........	72.0	Small Standard......	144.28	Collimation (mm).....	1.68
Height (cm).........	169	Low keV Air (cps)...	667477	Sample Size (mm).....	1.2x 1.2
Ethnic..............	White	High keV Air (cps)..	441867	Region height (mm)...	60.0
System..............	6254	Rvalue (%Fat).......	1.317(37.3)	Region width (mm)....	15.0
Side................	Right	Current (uA)........	750	Region angle (deg)...	55

NECK	: BMC[5] (grams)	= 3.16	AREA[5] (cm²)	= 4.82
WARDS	: BMC[5] (grams)	= 1.17	AREA[5] (cm²)	= 2.58
TROCH	: BMC[5] (grams)	= 8.73	AREA[5] (cm²)	= 13.68

REGION	BMD[1] g/cm²	Young Adult[2] %	Z	Age Matched[3] %	Z
NECK	0.657	67	-2.69	77	-1.62
WARDS	0.454	50	-3.51	63	-2.05
TROCH	0.638	81	-1.38	87	-0.89

1 - See appendix E on precision and accuracy. Statistically 68% of repeat scans will fall within 1 SD.
2 - UK Femur Reference Population, Ages 20-45. See Appendices.
3 - Matched for Age, Weight(males 50-100kg; females 35-80kg), Ethnic.
5 - Results for research purposes, not clinical use.

Figure 7.2 *continued* (b) Printout of a DXA scan (Lunar DPX instrument) of the proximal femur of a 60-year-old postmenopausal woman. Note that the BMD value for the femoral neck is more than 2.5 SD below the young adult value.

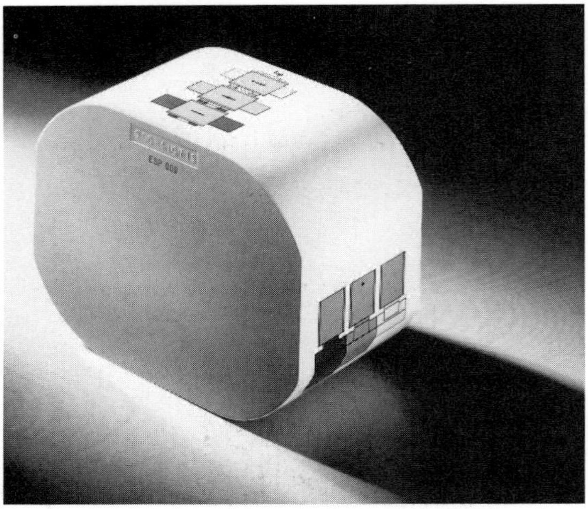

Figure 7.3 European Spine Phantom (ESP). This calibration standard for DXA and QCT instruments consists of three vertebral-shaped inserts of increasing bone mineral densities and thicknesses of cortical structure.

precision of <1% (Lees and Stevenson, 1992). These total body scans using dual-photon techniques provide information not only on bone mass but also on fat and lean tissue mass. Fat and lean tissue have different attenuation coefficients and therefore the relative amounts of fat and lean tissue can be calculated from the ratio of the attenuation coefficients in the pixels not containing bone (Mazess *et al.*, 1990). These data are then extrapolated over the entire body. The advantage of using DPA or DXA to measure body composition is that changes in the bone mineral component can be taken into account whereas some other methods of measuring body composition, such as hydrodensitometry, assume this to be a fixed entity (Heymsfield *et al.*, 1989). The correlations between measurements of total body bone mineral content and total body fat by dual-photon techniques and other methods such as neutron activation analysis, underwater weighing and total body ^{40}K are good (Heymsfield *et al.*, 1989; Haarbo *et al.*, 1991). A further advantage of measuring total body composition using DXA is that regional areas of interest on the total body scan can be selected for analysis (Ley *et al.*, 1992).

Advancements in the development of DXA software and high-resolution scanning permit selected regions of interest such as the forearm or calcaneus to be measured (Hagiwara *et al.*, 1994; Yamada *et al.*, 1995). The improvement in image quality has also allowed the measurement of hip biomechanical parameters such as 'hip axis length' which is defined as the distance along the femoral neck axis from the base of the greater trochanter to the inner pelvic brim. A recent study suggested that there is a relative risk of hip fracture of 1.8 per SD increase in hip axis length independent of hip BMD (Faulkner *et al.*, 1993).

Other special research applications have been developed for small animal research, paediatric studies and for measuring periprosthetic bone density. Similarly, software has been developed to measure the lumbar vertebral bodies in the lateral projection. Lateral DXA allows the highly trabecular vertebral body to be evaluated without the major influence of the cortical posterior elements, aortic calcification, osteophytes and other abnormalities encountered when scanning in the anteroposterior (AP) view. In the lateral decubitus position L1 and often L2 are affected by overlaying ribs while L4 is often obscured by the iliac crest. Precision error is increased compared with AP scanning but lateral BMD may be more sensitive for detecting vertebral loss than AP (Rupich *et al.*, 1990; Slosman *et al.*, 1990). Advances allowing lateral scanning in the supine position using a rotating gantry and an array of detectors and fan-beam source may incease the precision of lateral scanning (Figure 7.1) (Slosman *et al.*, 1992). In addition, the rotating gantry provides the potential to produce AP and lateral images of high quality which enable morphometric analysis to be performed.

Recently, imaging densitometry has been developed, which has greatly enhanced

WYNN DIVISION OF
METABOLIC MEDICINE
National Heart and Lung Institute

PATIENT ID: SCAN: 3.6z 22.09.94
NAME: S, F ANALYSIS: 3.6z 22.01.96

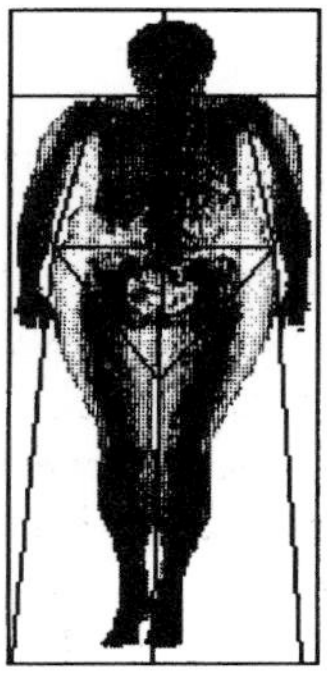

LUNAR®

IMAGE NOT FOR DIAGNOSIS

ID: SCAN DATE: 22.09.94

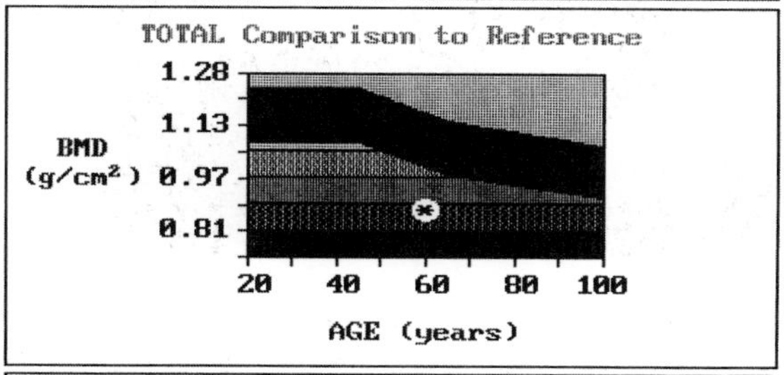

TOTAL BMD (g/cm²)1	0.871 ± 0.01
TOTAL % Young Adult2	77 ± 3
TOTAL % Age Matched3	81 ± 3

Age (years).........	60	Large Standard......	272.43	Scan Mode.......	Fast
Sex.................	Female	Medium Standard.....	205.25	Scan Type...........	DPX
Weight (Kg).........	72.0	Small Standard......	144.28	Collimation (mm).....	1.68
Height (cm).........	169	Low keV Air (cps)...	667477	Sample Size (mm).....	4.8x 9.6
Ethnic..............	White	High keV Air (cps)..	441867		
System..............	6254	Rvalue (%Fat).......	1.298(46.7)		
Current (uA)........	150				

REGION	BMD¹ g/cm²	Young Adult² %	Young Adult² Z	Age Matched³ %	Age Matched³ Z
HEAD	1.581	-	-	-	-
ARMS	0.621	74	-2.79	79	-2.10
LEGS	0.887	77	-2.98	81	-2.31
TRUNK	0.708	77	-3.02	79	-2.65
RIBS	0.554	-	-	-	-
PELVIS	0.863	78	-2.47	80	-2.11
SPINE	0.715	63	-3.04	67	-2.50
TOTAL	0.871	77	-3.17	81	-2.54

1 - See appendix E on precision and accuracy. Statistically 68% of repeat scans will fall within 1 SD.
2 - England Total Body Reference Population, Ages 20-45. See Appendices.
3 - Matched for Age, Weight(males 50-100kg; females 35-80kg), Ethnic.
- Extended Research Analysis.

Figure 7.4 Printout of a DXA scan (Lunar DPX instrument) of the total body of a 60-year-old post-menopausal woman. Note that in addition to measurements of bone, measurements of total and regional lean and fat tissue can also be made.

WYNN DIVISION OF
METABOLIC MEDICINE
National Heart and Lung Institute

PATIENT ID:	SCAN: 3.6z	22.09.94
NAME: S, F	ANALYSIS: 3.6z	22.01.96

BODY COMPOSITION**

Region of Interest	R Value	Tissue % Fat	Region % Fat	Tissue (g)	Fat (g)	Lean (g)	BMC (g)
LEFT ARM	1.301	45.3	44.0	3147	1426	1721	98
LEFT LEG	1.297	47.4	46.1	11151	5282	5868	317
LEFT TRUNK	1.294	48.8	48.3	19995	9760	10235	200
LEFT TOTAL	1.298	46.9	45.9	36676	17215	19461	831
RIGHT ARM	1.310	41.1	39.6	2834	1166	1669	106
RIGHT LEG	1.299	46.4	44.9	10059	4666	5393	327
RIGHT TRUNK	1.295	48.7	48.2	18305	8910	9395	197
RIGHT TOTAL	1.299	46.5	45.4	32735	15222	17513	776
ARMS	1.305	43.3	41.9	5981	2592	3389	204
LEGS	1.298	46.9	45.5	21210	9948	11261	644
TRUNK	1.294	48.7	48.2	38300	18670	19630	397
TOTAL	1.298	46.7	45.7	69412	32438	36974	1607

ANCILLARY TOTAL BODY RESULTS**

Total Bone Calcium (g)..	611
Air Points.............	11700
Tissue Points..........	11568
Bone Points............	4002
Total Points...........	23280
R-Value Points.........	4859

Name	Cut Locations Actual	Cut Locations Relative
Neck	25	25
Left Arm	-	-
Left Rib	54	-
Right Rib	66	-
Right Arm	-	-
Spine	58	58
Pelvis	69	69
Top of Head	0	
Center	-	

**Ancillary results for research purposes, not clinical use.
Extended Research Analysis.

Figure 7.4 *Continued*

spatial resolution compared to DXA. This technique uses solid-state detectors and a fan beam of X-rays. The k-edge radiation is produced by a rotating anode tube. The tube and detectors are mounted on a motorized C-arm which can be rotated for imaging in a variety of positions (Figure 7.5a). This allows the lateral spine to be scanned in the supine position and the potential for the hip to be scanned without the need for internal rotation. The improvements in spatial resolution provide near-radiographic quality images, allowing accurate morphometry of the lateral spine (Figure 7.5b) (Gowin *et al.*, 1995; Lang *et al.*, 1995). Improvements in precision and speed are also anticipated.

QUANTITATIVE COMPUTED TOMOGRAPHY (QCT)

The use of computed tomography (CT) for the measurement of BMD was first developed in the mid 1970s (Genant and Boyd, 1977).

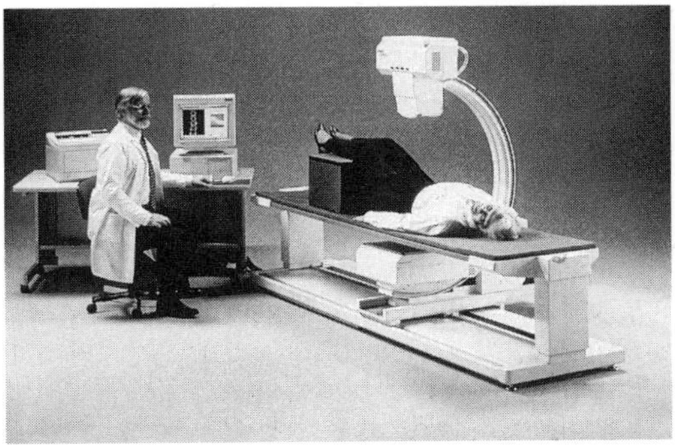

(a)

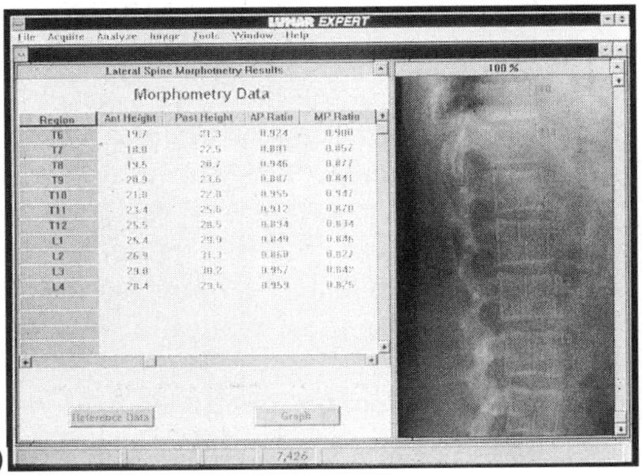

(b)

Figure 7.5 (a) Imaging densitometer. This system (Lunar Expert) uses a rotating anode tube and k-edge filter to produce relatively monoenergetic X-rays. The solid-state detector provides good spatial resolution and images of near radiographic quality. Courtesy of Lunar Corp. (b) Lateral spine scan using an imaging densitometer (Lunar Expert). The high-resolution images allow the identification of vertebral structure and accurate morphometry to be performed. Courtesy of Lunar Corp.

This was made possible with the development by EMI and Hounsfield (Hounsfield, 1973) of quantifiable cross-sectional images in the axial plane of the body. The image consists of attenuation coefficients measured in Hounsfield units (HU) which vary according to the type of tissue through which the X-ray beam passes. Since trabecular and cortical bone have different attenuation coefficients they can be clearly defined on a CT scan in both the axial and peripheral skeleton.

The development of quantitative CT (QCT) for the measurement of BMD has taken two directions. Firstly, CT scanners installed for general diagnosis have been used to measure vertebral BMD using dedicated bone density software and secondly, the construction of special CT equipment using a radionuclide source for the measurement of the forearm. With the conventional CT scanner, a region of interest (ROI) is defined from a transverse slice and quantitated to give measurements of BMD (Cann and Genant, 1980; Banks and Stevenson, 1986). Most QCT measurements are taken of the lumbar spine (Banks and Stevenson, 1990) but some investigators have looked at the radius and tibia (Stebler and Ruegsegger, 1983; Schneider *et al.*, 1988) and the proximal femur Gluer and Genant, 1987; Esses *et al.*, 1989).

In the standard protocol, the patient is scanned lying on a calibration phantom. Initially a lateral localization scan (scout view) of the lumbar spine is performed to select the scanning planes. A slice thickness of between 4 and 10 mm is used in the midplane of T12 to L4 vertebral bodies with strict adherence to a fixed table height (Banks and Stevenson, 1986). On the cross-sectional image a circular, elliptical, rectangular or manually drawn ROI in the trabecular area of each vertebral body is defined (Figure 7.6). Although a trabecular region is usually selected it is possible to measure the cortical and integral bone density of the vertebral body. The average HU is then determined in the region of interest. Using linear regression of HU obtained from the calibration phantom, which contains mineral equivalent of known density, the vertebral HU density is converted to a physical density in the same units as the calibration standard. The results are thus expressed as mg of mineral equivalent per cubic centimetre of trabecular bone volume (Genant *et al.*, 1982; Banks and Stevenson, 1990).

The first calibration standards contained liquid dipotassium hydrogen phosphate (Cann and Genant, 1980). However, these liquid phantoms can suffer with problems such as the development of gas bubbles and precipitation of the dissolved materials which affect their long-term stability. Therefore, more stable, solid calibration standards based on calcium hydroxyapatite in comparable concentrations have been developed (Reiser and Genant, 1984; Kalender *et al.*, 1987) (Figure 7.6).

Like DXA, there may be differences in QCT values between instruments, making the direct comparison of measurements difficult. This may be due to differences in instrument design between the CT manufacturers' e.g. solid state/zenon detectors, filtration materials and geometry as well as differences in calibration. The development of the European Spine Phantom (ESP) and the European Forearm Phantom (EFP) should allow the crosscalibration of instruments in the future (Kalender *et al.*, 1995).

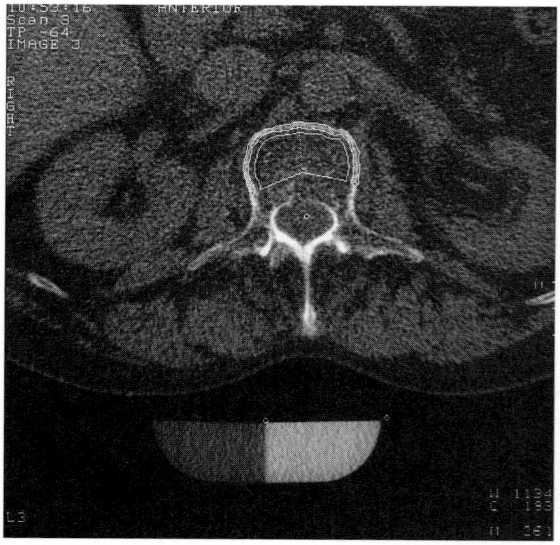

Figure 7.6 Quantitative computed tomography (QCT) (Siemens Somatom Plus instrument) image of a cross-sectional slice through a vertebral body showing regions of interest measured. The patient is lying on a solid calibration phantom.

The precision and accuracy of QCT are excellent (Banks and Stevenson, 1986) although the accuracy may be affected by the variable fat content in the vertebral body observed with ageing and some disease states, such that absolute trabecular density can be substantially underestimated with residual errors of 10–15% (Gluer and Genant, 1989). It has been suggested that this underestimation of bone mineral can be eliminated by using an age-related regression and including a fat variation within the estimated error of the mean (Genant *et al.*, 1985). However, in clinical practice this error due to marrow fat is only likely to be of importance in the elderly osteoporotic in whom a measurement may be of little practical value. The use of dual-energy QCT has been shown to reduce fat errors (Adams *et al.*, 1982) but although this increases the accuracy of the method, it is at the expense of an increase in precision error and possible radiation dose (Banks and Stevenson, 1986) and so it is not generally used for most clinical applications (Table 7.2).

Automatic selection of the ROI to minimize operator subjectivity and enhance precision has been introduced (Kalender *et al.*, 1987). Contour tracking algorithms trace the cortical walls of the vertebral body, the spinal cord and the posterior elements to select the optimum position and size of the ROI. Together with automatic selection of the midvertebral QCT slice on lateral localization digital radiographs (Kalender *et al.*, 1988), this can reduce the scanning and evaluation time.

QCT measures the absolute BMC of a specific volume of bone and therefore it is a true three-dimensional density as opposed to the 'areal' density measured by SPA, SXA, DPA and DXA. Another advantage of QCT is that it allows the isolation of purely trabecular bone of the vertebral body whereas SPA, SXA, DPA and DXA cannot distinguish between cortical and trabecular bone. This feature means that QCT may be a more sensitive technique for measuring bone loss. Several clinical studies (Heuck *et al.*, 1989; van Berkum *et al.*, 1989; Pacifici *et al.*, 1990) have confirmed the high sensitivity of the spinal trabecular site for documenting age and menopause-related bone loss and in discriminating osteoporotics from normals. In addition, because QCT is able to measure selectively trabecular bone within the vertebral body, artefacts that can affect bone density measurements by DPA and DXA such as osteophytes and aortic calcification are excluded from the measurement (Banks *et al.*, 1994).

The radiation dose is usually modest (approximately 60 μSv for a single energy QCT measurement of the spine) although not as low as with pencil-beam DXA (approximately 1 μSv) (Kalender, 1992). The main problem with using QCT for bone density measurements is that the majority of CT scanners are in constant use with clinical diagnostic work and most researchers cannot afford a CT scanner exclusively for bone mineral measurements.

PERIPHERAL QUANTITATIVE COMPUTED TOMOGRAPHY (PQCT)

A dedicated forearm CT scanner was first described by Ruegsegger *et al.* in 1976. CT forearm scanners usually use a ^{125}I photon source with a NaI scintillation detector but the most recent scanners employ an X-ray source (Butz *et al.*, 1994). A scout scan of the forearm is performed initially. This procedure permits the exact relocation of the measurement point with repeat measurements. Multiple thin slices of the forearm are taken at the distal end or in the midshaft. The software allows the selective quantification of trabecular and cortical bone. Although measurements of changes in trabecular bone at the forearm may not be as sensitive as those in the spine, the method has the advantages of a low radiation exposure and good precision and is rapid and simple to perform.

FUTURE DEVELOPMENTS USING QCT

The spatial resolution using conventional CT is in the order of 0.5–1.0 mm which is inadequate for highly accurate cortical measurements and for analysis of discrete trabecular morphological parameters, both important measurements in the assessment of bone strength. This has led to the development of high resolution CT scanners with the ability to perform *in vivo* measurements of the forearm or tibia with a spatial resolution of 100–200 μm. Although these scanners use a high radiation dose, they may yield important information on role of trabecular structure and cortical BMD on bone strength (Ruegsegger *et al.*, 1991). High resolution CT scanners have also been used to perform μCT measurements of very small bone samples where the spatial resolution of 60–100 μm allows a 3-D analysis of the trabecular network (Elliott and Dover, 1984; Kuhn *et al.*, 1990).

To date, there has been little research on the clinical utility of QCT of the hip (Sartoris *et al.*, 1986). However, recent developments in image-processing techniques have created the possibility of site-specific QCT of the hip (Gluer and Genant, 1987) where areas of trabecular, cortical or integral bone density can be measured by using two-dimensional or three-dimensional reformatting techniques. Recently QCT has been suggested as a suitable technique for measuring BMD changes around hip prostheses (Klotz *et al.*, 1994).

QCT studies of the spine and hip have

been used to create three-dimensional finite element models (FEM) to estimate vertebral strength. Vertebral geometry is derived from contiguous slice CT scans and material properties are based on the average bone mineral density of each vertebral element. Faulkner *et al.* (1991) used vertebral CT data to perform FEM analysis and found that it was more sensitive and specific than QCT alone at separating patients with and without osteoporotic fracture. Although these FEM studies are complex, future refinements may produce a clinically useful tool for accurately estimating skeletal strength *in vivo*.

NEUTRON ACTIVATION ANALYSIS (NAA)

Neutron activation analysis (NAA) is a technique which measures total body calcium. Since 99% of total body calcium is in the skeleton this measurement reflects total body bone calcium content.

Total body NAA was considered the 'gold standard' for total skeletal calcium measurement until the development of DPA and DXA. NAA uses a source of high-energy neutrons (provided by a reactor, neutron accelerator or radionuclide neutron source) to activate ^{48}Ca within the body to ^{49}Ca. The subsequent decay back to ^{48}Ca (the half-life of ^{49}Ca is approximately eight minutes) emits high-energy γ radiation which is convenient to measure with a γ radiation counter (Spinks, 1990). Total body irradiation time is 60 seconds after which the patient spends 20 minutes in a whole-body radioactivity monitor. The disadvantage of total body NAA is the high radiation dose (Table 7.2). Another disadvantage is that measurement of specific bony areas of interest is not possible as with DXA. Partial body NAA utilizes a radionuclide as the neutron source and regional sites, usually the hand, forearm or spine, are measured so the radiation dose is lower than with total body NAA. More recently a prompt-γ *in vivo* NAA method has been introduced for measuring total body calcium (Ryde *et al.*, 1987). The precision and dose equivalent compare favourably with the performance of the delayed-γ NAA technique. However, NAA is only available in specialist centres and therefore is not widely used to measure bone mass.

COMPTON SCATTERING

Bone density in the appendicular skeleton (radius and calcaneum) can be determined by a technique known as Compton scattering (Garnett *et al.*, 1973; Olkkonen and Karjalainen, 1975). Compton scatter refers to the radiation which changes direction and energy as it 'bounces off' an electron when it passes through matter. A radionuclide source (often 500 mCi ^{137}Cs) is used to provide the γ rays. The relation between transmitted and scattered radiation at specific angles is a measure of electron density and, indirectly, physical density and is therefore also an approximation of bone mineral content in a given volume of bone. One difficulty with this technique is to define a specific volume inside the body and to identify the same volume repeatedly. Currently Compton scattering techniques are used as research tools rather than in a clinical setting.

MAGNETIC RESONANCE IMAGING (MRI)

The feasibility of making direct assessments of trabecular density and structure using differences in magnetic susceptibility effects in magnetic resonance imaging (MRI) has recently been demonstrated (Majundar *et al.*, 1991; Majundar and Genant, 1992, 1995). Magnetic susceptibility is the ratio between the induced magnetic field of a tissue and the applied external field, i.e. it is a measure of the response of a tissue to an applied constant field. Magnetic field inhomogeneities due to differences in the magnetic susceptibility between trabecular bone and bone marrow affect the T2* relaxation time (a tissue parameter that may be measured using gradient echo MRI) of bone marrow. This change in T2* depends not only on the density of the surrounding trabeculae but also on their geometry. Although this work is in its early stages, gradient echo MRI may eventually provide unique morphologic information on trabecular structure and architecture which may be of potential use in assessing bone strength and predicting fracture risk.

ULTRASOUND

Ultrasound is a non-invasive technique that involves the transmission of sound waves (above the audible frequency) across bone (Langton *et al.*, 1984). The speed of sound (SOS) is a function of the mass, density and elastic modulus (Greenfield *et al.*, 1981). The elastic modulus is influenced by the spatial configuration of the trabeculae, biomechanical properties of bone and fatigue damage. In addition to the SOS, the attenuation of ultrasound signals during their passage through bone may be measured by determining the reduction in ultrasound signal amplitude. The broadband ultrasound attenuation (BUA) describes the increase in ultrasound attenuation over a particular frequency range, typically 0.2–0.6 MHz (Baran *et al.*, 1988). Scattering due to bone density and structure acts as a filter that selectively diminishes the frequency component across a transmission band, so that the number, spacing and orientation of the scattering elements determine the filtering effect on BUA. Ultrasound measurements may therefore provide information not only on bone mass but also bone quality (Gluer *et al.*, 1994).

Currently available commercial scanners usually perform ultrasound measurements across the os calcis. The heel is placed in a chamber between two ultrasonic transducers, one acting as the transmitter and the other as the receiver (Figure 7.7). Water or ultrasound gel is used as the coupling medium, depending on the system. The os calcis is chosen because it contains a high proportion of trabecular bone, a low amount of surrounding soft tissue and has approximately flat and parallel surfaces. Other sites that have been used for ultrasound measurements are the metacarpal, the phalanx, the patella, the proximal radius and the cortical part of the femur and tibia (Greenfield *et al.*, 1981; Heaney *et al.*, 1989; Grudi *et al.*, 1995; Kann *et al.*, 1995; Stegman *et al.*, 1995).

The manufacturers of some ultrasound instruments have combined SOS and BUA measurements into a term called 'stiffness' or 'quantitative ultrasound index' in an attempt to provide a clinically useful ultrasound measurement (Mazess *et al.*, 1992).

In vitro studies using excised calcanei have demonstrated a good correlation between BUA and QCT bone density measurements

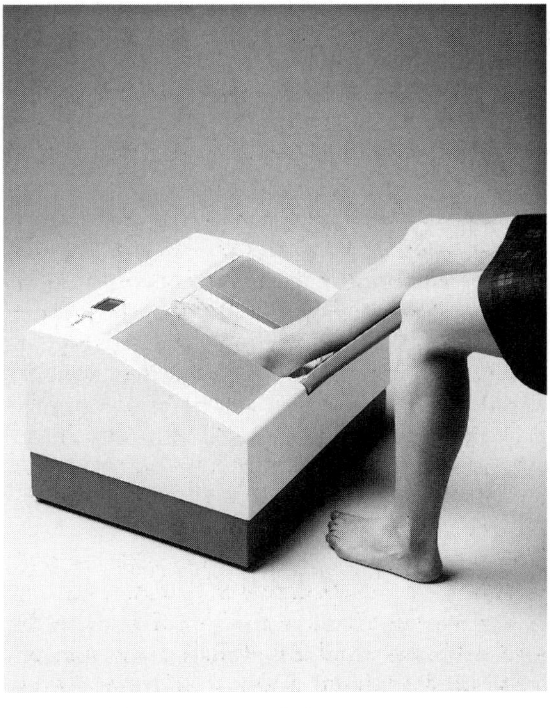

Figure 7.7 Ultrasound bone densitometer This system (Lunar Achilles) uses water as a medium for the ultrasound waves which are pulsed across the os calcis from an emitting transducer to a receiving tranducer. Courtesy of Lunar Corp.

(McKelvie *et al.*, 1989), indicating that bone density is an important determinant of BUA. Several studies have shown significant correlations between calcaneum SOS and BUA and spine or hip BMD by DPA and DXA (Baran *et al.*, 1988; Rossman *et al.*, 1989; McCloskey *et al.*, 1990; Agren *et al.*, 1991; Faulkner *et al.*, 1994), but the correlations are not sufficiently high to allow the use of ultrasound as a screening tool for low BMD as measured by DXA (Faulkner *et al.*, 1994). Waud *et al.* (1992) demonstrated a moderate correlation between BUA and SOS of the calcaneum and BMD of the calcaneum measured by DXA, but suggested that they measure properties of bone other than density and different from each other. Porter (Porter *et al.*, 1990) was the first to demonstrate prospectively a relationship between a reduction in BUA measurements and the risk of subsequent hip fracture in elderly women. This has been confirmed by two recent prospective studies which showed that BUA and SOS predicted hip fracture as well as BMD of the femoral neck by DXA and independently of BMD by DXA (Bauer *et al.*, 1995; Hans *et al.*, 1996). It has not been demonstrated whether ultrasound measurements add to the predictive value of DXA.

The ultrasonic measurement of bone is quick and simple to use and has good precision (Lees and Stevenson, 1993) with the additional advantage of avoiding ionizing radiation. It has not, as yet, been determined how ultrasound will be used clinically in the evaluation of osteoporosis.

POTENTIAL ERRORS IN THE MEASUREMENT OF BONE MASS

There are two main sources of error with the measurement of bone mass: instrument-induced errors and operator-induced errors. Instrument-induced errors may be reduced by the implementation of a quality control (QC) programme in addition to any daily calibration procedure required by the instrument. A QC programme should involve the regular scanning of a phantom allowing the performance of the instrument to be monitored and any drifts, surges or jumps in the BMD data noted and the instrument evaluated in a timely fashion (Orwoll *et al.*, 1993; Garland *et al.*, 1997).

Operator-induced error may be introduced during the acquisition of data (e.g. poor patient positioning) or may be due to analysis errors (e.g. incorrect regions of interest defined). To minimize both inter- and intra-operator variation it is important for all operators to be fully trained and to adhere to standardized protocols for both the acquisition and analysis of data. It is essential that measurements of BMD are as precise as possible because although instrument- and operator-induced errors may be small, perhaps in the region of a few percent, these can become significant, as any changes in BMD observed (as a result of treatment, ageing or disease) will be also probably be in the region of a few percent per year.

It is important to note that changes in software/hardware may affect BMD values and therefore if any changes are anticipated, appropriate cross calibration studies should be performed.

In addition to the absolute differences seen between instruments from different manufacturers, mainly due to the different assumptions made concerning the calibration of the instruments as well as differences in the bone area defined, there may be differences between instruments from the same manufacturer. The introduction of the ESP and the EFP should provide the opportunity for the crosscalibration of instruments for both DXA and QCT techniques (Kalender *et al.*, 1995).

The International DXA Standardization Committee has proposed the use of a standardized BMD (sBMD in mg/cm^2) for measurements of the lumbar spine based on the correlation of *in vivo* spinal BMD measurements among all DXA densitometers (Genant *et al.*, 1994). Work is in progress to provide a sBMD measurement of the proximal femur for use with all DXA densitometers.

It is also important to note that the normative ranges may not be comparable between instruments from different manufacturers and therefore it is possible that an individual's risk of fracture may appear to differ according to the instrument on which they are scanned (Laskey *et al.*, 1992). There may be country to country or even within-country variation in normal ranges and it is important for each centre to verify that its normative data are appropriate for use within its own population.

CONCLUSION

The main methods in current clinical use for the non-invasive measurement of bone mass are single-photon absorptiometry, single-energy X-ray absorptiometry, dual-energy X-ray absorptiometry, quantitative computed tomography and peripheral quantitative computed tomography. Dual-photon absorptiometry has been largely superseded by the introduction of dual-energy X-ray absorptiometry. Ultrasound and photodensitometry are techniques that are still being evaluated to determine their clinical usefulness. Other methods such as NAA and Compton scattering techniques are generally confined to a research setting. Radiogrammetry is not used routinely for the measurement of bone density, but radiographs are often essential to diagnose fracture and to perform morphometric measurements. The development of high-resolution imaging bone densitometers will enable the identification of vertebral abnormalities and provide the ability to perform spinal morphometry measurements.

Recent developments, such as the ultrasonic measurement of bone, structural analysis such as finite element analysis and the magnetic resonance imaging of bone, may provide information on the structure and quality of bone which may enhance the fracture prediction abilities of conventional densitometry.

Future methods are likely to take into consideration other factors that cause fragility besides reduced BMD, such as fatigue damage and trabecular connectivity on the microanatomic level and bone geometry and regional variations in BMD on the macrostructure level.

REFERENCES

Adami, S., Gatti, D., Rossini, M. *et al.* (1992) The radiological assessment of vertebral osteoporosis. *Bone* **13**: 533–6.

Adams, J.E., Chen, S., Adams, P.H. and Isherwood, I. (1982) Measurement of trabecular bone mineral by dual energy computed tomography. *J Comput Assist Tomogr* **6**: 601–7.

Agren, M., Karellas, A., Leahey, D., Marks, S. and Baran, D. (1991) Ultrasound attenuation of the calcaneus: a sensitive and specific discriminator of osteopenia in postmenopausal women. *Calcif Tissue Int* **48**: 240–4.

Aitken, M. (1984) Measurement of bone mass and turnover. In: *Osteoporosis in Clinical Practice*, (ed. Aitken, M.), Wright, Bristol, pp. 21–30.

Banks, L.M. and Read, W.S. (1993) New computer software for measuring spinal deformity on digitised X-rays. *Calcif Tissue Int* **52**: 173.

Banks, L.M. and Stevenson, J.C. (1986) Modified method of spinal computed tomography for trabecular bone mineral measurement. *J Comput Assist Tomogr* **10**: 463–7.

Banks, L.M. and Stevenson, J.C. (1990) Developments in computerised axial tomography scanning and its use in bone disease measurement. In: *New Techniques in Metabolic Bone Disease*, (ed. Stevenson, J.C.), Wright, London, pp. 138–56.

Banks, L.M., Lees, B., MacSweeney, J.E. and Stevenson, J.C. (1994) Effect of degenerative spinal and aortic calcification on bone density measurements in post-menopausal women: links between osteoporosis and cardiovascular disease? *Eur J Clin Invest* **24**: 813–17.

Baran, D.T., Kelly, A.M., Karellas, A. *et al.* (1988) Ultrasound attenuation of the os calcis in women with osteoporosis and hip fractures. *Calcif Tissue Int* **43**: 138–42.

Barnett, E. and Nordin, B.E.C. (1960) The radiological diagnosis of osteoporosis: a new approach. *Clin Radiol* **11**: 166–74.

Bauer, D.C., Gluer, C.C., Pressman, A.R. *et al.*

(1995) Broadband ultrasound attenuation (BUA) and the risk of fracture: a prospective study. *J Bone Miner Res* **10** (Suppl 1): S175.

Butz, S., Wuster, C., Scheidt-Nave, C. *et al.* (1994) Forearm BMD as measured by peripheral quantitative computed tomography (pQCT) in a German reference population. *Osteoporosis Int* **4**: 179–84.

Cameron, J.R. and Sorenson, J. (1963) Measurement of bone mineral *in vivo*: an improved method. *Science* **142**: 230–2.

Cameron, J.R., Mazess, R.B. and Sorenson, J.A. (1986) Precision and accuracy of bone mineral determination by direct photon absorptiometry. *Invest Radiol* **3**: 141–50.

Cann, C.E. and Genant, H.K. (1980) Precise measurement of vertebral mineral content using computed tomography. *J Comput Assist Tomogr* **4**: 493–500.

Colbert, C. and Bachtell, R.S. (1981) Radiographic absorptiometry (photodensitometry). In: *Non-Invasive Measurements of Bone Mass and Their Clinical Application*, (ed. Cohn, S.H.), CRC Press, Boca Raton, pp. 52–84.

Colbert, C., Mazess, R.B. and Sorenson, P.B. (1970) Bone mineral determination *in vitro* by radiographic densitometry and direct photon absorptiometry. *Invest Radiol* **5**: 336–40.

Consensus Development Conference (1991) Prophylaxis and treatment of osteoporosis. *Osteoporosis Int* **1**: 114–17.

Cosman, F., Herrington, B., Himmelstein, S. and Lindsay, R. (1991) Radiographic absorptiometry: a simple method for determination of bone mass. *Osteoporosis Int* **2**: 34–8.

Cummings, S.R., Black, D.M., Nevitt, M.C. *et al.* (1990) Appendicular bone density and age predict hip fracture in women. *J Am Med Assoc* **263**: 665–8.

Cummings, S.R., Black, D.M., Nevitt, M.C. *et al.* (1993) Bone density at various sites for prediction of hip fractures. *Lancet* **341**: 72–5.

Doyle, F.H. (1961) Ulnar bone mineral concentration in metabolic bone disease. *Br J Radiol* **34**: 698–712.

Eastell, R., Cedel, S.L., Wahner, H.W., Riggs, B.L. and Melton, L.J. (1991) Classification of vertebral fractures. *J Bone Miner Res* **6**: 207–15.

Elliott, J.C. and Dover, S.D. (1984) Three dimensional distribution of mineral in bone at a resolution of 15 um determined by X-ray microtomography. *Metab Bone Dis Rel Res* **5**: 219–21.

Esses, S.I., Lotz, J.C. and Hayes, W.C. (1989) Biomechanical properties of the proximal femur determined *in vitro* by single-energy quantitative computed tomography. *J Bone Miner Res* **4**: 715–22.

Faulkner, K.G., Cann, C.E. and Hanegawa, B.H. (1991) Effect of bone distribution on vertebral strength assessment with patient specific non-linear finite element analysis. *Radiology* **179**: 669–74.

Faulkner, K.G., Cummings, S.R., Black, D. *et al.* (1993) Simple measurement of femoral geometry predicts hip fracture: the study of osteoporotic fractures. *J Bone Miner Res* **8**: 1211–17.

Faulkner, K.G., McClung, M.R., Coleman, L.J. and Kingston-Sandahl, E. (1994) Quantitative ultrasound of the heel: correlation with densitometric measurements at different skeletal sites. *Osteoporosis Int* **4**: 42–7.

Garland, S.W., Lees, B. and Stevenson, J.C. (1997) DXA longitudinal quality control: a comparison of inbuilt quality assurance, visual inspection, multi-rule Shewhart charts and Cusum analysis. *Osteoporosis Int* **7**: 231–7.

Garn, S.M., Rohmann, C.G. and Nolen, P. (1963) The developmental nature of bone changes during aging. In: *Relations of Development and Aging*, (ed. Birren, J.E.), C.C. Thomas, Springfield.

Garnett, E.S., Kennett, T.J., Kenyon, D.B. and Webber, C.E. (1973) A photon scattering technique for the measurement of absolute bone density *in vivo*. *Radiology* **106**: 1209–12.

Genant, H.K. and Boyd, D.P. (1977) Quantitative bone mineral analysis using dual energy computed tomography. *Invest Radiol* **12**: 545–51.

Genant, H.K., Cann, C.E., Ettinger, B. and Gordon, G.S. (1982) Quantitative computer tomography of vertebral spongiosa: a sensitive method for measuring bone loss after oophorectomy. *Ann Intern Med* **97**: 699–705.

Genant, H.K., Ettinger, B., Cann, C.E. *et al.* (1985) Osteoporosis: assessment by quantitative computed tomography. *Orthop Clin North Am* **16**: 557–68.

Genant, H.K., Grampp, S., Gluer, C.G. *et al.* (1994) Universal standardization for dual energy X-ray absorptiometry: patient and phantom cross-calibration results. *J Bone Miner Res* **9**: 1503–14.

Gluer, C.G. and Genant, H.K. (1987) Quantitative computed tomography of the hip. In: *Osteoporosis Update 1987*, (ed. Genant, H.K.),

University of California Printing Services, San Francisco.

Gluer, C.G. and Genant, H.K. (1989) Impact of marrow fat on accuracy of quantitative CT. *J Comput Assist Tomogr* 13: 1023–35.

Gluer, C.C., Wu, C.Y., Jergas, J. *et al.* (1994) Three quantitative ultrasound parameters reflect bone structure. *Calcif Tissue Int* **55**: 46–52.

Gordan, G.S. and Vaughan, C. (1976) Evaluation of diagnostic methods in osteoporosis. In: *Clinical Management of the Osteoporoses*, (eds Gordan, G.S. and Vaughan, C.), Publishing Sciences Group, Aylesbury, p 59.

Gowin, W., Diessel, E., Mews, J. *et al.* (1995) Vertebral morphometry: a comparison of accuracy and reproducibility of radiographs with new DXA devices. *J Bone Miner Res* **10** (Suppl 1): S266.

Greenfield, M.A., Craven, R.D., Huddleston *et al.* (1981) Measurement of the velocity of ultrasound in human corticol bone *in vivo*. *Radiology* **138**: 701–10.

Grubb, S.A., Jacobsen, P.C., Aubrey, B.J. *et al.* (1984) Bone density in osteoporotic women: a modified distal radius density measurement procedure to develop an 'at risk' value for use in screening women. *J Orthop Res* **2**: 328–32.

Grudi, S., Malavolta, N., Ripamonti, C. and Cauderella, R. (1995) Ultrasound in the evaluation of osteoporosis: a comparison with bone mineral density at distal radius. *Br J Radiol* **68**: 476–80.

Haarbo, J., Gotfredsen, A., Hassager, C. and Christiansen, C. (1991) Validation of body composition by dual energy X-ray absorptiometry (DEXA). *Clin Physiol* **11**: 331–41.

Hagiwara, S., Engelke, K., Yang, S.O. *et al.* (1994) Dual x-ray absorptiometry forearm software: accuracy and intermachine relationship. *J Bone Miner Res* **9**: 1425–7.

Hans D., Dargent, P., Schott, A.M. *et al.* (1996) Ultrasonic heel measurements predict hip fracture in elderly women: the EPIDOS prospective study. *Lancet* **348**: 511–14.

Heaney, R.P., Aviolo, L.V., Chesnut, C.H. *et al.* (1989) Osteoporotic bone fragility. Detection by ultrasound transmission velocity. *J Am Med Assoc* **261**: 2986–90.

Heuck, A., Block, J.E., Gluer, C.G., Steiger, P. and Genant, H.K. (1989) Mild versus definite osteoporosis: comparison of bone densitometry techniques using different statistical models. *J Bone Miner Res* **4**: 891–900.

Heymsfield, S.B., Wang, J. Kehayias, J.J. and Pierson, R.N. (1989) Dual photon absorptiometry: comparison of bone mineral and soft tissue mass measurements *in vivo* with established methods. *Am J Clin Nutrition* **49**: 1283–9.

Hounsfield, G.N. (1973) Computerised transverse axial scanning (tomography). Part 1. Description of system. *Br J Radiol* **46**: 1016–22.

Hui, S.L., Slemenda, C.W. and Johnson, C.C. (1988). Age and bone mass as predictors of fracture in a prospective study. *J Clin Invest* **81**: 1804–9.

Kalender, W.A. (1992) Effective dose values in bone mineral measurements by photon absorptiometry and computed tomography. *Osteoporosis Int* **2**: 82–7.

Kalender, W.A., Klotz, E. and Suess, C. (1987) Vertebral bone mineral analysis: an integrated approach. *Radiology* **164**: 419–23.

Kalender, W.A., Brestowsky, H. and Felsenberg, D. (1988) Bone mineral measurement: automated determination of mid-vertebral CT section. *Radiology* **168**: 219–21.

Kalender, W.A., Felsenberg, D., Genant H.K. *et al.* (1995) The European Spine Phantom – a tool for standardization and quality control in spinal bone mineral measurements by DXA and QCT. *Eur J Radiol* **20**: 83–92.

Kann, P., Schultz, U., Kraus, D., Piepkom, B. and Beyer, J. (1995) *In-vivo* investigation of material quality of bone tissue by measuring apparent phalangeal ultrasound transmission velocity. *Clin Rheumatol* **14**: 26–34.

Kelly, T.L., Crane, G. and Baran, D.T. (1994) Single X-ray absorptiometry of the forearm: precision, correlation and reference data. *Calcif Tiss Int* **54**: 212–18.

Klotz, E., Hirchfleder, H., Salzer, F. and Kalender, W.A. (1994) Objective assessment of hip endoprothesis fit and precise measurement of periprosthetic bone mineral changes by CT. *Bone Mineral* **25**: Suppl 2 (25): S5.

Kotzski, P.O., Buyck, D., LeRoux, J.L. (1993) Measurement of the bone mineral density of the os calcis as an indicator of vertebral fracture in women with lumbar osteoarthritis. *Br J Radiol* **66**: 55–60.

Krolner, B. and Nielsen, P.S. (1980) Measurement of bone mineral content (BMC) of the lumbar spine. 1. Theory and application of a new two-dimensional dual-photon attenuation method. *Scand J Clin Lab Invest* **40**: 653–63.

Kuhn, J.L., Goldstein, S.A., Feldkamp, K.A. and Jesion, G. (1990) Evaluation of a microcomputed tomography system to study trabecular bone structure. *J Orthop Res* **8**: 833–42.

Lang, T., Fan, B., Wu, C. *et al.* (1995) Assessment of vertebral deformation with a high-resolution fan-beam densitometer. *J Bone Miner Res* **10** (Suppl 1): S367.

Langton, C.M., Palmer, S.B. and Porter, R.W. (1984) The measurement of broadband ultrasound attenuation in cancellous bone. *Eng Med* **13**: 89–91.

Laskey, A., Crisp, A.J. and Compston, J.E. (1992) Comparison of reference data of Lunar DPX and Hologic QDR-1000 dual energy X-ray absorptiometers. In: *Current Research in Bone Mineral Measurement II*, (ed. Ring, E.F.J.), British Institute of Radiology, London, p. 19.

LeBlanc, A.D., Evans, H.J., Marsh, C. *et al.* (1986) Precision of dual photon absorptiometry measurements. *J Nucl Med* **27**: 1362–5.

Lees, B. and Stevenson, J.C. (1992) An evaluation of dual energy X-ray absorptiometry and comparison with dual photon absorptiometry. *Osteoporosis Int* **2**: 146–56.

Lees, B., and Stevenson, J.C. (1993) Preliminary evaluation of a new ultrasound bone densitometer. *Calcif Tissue Int* **53**: 149–52.

Ley, C.J., Lees, B. and Stevenson, J.C. (1992) Sex and menopause associated changes in body fat distribution. *Am J Clin Nutrition* **55**: 950–4.

Lindsay, R. (1988) Pathogenesis, detection and prevention of post-menopausal osteoporosis. In: *The Menopause*, (eds Studd, J. and Whitehead, M.), Blackwell Scientific Publications, Oxford, pp. 156–67.

Lindsay, R., Fey, C. and Haboubi, A. (1987) Dual photon absorptiometric measurements of bone mineral density increase with source life. *Calcif Tissue Int* **41**: 293–4.

Mack, P.B., O'Brien, A.T., Smith, J.M. and Bauman, A.W. (1939) A method for estimating the degree of mineralisation of bones from tracings of roentgenograms. *Science* **89**: 467.

Madsen, M., Peppler, W. and Mazess, R.B. (1976) Vertebral and total body bone mineral content by dual photon absorptiometry. *Calcif Tissue Int* **21**: 361–4.

Majundar, S. and Genant, H.K. (1992) In vivo relationship betwen marrow T2* and trabecular bone density determined with a chemical shift-selective asymmetric spin-echo sequence. *J Magn Reson Imaging* **2**: 209–19.

Majundar, S. and Genant, H.K. (1995) A review of the recent advances in magnetic resonance imaging in the assessment of osteoporosis. *Osteoporosis Int* **5**: 79–92.

Majundar, S., Thomasson, D., Shimakawa, A. and Genant, H.K. (1991) Magnetic field inhomogeneity effects induced by the susceptibility differences between trabecular bone and bone marrow in gradient echo magnetic resonance imaging: experimental studies. *Magn Reson Med* **22**: 111–27.

Mazess, R.B. (1984) Advances in single and dual photon absorptiometry. In: *Osteoporosis*, (eds Arnaud, C.D., Nordin, B.E.C. *et al.*), Aslborg Stiftsbogtrykkeri, Glostrup, pp. 57–71.

Mazess, R.B., Collick, B., Trempe, J., Barden, H. and Hanson, J. (1989) Performance evaluation of a dual energy x-ray bone densitometer. *Calcif Tissue Int* **44**: 228–32.

Mazess, R.B., Barden, H.S., Bisek, J.P. and Hanson, J. (1990) Dual energy X-ray absorptiometry for total body and regional bone mineral and soft tissue composition. *Am J Clin Nutrition* **51**: 1106–12.

Mazess, R.B., Trempe, J. and Barden, H. (1992) Ultrasound bone densitometry of the os calcis. *J Bone Miner Res* **7** (Suppl 1): 186.

McCloskey, E.V., Murray, S.A., Miller, C. *et al.* (1990) Broadband ultrasound attenuation of the os calcis: relationship to bone mineral at other skeletal sites. *Clin Sci* **78**: 227–33.

McKelvie, M.L., Fordham, J., Clifford, C. and Palmer, S.B. (1989) *In vitro* comparison of quantitative computed tomography and broadband ultrasound attenuation of trabecular one. *Bone* **10**: 101.

Meema, H.E. (1962) The occurrence of cortical bone atrophy in old age and in osteoporosis. *J Can Assoc Radiol* **13**: 27.

Meema, H.E. and Meema, S. (1963) Measurable roentgenologic changes in some peripheral bones in osteoporosis. *J Am Geriatr Soc* **11**: 1170–82.

Meema, H.E. and Meema S. (1972) Comparison of microradiologic morphometric findings in hand bones with densitometric findings in the proximal radius in thyrotoxicosis and in renal osteodystrophy. *Invest Radiol* **7**: 88–96.

Morgan, D.B., Spiers, F.W., Pulvertaft, C.N. and Fourmia, P. (1967) The amount of bone in the metacarpal and the phalanx according to age and sex. *Clin Radiol* **18**: 101–8.

National Osteoporosis Foundation Working Group on Vertebral Fractures. (1995) Report assessing vertebral fractures. *J Bone Miner Res* **10**: 518–23.

Olkkonen, H. and Karjalainen, P. (1975) 170Tm gamma scattering technique for the determination of absolute bone density. *Br J Radiol* (**571**): 594–7.

Omnell, K.A. (1957) Quantitative roentgenologic studies on changes in mineral content of bone *in vivo*. *Acta Radiol* Suppl. 148: 1–86.

Orwoll, E.S., Oviatt, S.K. and Biddle, J. (1993) Precision of dual-energy x-ray absorptiometry: development of quality control rules and their application in longitudinal studies. *J Bone Miner Res* **8**: 693–9.

Orwoll, E.S., Oviatt, S.K. and Mann, T. (1990) The impact of osteophytic and vascular calcifications on vertebral mineral density measurements in men. *J Clin Endocrinol Metabol* **70**: 1202–7.

Ott, S.M., Kilcoyne, R.F. and Chesnut III, C.H. (1987) Ability of four different techniques of measuring bone mass to diagnose vertebral fractures in post-menopausal women. *J Bone Miner Res* **2**: 201–10.

Pacifici, R., Rupich, R., Griffin, M. *et al.* (1990) Dual energy radiography versus quantitative computer tomography for the diagnosis of osteoporosis. *J Clin Endocrinol Metab* **70**: 705–10.

Porter, R.W., Miller, C.G., Granger, D.E. and Palmer, S.B. (1990) Prediction of hip fracture in elderly women: a prospective study. *Br Med J* **301**: 638–41.

Price, W.A. (1901) The science of dental radiology. *Dent Cosmos* **43**: 484.

Reid, D.M., Lanham, S.A., McDonald, A.G. *et al.* (1990) Speed and comparability of 3 dual energy X-ray absorptiometer (DXA) models. Proceedings of the Third International Symposium on Osteoporosis, (eds Christiansen, C. and Overgaard, K.), Copenhagen, pp. 575–7.

Reid, I.R., Evans, M.C., Ames, R. and Wattie, D.J. (1991) The influence of osteophytes and aortic calcification on spinal mineral density in postmenopausal women. *J Clin Endocrinol Metab* **72**: 1372–4.

Reiser, U.J. and Genant, H.K. (1984) New water and bone equivalent solid material phantom materials used for calibration in quantitative computed tomography. *Radiology* **153**: 302.

Riggs, B.L., Wahner, H.W., Dunn, W.L. *et al.* (1981) Differential changes in bone mineral density of the appendicular and axial skeleton with aging. *J Clin Invest* **67**: 328–35.

Ross, P.D., Wasnich, R.D. and Vogel, J.M. (1988) Detection of prefracture spinal osteoporosis using bone mineral absorptiometry. *J Bone Miner Res* **3**: 1–11.

Rossman, P., Zagzebski, J., Mesina, C., Sorenson, T. and Mazess, R. (1989) Comparison of the speed of sound and ultrasound attenuation in the os calcis to bone density of the radius, femur and lumbar spine. *Clin Phys Physiol Meas* **10**: 353–60.

Ruegsegger, P., Elasser, U., Anliker, M. *et al.* (1976) Quantification of bone mineralisation using computerised tomography. *Radiology* **121**: 93–7.

Ruegsegger, P., Durand, E. and Dambacher, M.A. (1991) Localisation of regional forearm bone loss from high resolution computed tomographic images. *Osteoporosis Int* **1**: 76–80.

Rupich, R., Pacifici, R., Griffin, M. *et al.* (1990) Lateral dual energy radiography: a new method for measuring vertebral bone density. A preliminary study. *J Clin Endocrinol Metab* **70**: 1768–70.

Ryde, S.J.S., Morgan, W.D., Siryer, A., Evans, C. and Dutton, J. (1987) A clinical instrument for multi-element *in vivo* analysis by prompt, delayed and cyclic neutron activation using ^{252}Cf. *Phys Med Biol* **32**: 1257.

Sartoris, D.J., Andre, M., Resnick, C. and Resnick, D. (1986) Trabecular bone density in the proximal femur: quantitative CT assessment. *Radiology* **160**: 707–12.

Schneider, P., Borner, W., Mazess, R.B. and Barden, H. (1988) The relationship of peripheral to axial bone density. *Bone Mineral* **4**: 279–87.

Seeley, D.G., Browner, W.S., Cummings, S.R. and Genant, H.K. (1990) Which fractures are predicted with measurement of bone mineral density? *Radiology* **177**: 128.

Singh, M., Nagrath, A.R. and Mains, P.S. (1970) Changes in the trabecular pattern of the upper end of the femur as an index of osteoporosis. *J Bone Joint Surg* **52A**: 457–67.

Slosman, D.O., Rizzoli, R. Donarth, A. and Bonjour, J.P. (1990) Vertebral bone mineral density measured laterally by dual-energy X-ray absorptiometry. *Osteoporosis Int* **1**: 23–9.

Slosman, D.O., Rizzoli, R., Donarth, A. and Bonjour, J.P. (1992) Bone mineral density of lumbar vertebral body determined by supine and lateral decubitus. Study of precision and sensitivity. *J Bone Miner Res* **7** (Suppl 1): 192.

Sorenson, J.A. and Cameron, J.R. (1987) A reliable *in vivo* measurement of bone mineral content. *J Bone Joint Surg* **49A**: 491–7.

Spinks, T.J. (1990) The measurement of calcium and other body elements by *in vivo* NAA. In:

New Techniques in Metabolic Bone Disease, (ed. Stevenson, J.C.), Wright, London, pp. 157–71.

Stebler, B. and Ruegsegger, P. (1983) Special purpose CT system for quantitative bone evaluation in the appendicular skeleton. *Biomed Tech* (Berl) **28**: 196–205.

Stegman, M.R., Heaney, R.P., Travers-Gustafson, D. and Leist, J. (1995) Cortical ultrasound velocity as an indicator of bone status. *Osteoporosis Int* **5**: 349–53.

Stein, J.A., Hochberg, A.M. and Lazewatsky, L. (1987) Quantitative digital radiography for bone mineral analysis. In: *Bone Mineral Measurement by Photon Absorptiometry: Methodological Problems*, (eds Dequeker, J.V., Gawens, P. and Wahner, H.W.), Leuven University Press, Lourain, pp. 411–14.

Stevenson, J.C., Banks, L.M., Spinks, T.J. *et al.* (1987) Regional and total skeletal measurements in the early postmenopause. *J Clin Invest* **80**: 258–62.

Stevenson, J.C., Lees, B., Devenport, M., Cust, M.P. and Ganger, K.F. (1989) Determinants of bone density in normal women: risk factors for future osteoporosis. *Br Med J* **298**: 924–8.

Tothill, P. and Pye, D.W. (1992) Errors due to non-uniform distribution of fat in dual X-ray absorptiometry of the lumbar spine. *Br J Radiol* **65**: 807–13.

Tothill, P., Pye, D.W. and Teper, J. (1989) The influence of extra-skeletal fat on the accuracy of dual photon absorptiometry of the spine. In: *Osteoporosis and Bone Mineral Measurement*, (eds Ring, E.F.J., Evans, W.D. and Dixon, A.S.), IPSM, York, pp. 48–53.

Tothill, P., Smith, M.A. and Sutton, D. (1983) Dual photon absorptiometry of the spine with a low activity source of gadolinium 153. *Br J Radiol* **56**: 829–35.

Van Berkum FNR, Birkenhager, J.C., van Veen L.C.P. *et al.* (1989) Non-invasive axial and peripheral assessment of bone mineral content: a comparison between osteoporotic women and normal subjects. *J Bone Miner Res* **5**: 679–85.

Vose, G.P., Hoerster Jr, S.A. and Mack, P.B. (1964) New technique for the radiographic assessment of vertebral density. *Am J Med Electron* **3**: 181–8.

Wahner, H.W., Dunn, W.L., Brown, M.L., Morin, R.L. and Riggs, B.L. (1988) Comparison of dual energy X-ray absorptiometry and dual photon absorptiometry for bone mineral measurements of the lumbar spine. *Mayo Clin Proc* **63**: 1075–84.

Wasnich, R.D., Ross, P.D., Helbrun, L.K. and Vogel, J.M. (1985) Prediction of post-menopausal fracture risk with use of bone mineral measurements. *Am J Obstet Gynecol* **153**: 745–51.

Waud, C.E., Leu, R. and Baran, D.T. (1992) The relationship between ultrasound and densitometric measurements of bone mass at the calcaneus in women. *Calcif Tissue Int* **51**: 415–18.

WHO Study Group on Assessment of Fracture Risk and Its Application to Screening and Postmenopausal Osteoporosis (1994) Report of a WHO study group, Technical Report Series No. 843, World Health Organization, Geneva, p. 5.

Wilson, C.R. and Matson, M. (1977) Dichromatic absorptiometry of vertebral bone mineral content. *Invest Radiol* **12**: 188–94.

Yamada, M., Ito, M., Hayashi, K. *et al.* (1995) Dual energy x-ray absorptiometry of the calcaneus: comparison with other techniques to assess bone density and value in predicting risk of spine fracture. *Am J Roentgenol* **163**: 1435–40.

ESTROGEN AND OSTEOPOROSIS 8

R. Lindsay

INTRODUCTION

Fuller Albright originally described osteoporosis as a disease in which there was a high frequency of patients who had had ovariectomy performed in their premenopausal years (Albright *et al.*, 1940). Subsequently many studies have demonstrated that the loss of ovarian function is associated with increased bone turnover and consequently loss of bone mass (Lindsay, 1995). The comparatively recent demonstration that cells of the osteoblast lineage have functional estrogen receptors has improved our understanding of at least one of the mechanisms by which sex steroids may affect skeletal metabolism (Komm *et al.*, 1988; Eriksen *et al.*, 1988). In addition, it is clear that estrogens can influence calcium homeostasis, and thus indirectly modify skeletal metabolism (Cosman *et al.*, 1983). Thus it is not surprising that estrogens prevent postmenopausal bone loss and reduce the risk of osteoporotic fractures among older women.

THE EFFECT OF OVARIAN FAILURE

Irrespective of the cause, decline in the production of sex steroids and estrogen in particular leads to a series of changes in the metabolism of the skeleton (Recker *et al.*, 1988). As estrogen levels decline there is an increase in the frequency of activation of remodeling cycles in the skeleton. This can be observed by the increases that occur in markers of bone turnover in serum and urine (Christensen *et al.*, 1982; Fogelman *et al.*, 1984; Seibel *et al.*, 1993). Serum alkaline phosphatase and osteocalcin increase by 50% or more and the excretion of products of resorption of type 1 collagen, whether measured as hydroxyproline or the pyridinoline crosslinks of collagen, increase in some instances by greater amounts. Thus, with estrogen deficiency, there are increases in both bone formation and resorption.

Such increments in bone remodeling by themselves would only cause a small and reversible deficit in bone mass. However, when bone mass is measured among postmenopausal women there is a progressive decline that is greatest in the few years immediately after menopause and slows somewhat thereafter, but in many individuals may continue until old age (Aitken *et al.*, 1973; Lindsay *et al.*, 1979; Genant *et al.*, 1982; Mazess and Vatter, 1985; Nilas and Christiansen, 1988; Riggs and Wahner, 1988; Mazess, 1990; Wahner and Fogelman, 1994) (and may in fact accelerate at some skeletal sites in the older population). To produce such a decline in bone mass (or density) requires that bone resorption be increased to a greater extent than formation. It has been suggested, but never quite proven, that there is an increase in the aggressiveness of the osteoclast population with a consequent

Osteoporosis. Edited by John C. Stevenson and Robert Lindsay. Published in 1998 by Chapman & Hall, London.
ISBN 0 412 48870 1

deepening of the resorption lacuna that can only be partially filled by the osteoblast team. This imbalance between resorption and formation within each remodeling cycle could account for the progressive loss of bone mass.

Finally, at least one other feature probably accentuates the phenomenon. The increased frequency of remodeling sites increases the chances that trabeculae will have active remodeling occurring at the same time on opposite surfaces and thereby increases the chance of osteoclasts resorbing sufficient bone to completely transect the trabecula. This effect would be magnified by the deeper resorption cavities.

When that disconnection occurs (Figure 8.1) there is no remaining template upon which formation of new bone can build (Dempster *et al.*, 1986). Therefore net bone loss must occur. The consequence is loss of mass and the underlying architecture of normal cancellous bone. Thus, relatively small decrements in absolute mass can contribute large increments to the risk of fracture.

Prospective studies have demonstrated bone loss with ovarian failure at menopause or after ovariectomy in most if not all cultures in which it has been studied. In addition, ovarian failure from other causes also appears to cause bone loss (Rigotti *et al.*, 1984). Thus, bone mass is reduced in anorexia (Rigotti *et al.*, 1984; Warren *et al.*, 1989; Putukian, 1994) and hyperprolactinemia (Schlechte *et al.*, 1983; Koppelman *et al.*, 1984; Nystrome *et al.*, 1988), when reduced pituitary ovarian function is a feature, and is also low in exercise-induced amenorrhea (Sanborn *et al.*, 1982; Drinkwater *et al.*, 1984; Cann *et al.*, 1984; Lindberg *et al.*, 1984; Marcus *et al.*, 1988; Linnel *et al.*, 1989), although in the latter situation the effects may be attenuated by the positive effects of increased activity. Finally, the use of gonadotrophin agonists in the treatment of endometriosis, for example, also causes bone loss (Cann *et al.*, 1987).

These changes in bone remodeling can be measured using biochemical markers of bone turnover (Christensen *et al.*, 1982; Fogelman *et al.*, 1984; Seibel *et al.*, 1993). The newer immunoassays allow determination of markers commonly associated with resorption in urine samples and with formation in serum. Across the menopause, all increase usually by 50% or more and it has been suggested that a level above the upper limit of normal for premenopausal women should be considered as indicative of ongoing bone loss. At present, no data support that view. However, recent data do suggest that these higher values may represent, in themselves, risk factors for hip fracture, independent of bone mass (Nordin, 1986; Cummings *et al.*, 1996). It is assumed that those with higher values have higher rates of bone remodeling and consequently will be statistically more likely to produce trabecular penetration and disconnection, the microarchitectural problem that exaggerates the relationship between bone mass and fracture.

THE EFFECTS OF ESTROGEN

Intervention with estrogens reverses the effect of menopause and reduces the rate of bone loss (Albright, 1947; Lindsay *et al.*, 1976, 1978a, 1980, 1984; Horsman *et al.*, 1977; Recker *et al.*, 1977; Nachtigall *et al.*, 1979; Christiansen *et al.*, 1980; Ettinger *et al.*, 1985; Quigley *et al.*, 1987). Many prospective studies have demonstrated that estrogen intervention reduces bone remodeling to premenopausal levels and inhibits the loss of bone mass.

Several general statements may be made about the effect of estrogens. First, the dose of estrogen that is required produces circulating estrogen levels that are similar to those found in the early to midfollicular phase of the normal ovarian cycle. The route of administration appears to be irrelevant. Estrogens administered by mouth, across the skin (Need *et al.*, 1985; Aloia *et al.*, 1988; Ott and Chesnut, 1989) (transdermally, percutaneously or subcutaneously) or by vagina all seem to be

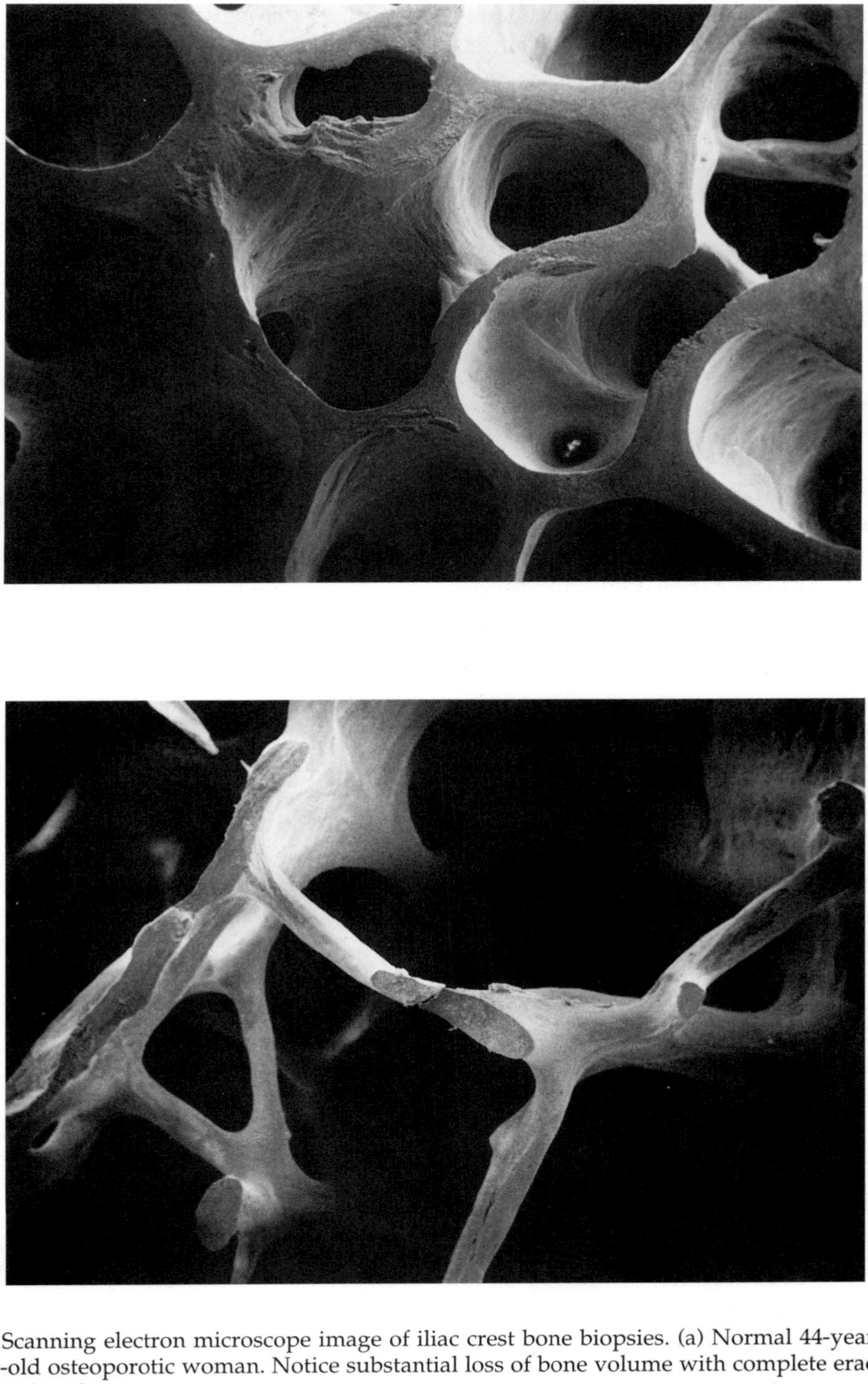

(a)

(b)

Figure 8.1 Scanning electron microscope image of iliac crest bone biopsies. (a) Normal 44-year-old man. (b) 47-year-old osteoporotic woman. Notice substantial loss of bone volume with complete eradication of many trabecular plates.

effective provided an adequate dose is administered. The use of transdermal estrogen has allowed closer evaluation of the effective dose (Need *et al.*, 1985). The administration of estradiol by skin patch results in relatively stable serum estradiol levels and a ratio of estrone to estradiol that is closer to the premenopausal ratio than that achieved when any estrogen is administered orally. Consequently, it has become evident from the recent transdermal data that estradiol levels of 50+ pg/ml are sufficient to produce a skeletal effect. Minimum doses for an adequate skeletal response have been determined for some estrogens given by the oral route.

Most of the original studies of estrogen utilized measurements of peripheral bone, either the metacarpal or radius. The study of longest duration used mestranol, a synthetic estrogen generally not used for postmenopausal women (Lindsay *et al.*, 1976, 1980) although ethinylestradiol, its close relative, is being re-evaluated. These early studies demonstrated conservation of peripheral bone mass and cross-sectional follow-up data confirmed that similar effects were seen in both spine and hip (Al-Azzawi *et al.*, 1987). Several controlled studies have been completed using bone density of the spine as the primary endpoint. These have demonstrated that the effect of estrogen on bone is a feature of all available estrogens, at generally recommended doses, with the exception of estriol which is inactive on bone up to 8 mg/day (Lindsay *et al.*, 1979).

There is more doubt about the effects of usual doses of estrogen on the femoral neck bone density. Only a few controlled studies have been completed and only one dose–response study. In that study of estrone sulfate, double the dose (1.25 mg/day) was required to obtain the effect on the hip as for the spine (Caniggia *et al.*, 1990). However, the largest prevention study completed, the PEPI study, found that the usually prescribed dose of conjugated equine estrogens, 0.625 mg/day, was almost equally effective at both spine and hip (Marcus *et al.*, 1995).

The biochemical consequences of estrogen administration are to be expected. There is a return of the biochemical markers of bone remodeling from postmenopausal to premenopausal levels (Seibel *et al.*, 1993). Indicators of both formation and resorption decline, consistent with reduction in the frequency of activation of new remodeling cycles. Since in most individuals, bone loss ceases or is significantly reduced (in fact, some individuals show a marked gain in bone mass), it must be assumed that the deficit between formation and resorption within each remodeling cycle is also corrected. Histologic confirmation of that, however, is not clearly evident in the literature.

The effects of estrogen persist for as long as therapy is given and long-term studies have shown effects lasting almost 20 years and have confirmed that the rate of bone remodeling remains at premenopausal levels as long as therapy is provided. When therapy is discontinued, bone remodeling increases again to postmenopausal levels and bone loss begins again (Lindsay *et al.*, 1978b; Christiansen *et al.*, 1981). A recent cross-sectional evaluation of older persons in the Framingham study has suggested that 10 years after stopping estrogen there is no apparent remaining effect on bone mass (Felson *et al.*, 1993).

EFFECTS OF ESTROGENS ON FRACTURES

A number of epidemiological studies have shown that estrogen intervention among postmenopausal women reduces the risk of both hip and Colles' fractures (Cameron and Sorenson, 1963; Burch *et al.*, 1974; Hutchinson *et al.*, 1979; Weiss *et al.*, 1979; Paganini-Hill *et al.*, 1981; Williams *et al.*, 1982; Kiel *et al.*, 1987). The general conclusion can be drawn that long-term estrogen use would result in about a 50% reduction in the risk of either fracture.

In several studies, 'any' estrogen exposure was used as the inclusion criterion, sometimes for as little as one year. One study of individuals over the age of 65 years suggests some protection for those who were currently on therapy, but maximum protection for those who started close to menopause and continued long term on treatment (Cauley *et al.*, 1994). Such epidemiological results can be equated with the bone density data which indicate resumption of loss of bone when estrogens are discontinued and with the Framingham study quoted above (Felson *et al.*, 1993). Ideally, a long-term controlled trial would answer such questions. With the long delay between menopause and the increase in hip fracture risk, such a study was thought unlikely, but the Women's Health Initiative sponsored by the National Institutes of Health has that as one of its goals. Shorter term studies introducing therapy among older subjects (>70 years) are currently ongoing to determine if estrogens can reduce the risk of hip fracture even if not initiated until the eighth decade.

Greater reductions in the risk of vertebral crush fracture may be expected in view of the greater vertebral responses in terms of bone mass changes. One long-term (10 year) controlled clinical trial of primary prevention suggested that perhaps 70–80% (Seibel *et al.*, 1993). In one other treatment study of established osteoporosis, in which transdermal estrogens were used, a reduction of 50% in recurrent vertebral fractures was observed (Aloia *et al.*, 1988).

TREATMENT OF ESTABLISHED OSTEOPOROSIS

Estrogen intervention also has a positive effect on osteoporosis even after the patient has presented with fracture. In a prospective controlled study we demonstrated that estrogen intervention stabilized skeletal mass and prevented further loss of bone both in the spine and hip in patients with postmenopausal osteoporosis (Lindsay and Tohme, 1990). Similar data have been reported for patients with steroid-induced osteoporosis (Lukert *et al.*, 1992). In a more recent study in which transdermal estrogens were administered to patients with postmenopausal osteoporosis, in addition to preservation of skeletal mass, a significant reduction in the risk of recurrent vertebral fracture was evident (Aloia *et al.*, 1988). Similar doses are generally used for both prevention and treatment.

INTERACTIONS WITH OTHER TREATMENT MODALITIES

CALCIUM

In almost all studies completed in the USA estrogens are given along with sufficient calcium to bring calcium intake up to 1000–1500 mg/day. Since calcium by itself has antiresorptive effects, somewhat weaker than estrogen, it is not surprising that an analysis of the published data suggests that there is some interaction between estrogen and calcium such that there may be an enhancement of the estrogen effect when calcium intake is raised to these levels (Nieves *et al.*, unpublished). This was also suggested in a small non-randomized study which demonstrated that 0.3 mg/day of conjugated equine estrogen, ineffective in preserving bone by itself, improved in efficacy when calcium intake was increased to at least 1500 mg/day (Ettinger *et al.*, 1987). Since such intakes of calcium are generally safe for most in the population, it seems reasonable to increase calcium intake above 1000 mg in anyone taking estrogen postmenopausally. It is general policy to suggest that the increase in calcium intake be achieved by dietary improvements. However, many individuals will not or cannot improve their intake by this mechanism and therefore supplemental calcium is usually provided. It should be remembered that the intent is to provide a *total* intake of 1000–1500 mg/day and in most circumstances, a 500 mg supplement will be enough to achieve this.

PROGESTINS

In women who have undergone a natural menopause, progestin therapy is usually added to the estrogen to protect the endometrium from the unopposed chronic effects of estrogen, which is known to increase the risk of endometrial hyperplasia and carcinoma (Lobo, 1994). The use of a progestin, given either cyclically for 10–12 days each calendar month or continuously with the estrogen, reverses the effects of estrogen on the endometrium. When medroxyprogesterone acetate is used in usual doses (5 mg/day for two weeks or 2.5 mg/day continuously), the addition of the progestin does not appear to influence the dominant effect of estrogen on the skeleton (Marcus *et al.*, 1995). However, there are some data that suggest that certain progestins, especially norethindrone, a 19-nortestoterone derivative, may in fact enhance the effects of estrogen on the skeleton (Christiansen and Riis, 1990). Confirmatory data for this effect are not yet available.

OTHER ANTIRESORPTIVE AGENTS

Almost no data have been published evaluating the effects of adding other antiresorptive agents, calcitonin and the bisphosphonates, to estrogen or vice versa. In one small study an additive effect on bone mass was found when estrogens and etidronate were prescribed together (Borali *et al.*, 1995). At present, studies are ongoing to determine if alendronate and estrogen can be prescribed together. It seems prudent to await the outcome of these studies before using both agents in the same patient.

ANABOLIC AGENTS

The first-line treatment for patients with osteoporosis at present is usually an agent that reduces bone turnover – estrogen, calcitonin or a bisphosphonate. Fluoride which stimulates bone formation is approved for the treatment of osteoporosis in some countries and PTH or PTHrp analogs are currently in clinical investigation (Libanati *et al.*, 1996). One retrospective review suggested that fluoride in conjunction with estrogen was more effective than either alone, but this has not been evaluated in prospective studies (Nagant de Deuxchaisnes *et al.*, 1990). Fluoride may cause *de novo* bone formation (i.e. without preceding bone resorption at the same site) or may induce increased formation by teams of osteoblasts following some resorption, consequently overfilling the cavity (Libanati *et al.*, 1996). If the latter is a feature then inhibition of resorption would have merit and if the former is more dominant, reduction in activation frequency would also have a beneficial effect. Since PTH seems to stimulate bone turnover and increase activation to produce its anabolic effect, a similar argument would hold for that agent. It is easy to hypothesize that the combination of an antiresorptive and anabolic agent would have greater effects on fracture recurrence than either alone, but no data are available. Indeed, there are limited data supporting the use of such anabolic agents by themselves, especially fluorides where conflicting data have been presented about their fracture effects.

GENERAL EFFECTS OF ESTROGENS

Estrogens are potent hormones with wide-ranging effects on a variety of tissues (Lobo, 1994). In addition to reducing the clinical sequelae of menopause (hot flushes and sweats), estrogens also affect the tissues of the urogenital tract. Vaginal dryness, often evident in postmenopausal women, is relieved and in some instances estrogens also reduce urinary incompetence that can occur not infrequently in the postmenopause. In addition to these effects on the genital organs, estrogens, which have specific receptors in many tissues, might be expected to have other more general effects. Indeed, considerable epidemiological evidence suggests that estrogens reduce the risk of cardiovascular disease among postmenopausal women (Spicer and Pike, 1994). Although no prospective clinical trials have been published, the epidemiological data are quite convincing. In general it appears as though estrogen use is associated with a reduction in risk of myocardial infarction of about 50%. The mechanism for these effects, like the mechanism for the effects of the skeleton, is not known in detail. Since estrogens increase HDL and reduce LDL in serum, it has been suggested that this might be the mechanism since it would improve the profile of lipids in circulation. However, more recent data, again from epidemiological studies, suggest that, at best, the effect of estrogen on lipids can account for no more than half of the observed effect on heart disease. Animal studies have pointed out that estrogens may have physiological effects on coronary blood flow, mediated by direct effects of estrogen on endothelium or smooth muscle. Estrogens may modulate the oxidation of cholesterol, reducing the uptake of cholesterol into the smooth muscle layer, one of the early occurrences in the development of atheromatous plaque. In addition, estrogen status may modulate the responses of the coronary artery to agents that normally control the state of vasodilation. For example, it has been suggested that in the absence of estrogen acetylcholine will produce vasoconstriction whereas in the presence of estrogen, the same agent produces vasodilation. In addition, the effects of estrogen on vasoactivity might be mediated by nitric oxide. Thus, local actions of estrogen may be responsible for modifing coronary artery disease among women. The effects, if any, of adding a progestin to the regimen are not known at this point.

As stated above, estrogens have multiple effects on tissues throughout the body. Perhaps the most concerning issue for women who require estrogen intervention after menopause is the relationship between breast disease and estrogen exposure (Spicer and Pike, 1994). The epidemiology of breast cancer suggests that the longer a woman has ovarian function (that is, the duration from menarche to menopause), the greater the risk of breast cancer. Ovariectomy in premenopausal years reduces the risk of breast cancer. It has been proposed that estrogen production by the ovary is the agent that increases risk. However, pregnancy, especially at a young age, appears protective and the mechanism is not clear.

Numerous epidemiological studies have examined the relationship between estrogen use among postmenopausal women and breast cancer (Spicer and Pike, 1994). The results vary considerably, with some studies showing an increase in risk while others do not. The meta-analyses that have been performed also reach conflicting conclusions (Spicer and Pike, 1994). Given the difficulty in interpreting the mechanism by which the presence or absence of ovaries influences breast cancer and the effect of pregnancy, it is perhaps not surprising that the epidemiological data for exogenous estrogen in postmenopausal women are variable. Since breast cancer is a disease whose incidence increases with age and one that can be a deadly and psychologically crippling disorder, perhaps the most important issue is to emphasize the important role of early detection. Mammography clearly is important for all postmenopausal women. Estrogen use, it must be emphasized to the patient, is not the criterion for mammography, but rather the knowledge that early diagnosis improves outcome in all patients.

ESTROGEN ANALOGS

There has been recent interest in harnessing the beneficial effects of estrogen while limiting its unwanted effects, especially on the uterus and breast. The demonstration that tamoxifen, an agent used for secondary prevention of breast cancer, was able to prevent bone loss among postmenopausal women (Turken *et al.*, 1989; Love *et al.*, 1992) has stimulated interest in the possibility that estrogen analogs might be found with skeletal and cardiovascular effects, but little if any effect on the uterus. The mechanism by which this might be achieved remains unclear. Since there appears to be only one estrogen receptor, at least in humans and outwith the CNS, differences in target tissue response must depend on the ligand interaction with the receptor and the postreceptor machinery. It has been suggested that an agent such as tamoxifen produces a different conformational change when it binds to the receptor, with the consequence that only one of the two transcription-activating sites is available. Alternatives to this include alterations in demineralization, phosphorylation or DNA binding, plus tissue differences in the many cofactors required for the transcription process (Lindsay, 1996).

At present several analogs are in development. The lead compound is raloxifene which in short-term data reduces bone turnover similarly to conjugated equine estrogens (Draper *et al.*, 1996). Animal and *in vitro* data support the concept that raloxifene does not stimulate the endometrium and may protect against breast cancer recurrence, like tamoxifen. Long-term clinical studies are under way.

CONCLUSION

Estrogen deprivation increases bone remodeling and accelerates bone loss. The consequence is an increase in the risk of osteoporotic fracture. The level of risk is inversely related to bone mass. Estrogen intervention reduces bone turnover and prevents bone loss. Long-term therapy has been associated with a reduction in the risk of osteoporotic fractures. Estrogens are potent hormones that have many effects throughout the body. An increase in the risk of endometrial hyperplasia and carcinoma has been associated with long-term estrogen use. For patients with a uterus, the addition of a progestin protects the endometrium. Some data suggest that long-term estrogen (>10 years) is associated with a small increase in the risk of breast cancer. However, other data have failed to confirm this. The effect of the progestin on breast tissue has yet to be evaluated fully. Estrogens have been shown in several epidemiological studies to reduce the risk of ischemic heart disease. The consequence is that for many postmenopausal women the benefits of estrogen probably outweigh the risks. Estrogen analogs with selective actions are currently in development.

REFERENCES

Aitken, J.M., Hart, D.M., Anderson, J.B., Lindsay, R. and Smith, D.A. (1973) Osteoporosis after oophorectomy for non-malignant disease. *Br Med J* **i**: 325–8.

Al-Azzawi F., Hart, D.M. and Lindsay, R. (1987) Long-term effect of oestrogen replacement therapy on bone mass as measured by dual photon absorptiometry. *Br Med J* **294**: 1261–2.

Albright, F. (1947) The effect of hormones on osteogenesis in man. *Recent Prog Horm Res* **1**: 293–353.

Albright, F., Bloomberg, F. and Smith, P.H. (1940) Postmenopausal osteoporosis. *Trans Assoc Am Phys* **55**: 298–305.

Aloia, J.F., Vaswani, A., Yeh, J.K. *et al.* (1988) Calcitriol in the treatment of postmenopausal osteoporosis. *Am J Med* **84**: 401–8.

Bovali, S.M., Wimalawansa, S.J. and Jolicoeur, F.B. (1995) Combined therapy with estrogen and etidronate has an additive effect on bone mineral density in the hip and vertebrae: 4 year randomized study. *Am J Med* **99**: 36–42.

Burch, J.C., Byrd, B.F. and Vaughn, W.K. (1974) The effects of long-term estrogen on hysterectomized women. *Am J Obstet Gynecol* **118**: 778–82.

Cameron, J.R. and Sorenson, J. (1963) Measurement of bone mineral *in vivo*: an improved method. *Science* **142**: 230–2.

Caniggia, A., Nuti, R., Lore, F. *et al.* (1990) Long-term treatment with calcitriol in post-menopausal osteoporosis. *Metabolism* **39** (Suppl. 1): 43–9.

Cann, C.E., Martin, M.C. and Genant, H.K. (1984) Decreased spinal mineral content in amenorrheic women. *J Am Med Assoc* **251**: 626–9.

Cann, C.E., Henzl, M.R., Burrk, K. *et al.* (1987) Reversible bone loss is produced by the GnRH agonist nafarelin. In: *Calcium Regulation and Bone Metabolism: Basic and Clinical Aspects*, (eds Cohn, D.V., Martin, T.J. and Meinier, P.J.), Elsevier, Amsterdam, pp. 123–7.

Cauley, J.A., Seeley, D.G., Ensrud, K. *et al.* (1994) Estrogen replacement therapy and fractures in older women. *Ann Intern Med* **122**: 9–16.

Christensen, M.S., Hagen, C., Christiansen, C. and Transbol, I. (1982) Dose–response evaluation of cyclic estrogen/gestagen in postmenopausal women: placebo controlled trial of its gynecologic and metabolic actions. *Am J Obstet Gynecol* **144**: 873–9.

Christiansen, C. and Riis, B.J. (1990) Beta-estradiol and continuous norethisterone: a unique treatment for established osteoporosis in elderly women. *J Clin Endocrinol Metab* **71**: 836–41.

Christiansen, C., Christiansen, M.S. and McNair, P. (1980) Prevention of early postmenopausal bone loss: conducted 2 years study in 315 normal females. *Eur J Clin Invest* **10**: 273–9.

Christiansen, C., Christiansen, M.S. and Transbol, I. (1981) Bone mass in postmenopausal women after withdrawal of estrogen/gestagen replacement therapy. *Lancet* **i**: 459–61.

Cosman, F., Shen, V., Xie, F. *et al.* (1983) A mechanism of estrogen action on the skeleton: protection against the resorbing effects of (1–34)hPTH infusion as assessed by biochemical markers. *Ann Intern Med* **118**: 337–43.

Cummings, S.R., Black, D., Ensrud, K. *et al.* (1996) Urine markers of bone resorption predict hip bone loss and fractures in older women: the study of osteoporotic fractures. *J Bone Miner Res* **11** (Suppl): S128 (abstract).

Dempster, D.W., Shane, E., Horbert, W. and Lindsay, R. (1986) A simple method for correlative light and scanning electron microscopy of human iliac crest bone biopsies: qualitative observations in normal and osteoporotic subjects. *J Bone Miner Res* **1**: 15–21.

Draper, M.W., Flowers, D.E., Huster, W.J. *et al.* (1996) A controlled trial of raloxifene (LY 139481) HCl: impact on bone turnover and serum lipid profile in healthy postmenopausal women. *J Bone Miner Res* **11**: 835–42.

Drinkwater, B.L., Nilson, K., Chestnut, C.H.I. *et al.* (1984) Bone mineral content of amenorrhea and eumenorrheic athletics. *N Engl J Med* **311**: 277–81.

Eriksen, EF, Colvard, D.S., Berg, N.J. *et al.* (1988) Evidence of estrogen receptors in normal human osteoblast-like cells. *Science* **241**: 84–6.

Ettinger, B., Genant, H.K. and Cann, C.E. (1985) Long-term estrogen therapy prevents bone loss and fracture. *Ann Intern Med* **102**: 319–24.

Ettinger, B., Genant, H.K. and Cann, C.E. (1987) Postmenopausal bone loss is prevented by treatment with low-dosage estrogen with calcium. *Ann Intern Med* **106**: 40–5.

Felson, D.T., Zhang, Y., Hannan, M.T. *et al.* (1993) The effect of postmenopausal estrogen therapy on bone density in elderly women. *N Engl J Med* **329**: 1141–6.

Fogelman, I., Poser, J.W., Smith, M.L., Hart, D.M. and Bevan, J.A. (1984) Alterations in skeletal metabolism following oophorectomy. In: *Osteoporosis*, (eds Christiansen, C. *et al.*), Aalborg Stiftsogtrykkeri, Glostrup pp. 519–22.

Genant, H.K., Cann, C.E., Ettinger, B. and Gordon, G.S. (1982) Quantitative computed tomography of vertebral spongiosa: a sensitive method for detecting early bone loss after oophorectomy. *Ann Intern Med* **97**: 699–705.

Horsman, A., Gallagher, J.C., Simpson, M. and Nordin, B.E.C. (1977) Prospective trial of estrogen and calcium in postmenopausal women. *Br Med J* **2**: 789–92.

Hutchinson, T.A., Polansky, J.M. and Feinstein, A.R. (1979) Postmenopausal oestrogens protect against fracture of hip and distal radius. *Lancet* **ii**: 705–9.

Kiel, D.P., Felson, D.T. and Anderson, J.J. (1987) Hip fracture and the use of estrogens in postmenopausal women. *N Engl J Med* **317**: 1169–74.

Komm, B.S., Terpening, C.M. and Benz, D.J. (1988) Estrogen binding, receptor mRNA, and biologic response in osteoblast-like osteosarcoma cells. *Science* **241**: 81–4.

Koppelman, M.C.S., Kurtz, D.W., Morrish, K.A. *et al.* (1984) Vertebral body bone mineral in hyperprolactinemic women. *J Clin Endocrinol Metab* **59**: 1050–3.

Libanati, C., Lau, K.W. and Baylink, D. (1996) Fluoride therapy for osteoporosis. In: *Osteoporosis*, (eds Marcus, R., Feldman, D. and Kelsey, J.), Academic Press, San Diego, pp. 1259–77.

Lindberg, J.S., Fears, W.B. and Hunt, M.M. (1984) Exercise induced amenorrhea and bone density. *Ann Intern Med* **101**: 747–49.

Lindsay, R. (1995) Estrogen deficiency. In: *Osteoporosis: Etiology, Diagnosis and Management*, (ed. Riggs, B.L.), Raven Press, New York, pp. 133–60.

Lindsay, R. (1996) The estrogen receptor in bone. Evolution of knowledge. *Br J Obstet Gynaecol* **13**: 16–19.

Lindsay, R. and Tohme, J. (1990) Estrogen treatment of patients with established postmenopausal osteoporosis. *Obstet Gynecol* **76**: 1–6.

Lindsay, R., Aitken, J.M., Anderson, J.B. *et al.* (1976) Long-term prevention of postmenopausal osteoporosis by oestrogen. *Lancet* **i**: 1038–41.

Lindsay, R., Hart, D.M., Purdie, P. *et al.* (1978a) Comparative effects of oestrogen and a progestogen on bone loss in postmenopausal women. *Clin Sci Mol M* **54**: 193–5.

Lindsay, R., Hart, D.M., MacLean, A. *et al.* (1978b) Bone response to termination of oestrogen treatment. *Lancet* **i**: 1325–7.

Lindsay, R., Hart, D.M., MacLean A, Garwood, J. and Kraszewski, A. (1979) Bone loss during oestrial therapy in postmenopausal women. *Maturitas* **1**: 279–85.

Lindsay, R., Hart, D.M., Forrest, C. and Baird, C. (1980) Prevention of spinal osteoporosis in oophorectomized women. *Lancet* **ii**: 1151–4.

Lindsay, R., Hart, D.M. and Clark, D.M. (1984) The minimum effective dose of estrogen for prevention of postmenopausal bone loss. *Obstet Gynecol* **63**: 759–63.

Linnel, S.L., Stager, M.M. and Blue, P.W. (1989) Bone mineral content and menstrual regularity in female runners. *Med Sci Sports Exer* **16**: 343–8.

Lobo, R. (ed.) (1994) *Treatment of the Postmenopausal Women. Basic and Clinical Aspects*, Raven Press, New York.

Love, R.R., Mazess, R.B., Barden, H.S. *et al.* (1992) Effects of tamoxifen on bone mineral density in postmenopausal women with breast cancer. *N Engl J Med* **326**; 852–6.

Lukert, P.B., Johnson, B.E. and Robinson, R.G. (1992) Estrogen and progesterone replacement therapy reduce glucocorticoid-induced bone loss. *J Bone Miner Res* **7**: 1063–9.

Marcus, R., Cann, C., Madorg, P. *et al.* (1988) Menstrual function and bone mass in elite women distance runners. *Ann Intern Med* **102**: 158–63.

Marcus, R. and the PEPI Trial Investigators. (1995) Effects of hormone replacement therapies on bone mineral density: results from the postmenopausal Estrogen and Progestin Interventions Trial. *J Bone Miner Res* **10** (Suppl 1): S30 (Abstract).

Mazess, R.B. (1990) Bone densitometry for clinical diagnosis and monitoring. In: *Osteoporosis: Physiological Basis, Assessment and Treatment*, (eds Deluca, H.F. and Mazess, R.B.), Elsevier, New York, pp. 63–85.

Mazess, R.B. and Vatter, J. (1985) The influence of marrow on measurement of trabecular bone using computed tomography. *Bone* **6**: 349–51.

Nachtigall L.E., Nachtigall, R.H. and Nachtigall R.D. (1979) Estrogen replacement therapy I: a 10-year prospective study in the relationship to osteoporosis. *Obstet Gynecol* **53**; 277.

Nagant de Deuxchaisnes, C., Devogelaer, J.P., Depresseux, G., Malghem, J. and Mardague, B. (1990) Treatment of the vertebral crush fracture syndrome with enteric-coated sodium fluoride tablets and calcium supplements. *J Bone Miner Res* **5**: 5–26.

Need, A.G., Horowitz, J.C., Philcox, J.C. and Nordin, B.E.C. (1985) Dihydroxycalciferol and calcium therapy in osteoporosis with calcium malabsorption. *Miner Electrolyte Metab* **11**: 35–40.

Nieves, J., Komar, L., Cosman, F. and Lindsay, R. Calcium potentiates the beneficial effect of antiresporptive therapy. Unpublished data.

Nilas, L. and Christiansen, C. (1988) Rates of bone loss in normal women: evidence of accelerated trabecular bone loss after the menopause. *Eur J Clin Invest* **18**: 529–34.

Nordin, B.E.C. (1986) Calcium. *J Food Nutrition* **42**: 67–82.

Nystrome, E., Leman, J., Lundberg, P.A. *et al.* (1988) Bone mineral content in normally menstruating women with hyperprolactinemia. *Horm Res* **29**: 214–17.

Ott, S.M. and Chesnut, C.H.I. (1989) Calcitriol treatment is not effective in postmenopausal osteoporosis. *Ann Intern Med* **110**: 267–74.

Paganini-Hill, A., Ross, R.K., Gerkins, V.R. *et al.* (1981) Menopausal estrogen therapy and hip fractures. *Ann Intern Med* **95**: 28–31.

Putukian, M. (1994) The female triad: eating disorders, amenorrhea, and osteoporosis. *Med Clin North Am* **78**: 345–56.

Quigley, M.E.T., Martin, B.L., Burnier, A.M. and

Brooks, P. (1987) Estrogen therapy arrests bone loss in elderly women. *Am J Obstet Gynecol* **156**: 1516–23.

Recker, R.R., Saville, P.D. and Heaney, R.P. (1977) The effect of estrogens and calcium carbonate on bone loss in postmenopausal women. *Ann Intern Med* **87**; 649–55.

Recker, R.R., Kimmel, D.B. and Parfitt, A.M. (1988) Static and tetracycline-base bone histomorphometric data from 34 normal postmenopausal females. *J Bone Miner Res* **3**: 133–44.

Riggs, B.L. and Wahner, H.W. (1988) Bone densitometry and clinical decision-making in osteoporosis. *Ann Intern Med* **108**: 293–4.

Rigotti, N.A., Nussbaum, S.R., Herzog, D.B. *et al.* (1984) Osteoporosis in women with anorexia nervosa. *N Engl J Med* **311**: 1601–6.

Sanborn, C.F., Martin, B.J. and Wagner, W.W. (1982) Is athletic amenorrhea specific to runners? *Am J Obstet Gynecol* **143**: 859–61.

Schlechte, J.A., Sherman, B. and Martin, R. (1983) Bone density in amenorrheic women with and without hyperprolactinemia. *J Clin Endocrinol Metab* **56**: 1120–3.

Seibel, M., Cosman, F., Shen, V. *et al.* (1993) Urinary hydroxypyridinium crosslinks of collagen as markers of bone resorption and estrogen efficacy in postmenopausal osteoporosis. *J Bone Miner Res* **8**: 881–9.

Spicer, D.V. and Pike, M.C. (1994) Epidemiology of breast cancer. In: *Treatment of the Postmenopausal Woman*, (ed. Lobo, R.), Raven Press, New York, pp. 315–24.

Turken, S., Siris, E., Seldin, D. and Lindsay, R. (1989) Effects of tamoxifen on spinal bone density. *J Natl Cancer Inst* **81**: 1086–8.

Wahner, H.W. and Fogelman, I. (1994) *The Evaluation of Osteoporosis in Dual Energy X-Ray Absorptiometry in Clinical Practice*, Martin Dunitz, London.

Warren, M.F., Shane, E., Lee, M.J. *et al.* (1989) Osteonecrosis of the hip associated with anorexia nervosa in a 20 year old ballet dancer. *Clin Orthop* **251**: 171–6.

Weiss, N.S., Szekely, D.R., Dalla, R. *et al.* (1979) Endometrial cancer in relation to patterns of menopausal estrogen use. *J Am Med Assoc* **242**: 261–4.

Williams, A.R., Weiss, N.S., Ure, C. *et al.* (1982) Effect of weight, smoking, and estrogen use on the risk of hip and forearm fractures in postmenopausal women. *Obstet Gynecol* **60:** 695.

THE USE OF BISPHOSPHONATES IN OSTEOPOROSIS 9

H. Fleisch

INTRODUCTION

The bisphosphonates are a new class of drugs developed in the past two decades for use in various diseases of bone and calcium metabolism. This chapter will deal with the chemistry, the effects and their mechanisms, the pharmacokinetics and the toxicology of these compounds, with emphasis on the parts relevant to their use in osteoporosis. Their clinical use in osteoporosis will then be reviewed. For a more complete update of the bisphosphonates and their clinical applications, also other than in osteoporosis, see Fleisch (1991, 1993, 1995) and Geddes *et al.* (1994). Their use in osteoporosis is the subject of three relatively recent reviews (Parfitt, 1991; Papapoulos *et al.*, 1992; Bijvoet *et al.*, 1993).

CHEMISTRY AND GENERAL CHARACTERISTICS

Bisphosphonates, previously erroneously called diphosphonates, are compounds characterized by two C-P bonds. If the two bonds are located on the same carbon atom, the compounds are called geminal bisphosphonates. They are therefore analogs of pyrophosphate, containing an oxygen instead of a carbon atom. For the sake of simplicity, they are usually just called bisphosphonates (Figure 9.1).

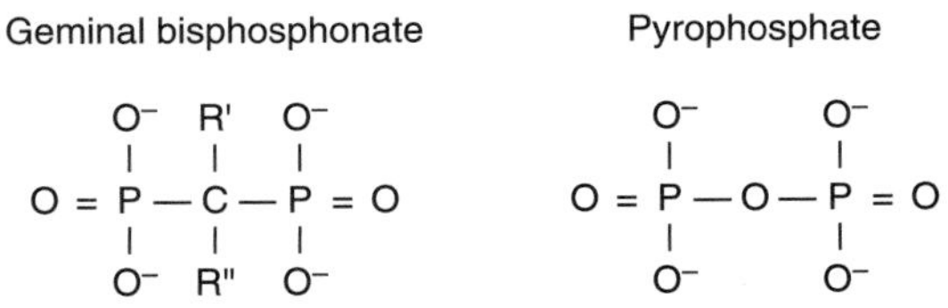

Figure 9.1 Structure of pyrophosphate and geminal bisphosphanate.

Since the first description of their biological effects on bone (Fleisch *et al.*, 1968), many different bisphosphonates have been synthesized and studied. The compounds listed in Figure 9.2, in order of their potency, have been investigated in humans with bone disease. Five are commercially available. Six of them have been studied in osteoporosis and of those, alendronate, clodronate, etidroonate and pamidronate are commercially available today for this indication.

Each bisphosphonate has its own physicochemical and biological characteristics. This is of interest in the light of future development of new compounds. It also means, however, that it is not possible to extrapolate from the results of one compound to others.

The P-C-P bond of the bisphosphonates is stable to heat and most chemical reagents and completely resistant to enzymatic hydrolysis. As a consequence, these compounds are not degraded in the body.

Osteoporosis. Edited by John C. Stevenson and Robert Lindsay. Published in 1998 by Chapman & Hall, London. ISBN 0 412 48870 1

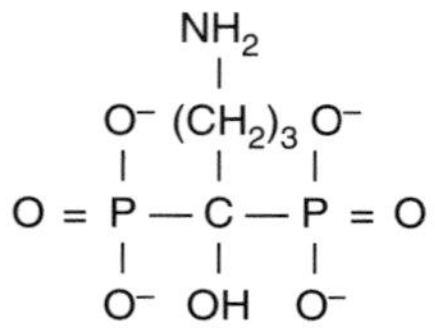

(4-Amino-1-hydroxybutylidene)-bis-phosphonate
Alendronate*
Gentili; Merck Sharp & Dohme

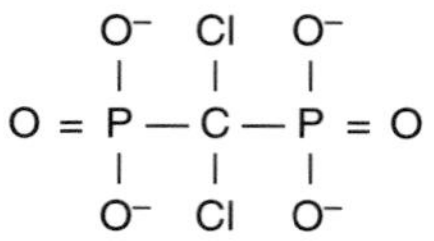

(Dichloromethylene)-bis-phosphonate
Clodronate*
Astra; Boehringer Mannheim; Gentili; Leiras; Rhône-Poulenc Rorer

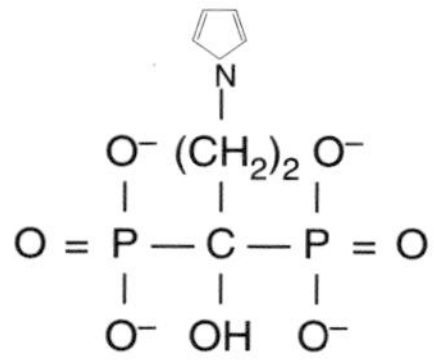

[1-Hydroxy-3-(1-pyrrolidinyl)-propylidene]bis-phosphonate
EB-1053
Leo

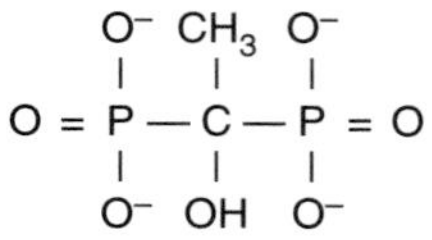

(1-Hydroxyethylidene)-bis-phosphonate
Etidronate*
Gentili; Procter & Gamble

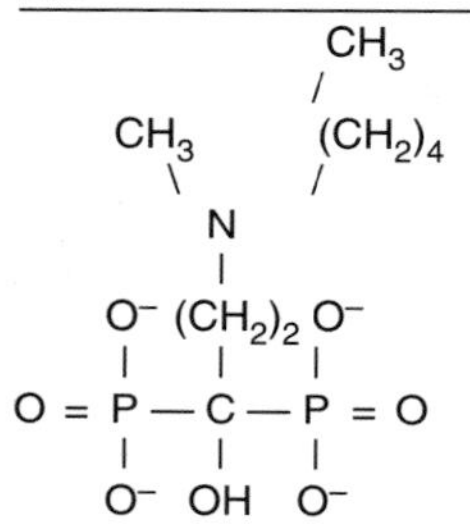

[1-Hydroxy-3-(methylpentylamino) propylidene]bis-phosphonate
Ibandronate*
Boehringer Mannheim

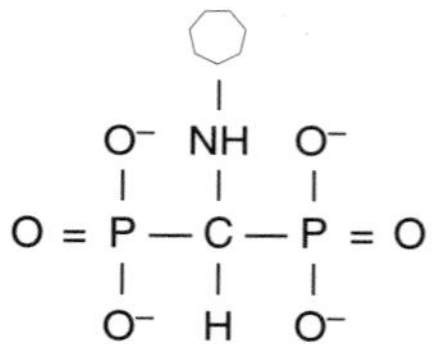

[(Cycloheptylamino)-methylene]bis-phosphonate
Incadronate
Yamanouchi

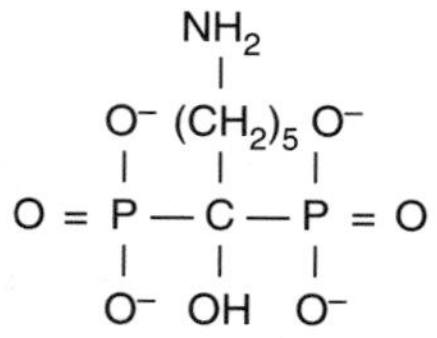

(6-Amino-1-hydroxyhexylidene)bis-phosphonate
Neridronate*
Gentili

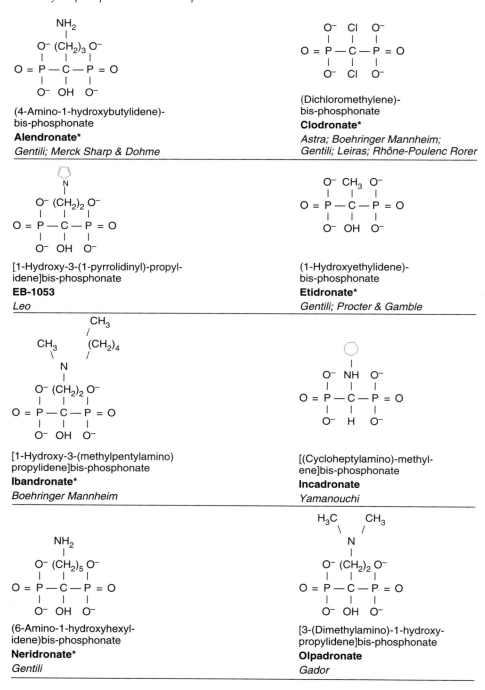

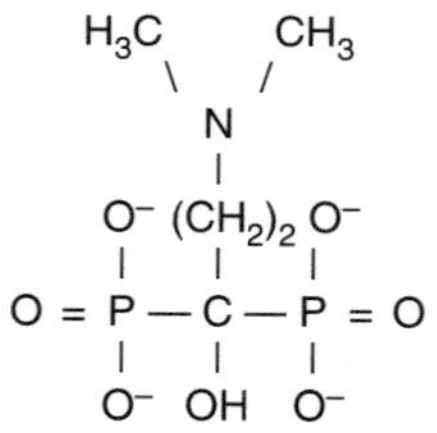

[3-(Dimethylamino)-1-hydroxypropylidene]bis-phosphonate
Olpadronate
Gador

Figure 9.2 Chemical structure of bisphosphonates investigated for their effect on bone in humans. *Commercially available.

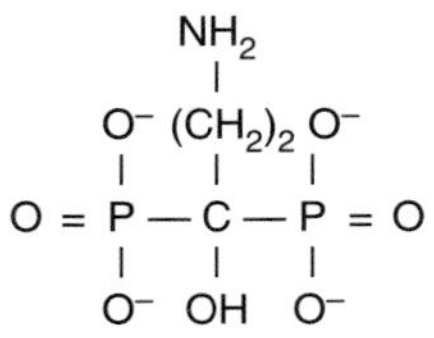

(3-Amino-1-hydroxypropy-
lidene)bis-phosphonate
Pamidronate*
Ciba-Geigy; Gador

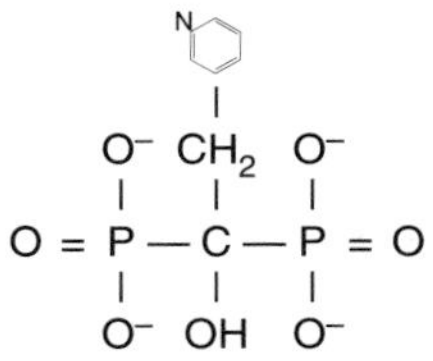

[1-Hydroxy-2-(3-pyridinyl)-
ethylidene]bis-phosphonate
Risedronate
Procter & Gamble

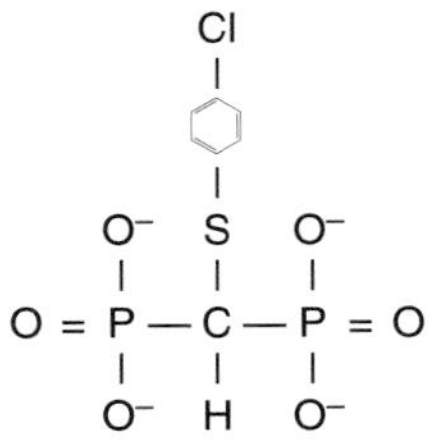

[[(4-Chlorophenyl)thio]-
methylene]bis-phosphonate
Tiludronate*
Sanofi

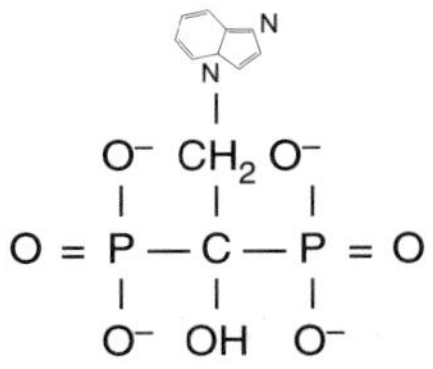

[1-Hydroxy-2-imidazo-(1,2-a) pyridin-
3-ylethylidene]bis-phosphonate
YH 529
Yamanouchi-Hoechst

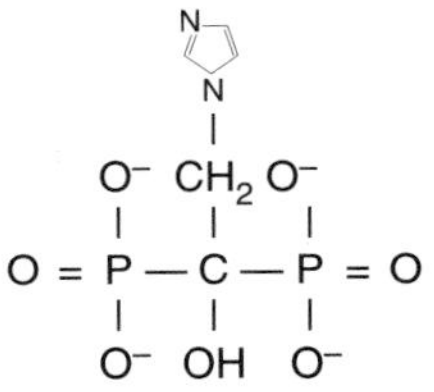

[1-Hydroxy-2-(1H-imidazde-1-yl)
ethylidene]bis-phosphonate
Zoledronate
Ciba-Geigy

Figure 9.2 *continued*

EFFECTS

PHYSICOCHEMICAL EFFECTS

The physicochemical effects are very similar to those of pyrophosphate, reflecting their chemical similarity. Thus, bisphosphonates have a marked affinity for solid-phase calcium phosphate. They bind to the crystal surface by chemisorption onto calcium (Jung *et al.*, 1973) and then act as crystal poisons of both growth and dissolution. Thus they can inhibit the formation of calcium phosphate crystals (Francis, 1969; Francis *et al.*, 1969; Fleisch *et al.*, 1970), as well as their aggregation (Hansen *et al.*, 1976), and slow down their dissolution (Fleisch *et al.*, 1969; Russell *et al.*, 1970).

INHIBITION OF BONE RESORPTION

Bisphosphonates are very powerful inhibitors of bone resorption, as shown both *in vitro* and *in vivo*.

In vitro they block bone resorption induced by various means in organ culture (Fleisch *et al.*, 1969; Reynolds *et al.*, 1972; Jung *et al.*, 1981; Boonekamp *et al.*, 1986). *In vivo* they are active both in normal animals and in experimentally induced resorption.

Normal animals

The inhibition of endogenous bone resorption can be visualized by various means. Thus, bisphosphonates block the destruction of the primary and secondary trabeculae, so that the metaphysis becomes club-shaped and radiologically more dense (Schenk *et al.*, 1973; Reitsma *et al.*, 1980). This effect, which is easily visualized morphologically, is used in the rat as a model to study the potency of new compounds (Schenk *et al.*, 1986). It can also be seen after long-term administration (Bijvoet *et al.*, 1980). In the mouse, it leads to a picture like that seen in gray-lethal congenital osteopetrotic mutants (Reynolds *et al.*, 1973). The inhibition of bone destruction is also visualized by other means, such as biochemical markers like urinary hydroxyproline excretion, as well as by ^{45}Ca kinetic studies (Gasser *et al.*, 1972).

The increase in bone mass observed in the metaphysis can also be detected by calcium balance. Thus etidronate (Gasser *et al.*, 1972) and, to a greater extent, clodronate (Gasser *et al.*, 1972), pamidronate (Reitsma *et al.*, 1980) and recently [1-hydroxy-3-(methylpentylamino)propylidene]bis-phosphonate (ibandronate) (Fleisch, 1996) are able to increase calcium balance by more than 25% when given to growing rats for 10 days. It is not known for how long this increase is sustained after discontinuing the drug. It is also unknown to what extent it is present in non-growing animals. If this uncoupling between bone resorption and bone formation is a general and durable effect, it would be relevant for the use of these compounds in osteoporosis. The increase in calcium balance is mediated through an increase in the intestinal absorption of calcium (Gasser *et al.*, 1972), as a result of an increase in $1{,}25(OH)_2D_3$ (Guilland *et al.*, 1975).

The effect on the balance is, however, less than would be expected considering the dramatic decrease in bone resorption. Studies with ^{45}Ca have shown that this is due to some decrease in bone formation (Gasser *et al.*, 1972; Reitsma *et al.*, 1980), which can be seen at the level of longitudinal growth (Schenk *et al.*, 1973) and midshaft expansion (Wink and Hill, 1988). Probably, at least for small doses, this is not due primarily to a direct effect of the bisphosphonates, but is secondary to the decrease in bone resorption, through the so-called 'coupling' between resorption and formation. In contrast, the decrease observed with high concentrations of some of the bisphosphonates may be direct. In the case of etidronate, it is also explained by the inhibition of mineralization.

Experimentally induced bone resorption in models other than osteoporosis

Bisphosphonates also impair bone resorption induced by various agents such as parathyroid hormone (Fleisch *et al.*, 1969; Russell *et al.*, 1970) and retinoids (Trechsel *et al.*, 1987). The latter effect has given a powerful screening assay for new compounds (Mühlbauer *et al.*, 1991). Furthermore, they are active in tumoral bone resorption where they can decrease or prevent hypercalcemia and hypercalciuria induced by subcutaneously implanted Walker 256 carcinomas (Johnson *et al.*, 1982; Kozak *et al.*, 1987) or Leydig tumors (Martodam *et al.*, 1983). Also bone resorption due to actual tumor invasion is slowed (Jung *et al.*, 1984). The bisphosphonates, however, do not inhibit the multiplication of tumor cells; they are therefore not active on the tumor itself but exert their action by inhibiting the osteolytic process.

Experimental osteoporosis

A number of bisphosphonates have been tested on various models of experimental osteoporosis. The results show that the compounds which inhibit bone resorption also inhibit bone loss in these models.

Sciatic nerve section

This model has been used by various groups, mostly in the rat. In general, the induced bone loss is completely inhibited and the contralateral non-immobilized paw even shows an increase in bone mass. Positive effects have been found with clodronate (Mühlbauer *et al.*, 1971; Michael *et al.*, 1971; Lane and Steinberg, 1973), etidronate (Mühlbauer *et al.*, 1971; Michael *et al.*, 1971; Cabanela and Jowsey, 1971; Hähnel *et al.*, 1973; Shiota, 1985), olpadronate (Lindenhayn *et al.*, 1979; Ferretti *et al.*, 1992) and tiludronate (Murakami *et al.*, 1994).

Spinal cord section

Pamidronate was found to inhibit bone loss in this model (Schoutens *et al.*, 1988).

Immobilization by other means

Immobilization by putting animals in very small cages or by suspending them by the tail to keep their back limbs unloaded also induces bone loss, which is inhibited by etidronate (Shvets *et al.*, 1986) and alendronate (Apseloff *et al.*, 1991, 1993) respectively.

Ovariectomy and male castration

Ovariectomy produces a significant bone loss in animals. This fact has, therefore, been used frequently as a model for human post-menopausal osteoporosis. Bisphosphonates are very effective in preventing this loss. In the past, most experiments were performed in the rat and the following bisphosphonates were found to be active in this model: alendronate (Seedor *et al.*, 1991), clodronate (Hannuniemi and Virtamo, 1992), etidronate (Shiota, 1985; Togari *et al.*, 1991; Wronski *et al.*, 1991, 1993), both when the compound was given immediately after ovariectomy or some months later, incadronate (Motoie *et al.*, 1995), risedronate (McOsker and Sietsema, 1990; Wronski *et al.*, 1991, 1993; Jee *et al.*, 1993) and tiludronate (Ammann *et al.*, 1993). Alendronate is also active in the ovariectomized baboon (Thompson *et al.*, 1992; Balena *et al.*, 1993) and tiludronate (De Vernejoul *et al.*, 1990), ibandronate (Monier-Faugere *et al.*, 1993) and incadronate (Motoie *et al.*, 1995) in the dog.

Furthermore, the loss induced by castration in males is attenuated by bisphosphonates, as shown for clodronate (Wink *et al.*, 1985) and tiludronate (Barbier *et al.*, 1990).

It is of interest that bisphosphonates, particularly risedronate, also protect new bone induced by a bone-forming agent such as prostaglandins from destruction (Jee *et al.*, 1993).

Corticosteroids

Corticosteroids can produce bone loss in animals. This loss was inhibited by clodronate in the rabbit (Jee *et al.*, 1981), while etidronate was ineffective in one study in the rat (Cabanela and Jowsey, 1971).

Thyroid hormones

Bone loss induced in rats with tri-iodothyronine was prevented by the administration of pamidronate (Rosen *et al.*, 1993a) and loss induced with thyroxine by alendronate (Yamamoto *et al.*, 1993).

Low-calcium diet

The results with low-calcium diet are ambiguous. Both etidronate and clodronate were unable to alter the bone loss in the rat in one study (Jowsey and Holley, 1973), while etidronate was active in another (Shiota, 1985). Clodronate was active in the lactating rat fed low calcium (Brommage and Baxter, 1990).

Heparin

The bone loss induced by heparin is inhibited by etidronate (Hähnel *et al.*, 1973).

Many of these studies were performed in growing animals, in which the bisphosphonates increased bone mass conspicuously by inhibiting the resorption of the metaphyseal bone. Therefore, it is generally not possible to know whether an inhibition of the bone loss induced by the various procedures is due only to the effect of the compound on the induced bone loss or also to a general effect on endogenous bone resorption. This is especially true since the proper controls, namely non-osteoporotic animals, are often not available.

Effect of bisphosphonates on bone strength

Although it is generally accepted that bone strength usually correlates well with bone density, it is nevertheless necessary to prove that this is indeed true when testing a pharmacological treatment. This is even more so in the case of the bisphosphonates, since some of them, like etidronate, can inhibit mineralization if given in high doses. Furthermore, one study indicates that when bisphosphonates are given at very high doses, they can inhibit bone resorption to such an extent that bone may become fragile due to an excessively low turnover, thus resembling bones seen in osteopetrosis (Flora *et al.*, 1980). It is only recently that this issue has been addressed extensively. The results available show that the increase in bone mass is accompanied by an increase in biomechanical strength, unless very high doses are administered.

Normal animals

Alendronate, when given daily to rats over 100 weeks, increased the ultimate femoral bending load and the vertebral ultimate compressive load (Guy *et al.*, 1993).

In one study, etidronate had either no effect or, when given in large doses which inhibit mineralization, decreased the torsional torque of chicken femur diaphyses (Chan *et al.*, 1977). A similar decrease in mechanical strength when administering high doses was observed in rats (Kawamuki *et al.*, 1990).

Positive effects have also been seen with incadronate, which increases the maximum compressive strength (Kawamuki *et al.*, 1990).

Olpadronate also induced an increase in the ultimate bending strength (Ferretti *et al.*, 1992). Pamidronate improved the ultimate bending strength, also called ultimate load, that is the load necessary for fracture of femur diaphyses in mice (Glatt *et al.*, 1986). In rat femurs, it increased the maximum elastic strength where plastic deformation starts to occur, as well as the ultimate bending strength, when given in daily doses of up to 0.45 mg/kg i.p. for 25 days (Ferretti *et al.*, 1990). Young's module of elasticity was also increased. In contrast, higher doses decreased these parameters. In dogs, a one-year administration of pamidronate increased the elastic modulus of spongious bone in the sternum as measured by an ultrasonic pulse transmission method (Grynpas *et al.*, 1992).

Lastly, tiludronate given in doses of 10–126 mg/kg daily for one year to normal and ovariectomized baboons enhanced the transversal and torsional stiffness of the radius (Geusens *et al.*, 1992).

Experimental osteoporosis

Bisphosphonates also display positive effects on mechanical properties in experimental osteoporosis models.

Thus, alendronate given daily for 14 days attenuated or completely prevented the decrease in the ultimate bending strength as well as the stiffness in the tibia of rats submitted to weightlessness by tail suspension (Apseloff *et al.*, 1991, 1993). It also prevented the reduction in stiffness and ultimate load of vertebrae in ovariectomized rats (Toolan *et al.*, 1992). The effect was improved by the administration of prostaglandins (Lauritzen *et al.*, 1993). In the baboon, this compound given every two weeks for two years prevented the decrease of ovariectomy-induced vertebral strength as assessed by the breaking force of trabecular bone (Balena *et al.*, 1993).

Etidronate given parenterally at 0.5–2 mg/kg daily for six months increased the ultimate bending strength in oophorectomized rats (Shiota, 1985). Administration for two weeks showed a small effect with daily doses up to 10 mg/kg, while 30 mg/kg had a negative effect, probably due to the inhibition of mineralization (Kawamuki *et al.*, 1990). This bisphosphonate also partly prevents the decrease of diaphyseal stiffness induced by corticosteroids (Ferretti *et al.*, 1993).

Pamidronate and olpadronate had a beneficial effect on the elastic and ultimate strength of bones in rats immobilized by sciatic nerve section, as well as in ovariectomized animals (Ferretti *et al.*, 1992), while pamidronate was also active on corticosteroid-induced femoral stiffness but not strength (Ferretti *et al.*, 1993).

Finally, other bisphosphonates such as YM 529 also prevented the changes induced by immobilization and ovariectomy (Kudo *et al.*, 1992).

It appears, therefore, that the bisphosphonates are able to increase the mechanical strength of bones in normal animals and to prevent the decrease induced in various experimental models of osteoporosis.

Activity of various bisphosphonates

The activity of bisphosphonates on bone resorption varies greatly from compound to compound (Shinoda *et al.*, 1983). The first compounds described had relatively little activity, especially etidronate, clodronate being somewhat more potent (Fleisch *et al.*, 1969). A large number of compounds have since been synthesized with increasing potency in their activity on bone resorption.

Up to now, no clearcut structure–activity relationship could be worked out. The length of the aliphatic carbon is important and adding a hydroxyl group to the carbon atom at position 1 increases potency (Shinoda *et al.*, 1983). Derivatives with an amino group at the end of the side chain are very active. The first of these compounds to be described was pamidronate (Bijvoet *et al.*, 1978; Reitsma *et al.*, 1980). The activity increases when the backbone has four carbons (alendronate) (Schenk *et al.*, 1986), but decreases again with longer compounds. Alkylation of the amino group increases activity. Thus, if the amino group of pamidronate is dimethylated, the efficacy is enhanced (Boonekamp *et al.*, 1987). Addition of larger alkyl groups results in even greater enhancement, as shown with ibandronate which is even more active (Mühlbauer *et al.*, 1991). Cyclic bisphosphonates are also very active, especially those containing a nitrogen atom in the ring, such as risedronate and zoledronate (Green *et al.*, 1994), which seems to be the most potent compound described up to now. This effect of nitrogen is very intriguing and not yet explained.

Mechanisms of action of bone resorption inhibition

Effects on osteoclasts

There is no doubt that the action *in vivo* is mediated through mechanisms other than the physicochemical inhibition of crystal dissolution, which was initially postulated. The nature of these mechanisms is, however, still unclear and it may well be that more than one is operating. The fact that the bisphosphonates alter the morphology of osteoclasts both *in vitro* and when administered *in vivo* (Schenk *et al.*, 1973; Miller and Jee, 1979) suggests an effect on the activity of these cells. This is supported by the finding that the addition of bisphosphonates *in vitro* to osteoclasts exposed to a mineralized tissue leads to an inhibition of their resorbing activity (Flanagan and Chambers, 1989; Sato and Grasser 1990; Sato *et al.*, 1991). The inhibition is still present when only the mineralized tissue is exposed to the bisphosphonates before the osteoclasts are added. This suggests that the osteoclasts are inhibited when they come in contact with bone containing bisphosphonate (Flanagan and Chambers, 1989).

However, the fact that bisphosphonates with an activity up to 1000-fold different in the living animal show the same activity on the osteoclasts *in vitro* in these experiments (Sato and Grasser, 1990) casts serious doubt on the above explanation representing the only mechanism of action. Very recently, it was found that only when the osteoclast-containing cell population was exposed to the bisphosphonates before being incubated with the hard tissues did the activity of various compounds correlate well with the activity *in vivo* (Sahni *et al.*, 1993). This was not the case if the bisphosphonates were added to the tissues together with the osteoclasts or to the mineral before the osteoclasts. These results suggest that the bisphosphonates act on these cells before they adhere to the bone. In a continuation of these studies, it was then shown that the effect was primarily not on the osteoclasts, but on the osteoblasts which are always present in this system. The inhibition is due to a decrease in the production by the osteoblasts of osteoclast-activating activity (Sahni *et al.*, 1993). More recently, it was found that the bisphosphonates induce the osteoblasts to produce an inhibitor of osteoclastic resorption (Vitté *et al.*, 1996).

Another possibility is that the decrease in resorption is also due to a decrease in the number of osteoclasts, either because cells already present are destroyed when they come into contact with bone containing the compounds, or because recruitment of new cells is inhibited. Indeed, in humans the number of osteoclasts is decreased after long-term treatment with various bisphosphonates. The possibility of an enhanced destruction of the osteoclasts has recently been strengthened by the finding that bisphosphonates induce earlier apoptosis of these cells, both *in vitro* and *in vivo* (Hughes *et al.*, 1995). An effect through recruitment is suggested by the fact that in culture, a correlation between the *in vitro* and *in vivo* effects is not detectable in models where osteoclasts are already present, such as newborn calvaria (Shinoda *et al.*, 1983; Boonekamp *et al.*, 1986); however, this is not the case in systems where resorption depends upon formation of new osteoclasts (Boonekamp *et al.*, 1986; Löwik *et al.*, 1988). The effect on the osteoclast recruitment appears to be at the terminal steps of differentiation (van der Pluijm *et al.*, 1991). Moreover, in long-term bone marrow culture, the formation of multinuclear cells is inhibited by bisphosphonates, the activity of various compounds being parallel to their potency *in vivo* (Hughes *et al.*, 1989).

Lastly, the inhibitory activity of bone resorption produced by the osteoblasts under the influence of bisphosphonates does not decrease the activity of the osteoclasts but only their formation (Vitté *et al.*, 1996). In contrast, the finding that in the animal, the number of osteoclasts is often increased in spite of the fact that bone resorption is blocked (Schoutens *et al.*, 1988; Mühlbauer *et al.*, 1991) does not support this theory. Therefore, in this condition, multinuclear cells are formed in the presence of bisphosphonates, but these are not active.

It appears likely that several mechanisms are operating. These may include:

1. an inhibition of the recruitment of active osteoclasts, possibly via an effect on the osteoblasts;
2. an inhibition of the activity of already formed osteoclasts following the uptake of bisphosphonate-containing mineral, or following the exposure to high concentrations of bisphosphonates which deposit under these cells;
3. earlier apoptosis or a toxic destruction of osteoclasts.

Biochemical and cellular effects

A great number of different biochemical effects have been described. Some may be relevant to bone resorption, such as the reduction of lactic acid production (Morgan *et al.*, 1973; Fast *et al.*, 1978) and of proton accumulation (Carano *et al.*, 1990) and extrusion (Zimolo *et al.*, 1995), the inhibition of lysosomal enzymes (Morgan *et al.*, 1973; Felix *et al.*, 1976; Ende, 1979; Delaissé *et al.*, 1985), the inhibition of pyrophosphatases (Felix and Fleisch, 1975; Smirnova *et al.*, 1988), the inhibition of prostaglandin synthesis (Felix *et al.*, 1981; Ohya *et al.*, 1985), the inhibition of LPS-stimulated production of IL-1 by macrophages (Matsuda *et al.*, 1991) and a change in cellular calcium handling (Guilland *et al.*, 1974; Plasmans *et al.*, 1980). The fact that these effects are usually found with high bisphosphonate concentrations does not invalidate them, since it has been calculated that under the osteoclasts these concentrations may reach nearly 1 mM (Sato *et al.*, 1991).

It is also possible that the inhibitory effect is partly mediated through other cells. Besides the osteoblasts mentioned above, macrophages may play a role, since they are especially sensitive to bisphosphonates which inhibit their activity (Chambers, 1980; Stevenson and Stevenson, 1986) as well as their multiplication (Cecchini *et al.*, 1987; Cecchini and Fleisch, 1990). Since macrophages produce a variety of bone-resorbing cytokines, it is possible that the inhibition of resorption is partly mediated through them.

These findings suggest that bisphosphonates enter mammalian cells. This has been confirmed by studies *in vitro*, both for etidronate and clodronate (Fast *et al.*, 1978). The cellular uptake is mostly in the cytosol and the concentration expressed in terms of cellular water can be several-fold higher than in the medium (Felix *et al.*, 1984). Cells with phagocytic properties display special avidity if the compounds are bound to apatite crystals (Chambers, 1980).

EFFECT ON CALCIFICATION *IN VIVO*

Bisphosphonates, when given in sufficiently high doses, inhibit mineralization *in vivo*. This is true not only for experimentally induced calcification of soft tissues such as arteries, kidneys, skin and heart (Fleisch *et al.*, 1970; Rosenblum *et al.*, 1977), but also for ectopic ossification (Plasmans *et al.*, 1978; Ahrengart and Lindgren, 1986). However, they can also impair the mineralization of normal calcified tissues. Most experiments have been performed with etidronate. Other bisphosphonates probably have similar effects, but they are difficult to visualize since these compounds cannot be administered at high enough doses due to their toxicity. Etidronate inhibits the mineralization of bone (Jowsey *et al.*, 1970; King *et al.*, 1971; Schenk *et al.*, 1973) and cartilage (Schenk *et al.*, 1973). The inhibition is eventually reversed after discontinuation of the drug (Flora *et al.*, 1980). The doses required to induce the block of mineralization vary according to the animal species and the length of treatment, but start at about 5 mg P/kg. The inhibition is not corrected by 1,25 $(OH)_2D_3$ or $24,25(OH)_2D_3$ (Atkin *et al.*, 1988). Hypomineralization is also observed in dentine and in enamel (Larsson, 1974; Ogawa *et al.*, 1989). There is a close relationship between the ability of an individual bisphosphonate to inhibit the formation of calcium phosphate *in vitro* and its effectiveness on ectopic calcification *in vivo* (Fleisch *et al.*, 1970; Shinoda *et al.*, 1983), suggesting that the inhibition *in vivo* is explained in terms of a physicochemical mechanism. However, it cannot be entirely excluded that some effect on matrix formation is also involved.

PHARMACOKINETICS

Bisphosphonates are synthetic compounds which have not yet been found to occur naturally in animals or humans. The compounds investigated to date, namely alendronate, clodronate, etidronate, pamidronate and tiludronate, appear to be absorbed, stored and excreted unaltered in the body and therefore to be non-biodegradable. However, it cannot be excluded that other bisphosphonates may be altered in their side chain.

Relatively few pharmacokinetic studies are available at present, partly because of the lack of sensitive chemical methods to measure the relevant compounds. Results with ^{99m}Tc compounds have to be interpreted with caution since they do not necessarily reflect the kinetics of the compound without technetium (Daley-Yates and Bennett, 1988). Most of the data on bisphosphonates have been obtained with alendronate, clodronate, etidronate, pamidronate and tiludronate. The intestinal absorption lies between 1% or even less and 10% of an oral dose, is generally higher in the young and shows a great inter- and intraspecies variation (Michael *et al.*, 1972; Recker and Saville, 1973; Gural, 1975; Yakatan *et al.*, 1982; Lin *et al.*, 1991). The fact that the absorbed fraction increases when the absolute ingested amount is higher explains why the absorption of the newer, more potent bisphosphonates is relatively small. Absorption is diminished when the drug is given with meals and in the presence of calcium (Francis and Martodam, 1983; Lin *et al.*, 1991) or iron (Österman *et al.*, 1994), while EDTA increases it (Janner *et al.*, 1991). Therefore, bisphosphonates always have to be given between meals and never together with milk products, calcium or iron supplements, which have to be administered at another time of the day. Also orange juice and coffee decrease the absorption.

Between 20% and 60% of the absorbed etidronate is localized in bone, the remainder being rapidly excreted in the urine (Michael *et al.*, 1972; Conrad and Lee, 1981; Yakatan *et al.*, 1982; Hanhijärvi *et al.*, 1989; Lin *et al.*, 1991).

Bisphosphonates, especially pamidronate, can occasionally deposit in other organs such as the stomach (Larsson and Rohlin, 1980), liver and spleen (Wingen and Schmähl, 1987; Mönkkönen, 1988; Mönkkönen *et al.*, 1989). The deposition is increased percentually when large amounts of compounds are given (Wingen and Schmähl, 1987; Mönkkönen *et al.*, 1989). This is explained by the formation of complexes and aggregates with divalent cations, especially calcium (Mönkkönen and Ylitalo, 1990), which are then phagocytosed by the macrophages of the reticuloendothelial system. Thus, results obtained with large amounts of labeled compounds given rapidly intravenously have to be interpreted with caution.

The half-life of circulating bisphosphonates is short, in the rat only in the order of minutes (Bisaz *et al.*, 1978). In humans it is somewhat longer, about two hours (Conrad and Lee, 1981; Yakatan *et al.*, 1982; Hanhijärvi *et al.*, 1989). The rate of entry into bone is very fast, similar to that of calcium and phosphate. It has been calculated that the bone clearance is compatible with a complete extraction from the skeleton after the first passage, so that skeletal uptake might be determined above all by the vascularization of the bone and its turnover (Bisaz *et al.*, 1978). The areas of deposition are mostly those of bone formation. However, a recent study showed that at least alendronate deposits preferentially under the osteoclasts (Sato *et al.*, 1991). The repartition between bone-forming and bone-resorbing areas depends upon the amount of bisphosphonate and the type of compound administered. Lower amounts will favor deposition in resorptive areas and alendronate seems to show a somewhat greater tendency for the latter than etidronate (Masarachia *et al.*, 1996). In view of the rapid extraction by bone, soft tissues are exposed to the bisphosphonates for short periods only, which explains why, despite the many cellular effects described *in vitro*, practically, only bone is affected *in vivo*.

Once buried in the skeleton, the largest part of the bisphosphonates incorporated is probably liberated again only when the bone in which they are deposited is destroyed in the course of bone turnover. As the bisphosphonates slow down the resorption of the bone where they are embedded, their half-life will be even longer than that of the rest of the skeleton and it is possible that part of the administered bisphosphonates remain in the human body for life. Half-life has been evaluated at up to a year in mice, rats and dogs (Wingen and Schmähl, 1987; Mönkkönen, 1988; Mönkkönen *et al.*, 1989; Lin *et al.*, 1991). Etidronate and pamidronate have a similar retention time, while clodronate is cleared somewhat more rapidly (Mönkkönen *et al.*, 1989). This long retention explains why one administration of bisphosphonates can be active for long periods of time, both in animals (Stutzer *et al.*, 1988) and in humans (Thiébaud *et al.*, 1986).

The renal clearance of bisphosphonates is high, often around that of inulin (Conrad and Lee, 1981; Hanhijärvi *et al.*, 1989). If the conspicuous plasma protein binding is taken into account, the clearance is above that of inulin, suggesting the presence of a secretory pathway (Troehler *et al.*, 1975; Lin *et al.*, 1992).

ANIMAL TOXICOLOGY

Published toxicological animal studies reported to date are scanty and deal mostly with etidronate and clodronate. Acute, subacute and chronic administration in several animal species have revealed little toxicity. Teratogenic, mitogenic and carcinogenic tests were negative (Nolen and Buehler, 1971; Nixon *et al.*, 1972). The acute toxicity appears to be due to the formation of complexes with calcium, leading to hypocalcemia and the formation of insoluble aggregates. When the compound is administered intravenously, toxicity varies with the speed of infusion (Francis and Slough, 1984). This is another reason why great care has to be taken when administering bisphosphonates intravenously. Such administration should be done by slow infusion only, especially when large amounts are given.

For etidronate, the first chronic adverse event is the inhibition of bone calcification described above. Fractures can occur, but they can also be induced when mineralization is not impaired, since a long-term decrease of bone turnover itself can lead to an increased fragility (Flora *et al.*, 1980). At higher doses, renal lesions appear with various bisphosphonates (Hintze and D'Amato, 1980; Alden *et al.*, 1989; Cal and Daley-Yates, 1990). This is a property of many phosphate compounds. Atrophy of the thymus and some immunological alterations can occur after very high doses of clodronate in newborn animals (Milhaud *et al.*, 1983; Labat *et al.*, 1983, 1984). It is, however, not known whether they are secondary to the inhibition of bone resorption and therefore of marrow expansion.

Bisphosphonates cross the placenta and can affect the fetus. Thus, large doses (200 mg/kg s.c.) of etidronate given to pregnant rats daily from day 7–11 of pregnancy lead to fetal abnormalities involving weight, skeleton and skin and induce malformations and hemorrhages (for references, see Fleisch, 1993).

As mentioned above, the results with one bisphosphonate cannot necessarily be extrapolated to others, since toxicity both in culture and *in vivo* varies greatly from one compound to another, so that great caution has to be applied when using new compounds clinically.

ADVERSE EVENTS IN THE HUMAN

As in animals, studies in humans have revealed only a few important adverse events.

Caution must be taken with the intravenous administration of bisphosphonates, since rapid injection has led to renal failure (Bounameaux *et al.*, 1983), possibly because of the formation of insoluble calcium bisphosphonate in the blood which is then retained in the kidney. No further events of this kind have been observed since care has been taken to administer all bisphosphonates by slow infusion in a large volume of fluid if given intravenously in larger amounts. For exact indications, the package insert should be consulted.

Sometimes bisphosphonates can induce a certain degree of hypocalcemia, especially when given intravenously in large amounts. Since severe hypocalcemia has been reported in a patient who received aminoglycoside antibiotic therapy, the two drugs should not be administered together.

When given orally, the bisphosphonates have a tendency to produce gastrointestinal effects, such as nausea, dyspepsia, vomiting, gastric pain and diarrhea and sometimes even ulcerations. These effects can be diminished or avoided by administering the compounds with a large amount of fluid, dividing the dose and avoiding administration in a recumbent position.

ALENDRONATE

In clinical studies alendronate is usually well tolerated up to a daily dose of 20 mg, although signs of upper gastrointestinal intolerance may occur.

A recent postmarketing analysis performed by the manufacturer reported that about 0.1‰ of patients who had received 10 mg of alendronate daily *per os* displayed serious or severe adverse esophageal effects. These included symptoms like esophagalgia, odynophagia and dysphagia, and structural alterations like esophagitis, erosions and ulcerations (De Groen *et al.*, 1996).

An analysis of these patients showed that the majority of the more severely affected patients did not follow the recommendations in the product label to take the drug with a full glass of water and not to recline afterwards. In response to these facts, the instructions in the product label were strengthened by the manufacturer and include that the patients should stop taking their medication if they develop esophageal symptoms. Since the dosing instructions were reinforced, the number of reports of the above-mentioned events has declined, and this despite a substantial increase in the number of patients treated.

CLODRONATE

No proven side effects have been described as yet for clodronate, except for a mild diarrhea when given orally. In contrast to etidronate, this compound does not inhibit mineralization of bone at the dosage used. In the course of the clinical evaluation of this compound, some of the treated patients developed acute leukemia. However, an extremely careful further evaluation over many years led to the conclusion that causes other than the drug, especially preselection of patients, were as likely or more likely to have been the cause of this finding.

ETIDRONATE

Etidronate has now been used in humans for more than 15 years and has proven to be very well tolerated if not administered in excessive amounts. The first and major complication is the inhibition of normal skeletal mineralization. This effect appears at daily oral doses between 800 and 1600 mg and has been described by many investigators, mostly in patients with Paget's disease (for reference, see Fleisch, 1993). The inhibition regresses after discontinuation of therapy. A focal osteomalacia has been described at areas of high bone turnover at doses as low as 400 mg p.o. (Nagent de Deuxchaisnes *et al.*, 1981; Boyce *et al.*, 1984).

The effect of smaller doses in long-term therapy is more difficult to assess. There is a consensus that intermittent treatment with 400 mg for two weeks every three months over a period of three years does not lead to any clinical or morphological alterations of mineralization. The situation is less clear when therapy is pursued over a longer period. One study showed no histological changes after seven years, while in a large multicenter study performed in the US, areas of widening of the osteoid borders, suggestive of a certain degree of inhibition of mineralization, were seen in some patients.

Fractures have occurred in children treated

with long-term oral doss of 20 mg/kg daily for fibrodysplasia ossificans progressiva (Reiner *et al.*, 1980). In these children, a proximal muscular weakness leading to abnormal gait, similar to that seen in rickets, also appeared (Reiner *et al.*, 1980). Fractures possibly also occur in adults in Paget's disease when high doses are given over longer periods. However, fractures are also more frequent in untreated patients in this disease, so that the role of treatment is difficult to assess (Johnston *et al.*, 1983).

Etidronate also causes a conspicuous rise in plasma phosphate, often to high levels, both in healthy persons and in patients. The change is associated with an increase in renal tubular reabsorption of phosphate (Recker *et al.*, 1973; Walton *et al.*, 1975).

Finally, some gastrointestinal disturbances can occur occasionally when the compound is given orally, which can, however, be overcome in most cases by dividing the dose. Intravenous infusions can induce a transient loss or alteration of taste, with a metallic flavor (Jones and Henderson, 1987; Singer *et al.*, 1991).

PAMIDRONATE

Pamidronate does not usually inhibit bone mineralization at doses active on bone resorption. However, recent results have shown that large doses administered intravenously to pagetic patients induced an inhibition of mineralization both in pagetic and normal bone (Adamson *et al.*, 1993). Furthermore, in a child with fibrodysplasia, a radiologically visible inhibition occurred at the femoral growth plate (Liens *et al.*, 1994). When given orally, this bisphosphonate can induce gastrointestinal disturbances such as nausea, vomiting, pain and diarrhea, especially at a dose of 600 mg or more daily (van Breukelen *et al.*, 1982; Harinck *et al.*, 1987; Dodwell *et al.*, 1990). In some cases esophagitis occurred. However, these effects seem to depend upon the preparation used and can apparently be avoided by using improved galenic forms, by refraining from administering the drug before going to bed and by using moderate doses.

The intravenous administration of pamidronate induces a transient pyrexia in about 10% of the patients or more in some studies. This is also the case with other aminobisphosphonates, but contrasts with clodronate and etidronate which have no such effect. The pyrexia is maximal within 24–48 hours and disappears after approximately three days, even when treatment is continued (van Breukelen *et al.*, 1979; Bijvoet *et al.*, 1980; Adami *et al.*, 1987). The effect is dose dependent and is only observed once, even if treatment is discontinued and restarted later. At the same time there is a decrease in peripheral lymphocytes, an increase in serum C-reactive protein and a decrease in serum zinc (Adami *et al.*, 1987). The mechanism of these changes, which resemble an acute-phase response, is still not understood but it might involve the stimulation of macrophages to release cytokines such as IL-1 and IL-6 (Schweitzer *et al.*, 1995).

Lastly, it was reported that on rare occasions, adverse ocular reactions, such as anterior uveitis, episcleritis, scleritis and conjunctivitis, occurred (Marcarol and Fraunfelder, 1994).

TILUDRONATE

Tiludronate appears to be well tolerated. One patient with personal and family history of allergies developed a condition first diagnosed as toxidermia, later possibly as pemphigus (Roux *et al.*, 1992).

No results are available for the other bisphosphonates.

CONTRAINDICATIONS

To date, no absolute contraindications have been described. The question is often raised whether bisphosphonates can be administered in renal failure. Since these compounds are cleared from blood to a large extent by the skeleton, there is no theoretical reason to avoid them in this condition. In fact, pamidronate has been successfully used for hypercalcemia in patients with renal failure (Yap *et al.*, 1990). However, plasma levels are likely to be higher, so that the dosage should be reduced. The extent of this reduction will only be known as plasma data become available. However, since on the average only about 50% of the bisphosphonate is excreted in the urine, cutting the dose by up to 75% according to the degree of renal failure should theoretically be sufficient.

Another open question is whether bisphosphonates should be given during fracture healing. Unfortunately, only very few data are available on this question. It is obvious that large doses of etidronate which inhibit mineralization should be avoided since they can lead to an impairment of fracture healing (Lenehan *et al.*, 1985). In contrast, there is no evidence that lower doses of this bisphosphonate or others are harmful. Similar considerations can be made in patients with cementless implantation of porous devices which depend on osseous ingrowth for stabilization. Indeed, etidronate administered in dogs at a dose which inhibits mineralization led to a decrease of bone implant interfacial shear strength (Rivero *et al.*, 1987).

USE IN OSTEOPOROSIS IN HUMANS

Clinical applications in medicine have focused upon three main areas:

1. use as skeletal markers in the form of ^{99m}Tc derivatives for diagnostic purposes in nuclear medicine;
2. therapautic use in patients with ectopic calcification and ossification;
3. use in patients with increased bone destruction, especially Paget's disease (for review, see Kanis, 1991), tumoral bone disease (for review, see Fleisch, 1991) and recently osteoporosis.

Only the latter application will be reviewed here.

Until recently there have been few controlled studies using bisphosphonates in patients with osteoporosis. This has changed only in the past few years and led very recently to the registration of etidronate for this disease in various countries, as well as that of alendronate and clodronate in Italy.

ETIDRONATE

The first controlled studies with a bisphosphonate were performed with etidronate, so this compound will be discussed first.

Bone mass and calcium metabolism

Etidronate was first administered at a dose of 20 mg/kg daily p.o. for six months in women with senile osteoporosis back in the 1970s (Heaney and Saville, 1976). The results were not very encouraging, since bone resorption and formation decreased approximately to the same extent, so that the effect on Ca balance was only small. Intestinal Ca absorption as well as urinary Ca were increased. However, at this dose an inhibition of mineralization was likely to occur. Thus, a positive effect on bone balance, if present, would have been obscured. Later studies confirmed the increase in intestinal Ca absorption (Nuti *et al.*, 1981), probably through an increase in $1,25(OH)_2D_3$.

In uncontrolled bed rest studies lasting 20 weeks, oral etidronate administered daily also at 20 mg/kg appeared to diminish the negative balance induced by the immobilization. However, calcaneal loss assessed by γ absorptiometry was not altered. In contrast, 5 mg/kg had no effect (Lockwood *et al.*, 1975; Schneider and McDonald, 1984).

A series of studies used so-called coherence therapies, namely multiple cycles of short periods of etidronate, preceded by a short course of an activator of bone resorption and followed by a period without treatment.

The results are in general difficult to interpret since the investigations were often inadequately controlled. The first of these studies (Anderson *et al.*, 1984) was performed on five patients between 62 and 77 years of age who received 3–6 cycles, starting with three days of oral phosphate administration, followed by 15 days of 5 mg/kg of etidronate and 70 days without therapy. The treatment appeared to increase the trabecular bone volume as assessed by histomorphometry and also to increase bone turnover; however, an extension of this study on 37 patients treated with a similar protocol over two years, but receiving phosphate for four days and an increased dose of etidronate to 7.5 mg/kg, showed no significant change in trabecular bone volume measured histomorphometrically and a decrease in turnover (Hodsman, 1989). The treatment, however, induced an increase in lumbar bone mineral density assessed by dual-photon absorptiometry. Both studies had no placebo control group.

Another coherence study (Hesch *et al.*, 1988) used 400 U of PTH given daily for two weeks and 5 mg/kg/day of etidronate given orally for two weeks starting the second week, followed by six weeks without therapy. The cycle was repeated six times. Again, the results are difficult to interpret because of lack of controls and because it is known that PTH has an effect on its own. Calcium balance, which was measured once after the first cycle, became positive in four of the eight patients and there was no change in iliac trabecular bone as assessed by histomorphometry.

In another study (Silberstein and Schnur, 1992), the effect of a regimen with phosphate for three days followed by 10 mg/kg for 14 days and 12 weeks without treatment, over four cycles, was investigated in postmenopausal osteoporotic women. The treatment was then continued over three years but with 5 mg/kg of etidronate. Unfortunately, the controls were obtained retrospectively. While all the patients in the control group showed a decrease in bone mineral density of the lumbar spine, the femoral neck, Ward's triangle and greater trochanter, a majority of the treated patients showed an increase.

Another study (Pacifici *et al.*, 1988) on 30 women, now controlled with groups of patients receiving either estrogens and calcium or calcium alone, used three days of phosphate followed by 14 days of 400 mg/day of etidronate and eight weeks without drugs. All patients received 1 g of calcium a day. The treatment lasted 1–2 years. No effect from etidronate was detected on spinal bone density and on proximal and distal radius density. However, it is not clear whether the etidronate and calcium were given simultaneously or at different times. If given together, a low absorption of the drug due to the calcium may explain the negative results.

Finally, a preliminary study on eight patients (Mallette *et al.*, 1989) used cycles of seven days of phosphate, followed by five days of etidronate at 1800 mg daily and then 48 days of 1 g of calcium. No controls were available. There was an increase of lumbar bone mineral density of 7.2% at six months and 8.2% at 12 months.

More recently, a controlled double-blind study on 423 patients, 363 of which completed two years, investigated the effect of etidronate over a period of up to three years in osteoporotic postmenopausal women (Watts *et al.*, 1990). Four treatment regimens were used:

1. 1 g of oral phosphate daily for three days, followed by 14 days of oral etidronate daily and 74 days without drug but with 500 mg of calcium daily;
2. the same but without phosphate;
3. the same but without etidronate;
4. the same but without etidronate and without phosphate.

The patients were on average 65 years old and 16–19 years past the menopause. They had 1–4 vertebral compression fractures and evidence of slight vertebral osteopenia.

After two years, there was no difference in bone mineral density of the lumbar spine between the patients receiving phosphate or not, so that the results were pooled for some of the statistical analyses into two groups, one receiving etidronate and one a placebo. The groups treated with etidronate showed a statistical increase from baseline and a statistical difference from the controls in lumbar bone mineral density after 12, 18 and 24 months. The groups receiving no etidronate showed no change, which means that these patients were not in a stage of progressing osteoporosis. The results of bone density in the hip were more heterogeneous. However, the fact that there was no change from baseline in most groups allowed the conclusion that the increase in the spine was not at the expense of the hip.

The double-blind study was then extended to a third year in 357 patients. In a fourth year, 277 patients received only the etidronate treatment without phosphate and a placebo group was no longer followed (Harris *et al.*, 1993).

In the third year, the etidronate patients maintained the significant increase in spinal density and the values in the femur tended to increase. The femoral neck, trochanter and Ward's triangle displayed a significant increase in bone density, as well as a significant difference compared to the untreated controls. In the fourth year, the patients who had previously received etidronate still did not show any further change, indicating that the effect had reached a plateau. The previous placebo patients now showed a sharp increase similar to that observed with etidronate three years earlier (Harris *et al.*, 1993).

It was reported recently that when some of the patients in the above study were further treated for up to seven years, there was still a small but significant increase in lumbar bone density. However, bone turnover rates assessed histologically returned towards baseline. If confirmed with biochemical markers of bone turnover, this result would allay the concern that long-term bisphosphonate therapy diminishes turnover to an extent which may be associated with increased skeletal fragility.

A similar double-blind, placebo-controlled study was performed on fewer patients who had, however, a more marked osteoporosis (Storm *et al.*, 1990). The study had a similar protocol, but no oral phosphate was given. The period without treatment consisted of 13 weeks instead of 10. The trial started on 66 patients with a mean age of 68 years, 40 of whom finished the study. Etidronate treatment resulted in an increase of the lumbar bone mineral content which became significant after 90 weeks of therapy and reached a value of 5.3% after 150 weeks. In contrast, the placebo patients decreased by 2.7% during the same period of time. The changes between the two groups were significantly different. In the distal forearm, there was a difference of 5.1% between the groups which was, however, not significant. A histomorphometric investigation of the transiliac crest showed no signs of osteomalacia.

The study was extended for another two years, during which all patients then received the etidronate treatment (Sorensen 1992). In the patients who had previously received etidronate, the density of the lumbar spine maintained its plateau of +7%, which had been reached after 120 weeks. The former placebo patients now also showed an increase.

A study performed on 36 healthy women three years after their menopause showed that a similar regimen of etidronate induced a gain of 3.1% of spinal bone mineral density instead of a loss of 4.7% (Evans *et al.*, 1993).

Finally, a daily dose of 400 mg of etidronate for three months was also used in a double-blind study in patients following a surgical menopause (Smith *et al.*, 1989). The treatment reduced to some extent the increase in bone turnover induced by the oophorectomy, as assessed by whole-body retention of ^{99m}Tc-etidronate, as well as by serum and urine calcium and plasma osteocalcin.

Fractures

Unfortunately, only few studies deal adequately with the question of whether treatment alters the occurrence of fractures. This is due to the fact that the evalation of vertebral fractures is difficult and that a successful study implies an excellent placebo group and a large number of patients in order to obtain significant results.

Two studies using coherence therapy were difficult to interpret (Hodsman, 1989; Silberstein and Schnur, 1992) because of inadequate control. In the first study, a decrease in the vertebral fracture rate, defined as a 15% decrease in the height of any vertebra, showed a significantly lower rate in the period of 15–35 months of treatment than in the first 15 months (Hodsman, 1989). No controls were included. In the second study (Silberstein and Schnur, 1992), which was also not adequately controlled, three fractures, defined as a 20% decrease in lumbar vertebral height, were observed in the treated group against nine in a historical control group.

The only controlled studies of etidronate are those described above (Watts *et al.*, 1990; Storm *et al.*, 1990; Harris *et al.*, 1993). In the former, new fractures were measured in the thoracic and lumbar spine. A fracture was defined as a reduction of 20% or more of either the anterior, middle or posterior vertebral height, accompanied by a reduction of 10% or more in the total area in a previously unfractured vertebra. Using these criteria, it appears that the number of new fractures was unusually small, showing that the patients used in this study had only mild osteoporosis. This made the statistical analysis difficult. Only the group receiving phosphate and etidronate showed a significantly lower incidence of fractures when compared to the group receiving placebo alone, when either all vertebral fractures or only new fractures were considered. When the two etidronate groups and the two groups not receiving etidronate were combined, the difference was not significant, both when only new vertebral fractures were considered (29.5 per 1000 patient-years against 62.9 for the controls) as well as when all vertebral fractures were considered (50 per 1000 patient-years against 107 for controls). The results became significant if only patients with low bone mass were selected (42.3 new fractures per 1000 patient-years against 132.7). In contrast, there was no significant difference among non-vertebral fractures.

It was subsequently reported, however, that in the third year the number of new fractures was somewhat higher in the treated group, this despite the fact that bone density was still further increased. The total rate of new fractures in the three years was no longer significantly lower in the treated group (61 per 1000 patient-years for the treated group against 71 per 1000 patient-years for the controls). The same was true for the total number of fractures, that is, both in vertebrae which showed no previous fracture and in those which had already sustained one (86 fractures per 1000 patient-years in the treated group against 117 for the control group). However, when the higher risk patients with a low bone density were analyzed, the difference again became significant (219 versus 412 fractures per 1000 patient-years) (Harris *et al.*, 1993).

In the fourth year, the fractures in the treated patients were again lower than in the third year, lower even than in any other study period (Harris *et al.*, 1993). No placebo patients were present in this last year, so that the results are difficult to interpret. It is, however, most likely that the increase in fractures observed in the third year was fortuitous and not due to a detrimental effect of the treatment, such as osteomalacia, or a decrease in bone strength because of a slower turnover.

In the second study (Storm *et al.*, 1990), not only the new vertebral fractures but also the spinal deformity as well as changes in height were investigated. A spinal deformity index was made by assessing semiquantitatively the anterior, middle and proximal deformity of the thoracic and lumbar vertebrae, as well as their total area. A similar rate of decrease in the spinal deformity index was observed in the two groups in the first 60 weeks. Thereafter, the placebo group continued to decrease while the treated group stabilized, the difference being significant after 150 weeks. In analogy, the rate of new vertebral fractures was similar in the first 60 weeks, but significantly lower (6 versus 54 per 100 patient-years) if calculated from week 60 to week 150; in contrast, if calculated over the entire 150-week period, the difference was not significant. Finally, there was a small, insignificant difference in the decrease of body height of the patients.

In the last two years of treatment, the low fracture rate was maintained (17 versus 18 per 100 patient-years) in the patients with continued etidronate treatment. The rate of new vertebral fractures decreased from 46 to 16 per 100 patient-years in the former placebo patients who had then begun treatment. Similar results were obtained when all fractures were assessed (Storm *et al.*, 1992).

Although these results do not allow the conclusion that etidronate decreases the fracture incidence in osteoporosis, they nevertheless look very promising and suggest that such an effect might be seen if a large enough population with actively developing osteoporosis is investigated.

ALENDRONATE

Bone mass

Until recently, few studies have investigated the effect of alendronate on osteoporosis. In an open study, 40 patients with postmenopausal osteoporosis (between one and three fractures and low bone mass) received either 5 mg/day of alendronate for two days intravenously every three months for one year or 1 g of calcium (Passeri *et al.*, 1991). Bone mineral density of the lumbar spine increased with alendronate treatment and decreased slightly in the controls, with a significant difference betweeen the two groups after one year. The same occurred in the distal radius, although at this site there was no significant difference after one year, but a difference in the linear trend. Interestingly, the alendronate patients had significantly less back pain after six months.

More recently, in a double-blind study on 285 postmenopausal osteoporotic women aged 46–66 years with a mean age of 59 years, 10 mg and 20 mg daily of alendronate, administered orally for two years, led to an increase in bone mineral density of 4–6% in the lumbar spine, 3% in the femoral neck and about 4% in the trochanter. Patients receiving a placebo or 100 U of intranasal calcitonin showed no changes (Adami *et al.*, 1993).

In two other studies, both multicenter, randomized and placebo controlled, performed on postmenopausal women with osteoporosis defined as a bone mineral density of the lumbar spine at least 2.5 SD below the mean value in premenopausal women (T score), alendronate was given orally at 5 mg, 10 mg, 20 mg and 40 mg for two years (Chesnut *et al.*, 1995; Liberman *et al.*, 1995). Both studies have shown an increase in bone density both in the vertebrae and in the hip, instead of a drop or no change in the controls. Since 10 mg was more active than 5 mg, but not less active than 20 mg, 10 mg appears to be the most favorable dose. A prolongation to three years and combination of the two studies showed similar results. There was an increase of about 8% in the lumbar spine, 5% in the femoral neck, 7% in the trochanter and 1–2% in the whole body, instead of a loss of about 1%. The plateau does not seem to have been reached yet (Liberman *et al.*, 1995).

It is interesting that, in analogy to what has been seen in rats and baboons, the inhibitory effect on bone destruction reaches a plateau even if the administration is continued and this plateau is dependent on the dose administered. With appropriate dosage of 10 mg daily premenopausal levels were reached (Garnero *et al.*, 1994). Furthermore, the inhibition of resorption disappears when the drug is discontinued (Gertz *et al.*, 1994). These results suggest that the bisphosphonate buried in the bone is inactive and that there is no danger of a continuous decrease in bone turnover with an increase in bone fragility.

Fractures

The above-mentioned three-year study also showed a significant decrease in vertebral fractures when all patients with all dosages were pooled. Thus, 6.2% of 355 placebo patients and 3.2% of the treated patients showed new vertebral fractures, the difference being highly significant. The decreased risk was present in all dosage groups. The proportion of patients displaying two or more fractures was even more pronounced, namely 0.6% versus 4.2%. If the total number of fractures were analyzed, treated patients showed 4.2 fractures per 100 women against 11.3 for the placebo group.

These results are supported by investigations on the spine deformity index which increased in 33% of the treated women against 41% in the placebo group ($p = 0.028$). Furthermore, the loss of height was 35% less in the treated group than in the placebo patients (3.0 mm versus 4.6 mm, $p = 0.005$).

Not only vertebral but also non-vertebral fractures were decreased to some extent. The cumulative incidence was 8.5% with an overall rate of 3.0 women with fractures per 100 patient-years at risk for the treated group, against 10.7% and 3.7 women respectively in the placebo group.

These results were confirmed recently in a study on 2027 women between the ages of 55 and 80, with low BMD of the femoral neck and with at least one vertebral fracture. The oral administration of 5 mg daily for 2 years followed by approximately 1 year at 10 mg reduced the risk of vertebral fractures by about 50% and the risk of sustaining more than one fracture by 89%. Furthermore, both hip and wrist fractures were significantly decreased by 51% and 44%, respectively. The effect was independent of age, initial bone mineral density and the number of pre-existing fractures (Black *et al.*, 1996).

CLODRONATE

Many studies have shown the efficacy of clodronate in decreasing bone destruction and hypercalcemia in tumoral bone disease (for review, see Fleisch, 1991) and this compound is commercially available in various countries for this indication. Fewer studies have been carried out in osteoporosis.

The first results were encouraging. Approximately 11 months of continuous oral administration of 1200–1600 mg of this compound to 24 patients with postmenopausal osteoporosis led to an increase of as much as 6% in total body Ca measured by neutron activation, as compared to a decrease of 2% in 22 patients given placebo (Chesnut, 1988).

A study in 21 paraplegic patients showed that daily oral doses of 400 and 1600 mg given for 3.5 months prevented the bone loss occurring in the lower end of the tibia which occurred in seven placebo patients (Minaire *et al.*, 1981). It also prevented the increase in serum and urinary calcium and in urinary hydroxyproline.

Recently, clodronate administered orally at a dose of 400 mg per day for 30 consecutive days every three months for one year was investigated in 60 postmenopausal women between the ages of 42 and 79 years, mean age 59 years (Giannini *et al.*, 1993). Placebo-treated patients lost 2.3% of lumbar bone density, while the clodronate-treated patients gained 3.9%. Addition of calcitriol to the clodronate patients added no further effect.

Very recently ibandronate has also been found to increase bone mineral density instead of the usual loss in placebo patients. Of interest is the fact that this compound is active both when given orally at 0.5–5 mg daily, as well as when given discontinuously in intravenous injections of 0.25–2.0 mg, once every 3 months (Ravn *et al.*, 1996; Thiébaud *et al.*, 1996).

PAMIDRONATE

This compound is used in various diseases with high bone turnover, such as Paget's disease (for review, see Kanis, 1991) and tumoral bone disease (for review, see Fleisch, 1991). It is currently commercially available in various countries for the latter indication. Some information is also available in osteoporosis.

One publication reported several investigations, some of them with controls (Valkema *et al.*, 1989). Seven osteoporotic patients of both sexes receiving 600 mg of oral pamidronate daily for 10 days showed an increase of Ca balance of over 200 mg per day. The administration of 150 mg daily for one year still induced a rise of 80 mg after this period. For both these studies the patients were used as their own controls. These findings were supported by bone mineral measurements of the lumbar spine in osteoporotic patients of both sexes treated for between one and six years with 150 mg of oral pamidronate daily. The treated patients showed a mean annual increase of about 3% as compared to an insignificant change in 19 non-treated patients. However, the latter were not investigated during the same time and are therefore not entirely valid controls. Furthermore, the study included an increasing number of patients over the years, making an interpretation difficult. The authors believe, however, that the increase in bone mass does continue over some years.

Oral treatment with 250–300 mg daily two months on, two months off, showed an increase in bone mass in the lumbar spine of 2.4% in the first year and 2.5% in the second year, against a 2.4% loss in a simultaneous control group (Devogelaer and Nagant de Deuxchaisnes, 1990). The increase reached a plateau after two years and was apparently not obtained at the expense of the appendicular bone.

An increase of 3–5% in bone density of the lumbar spine and the femoral neck and in the whole-body mineral content was also seen when 200 mg per day was given orally for 14 months to 36 postmenopausal osteoporotic patients; 20 controls displayed a small decrease (Zanchetta *et al.*, 1990). However, the results did not seem to reach significance.

Daily oral administration of 4.8–6 mg/kg in 35 osteoporotic postmenopausal women with a mean age of 64 years also induced a significant increase in bone mineral density of the lumbar spine of 5.3% after a year and 7.5% after 18 months, the patients being taken as their own controls (Fromm *et al.*, 1991). Some increase was also seen in the femoral neck, Ward's triangle and trochanter, although only the latter was significant.

More recently, daily oral administration over two years of 150 mg of pamidronate in patients with postmenopausal osteoporosis increased lumbar bone mineral density by about 7% against no change in the placebo group (Reid *et al.*, 1994).

Lastly, a single intravenous administration of 30 mg of pamidronate every three months to osteoporotic women with a mean age of 64 years significantly increased bone mineral density of the lumbar spine, the femoral neck and the distal forearm, more than when fluoride was administered (Thiébaud *et al.*, 1994). No untreated controls were included in this study.

Pamidronate is active in steroid-induced osteoporosis. In a prospective, randomized, placebo-controlled trial (Reid *et al.*, 1988), 150 mg per day was given orally for 12 months to 20 patients receiving long-term supraphysiological doses of glucocorticoids. Whilst in the placebo group both lumbar vertebral mineral density and metacarpal cortical area decreased by 8.8% and 1.2% respectively in one year, the treated group showed an increase of

19.6% and 1.2%. The changes were significant in both instances. The biochemical parameters showed a decrease in bone turnover (Reid *et al.*, 1990). Pamidronate also normalized calcemia in acute spinal injury (Gallacher *et al.*, 1990; Varache *et al.*, 1991).

Ten mg daily of pamidronate given intravenously for 18 days, followed by 300 mg daily given orally for another 42 days dramatically reduced bone resorption and increased radiological density in the metaphyses of long bones in one case of juvenile osteoporosis (Hoekman *et al.*, 1985). In this patient, bone turnover relapsed within one month of cessation of therapy.

Pamidronate also prevents the increase in bone turnover induced by tri-iodothyronine administration (Rosen *et al.*, 1993b).

TILUDRONATE

Currently, only one study is available for this compound (Reginster *et al.*, 1989). Seventy-six healthy women, 3–10 years after menopause, were given either tiludronate at an oral dose of 100 mg daily for six months and a placebo for another six months or a placebo during the whole time. Whilst the control patients showed a significant decrease of 2.1% in the mineral density of the lumbar spine after one year, the treated group increased insignificantly by 1.3%. The difference between the two groups was significant and remained the same after two years.

MODE OF ACTION OF BISPHOSPHONATES IN OSTEOPOROSIS

The bone loss which leads to the diminished bone mass and the increase in fragility of the skeleton in osteoporosis is due to two main mechanisms. The first is an imbalance between bone resorption and bone formation during remodeling and modeling, so that each new bone structural unit (BSU) will be smaller than the one it replaces. This imbalance is caused by either a decrease in the new

Devogelaer and Nagant de D 1990; Storm *et al.*, 1990; Wat Adami *et al.*, 1993; Ches Thiébaud *et al.*, 1994; Lib This apparently para have several explana between resorptio occur immediat certain time, while the n erosion are al thei

this parameter, markers such as urinary calcium, hydroxyproline and pyridinoline crosslinks for resorption (Reid *et al.*, 1988; Reginster *et al.*, 1989; Valkema *et al.*, 1989; Passeri *et al.*, 1991) and plasma alkaline phosphatase and osteocalcin for formation (Reid *et al.*, 1988; Storm *et al.*, 1990; Watts *et al.*, 1990; Passeri *et al.*, 1991). As mentioned above, the effect is primarily on the resorption, the decrease in formation most probably being secondary.

The decrease in turnover is substantiated by histomorphometric data which show that the bisphosphonates decrease both the activation frequency (Hodsman, 1989; Pallot-Prades *et al.*, 1991; Steiniche *et al.*, 1991; Storm *et al.*, 1993) and the resorption depth, that is, the depth of bone eroded by the osteoclasts (Steiniche *et al.*, 1991; Storm *et al.*, 1993). Interestingly, it would appear that the bisphosphonates decrease the number of trabecular osteoclasts but not the cortical ones (Chappard *et al.*, 1991). Thus, the bisphosphonates act at both steps, namely rate of formation and erosion depth of the BMUs.

It has been observed that the bisphosphonates, as well as other inhibitors of bone resorption, can not only prevent bone loss, but actually induce an increase in bone mass (Reginster *et al.*, 1989; Valkema *et al.*, 1989;

[illegible] euxchaisnes, [illegible] s *et al.*, 1990; [illegible] ut *et al.*, 1995; [illegible] erman *et al.*, 1995). [illegible] doxical increase can [illegible] tions. First, the coupling [illegible] n and formation does not [illegible] ely but operates only after a [illegible] usually some months. Thus, [illegible] umber of new BMUs, that is new [illegible] pots, is decreased, the BMUs which [illegible] eady on their way will still complete [illegible] refilling with new bone. The amount [illegible] presented by this mechanism, called the remodeling space, is in the order of a few percent and is proportional to the rate of turnover. Secondly, the increase in bone mass can also be explained in part by the fact that, due to the decrease in turnover, the bone will become older and therefore more heavily mineralized. Theoretically, the increase induced by these two mechanisms should reach a plateau when a new steady rate is obtained and remain as long as the treatment is continued. This appears to be the case in most studies, although the timing of the new steady state is not clear but is probably longer than three years (Reginster *et al.*, 1989; Devogelaer and Nagant de Deuxchaisnes, 1990; Watts *et al.*, 1990; Storm *et al.*, 1992; Harris *et al.*, 1993; Adami *et al.*, 1993). Only one study suggests an increase over several years (Valkema *et al.*, 1989), but the results are questionable.

The question of whether bisphosphonates also improve the balance at the level of each BMU is not yet answered definitively, although it seems that it is the case. Resorption depth is difficult to measure precisely. It seems, however, that a decrease does occur (Steiniche *et al.*, 1991; Storm *et al.*, 1993). The results available on mean wall thickness do not yet allow a definitive conclusion either. Some results show no change (Ott *et al.*, 1994; Steniche *et al.*, 1991) or possibly a decrease, at least with etidronate after one year (Pallot-Prades *et al.*, 1991). In contrast, alendronate was recently found to increase mean wall thickness in ovariectomized baboons, suggesting a stimulation of bone formation (Balena *et al.*, 1993). Even if the bisphosphonates are not able to increase bone formation, the net balance at each BMU could still be increased if the resorption depth was indeed smaller. If true, this would be of considerable interest, since total bone mass could be gradually increased by a mechanism other than the one described above. It should be noted that if this occurred, the decrease in bone turnover would actually be counterproductive.

One question is why such small changes in bone density result in the relatively large improvement in fracture rate, if the latter is real. One explanation is that the incidence of fractures is closely related to the perforation of trabeculae, resulting in a change of the architectural structure and a decrease in resistance to mechanical stress. A decrease in turnover will lead to a change in these events, even without an appreciable change in bone density (Parfitt, 1991).

GENERAL CONSIDERATIONS

Much has been learned about the effects of the bisphosphonates, both in general and in osteoporosis. However, many questions remain still open.

There is now enough evidence to draw the conclusion that bisphosphonates can stop the decrease in bone mass in various forms of osteoporosis. Furthermore, they are even able to induce a small increase of a few percent of bone mineral density. However, it is not definitely known yet whether long-term treatment can lead to a progressive increase or whether, as is more probable, the latter reaches a plateau after a few years, as seen with other inhibitors of bone resorption.

Little is known yet about the best mode of administration of these compounds. Is there any advantage in discontinuous versus continuous administration? One study in rats showed no difference when tiludronate was given over a period of 16 weeks at the same total dose for five days every four weeks or five days a week (Ammann *et al.*, 1993). If discontinuous treatment was used, what would be the best regimen? There is no proof that the regimen prescribed for etidronate is optimal. Indeed, the ADFR theory, if it is applicable at all, may well be inapplicable to a drug with a long-term action. A single administration of pamidronate every three months actively increased bone mineral density in various sites (Thiébaud *et al.*, 1994). Recently it was shown that 10 mg of alendronate infused over five days was effective on bone turnover for >720 days in Paget's disease, >120 days in metastatic bone disease, 124 ± 82 days in postmenopausal osteoporosis, 28 ± 32 days in primary hyperparathyroidism and only 12 ± 9 days in humoral hypercalcemia of malignancy (Adami *et al.*, 1992). This might raise the possibility of a biannual treatment in osteoporosis and, since the duration probably depends on the dose, a less frequent treatment may even be envisaged. However, since the total dose is most probably the relevant one, the less frequent the administration, the higher the individual dose, which might present drawbacks, the continuous administration having the advantage of lower peak blood levels.

The optimal dose will have to be determined for each bisphosphonate. It should be chosen such that bone turnover is not decreased excessively, but bone loss is still inhibited adequately or, better yet, bone is gained.

Many other questions remain. For example, do differences exist between various bisphosphonates? Will it be of advantage to administer the bisphosphonates together with a compound which increases bone formation, such as fluoride? Should these compounds be used both for treatment and for prevention of the disease?

All these questions will have to be answered in the future. Whatever the answers, it seems most probable that the class of bisphosphonates will have an important place in the treatment of osteoporosis.

CONCLUSION

Bisphosphonates are non-biodegradable compounds characterized by a P-C-P bond. They have the property to inhibit bone resorption through a cellular mechanism which is still not completely understood. When given in large amounts, some bisphosphonates also inhibit normal and ectopic mineralization.

The bisphosphonates are rapidly cleared from plasma, 20–50% going to bone, the rest being excreted in the urine. In contrast, the half-life in bone is very long. The reason for their low toxicity is probably their rapid plasma and soft tissue clearance.

Bisphosphonates are used successfully in diseases with increased bone turnover, such as Paget's disease, tumoral bone disease and recently also osteoporosis. Most results in osteoporosis have been obtained with alendronate, clodronate, etidronate, pamidronate and tiludronate. The first four are now registered for this use in some countries. All bisphosphonates investigated inhibit bone loss and, to a certain degree, increase bone mass. Alendronate in particular decreases vertebral and non-vertebral fractures.

In view of the results currently available, it appears that the class of bisphosphonates is becoming a most important addition to the therapeutic options available for the treatment and possibly the prevention of osteoporosis.

REFERENCES

Adami, S., Bhalla, A.K., Dorizzi, R. *et al.* (1987) The acute-phase response after bisphosphonate administration. *Calcif Tissue Int* **41**: 326–31.

Adami, S., Rosini, M., Bertolo, F. *et al.* (1992) Duration of pharmacological activity of bisphosphonates. *Bone Mineral* **17** (Suppl 1): S14.

Adami, S., Baroni, M.C., Broggini, M. *et al.* (1993) Treatment of postmenopausal osteoporosis with continuous daily oral alendronate in comparison with either placebo or intranasal salmon calcitonin. *Osteoporosis Int* **3**: S21–7.

Adamson, B.B., Gallacher, S.J., Byars, J. *et al.* (1993) Mineralisation defects with pamidronate therapy for Paget's disease. *Lancet* **342**: 1459–60.

Ahrengart, L. and Lindgren, U. (1986) Prevention of ectopic bone formation by local application of ethane-1-hydroxy-1,1-diphosphonate (EHDP): an experimental study in rabbits. *J Orthop Res* **4**: 18–26.

Alden, C.L., Parker, R. and Eastman, D.F. (1989) Development of an acute model for the study of chloromethanediphosphonate nephrotoxicity. *Toxicol Pathol* **17**: 27–32.

Ammann, P., Rizzoli, R., Caverzasio, J. *et al.* (1993) Effects of the bisphosphonate tiludronate on bone resorption, calcium balance, and bone mineral density. *J Bone Miner Res* **8**(12): 1491–8.

Anderson, C., Cape, R.D.T., Crilly, R.G. *et al.* (1984) Preliminary observations of a form of coherence therapy for osteoporosis. *Calcif Tissue Int* **36**: 341–3.

Apseloff, G., Girten, B., Walter, M. *et al.* (1991) Aminohydroxybutane bisphosphonate prevents one loss in a rat model of simulated weightlessness. *Curr Ther Res* **50**: 794–803.

Apseloff, G., Girten, B., Steven, E. *et al.* 1993) Effects of amino-hydroxybutane bisphosphonate on bone growth when administered after hind-limb bone loss in tail-suspended rats. *J Pharmacol Exp Ther* **257**(1): 515–21.

Atkin, I., Ornoy, A., Pita, J.C. *et al.* (1988) EHDP-induced rachitic syndrome in rats is not reversed by vitamin D metabolites. *Anat Rec* **220**: 22–30.

Balena, R., Toolan, B.C., Shea, M. *et al.* (1993) The effects of 2-year treatment with the aminobisphosphonate alendronate on bone metabolism, bone histomorphometry, and bone strength in ovariectomized nonhuman primates. *J Clin Invest* **92**: 2577–86.

Barbier, A., Edmonds-Alt, X., Brelière, J.C. *et al.* (1990) *In vitro* and *in vivo* osseous pharmacological profile of tiludronate. Implication for osteoporosis treatment. Third International Symposium on Osteoporosis, (eds Christiansen, C. and Overgaard, K.), Osteopress ApS, Copenhagen, pp. 1127–30.

Bijvoet, O.L.M., Hosking, D.J., Lemkes, H.H.P.J., Reitsma, P.H. and Frijlink, W. (1978) Development in the treatment of Paget's disease. In: *Endocrinology of Calcium Metabolism*, (eds Copp, D.H. and Talmage, R.V.), Excerpta Medica, Amsterdam pp. 48–54.

Bijvoet, O.L.M., Frijlink, W.B., Jie, K. *et al.* (1980) APD in Paget's disease of bone. Role of the mononuclear phagocyte system? *Arthrit Rheum* **23**: 1193–204.

Bijvoet, O.L., Valkema, R., Löwik, C.W.GM and Papapoulos, S.E. (1993) Bisphosphonates in osteoporosis? *Osteoporosis Int* **S1**: 230–6.

Bisaz, S., Jung, A. and Fleisch, H. (1978) Uptake by bone of pyrophosphate, diphosphonates and their technetium derivatives. *Clin Sci Mol Med* **54**: 265–72.

Black, D.M., Cummings, S.R., Karpf, D.B. *et al.* (1996) Randomised trial of effect of alendronate on risk of fracture in women with existing vertebral fractures. Fracture Intervention Trial Research Group. *Lancet* **348**: 1535–41.

Boonekamp, P.M., Van der Wee-Pals, L.J.A., Van Wijk-Lennep, M.M.L. *et al.* (1986) Two modes of action of bisphosphonates on osteoclastic resorption of mineralized matrix. *Bone Miner* **1**: 27–39.

Boonekamp, P.M., Löwik, C.W.G.M., van der Wee-Pals, L.J.A., van Wijk-Lennep, M.L.L. and Bijvoet, O.L.M. (1987) Enhancement of the inhibitory action of APD on the transformation of osteoclast precursors into resorbing cells after dimethylation of the amino group. *Bone Miner* **2**: 29–42.

Bounameaux, H.M., Schifferli, J., Montani, J.P., Jung, A. and Chatelanat, F. (1983) Renal failure associated with intravenous diphosphonate. *Lancet* **i**: 47.

Boyce, B.F., Fogelman, I., Ralston, S. *et al.* (1984) Focal osteomalacia due to low-dose diphosphonate therapy in Paget's disease. *Lancet* **i**: 821–4.

Brommage, R. and Baxter, D.C. (1990) Inhibition of bone mineral loss during lactation by Cl_2MBP. *Calcif Tissue Int* **47**: 169–72.

Cabanela, M.E. and Jowsey, J. (1971) The effects of phosphonates on experimental osteoporosis. *Calcif Tissue Res* **8**: 114–20.

Cal, J.C. and Daley-Yates, P.T. (1990) Disposition and nephrotoxicity of 3-amino-1-hydroxypropylidene-1,1-bisphosphonate (APD), in rats and mice. *Toxicology* **65**: 179–97.

Carano, A., Teitelbaum, S.L., Konsek, J.D. *et al.* (1990) Bisphosphonates directly inhibit the bone resorption activity of isolated avian osteoclasts *in vitro*. *J Clin Invest* **85**: 456–61.

Cecchini, M. and Fleisch, H. (1990) Bisphosphonates *in vitro* specifically inhibit, among the hematopoietic series, the development of the mouse mononuclear phagocyte lineage. *J Bone Miner Res* **5**: 1019–27.

Cecchini, M., Felix, R., Cooper, P.H. and Fleisch, H. (1987) Effect of bisphosphonates on proliferation and viability of mouse bone marrow-derived macrophages. *J Bone Miner Res* **2**: 135–42.

Chambers, T.J. (1980) Diphosphonates inhibit bone resorption by macrophages *in vitro*. *J Pathol* **132**: 255–62.

Chan, M.M., Riggins, R.S. and Rucker, R.B. (1977) Effect of ethane-1-hydroxy-1,1-diphosphonate (EHDP) and dietary fluoride on biomechanical and morphological changes in chick bone. *J Nutrition* **107**: 1747–54.

Chappard, D., Petitjean, M., Alexandre, C. *et al.* (1991) Cortical osteoclasts are less sensitive to etidronate than trabecular osteoclasts. *J Bone Miner Res* **6**(7): 673–80.

Chesnut III, C.H. (1988) Drug therapy: calcitonin, bisphosphonates, anabolic steroids, and hPTH (1–34. In: *Osteoporosis: Etiology, Diagnosis, and Management*, (eds Riggs, B.L. and Melton III, L.J.), Raven Press, New York, pp. 403–14.

Chesnut III, C.H., McClung, M.R., Ensrud, K.E. *et al.* (1995) Alendronate treatment of the postmenopausal osteoporotic women: effect of multiple dosages on bone mass and bone remodeling. *Am J Med* **99**: 144–52.

Conrad, K.A. and Lee, S.M. (1981) Clodronate kinetics and dynamics. *Clin Pharmacol Ther* **30**: 114–20.

Daley-Yates, P.T. and Bennett, R. (1988) A comparison of the pharmacokinetics of ^{14}C-labelled APD and ^{99m}Tc-labelled APD in the mouse. *Calcif Tissue Int* **43**: 125–7.

de Groen, P.C., Lubbe, D.F., Hirsch, L.J. *et al.* (1996) Esophagitis associated with the use of alendronate. *N Engl J Med* **335**: 1958–9.

Delaissé, J-M., Eeckhout, Y. and Vaes, G. (1985) Bisphosphonates and bone resorption: effects on collagenase and lyosomal enzyme excretion. *Life Sci* **37**: 2291–6.

de Vernejoul, M.C., Jiang, Y., Lacheretz, F. *et al.* (1990) Prevention of bone loss following tiludronate administration to ovariectomized beagle dogs. Third International Symposium on Osteoporosis, (eds Christiansen, C. and Overgaard, K.), Osteopress ApS, Copenhagen, pp. 1119–22.

Devogelaer, J.P. and Nagant de Deuxchaisnes, C. (1990) Treatment of involutional osteoporosis with the bisphosphonate APD (disodium pamidronate): non-linear increase of lumbar bone mineral density. *Third International Symposium on Osteoporosis*, (eds Christiansen, C. and Overgaard, K.), Osteopress ApS, Copenhagen, pp. 1507–9.

Dodwell, D.J., Howell, A. and Ford, J. (1990) Reduction in calcium excretion in women with breast cancer and bone metastases using the oral bisphosphonate pamidronate. *Br J Cancer* **61**: 123–5.

Ende, J.J. (1979) Effects of some diphosphonates on the metabolism of bone *in vivo* and *in vitro*. Thesis, University of Leiden.

Evans, R.A., Somers, N.M., Dunstan, C.R., Royle, H. and Kos, S. (1993) The effect of low-dose cyclical etidronate and calcium on bone mass in early postmenopausal women. *Osteoporosis Int* **3**: 71–5.

East, D.K., Felix, R., Dowse, C. *et al.* (1978) The effect of diphosphonates on the growth and glycolysis of connective-tissue cells in culture. *Biochem J* **172**: 97–107.

Felix, R. and Fleisch, H. (1975) Properties of inorganic pyrophosphatase of pig scapula cartilage. *Biochem J* **147**: 111–18.

Felix, R., Russell, R.G.G. and Fleisch, H. (1976) The effect of several diphosphonates on acid phosphohydrolases and other lysosomal enzymes. *Biochim Biophys Acta* **429**: 429–38.

Felix, R., Bettex, J.D. and Fleisch, H. (1981) Effect of diphosphonates on the synthesis of prostaglandins in cultured calvaria cells. *Calcif Tissue Int* **33**: 549–52.

Felix, R., Guenther, H.L. and Fleisch, H. (1984) The subcellular distribution of ^{14}C dichloromethylenebisphosphonate and ^{14}C 1-hydroxyethylidene-1,1-bisphosphonate in cultured calvaria cells. *Calcif Tissue Int* **36**: 108–13.

Ferretti, J.L., Cointry, G., Capozza, R. *et al.* (1990) Biomechanical effects of the full range of useful doses of (3-amino-1-hydroxypropylidene)-1,1-bisphosphonate (APD) on femur diaphyses and cortical bone tissue in rats. *Bone Mineral* **11**: 111–22.

Ferretti, J.L., Mondelo, N., Capozza, R. *et al.* (1992) Pamidronate and dimethyl-pamidronate effects on femur biomechanics in ovariectomized-hemisciaticectomized rat. *Bone Mineral* 17(S1): A5.

Ferretti, J.L., Delgado, C.J., Capozza, R.F. *et al.* (1993) Protective effects of disodium etidronate and pamidronate against the biomechanical repercussion of betamethasone-induced osteopenia in growing rat femurs. *Bone Mineral* **20**: 265–76.

Flanagan, A.M. and Chambers, T.J. (1989) Dichloromethylenebisphosphonate (Cl_2MBP) inhibits bone resorption through injury to oesteoclasts that resorb Cl_2MBP-coated bone. *Bone Mineral* **6**: 33–43.

Fleisch, H. (1991) Bisphosphonates. Pharmacology and use in the treatment of tumor-induced hypercalcaemic and metastatic bone disease. *Drugs* **42**: 919–44.

Fleisch, H. (1993) Bisphosphonates: mechanisms of action and clinical use. In: *Handbook of Experimental Pharmacology*, Vol. 107, *Physiology and Pharmacology of Bone*, (eds Mundy, G.R. and Martin, T.J.), Springer Verlag, Berlin, pp. 377–418.

Fleisch, H. (1995) *Bisphosphonates in Bone Disease – From the Laboratory to the Patient*, Parthenon Publishing Group, New York.

Fleisch, H. (1996) The bisphosphonate ibandronate, given daily as well as discontinuously, decreases bone resorption and increases calcium retention as assessed by Ca^{45} kinetics in the intact rat. *Osteoporosis* **6**: 166–70.

Fleisch, H., Russell, R.G.G., Bisaz, S. *et al.* (1968) The influence of pyrophosphate analogues (diphosphonates) on the precipitation and dissolution of calcium phosphate *in vitro* and *in vivo*. *Calcif Tissue Res* **2** (Suppl): 10–10A.

Fleisch, H., Russell, R.G.G. and Francis, M.D. (1969) Diphosphonates inhibit hydroxyapatite dissolution *in vitro* and bone resorption in tissue culture and *in vivo*. *Science* **165**; 1262–4.

Fleisch, H., Russell, R.G.G., Bisaz, S. *et al.* (1970) The inhibitory effect of phosphonates on the formation of calcium calcification *in vivo*. *Eur J Clin Invest* **1**: 12–18.

Flora, L., Hassing, G.S., Parfitt, A.M. and Villanueva, A.R. (1980) Comparative skeletal effects of two diphosphonates in dogs. *Metab Bone Dis Rel Res*. **2**: 389–407.

Francis, M.D. (1969) The inhibition of calcium hydroxyapatite crystal growth by polyphosphates. *Calcif Tissue Res* **3**: 151–62.

Francis, M.D. and Martodam, P.R. (1983) Chemical, biochemical, and medicinal properties of the diphosphonates: in: *The Role of Phosphonates in Living Systems*, (ed. Hilderbrand, R.L.), CRC Press, Boca Raton, p. 55.

Francis, M.D. and Slough, C.L. (1984) Acute intravenous infusion of disodium dihydrogen (1-hydroxyethylidene)diphosphonate: mechanism of toxicity. *J Pharmaceut Sci* **73**: 1097–100.

Francis, M.D., Russell, R.G.G. and Fleisch, H. (1969) Diphosphonates inhibit formation of calcium phosphate crystals *in vitro* and pathological calcification *in vivo*. *Science* **165**: 1264–6.

Fromm, G.A., Vega, E., Plantalech, L., Galich, A.M. and Mautalen, C.A. (1991) Differential action of pamidronate on trabecular and cortical bone in women with involutional osteoporosis. *Osteoporosis Int* **1**: 129–33.

Gallacher, S.J., Ralston, S.H., Dryburgh, F.J. *et al.* (1990) Immobilization-related hypercalcaemia – a possible novel mechanism and response to pamidronate. *Postgrad Med J* **66**: 918–22.

Garnero, P., Shih, W.J., Gineyts, E., Karpf, D.B. and Delmas, P.D. (1994) Comparison of new biochemical markers of bone turnover in late postmenopausal osteoporotic women in response to alendronate treatment. *J Clin Endocrinol Metab* **79**: 1693–700.

Gasser, A.B., Morgan, D.B., Fleisch, H.A. and Richelle, L.J. (1972) The influence of two diphosphonates on calcium metabolism in the rat. *Clin Sci* **43**: 31–45.

Geddes, A.D., D'Souza, S.M., Ebetino, F.H. and Ibbotson, K.J. (1994) Bisphosphonates: structure–activity relationships and therapeutic implications. In: *Bone and Mineral Research*, (eds Heersche, J.M. and Kanis, J.A.), Elsevier, Amsterdam, pp. 265–306.

Gertz, B.J., Shao, P., Hanson, D.A. *et al.* (1994) Monitoring bone resorption in early postmenopausal women by an immunoassay for cross-linked collagen peptides in urine. *J Bone Miner Res* **9**: 135–42.

Geusens, P., Nijs, G., van der Perre, G. *et al.* (1992) Longitudinal effect of tiludronate on bone mineral density, resonant frequency, and strength in monkeys. *J Bone Miner Res* **7**(6): 599–608.

Giannini, S., D'Angelo, A., Malvasi, L. *et al.* (1993) Effects of one-year cyclical treatment with clodronate on postmenopausal bone loss. *Bone* **14**: 137–41.

Glatt, M., Pataki, A., Blätter, A. and Reife, R. (1986) APD longterm treatment increases bone mass and mechanical strength of femora of adult mice. *Calcif Tissue Int* **39**, A72.

Green, J.R., Müller, K. and Jaeggi, K.A. (1994) Preclinical pharmacology of CGP 42'446, a new, potent, heterocyclic bisphosphonate compound. *J Bone Miner Res* **9**(5): 745–51.

Grynpas, M.D., Acito, A., Dimitriu M. *et al.* (1992) Changes in bone mineralization, architecture and mechanical properties due to long-term (1 year) administration of pamidronate (APD) to adult dogs. *Osteoporosis Int.* **2**: 74–81.

Guilland, D.F., Sallis, J.D. and Fleisch, H. (1974) The effect of two diphosphonates on the handling of calcium by rat kidney mitochondria *in vitro. Calcif Tissue Res* **15**: 303–14.

Guilland, D., Trechsel, U., Bonjour, J.P. and Fleisch, H. (1975) Stimulation of calcium absorption and apparent increased intestinal, 1,25-dihydroxycholecalciferol in rats treated with low doses of ethane-1-hydroxy-1,1-diphosphonate. *Clin Sci Mol Med* **48**: 157–60.

Gural, R.P. (1975) Pharmacokinetics and gastrointestinal absorption behavior of etidronate. Dissertation, University of Kentucky.

Guy, J.A., Shea, M., Peter, C.P., Morrissey, R. and Hayes, W.C. (1993) Continuous alendronate treatment throughout growth, maturation, and aging in the rat results in increases in bone mass and mechanical properties. *Calcif Tissue Int* **53**: 283–8.

Hähnel, H., Mühlbach, R., Lindenhayn, K. *et al.* (1973) Zum Einfluss von Diphosphonat auf die experimentelle Heparinosteopathie. *Zeitschr Alternsforschung* **28**: 289–92.

Hanhijärvi, H., Elomaa, I., Karlsson, M. and Lauren, L. (1989) Pharmacokinetics of disodium clodronate after daily intravenous infusions during five consecutive days. *Int J Clin Pharmacol Ther Toxicol* **27**: 602–6.

Hannuniemi, R. and Virtamo, T. (1992) Clodronate has an inhibitory effect on bone loss in ovariectomized rats. *Bone Mineral* **17** (Suppl 1), S13.

Hansen, Jr, N.M., Felix, R., Bisaz, S. and Fleisch, H. (1976) Aggregation of hydroxyapatite crystals. *Biochim Biophys Acta* **451**: 549–59.

Harinck, H.I.J., Papapoulos, S.E., Blanksma, H.J. *et al.* (1987) Paget's disease of bone: early and late responses to three different modes of treatment with aminohydroxypropylidene bisphosphonate (APD). *Br Med J* **295**: 1301–5.

Harris, S.T., Watts, N.B., Jackson, R.D. *et al.* (1993) Four-year study of intermittent cyclic etidronate treatment of postmenopausal osteoporosis: three years of blinded therapy followed by one year of open therapy. *Am J Med* **95**: 557–67.

Heaney, R.P. and Saville, P.D. (1976) Etidronate disodium in postmenopausal osteoporosis. *Clin Pharmacol Ther* **20**: 593–604.

Hesch, R.D., Heck, J., Delling, G. *et al.* (1988) Results of a stimulatory therapy of low bone metabolism in osteoporosis with (1–38) hPTH and diphosphonate EHDP. Protocol of study I, osteoporosis trial Hannover. *Klin Wochenschr* **66**: 976–84.

Hintze, K.L. and D'Amato, R.A. (1980) Comparative toxicity of two bisphosphonates. *Toxicology* **2**: 192.

Hodsman, A.B. (1989) Effects of cyclical therapy for osteoporosis using an oral regimen of inorganic phosphate and sodium etidronate: a clinical and bone histomorphometric study. *Bone Mineral* **5**: 201–12.

Hoekman, K., Papapoulos, S.E., Peter, A.C.B. and Bijvoet, O.L.M. (1985) Characteristics and bisphosphonate treatment of a patient with juvenile osteoporosis. *J Clin Endocrinol Metab* **61**: 952–6.

Hughes, D.E., MacDonald, B.R., Russell, R.G.G. and Gowen, M. (1989) Inhibition of oseoclast-like cell formation by bisphosphonates in long-term cultures of human bone marrow. *J Clin Invest* **83**: 1930–5.

Hughes, D.E., Wright, K.R., Uy, H.L. *et al.* (1995) Bisphosphonates promote apoptosis in murine osteoclasts *in vitro* and *in vivo. J Bone Miner Res* **10**: 1478–87.

Janner, M., Mühlbauer, R.C. and Fleisch, H. (1991) Sodium EDTA enhances intestinal absorption of two bisphosphonates. *Calcif Tissue Int* **49**: 280–3.

Jee, W.S.S., Black, H.E. and Gotcher, J.E. (1981) Effect of dichloromethane diphosphonate on cortisol-induced bone loss in young adult rabbits. *Clin Orthop Res* **158**: 39–51.

Jee, W.S.S., Tang, L., Ke, H.Z., Setterberg, R.B. and Kimmel, D.B. (1993) Maintaining restored bone with bisphosphonate in the ovariectomized rat skeleton: dynamic histomorphometry of changes in bone mass. *Bone* **14**: 493–8.

Johnson, K.Y., Wesseler, M.A., Olson, H.M. *et al.* (1982) The effects of diphosphonates on tumor-induced hypercalcemia and osteolysis in Walker carcinosarcoma 256 (W-256) of rats. In: *Diphosphonates and Bone*, (eds Donath, A. and Courvoisier, B.), Editions Médecine et Hygiène, Geneva, pp. 386–9.

Johnston Jr, C.C., Altman, R.D., Canfield, R.E. *et al.* (1983) Review of fracture experience during treatment of Paget's disease of bone with etidronate disodium (EHDP). *Clin Orthop* **172**: 186–94.

Jones, R.G. and Henderson, M.J. (1987) Transient taste-loss during treatment with etidronate. *Lancet* **12**: 637.

Jowsey, J. and Holley, K.E. (1973) Influence of

diphosphonates on progress of experimentally induced osteoporosis. *J Lab Clin Med* **82**(4): 567–75.

Jowsey, J., Holley, K.E. and Linman, J.W. (1970) Effect of sodium etidronate in adult cats. *J Lab Clin Med* **76**: 126–33.

Jung, A., Bisaz, S. and Fleisch, H. (1973) The binding of pyrosphosphate and two diphosphonates on hydroxyapatite crystals. *Calcif Tissue Res* **11**: 269–80.

Jung, A., Mermillod, B., Barras, C. *et al.* (1981) Inhibition by two disphosphonates of bone lysis in tumor conditioned media. *Cancer Res* **41**: 3233–7.

Jung, A., Bornand, J., Mermillod, B. *et al.* (1984) Inhibition by diphosphonates of bone resorption induced by the Walker tumor in the rat. *Cancer Res* **44**: 3007–11.

Kanis, J.A. (1991) Drugs used for the treatment of Paget's disease. In: *Pathophysiology and Treatment of Paget's Diseases*, (ed. Kanis, J.A.) Martin Dunitz, London, Ch. 7.

Kawamuki, K., Abe, T., Kudo, M. *et al.* (1990) Effect of YM175 on bone positively correlates with its concentraton in bone. *J Bone Miner Res* **5**(Suppl2): S245.

King, W.R., Francis, M.D. and Michael, W.R. (1971) Effect of disodium ethane-1-hydroxy-1,1-diphosphonate on bone formation. *Clin Orthop Rel Res* **78**: 251–70.

Kozak, S.T., Rizzoli, R., Trechsel, U. and Fleisch, H. (1987) Effect of a single injection of two new bisphosphonates on the hypercalcemia and hypercalciuria induced by Walker carcinosarcoma 256/B in thyroparathyroidectomized rats. *Cancer Res* **47**: 6193–7.

Kudo, M., Abe, T., Motoie, H. *et al.* (1992) Pharmacological profile of new bisphosphonate, 1-hydroxy-2-(imidazo[1,2-a]pyridin-3-yl) ethane-1,1-bis(phosphonic acid). *Bone Mineral* **17**(Suppl 1), S13.

Labat, M.L., Tzehoval, E., Moricard, Y. *et al.* (1983) Lack of a T-cell dependent subpopulation of macrophages in (dichloromethylene) diphosphonate-treated mice. *Biomed Pharmacother* **37**: 270–6.

Labat, M.L., Florentin, I., Davigny, M. *et al.* (1984) Dichloromethylene diphosphonate (Cl2MDP) reduces natural killer (NK) cell activity in mice. *Metab Bone Dis Rel Res* **5**: 281–7.

Lane, J.M. and Steinberg, M.E. (1973) The role of diphosphonates in osteoporosis of disuse. *J Trauma* **13**(10): 863–9.

Larsson, A. (1974) The short-term effects of high doses of ethylene-1-hydroxy-1,1-diphosphonates upon early dentine formation. *Calcif Tissue Res* **16**: 109–27.

Larsson, A. and Rohlin, M. (1980) *In vivo* distribution of ^{14}C-labeled ethylene-1-hydroxy-1,1-diphosphonate in normal and treated young rats. An autoradiographic and ultrastructural study. *Toxicol Appl Pharmacol* **52**: 391–9.

Lauritzen, D.B., Balena, R., Shea, M. *et al.* (1993) Effects of combined prostaglandin and alendronate treatment on the histomorphometry and biomechanical properties of bone in ovariectomized rats. *J Bone Miner Res* **8**(7): 871–9.

Lenehan, T.M., Balligand, M., Nunamaker, D.M. and Wood Jr, F.E. (1985) Effect of EHDP on fracture healing in dogs. *J Orthop Res* **3**: 499–507.

Liberman, U.A., Weiss, S.R., Bröll, J. *et al.* (1995) Effect of oral alendronate on bone mineral density and the incidence of fractures in postmenopausal osteoporosis. *N Engl J Med* **333**: 1437–43.

Liens, D., Delmas, P.D. and Meunier, P.J. (1994) Long-term effects of intravenous pamidronate in fibrous dysplasia of bone. *Lancet* **343**: 953–4.

Lin, J.H., Duggan, D.E., Chen, I-W. and Ellsworth, R.L. (1991) Physiological disposition of alendronate, a potent anti-osteolytic bisphosphonate, in laboratory animals. *Drug Metab Disposition* **19**(5): 926–32.

Lin, J.H., Chen, I-W., Deluna, F.A. and Hichens, M. (1992) Renal handling of alendronate in rats – an uncharacterized renal transport system. *Drug Metabol Disposition* **20**(4): 608–13.

Lindenhayn, K., Hähnel, H., Schmidt, U.J. and Kalbe, I. (1979) Effect of dimethylamino methylendiphosphonate on the immobilisation osteoporosis in rats. *Zeitschr Alternsforschung* **34**: 173–6.

Lockwood, D.R., Vogel, J.M., Schneider, V.S. and Huley, S.B. (1975) Effect of the diphosphonate EHDP on bone mineral metabolism during prolonged bed rest. *J Clin Endocrinol Metab* **41**: 533–41.

Löwik, C.W.G.M., Vander Pluijm, G. van der Wee-Pals, L.J.A. *et al.* (1988) Migration and phenotypic transformation of osteoclast precursors into mature osteoclasts: the effect of a bisphosphonate. *J Bone Miner Res* **3**: 185–91.

Mallette, L.E., LeBlanc, A.D., Pool, J.L. and Mechanick, J.I. (1989) Cyclic therapy of osteoporosis with neutral phosphate and brief, high dose pulses of etidronate. J Bone Miner Res **4**(2): 143–8.

Marcarol, V. and Fraunfelder, F.T. (1994) Pamidronate disodium and possible ocular adverse drug reactions. *Am J Ophthalmol* **118**: 220–4.

Martodam, R.R., Thornton, K.S., Sica, D.A. *et al.* (1983) The effects of dichloromethylene diphosphonate on hypercalcemia and other parameters of the humoral hypercalcemia of malignancy in the rat Leydig cell tumor. *Calcif Tissue Int* **35**: 512–19.

Masarachia, P., Weinrieb, M., Balena, R. and Rodan, G.A. (1996) Comparison of the distribution of 3H-alendronate and 3H-etidronate in rat and mouse bones. *Bone* **19**: 281–90.

Matsuda, T., Matsui, K., Shimakoshi, Y. *et al.* (1991) 1-Hydroxyethylidene-1,1-bisphosphonate decreases the postovariectomy enhanced interleukin 1 secretion from peritoneal macrophages in adult rats. *Calcif Tissue Int* **49**: 403–6.

McOsker, J.E. and Sietsema, W.K. (1990) Preclinical pharmacology of risedronate, a novel bisphosphonate. Third International Symposium on Osteoporosis, (eds Christiansen, C. and Overgaard, K.), Osteopress ApS, Copenhagen.

Michael, W.R., King, W.R. and Francis, M.D. (1971) Effectiveness of diphosphonates in preventing 'osteoporosis' of disuse in the rat. *Clin Orthop* **78**: 271–6.

Michael, W.R., King, W.R. and Wakim, J.M. (1972) Metabolism of disodium ethane-1-hydroxy-1,1-diphosphonate (disodium etidronate) in the rat, rabbit, dog and monkey. *Toxicol Appl Pharmacol* **21**: 503–15.

Milhaud, G., Labat, M.L. and Moricard, Y. (1983) (Dichloromethylene) diphosphonate-induced impairment of T-lymphocyte function. *Proc Natl Acad Sci USA* **80**: 4469–73.

Miller, S.C. and Jee, W.S.S. (1979) The effect of dichloromethylene-diphosphonate, a pyrophosphate analog, on bone and bone cell structure in the growing rat. *Anat Rec* **193**: 439–62.

Minaire, P., Bérard, E., Meunier, P.J. *et al.* (1981) Effects of disodium dichloromethylene diphosphonate on bone loss in paraplegic patients. *J Clin Invest* **68**: 1086–92.

Monier-Faugere, M-C., Friedler, R.M., Bauss, F. and Malluche, H.H. (1993) A new bisphosphonate, B 21.0955, prevents bone loss associated with cessation of ovarian function in experimental dogs. *J Bone Miner Res* **8**(11): 1345–55.

Mönkkönen, J. (1988) A one year follow-up study of the distribution of ^{14}C-clodronate in mice and rats. *Pharmacol Toxicol* **62**: 51–3.

Mönkkönen, J. and Ylitalo, P. (1990) The tissue distribution of clodronate (dichloromethylene bisphosphonate) in mice. The effects of vehicle and the route of administration. *Eur J Drug Metab Pharmacokinet* **15**: 239–94.

Mönkkönen, J., Koponen, H.M. and Ylitalo, P. (1989) Comparison of the distribution of three bisphosphonates in mice. *Pharmacol Toxicol* **65**: 294–8.

Morgan, D.B., Monod, A., Russell, R.G.G. and Fleisch, H. (1973) Influence of dichloromethylene diphosphonate (Cl_2MDP) and calcitonin on bone resorption, lactate production and phosphatase and pyrophosophatase content of mouse calvaria treated with parathyroid hormone *in vitro*. *Calcif Tissue Res* **13**: 287–94.

Motoie, H., Nakamura, T., O'Uchi, N. *et al.* (1995) Effects of the bisphosphonate YM175 on bone mineral density, strength, structure, and turnover in ovariectomized beagles on concomitant dietary calcium restriction. *J Bone Miner Res* **10**: 910–20.

Mühlbauer, R.C., Russell, R.G.G., Williams, D.A. and Fleisch, H. (1971) The effects of diphosphonates, polyphosphonates, and calcitonin on immobilisation osteoporosis in rats. *Eur J Clin Invest* **1**: 336–44.

Mühlbauer, R.C., Bauss, F., Schenk, R. *et al.* (1991) BM 21.0955 – a potent new bisphosphonate to inhibit bone resorption. *J Bone Miner Res* **6**: 1003–11.

Murakami, H., Nakamura, T., Tsurukami, H. *et al.* (1994) Effects of tiludronate on bone mass, structure, and turnover at the epiphyseal, primary, and secondary spongiosa in the proximal tibia of growing rats after sciatic neurectomy. *J Bone Miner Res* **9**: 1355–64.

Nagant de Deuxchaisnes, C., Rombouts-Lindemans, C., Huaux, J.P. *et al.* (1981) Paget's disease of bone. *Br Med J* **283**: 1054–5.

Nixon, G.A., Buehler, E.V. and Newmann, E.A. (1972) Preliminary safety assessment of disodium etidronate as an additive to experimental oral hygiene products. *Toxicol Appl Pharmacol* **22**: 661–71.

Nolen, G.A. and Buehler, E.V. (1971) The effects of disodium etidronate on the reproductive functions and embryogeny of albino rats and New Zealand rabbits. *Toxicol Appl Pharmacol* **18**: 548–61.

Nuti, R., Righi, G., Turchetti, V. and Vattimo, A. (1981) Etidronato sodico (EHDP) ed osteoporosi. *Clin Therapeut* **99**: 33–42.

Ogawa, Y., Adachi, Y., Hong, S. and Yagi, T. (1989) 1-hydroxyethylidene-1,1-bisphosphonate (HEPB) simultaneously induces two distinct types of hypomineralization in the rat incisor dentine. *Calcif Tissue Int* **44**: 46–60.

Ohya, K., Yamada, S., Felix, R. and Fleisch, H. (1985) Effect of bisphosphonates on prostaglandin synthesis by rat bone cells and mouse calvaria in culture. *Clin Sci* **69**: 403–11.

Österman, T., Juhakoski, A., Laurén, L. and Sellman, R. (1994) Effect of iron on the absorption and distribution of clodronate after oral administration in rats. *Pharmacol Toxicol* **74**: 267–70.

Ott, S.M., Woodson, G.C., Huffer, W.E., Miller, P.D. and Watts, N.B. (1994) Bone histomorphometric changes after cyclic therapy with phosphate and etidronate disodium in women with post menopausal osteoporosis. *J Clin Endocrinol Metab* **78**: 968–72.

Pacifici, R., McMurtry, C., Vered, I. *et al.* (1988) Coherence therapy does not prevent axial bone loss in osteoporotic women: a preliminary comparative study. *J Clin Endocrinol Metab* **88**: 747–53.

Pallot-Prades, B., Chappard, D., Tavan, P. *et al.* (1991) Etude histomorphométrique osseuse dans l'ostéoporose fracturaire d'involution traitée par l'éthane-1,hydroxy-1,1-bisphosphonate (étidronate) pendant un an. *Rev Rhum Mal Ostéoartic* **58**(11): 771–6.

Papapoulos, S.E., Landman, J.O., Bijvoet, O.L.M. *et al.* (1992) The use of bisphosphonates in the treatment of osteoporosis. *Bone* **13**: S41–S49.

Parfitt, A.M. (1990) The three organizational levels of bone remodeling: implications for the interpretation of biochemical markers and the mechanisms of bone loss. Third International Symposium on Osteoporosis, (eds Christiansen, C. and Overgaard, K.), Osteopress ApS, Copenhagen.

Parfitt, A.M. (1991) Use of bisphosphonates in the prevention of bone loss and fractures. *Am J Med* **91** (Suppl 5B): 42S–46S.

Parfitt, A.M. (1992) The physiologic and pathogenic significance of bone histomorphometric data. In: *Disorders of Bone and Mineral Metabolism*, (eds Coe, F.L. and Favus, M.J.), Raven Press, New York, pp. 475–98.

Passeri, M., Baroni, M.C., Pedrazzoni, M. *et al.* (1991) Intermittent treatment with intravenous 4-amino-1-hydroxybutylidene-1,1-bisphosphonate (AHBuBP) in the therapy of postmenopausal osteoporosis. *Bone Mineral* **15**: 237–48.

Plasmans, C.M.T., Kuypers, W. and Slooff, T.J.J.H. (1978) The effect of ethane-1-hydroxy-1,1-diphosphonic acid (EHDP) on matrix induced ectopic bone formation. *Clin Orthop Rel Res* **132**: 233–43.

Plasmans, C.M.T., Jap, P.H.K., Kujipers, W. and Slooff, T.J.J.H. (1980) Influence of diphosphonate on the cellular aspect of young bone tissue. *Calcif Tissue Int* **32**: 247–56.

Ravn, P., Clemmesen, B., Riis, B.J. and Christiansen, C. (1996) The effect on bone mass and bone markers of different doses of ibandronate, a new bisphosphonate for prevention and treatment of postmenopausal osteoporosis: a 1-year, randomized, double-blind, placebo-controlled dose-finding study. *Bone* **19**: 527–33.

Recker, R.R. and Saville, P.D. (1973) Intestinal absorption of disodium ethane-1-hydroxy-1,1-diphosphonate (disodium etidronate) using a deconvolution technique. *Toxicol Appl Pharmacol* **24**: 580–9.

Recker, R.R., Hassing, G.S., Lau, J.R. and Saville, P.D. (1973) The hyperphosphatamic effect of disodium ethane-1-hydroxy-1,1-diphosphonates (EHDPTM): renal handling of phosphorus and the renal response to parathyroid hormone. *J Lab Clin Med* **81**: 258–66.

Reginster, J.Y., Deroisy, D., Denis, D. *et al.* (1989) Prevention of postmenopausal bone loss by tiludronate. *Lancet* **23**(30), 1469–71.

Reid, I.R., Alexander, C.J., King, A.R. and Ibbertson, H.K. (1988) Prevention of steroid-induced osteoporosis with (3-amino-1-hydroxypropylidene)-1,1-bisphosphonate (APD). *Lancet* **i**: 143–6.

Reid, I.R., Schooler, B.A. and Stewart, A.W. (1990) Prevention of glucocorticoid-induced osteoporosis. *J Bone Miner Res* **5**(6): 619–23.

Reid, I.R., Wattie, D.J., Evans, M.C. *et al.* (1994) Continuous therapy with pamidronate, a potent bisphosphonate, in postmenopausal osteoporosis. *J Clin Endocrinol Metab* **79**: 1595–9.

Reiner, M., Sautter, V., Olah, A. *et al.* (1980) Diphosphonate treatment in myolitis ossificans progressiva. In: *Etidronate*, (ed. Caniggia, A.), Istituto Gentili, Pisa, p. 237.

Reitsma, P.H., Bijvoet, O.L.M., Verlinden-Ooms, H, Van der Wee-Pals, L.J.A. (1980) Kinetic studies of bone and mineral metabolism during treatment with (3-amino-1-hydroxy-propylidene)-1,1-bisphosphonate (ADP) in rats. *Calcif Tissue Int* **32**: 145–7.

Reynolds, J.J., Minkin, C., Morgan, D.B. *et al.* (1972) The effect of two diphosphonates on the resorption of mouse calvaria *in vitro*. *Calcif Tissue Res* **19**: 302–13.

Reynolds, J.J., Murphy, H., Mühlbauer, R.C. *et al.* (1973) Inhibition by diphosphonates of bone resorption in mice and comparison with grey lethal osteopetrosis. *Calcif Tissue Res* **12**: 59–71.

Rivero, D.P., Skipor, A.K., Singh, M. *et al.* (1987) Effect of disodium etidronate (EHDR) on bone ingrowth in a porous material. *Clin Orthop* **215**: 279–86.

Rosen, H.N., Sullivan, E.K., Middlebrooks, V.L. *et al.* (1993a) Parenteral pamidronate prevents thyroid hormone-induced bone loss in rats. *J Bone Miner Res* **8**(10): 1255–61.

Rosen, H.N., Moses, A.C., Gundberg, C. *et al.* (1993b) Therapy with parenteral pamidronate prevents thyroid hormone-induced bone turnover in humans. *J Clin Endocrinol Metab* **77**(3): 664–9.

Rosenblum, I.Y., Black, H.E. and Ferrell, J.F. (1977) The effects of various diphosphonates on a rat model of cardiac calciphylaxis. *Calcif Tissue Res* **23**: 151–9.

Roux, C., Listrat, V., Villette, B. *et al.* (1992) Long-lasting dermatological lesions after tiludronate therapy. *Calcif Tissue Int* **50**: 378–80.

Russell, R.G.G., Mühlbauer, R.C., Bisaz, S. *et al.* (1970) The influence of pyrophosphate, condensed phosphates, phosphonates and other phosphate compounds on the dissolution of hydroxyapatite *in vitro* and on bone resorption induced by parathyroid hormone in tissue culture and in thyroparathyroidectomised rats. *Calcif Tissue Res* **6**: 183–96.

Sahni, M., Guenther, H.L., Fleisch, H., Collin, P. and Martin, T.J. (1993) Bisphosphonates act on rat bone resorption through the mediation of osteoblasts. *J Clin Invest* **91**: 2004–11.

Sato, M. and Grasser, W. (1990) Effects of bisphosphonates on isolated rat osteoclasts as examined by reflected light microscopy. *J Bone Miner Res* **5**: 31–40.

Sato, M., Grasser, W., Endo, N. *et al.* (1991) Bisphosphonate action: alendronate localization in rat bone and effects on osteoclast ultrastructure. *J Clin Invest* **88**(6): 2095–105.

Schenk, R., Merz, W.A, Mühlbauer, R. *et al.* (1973) Effect of ethane-1-hydroxy-1,1-diphosphonate (EHDP) and dichloromethylene diphosphonate (Cl_2MDP) on the calcification and resorption of cartilage and bone in the tibial epiphysis and metaphysis of rats. *Calcif Tissue Res* **11**: 196–214.

Schenk, R., Eggli, P., Felix, R. *et al.* (1986) Quantitative morphometric evaluation of the inhibitory activity of new aminobisphosphonates on bone resorption in the rat. *Calcif Tissue Int* **28**: 342–9.

Schneider, V.S. and McDonald, J. (1984) Skeletal calcium homeostasis and countermeasures to prevent disuse osteoporosis. *Calcif Tissue Int* **36**(1): 151–4.

Schoutens, A., Verhas, M., Dourov, N. *et al.* (1988) Bone loss and bone blood flow in paraplegic rats treated with calcitonin, diphosphonate, and indomethacin. *Calcif Tissue Int* **42**: 136–42.

Schweitzer, D.H., Oostendorp-van de Ruit, M., van der Pluijm, G., Löwik, C.W.G.M. and Papapoulos, S.E. (1995) Interleukin-6 and the acute phase response during treatment of patients with Paget's disease with the nitrogen-containing bisphosphonate dimethylamino-hydroxypropylidene bisphosphonate. *J Bone Miner Res* **10**: 956–62.

Seedor, J.G., Quartuccio, H.A. and Thompson, D.D. (1991) The bisphosphonate alendronate (MK-217) inhibits bone loss due to ovariectomy in rats. *J Bone Miner Res* **6**: 339–46.

Shinoda, H., Adamek, G., Felix, R. *et al.* (1983) Structure–activity relationship of various bisphosphonates. *Calcif Tissue Int* **35**: 87–99.

Shiota, E. (1985) Effects of diphosphonate on osteoporosis induced in rats. Roentgenological, histological and biomechanical studies. *Fukuoka Acta Med* **76**(6): 317–42.

Shvets, V.N., Pankova, A.S., Kabitskaya, O.E. *et al.* (1986) Diphosphonate effects on bones of hypokinetic rats. *Kosmiceskaja Biologija Aviakosmiceskaja Medidina, Moscow*, **20**: 45–9.

Silberstein, E.B. and Schnur, W. (1992) Cyclic oral phosphate and etidronate increase femoral and lumbar bone mineral density and reduced lumbar spine fracture rate over three years. *J Nucl Med* **33**(1): 1–5.

Singer, F.R., Ritch, P.S., Lad, T.E. *et al.* (1991) Treatment of hypercalcemia of malignancy with intravenous etidronate. *Arch Intern Med* **1151**: 471–6.

Smirnova, I.N., Kudryavtseva, N.A., Komissarenko, S.V. *et al.* (1988) Diphosphontes are potent inhibitors of mammalian inorganic pyrophosphatase. *Arch Biochem Biophys* **267**: 280–4.

Smith, M.L., Fogelman, I., Hart, D.M. *et al.* (1989) Effect of etidronate disodium on bone turnover following surgical menopause. *Calcif Tissue Int* 44: 74–9.

Sorenson, O.H. (1992) Osteoporosis: a review of the current clinical *data on etidronate – the European study. Bisphosphonates, State-of-the-Art in Research and Potential Clinical Applications.* International Conference, London, June 18–19.

Steiniche, T., Hasling, C., Charles, P. *et al.* (1991) The effects of etidronate on trabecular bone remodeling in postmenopausal spinal osteoporosis: a randomized study comparing intermittent treatment and an ADFR regime. *Bone* **12**: 155–63.

Stevenson, P.H. and Stevenson, J.R. (1986) Cytotoxic and migration inhibitory effects of bisphosphonates on macrophages. *Calcif Tissue Int* **38**: 227–33.

Storm, T., Thamesborg, G, Steiniche, T. *et al.* (1990) Effect of intermittent cyclical etidronate therapy on bone mass and fracture rate in women with postmenopausal osteoporosis. *N Engl J Med* 322(18): 1265–71.

Storm, T., Thamsborg, G., Kollerup, H.A. *et al.* (1992) Five years of intermittent, cyclical etidronate therapy increases bone mass and reduces vertebral fracture rate in postmenopausal osteoporosis. *Bone Miner* **17**(Suppl 1): S24.

Storm, T., Steiniche, T., Thamsborg, G. and Melsen, F. (1993) Changes in bone histomorphometry after long-term treatment with intermittent, cyclic etidronate for postmenopausal osteoporosis. *J Bone Miner Res* **8**(2): 199–208.

Stutzer, A., Fleisch, H. and Trechsel, U. (1988) Short- and long-term effects of a single dose of bisphosphonates on retinoid-induced bone resorption in thyroparathyroidectomized rats. *Calcif Tissue Int* **43**: 294–9.

Thiébaud, D., Jaeger, P., Jacquet, A.F. and Burckhardt, P. (1986) A single-day treatment of tumor-induced hypercalcemia by intravenous amino-hydroxypropylidene bisphosphonate. *J Bone Miner Res* **1**: 555–62.

Thiébaud, D., Burckhardt, P., Melchior, J. *et al.* (1994) Two years' effectiveness of intravenous pamidronate (APD) versus oral fluoride for osteoporosis occurring in the postmenopause. *Osteoporosis Int* **4**: 76–83.

Thiébaud, D., Kriegbaum, H., Huss, H., Christiansen, C. and Burckhardt, P. (1996) Intravenous injections of ibandronate in the treatment of postmenopausal osteoporosis. *Osteoporosis* 1996: 321–5.

Thompson, D.D., Seedor, J.G., Quartuccio, H. *et al.* (1992) The bisphosphonate, alendronate, prevents bone loss in ovariectomized baboons. *J Bone Miner Res* **7**(8): 951–60.

Togari, A., Arai, M., Hironaka, M. *et al.* (1991) Effect of HEBP (1-hydroxyethylidene-1,1-bisphosphonate) on experimental osteoporosis induced by ovariectomy in rats. *Japan J Pharmacol* **56**: 177–85.

Toolan, B.C., Shea, M., Myers, E.R. *et al.* (1992) Effects of 4-amino-1-hydroxybutylidene bisphosphonate on bone biomechanics in rats. *J Bone Miner Res* **7**(12): 1399–406.

Trechsel, U., Stutzer, A. and Fleisch, H. (1987) Hypercalcemia induced with an arotinoid in thyroparathyroidectomized rats. A new model to study bone resorption *in vivo. J Clin Invest* **80**: 1679–86.

Troehler, U., Bonjour, J-P. and Fleisch, H. (1975) Renal secretion of diphosphonates in rats. *Kidney Int* **8**: 6–13.

Valkema, R., Vismans F-J.F.E., Papapoulos, S.E. *et al.* (1989) Maintained improvement in calcium balance and bone mineral content in patients with osteoporosis treated with the bisphosphonate APD. *Bone Mineral* **5**: 183–92.

Van der Pluijm, G., Löwik, C.W.G.M., de Groot, H. *et al.* (1991) Modulation of PTH-stimulated osteoclastic resorption by bisphosphonates in fetal mouse bone explants. *J Bone Miner Res* **6**(11): 1203–10.

Van Breukelen, F.J.M., Bijvoet, O.L.M. and von Oosterom, A.T. (1979) Inhibition of osteolytic bone lesions by (3-amino-1-hydroxypropylidene)-1,1-bisphosphonate (A.P.D.). *Lancet* **i**: 803–5.

Van Breukelen, F.J.M., Bijvoet, O.L.M., Frijlink, W.B. *et al.* (1982) Efficacy of amino-hydroxypropylidene bisphosphonate in hypercalcemia: observations on regulation of serum calcium. *Calcif Tissue Int* **34**: 321–7.

Varache, M., Audran, P., Clochon, A. *et al.* (1991) Aminohydroxypropylidene bisphosphonate (AHPrBP) treatment of severe immobilization hypercalcaemia in a young patient. *Clin Rheumatol* **10**(3): 328–32.

Vitté, C., Fleisch, H. and Guenther, H.L. (1996) Bisphosphonates induce osteoblasts to secrete an inhibitor of osteoclast-mediated resorption. *Endocrinology* **137**: 2324–33.

Walton, R.J., Russell, R.G.G. and Smith, R. (1975)

Changes in the renal and extrarenal handling of phosphate induced by disodium etidronate (EHDP) in man. *J Clin Sci Mol Med* **49**: 45–56.

Watts, N.B., Harris, S.T., Genant, H.K. *et al.* (1990) Intermittent cyclical etidronate treatment of postmenopausal osteoporosis. *N Engl J Med* **323**(2): 73–9.

Wingen, F. and Schmähl, D. (1987) Pharmaco-kinetics of the osteotropic diphosphonate 3-amino-1-hydroxypropane-1,1-diphosphonic acid in mammals. *Arzneimittelforschung* **37**: 1037–42.

Wink, C.S., Onge, M.S. and Parker, B. (1985) The effects of dichloromethylene bisphosphonate on osteoporotic femora of adult castrated male rats. *Acta Anat* **124**: 117–21.

Wink, C.S. and Hill, E.M. (1988) Dichloro-methylene bisphosphonate retards femoral expansion in normal and castrated adult male rats. *Acta Anat* **132**: 321–3.

Wronski, T.J., Yen, C-F. and Scott, K.S. (1991) Estrogen and diphosphonate treatment provide long-term protection against osteopenia in overiectomized rats. *J Bone Miner Res* **6**: 387–94.

Wronski, T.J., Dann, L.M., Qi, H. and Yen, C.-F. (1993) Skeletal effects of withdrawal of estrogen and diphosphonate treatment in ovariectomized rats. *Calcif Tissue Int* **53**: 210–16.

Yakatan, G.J., Poynor, W.J., Talbert, R.L. *et al.* (1982) Clodronate kinetics and bioavailability. *Clin Pharmacol Therapeut* **31**: 402–10.

Yamamoto, M., Markatos, A., Seedor, J.G. *et al.* (1993) The effects of the aminobisphosphonate alendronate of thyroid hormone-induced osteopenia in rats. *Calcif Tissue Int* **53**: 278–82.

Yap, A.S., Hockings, G.I., Fleming, S.J. and Khafagi, F.A. (1990) Use of aminohydroxypropylidene bisphosphonate (AHPrBP, 'APD') for the treatment of hypercalcemia in patients with renal impairment. *Clin Nephrol* **34**: 225–9.

Zanchetta, J.R., del Valle, E., Bogado, C.E. *et al.* (1990) Improvement in bone mineral content in patients with osteoporosis treated with the bisphosphonate APD. Third International Symposium on Osteoporosis, (eds Christiansen, C. and Overgaard, K.), Osteopress ApS, Copenhagen, pp. 1461–3.

Zimolo, Z., Wesolowski, G. and Rodan, G.A. (1995) Acid extrusion is induced by osteoclast attachment to bone. *J Clin Invest* **96**: 2277–83.

CALCITONIN THERAPY IN OSTEOPOROTIC SYNDROMES 10

L.V. Avioli

Calcitonin is a hormone which, like insulin, cortisone and estrogen, is normally synthesized and secreted by a specific endocrine gland. The thyroid gland produces calcitonin in addition to the thyroid hormones thyroxine (T4) and tri-iodothyronine (T3). Whereas thyroid-stimulating hormone of the pituitary gland (TSH) controls thyroid hormone production and secretion, the circulating level of ionized calcium controls calcitonin release low values decreasing calcitonin secretion and high values stimulating the release of the hormone. Calcitonin appears to respond to changes in dietary calcium in a manner which is consistent with its primary biological activity, i.e. preventing osteoclastic-stimulated bone resorption. In this regard, the effect of calcitonin on the skeleton is opposite to that of parathyroid hormone which stimulates osteoclastic-regulated bone resorption. Whereas diets which are consistently low in elemental calcium content result in increased parathyroid hormone secretion and stimulated bone resorption, calcium feeding results in a decrease in parathyroid hormone production and an increase in calcitonin production. The calcitonin response to calcium feeding is much more pronounced in men than in women (Body and Heath, 1983). As a result, females are considered to have a lifelong relative deficiency in calcitonin production on a daily basis (Heath and Sizemore, 1977). A significant correlation between circulating plasma estrone and calcitonin values has been documented and decreased calcitonin reserve (Zseli *et al.*, 1985) and production rates (Reginster *et al.*, 1989) noted in osteoporotic postmenopausal women when compared to an age-matched non-osteoporotic population.

Salmon calcitonin has been approved by the United States FDA for the treatment of Paget's disease of bone, hypercalcemia and postmenopausal osteoporotic syndromes. Since the discovery of this hormone in 1961, it has also been used to effectively reverse the bone loss observed in immobilized paraplegic patients (Minaire *et al.*, 1984), in Sudeck's atrophy of bone (Bisson *et al.*, 1982), in patients treated with glucocorticoid medications (Eufemio, 1990; Luengo *et al.*, 1990; Montemurro *et al.*, 1991) and in malignant diseases such as multiple myeloma (Rico *et al.*, 1990).

The efficacy of calcitonin therapy in steroid-induced osteoporosis led the American College of Rheumatology to propose that calcitonin be used in patients at risk for steroid-induced osteoporosis at its 53rd Annual Meeting in 1989 (Eufemio, 1990). Therapeutic responses of patients with Paget's disease include a general suppression of the osteoclastic-induced osteolytic bone

Osteoporosis. Edited by John C. Stevenson and Robert Lindsay. Published in 1998 by Chapman & Hall, London.
ISBN 0 412 48870 1

disease, reversal of neural entrapment syndromes in patients with vertebral involvement, increased motility and amelioration of cardiac 'high-turnover' failure in others with more extensive skeletal disease (Nagant de Deuxchaisnes *et al.*, 1977; Woodhouse *et al.*, 1977; Herzberg and Bayless, 1980; Ravichandran, 1981; Nagant de Deuxchaisnes, 1983) and a halt in the progression of the hearing loss (Samaa *et al.*, 1986). Following the cessation of the osteoclastic bone loss, continued treatment of pagetic patients with calcitonin leads to a gradual remodeling of the involved area with new bone production and a gradual restoration of normal bone content in the original osteolytic areas (Nagant de Deuxchaisnes *et al.*, 1977; Woodhouse *et al.*, 1977). Pain relief has also been documented in over 75% of those pagetic patients treated with calcitonin (Nagant de Deuxchaisnes, 1983), as well as in patients with malignancies (Hindley *et al.*, 1982). This analgesic effect of calcitonin has been an unexpected bonus. Recent studies reveal that the analgesic effect may be mediated via the endogenous opiate system since pain relief in calcitonin-treated patients is associated with an increase in circulating β-endorphin (Graf *et al.*, 1985). The analgesia is probably also the result of a direct effect of calcitonin on pain threshold centers in the central nervous system since sustained analgesic effects have been observed with epidural and subarachnoid injections of salmon calcitonin (Fiore *et al.*, 1983).

Calcitonin has been evaluated in therapeutic trials in osteoporotic women in both the United States and abroad for more than 20 years. Reports of therapeutic responses vary from those demonstrating simple suppression of annual bone loss rates, as observed in the past with estrogen treatment, to others which reveal striking dose-related increments in bone mass of the vertebral and long bones (Gennari *et al.*, 1985; Mazzuoli *et al.*, 1986; Civitelli *et al.*, 1988; MacIntyre *et al.*, 1988; Overgaard *et al.*, 1989a, b), a decrease in vertebral fracture rates (Overgaard *et al.*, 1992; Rico *et al.*, 1992; Stock *et al.*, 1997) and, comparable to results obtained in Paget's disease, relief of bone pain syndromes (Lyritis *et al.*, 1991).

The skeletal response to calcitonin therapy is related to the rate of bone turnover. There are at least two histological variants of postmenopausal osteoporosis, i.e. high turnover and low/normal turnover forms, also known as the active and inactive forms respectively (Whyte *et al.*, 1982). In high-turnover or active osteoporosis, a bone biopsy specimen will demonstrate an abundance of bone cells, i.e. osteoblasts and osteoclasts (Whyte *et al.*, 1982). Patients with this form of the postmenopausal osteoporotic syndrome respond rapidly and very well to calcitonin treatment (Overgaard *et al.*, 1989a, 1990). The patients can also be identified by measuring the level of circulating bone gla protein (BGP), the concentration of urinary markers of bone resorption such as hydroxyproline (Table 10.1) or the retention of a bolus of radioactive technetium (Civitelli *et al.*, 1988). Since technetium retention and bone biopsy analyses are expensive procedures, it appears prudent to utilize urinary markers of bone resorption as an index of bone turnover. If these values are elevated, the physician should anticipate a rapid and progressively favorable response

Table 10.1 Blood bone gla protein (BGP) and urinary hydroxyproline/creatinine (OH-Pr/Cr) in postmenopausal women with high turnover osteoporosis (HTOP) and normal turnover osteoporosis (NTOP). Adapted from Civitelli *et al.* (1988)

	NTOP ($n = 36$)	*HTOP* ($n = 17$)
BGP (ng/ml)	6.46 ± 3.0	11.6 ± 6.2*
OH-Pr/Cr (mg/g)	16.3 ± 5.5	30.44 ± 8.8*

*Values are represented as the mean ± SD; differences between NTOP and HTOP significant at $p < 0.001$.

to calcitonin treatment as also noted for estrogen therapy (Rosen *et al.*, 1997).

Osteoporotic patients treated with calcitonin respond in a variable fashion not unlike those treated with diets enriched with either calcium or estrogens or both (Ettlinger *et al.*, 1987; Rosen *et al.*, 1997). Some osteoporotic patients on daily calcitonin treatment regimens respond within one year with a substantial increase in bone mass and no progressive deteriorating anatomical vertebral changes (Mazzuoli *et al.*, 1986; Civitelli *et al.*, 1988; Avioli, 1996). Others may manifest a delayed skeletal response with a decrease in the annual rate of bone loss but no increments in bone mass demonstrable for 18–24 months (Avioli, 1988; Candona and Pastur, 1997). Subclinical forms of vitamin D deficiency (blood 25-OHD below 10 ng/ml), which are not uncommon in the more elderly female patient (Bouillon *et al.*, 1987; Villareal *et al.*, 1991), may blunt the skeletal response to calcitonin (Avioli, 1988). For this reason a blood specimen for measurement of the vitamin D metabolite, 25-OHD, is obtained before initiating treatment, especially in the more advanced forms of postmenopausal osteoporosis usually seen in elderly female populations. It has been well established that circulating 25-OHD, which is a readily available commercial assay, reflects the state of vitamin D economy in humans (Villareal *et al.*, 1991).

Elderly individuals with what used to be known as a 'Type II' form of osteoporosis are also excellent candidates for calcitonin therapy since, as noted in Table 10.2, they usually have abnormally high blood parathyroid hormone levels (Johnston *et al.*, 1985) which normally accentuate the bone loss of the osteoporotic syndrome. Unlike osteoporosis in the early postmenopausal female (i.e. 'Type I'), which is characterized by a decrease in vertebral trabecular bone and vertebral fractures, osteoporosis of the elderly individual is characterized by a loss of both trabecular and cortical bone and presents clinically with hip fractures as well as fractures of the pelvis, proximal femur and proximal tibia in elderly individuals (Riggs and Melton, 1983). As many physicians have observed in postmenopausal osteoporotic patients on estrogen therapy, there are individuals who do not respond to theory (Rosen *et al.*, 1997) and who will continue to sustain vertebral fractures during the early phase of calcitonin treatment (Avioli, 1988) either because the bone mass has not yet achieved that critical threshold essential to minimize the potential of a traumatic vertebral fracture incident or because the analgesic effects of the medication result in greater mobility and the imposition of increased skeletal stress before the bone mass has increased sufficiently to sustain the insult.

Table 10.2 Circulating calcium and parathyroid hormone (IPTH) levels in patients with type I and type II osteoporosis. Adapted from Johnston *et al.* (1988)

	*'Type I'** *osteoporosis*	*'Type II'** *osteoporosis*
Calcium (mg/dl)	9.5 ± 0.5	8.6 ± 1.0†
IPTH (pg/ml)	550 + 398	852 + 674†

*'Type I' and 'Type II' are no longer considered simple classifications since the osteoporotic syndrome in the postmenopausal female is currently considered a continuous spectrum of various degrees of bone turnover with elevations in circulating IPTH conditioned by levels of vitamin D intake.
† Values are represented as the mean ± SD; differences between 'type I' and 'type II' are significant for calcium ($p < 0.001$) and IPTH ($p < 0.05$).

Although some have noted that alternate day calcitonin therapy is therapeutic (Overgaard *et al.*, 1989a,b; Meunier *et al.*, 1990) this has not been a universal observation (Ellerington *et al.*, 1996). Following ovariectomy, calcitonin is as effective as estrogens in preventing early postmenopausal bone loss (Mazzuoli *et al.*, 1986; MacIntyre *et al.*, 1988; Overgaard *et al.*, 1989b; Meunier *et al.*, 1991). These results are helpful for osteoporotic individuals with established vertebral fracture or others who are either decidedly osteopenic by bone mass analysis or confronted with the need for preventive therapy because of an accumulation of detrimental risk factors such as chronic thyroid hormone (Paul *et al.*, 1988) or glucocorticoid (Adinoff and Hollister, 1983) therapy treatment regimens. Many of these females are uncomfortable with estrogen therapy either because of the requirements for gynecological surveillance which may entail periodic endometrial biopsies (Quigley and Hammond, 1979; Weinstein, 1980; Bergkvist *et al.*, 1989), an increased risk of cancer syndromes (Quigley and Hammond, 1979; Judd *et al.*, 1983; Bergkvist *et al.*, 1989) and/or the simple matter of dealing with the inconvenience of recurrent monthly menstruation. Many females also shy away from estrogen treatment regimens because of contradictions and paradoxical statements often published in feature articles of tabloids, especially those directed primarily toward female populations (Graber and Barber, 1975; Nachtigall and Heilman, 1986; Eagan, 1989).

Physicians are also confronted with the gradual emergence of a specific premenopausal osteoporotic-prone female population for whom estrogen therapy is contraindicated because of a history of metastatic breast cancer. These females have been rendered 'menopausal' prematurely by adjuvant chemotherapy (Warne *et al.*, 1973; Rivkees and Crawford, 1988; Ludwig Breast Cancer Study Group, 1988). Antiestrogen therapeutic regimens such as GnRH agonist or antagonist therapy for polycystic ovarian syndromes or endometriosis can also result in accelerated bone loss in unsuspecting females (Steingold *et al.*, 1986, 1987). The availability of an alternative FDA-approved therapeutic mode such as nasal spray calcitonin, which is not contraindicated in these patients and is also an effective estrogen substitute for suppressing early bone loss in ovarian-deficit states (MacIntyre *et al.*, 1988; Overgaard *et al.*, 1989b; Meunier *et al.*, 1991), should now prove comforting for both the physician and those patients with chemotherapy-induced 'medical' oophorectomy syndromes.

Since vertebral bone mass can be increased by salmon calcitonin therapy, calcitonin treatment regimens should also be considered for young amenorrheic athletic individuals with low bone mineral density (Jones *et al.*, 1990; Joyce *et al.*, 1990; Drinkwater *et al.*, 1990), even after they resume a normal menstrual pattern, since the bone mass is often still well below the normal average for their age many years after resumption of normal menses (Joyce *et al.*, 1990; Drinkwater *et al.*, 1990). Moreover, many amenorrheic athletes shy away from estrogen therapeutic regimens because of unwanted problems of associated weight gain, breast engorgement and/or the resumption of inconvenient monthly menstrual function.

Although the skeletal response to either injectable or nasal spray forms of salmon calcitonin treatment is dose related (Overgaard and Christiansen, 1991; Thamsborg *et al.*, 1991), the analgesic response is not. Osteoporotic patients with skeletal pain should be treated with 50–100 units of salmon calcitonin subcutaneously daily for five days a week. If pain is not a factor, as may be the case in young postmenopausal women or young premenopausal females with 'medical' oophorectomy syndromes, the recommended therapy for injectable forms of the calcitonin is 50 units, thrice weekly. The greatest effect of nasal spray forms is 200 IU daily in women more than five years postmenopausal (Overgaard and Riis, 1994). Beneficial effects have also been obtained using 50 units on alternate days for two weeks of every month (Szucs *et al.*, 1992) or 100 units for 10 consecutive days of each month (Rico *et al.*, 1992). Nasal spray doses of 200–400 IU in the immediate postmenopausal period can decrease vertebral bone loss during the first year of treatment, in addition to decreasing bone turnover (Overgaard, 1994). Intermittent regimens allow the patient to adjust to the subcutaneous treatment regimen gradually and also to realize that self-administration of the drug is neither difficult nor hazardous. However, as noted above, some patients do require daily dosing (Ellerington *et al.*, 1996) for maximal effect. The skeletal response to intermittent or discontinuous calcitonin therapy is usually observed within the first 6–8 months of therapy with significant decreases in vertebral fracture rates noted as early as 24 months (Rico *et al.*, 1992). Patients with high-turnover osteoporotic syndromes characteristically respond much quicker to lower calcitonin dose regimens (Overgaard *et al.*, 1989a, 1990; Overgaard and Christiansen, 1991). Therapy can be interrupted after 18–24 months and the vertebral bone mass followed semiannually with non-invasive techniques which offer a precision greater than 1% (Gutteridge *et al.*, 1984; Mazess *et al.*, 1989; Pacifici *et al.*, 1990). If the bone mass value decreases substantially (greater than 2–3%) or if another risk factor complicates the patient's clinical course, such as the initiation of glucocorticoid or thyroid treatment regimens (Adinoff and Hollister, 1983; Paul *et al.*, 1988), calcitonin therapy should be reinstituted.

As a potent antiosteoclastic drug, calcitonin appears relatively innocuous when compared to the potential hazards of pharmacological doses of bisphosphonates, estrogens, androgens, sodium fluoride or non-steroid anti-inflammatory agents, especially in the elderly postmenopausal osteoporotic women (Wimalawansa, 1993). Nasal spray forms are also more appropriate for the elderly who, because of multidrug regimens, are often unable to follow their prescribed dosages in a rigid fashion, as is essential for some therapies, e.g. the bisphosphonate alendronate. Nausea and mild gastric discomfort characteristically manifest at the initiation of subcutaneous therapy and either decrease in severity or disappear completely during the therapeutic interval. Facial flushing, dermatologic hypersensitivity and local pruritic reactions at injection sites are usually mild. They also tend to disappear with continued administration of the drug. Since salmon calcitonin is a potent inhibitor of free acid production, gastrointestinal side effects such as bloating or mild epigastric fullness can be minimized if the drug is administered 4–5 hours following the evening meal, i.e. preferably at bedtime. Only rarely are urinary frequency and diarrhea encountered with the injectable forms of calcitonin.

As expected, the 'side effects' of therapy are more severe when calcitonin is administered intramuscularly and minimized when given subcutaneously because of the higher peak blood levels achieved following intramuscular injections. Of note is the fact that the side effects observed in the past with injectable forms of calcitonin are allayed considerably when salmon calcitonin is administered by the nasal spray form of the drug (Overgaard *et al.*, 1989a, b, 1990; Montemurro *et al.*, 1991; Wimalawansa, 1993). Considerable experience has also been accumulated for at least 20 years in treating patients with Paget's disease (which characteristically occurs in the elderly) or osteoporotic disorders many of whom were on 'polypharmacy' drug regimens for cardiovascular diseases, gout, diabetes, rheumatoid arthritis and osteoarthritis. The lack of any documented adverse drug interaction report(s) for this relatively older population when treated with calcitonin is also gratifying.

One should not confuse the increments in bone mass observed during calcitonin therapy with changes seen in patients on sodium fluoride regimens, which are still not approved by the United States FDA. Whereas salmon calcitonin increases bone mass in both the vertebrae and long bones of the skeleton, and decreases fracture incidence (Stock *et al.*, 1997), sodium fluoride increases vertebral bone mass with no well-documented change in fracture incidence (Riggs *et al.*, 1990). An associated decrease in the bone mass of the long bones of the extremities has also been observed in some studies (Riggs *et al.*, 1990).

These findings, together with reports of increased incidences of arthralgia and lower extremity 'bone pain', stress fractures, anemia and gastrointestinal bleeding (Mamell *et al.*, 1988; Hedlund and Gallagher, 1989; Riggs *et al.*, 1990) in women receiving sodium fluoride, should lead the physician to be extremely cautious in recommending this form of therapy for osteoporotic patients who are either non responsive to or poor candidates for calcitonin therapy.

REFERENCES

Adinoff, A.D. and Hollister, J.R. (1983) Steroid-induced fractures and bone loss in patients with asthma. *N Engl J Med* **309**: 365–8.

Avioli, L.V. (1988) Rationale for the use of calcitonin in postmenopausal osteoporosis. *Ann Chir Gynaecol* **77**: 224–8.

Avioli, L.V. (1996) Salmon calcitonin nasal spray. *Endocrine* **5**: 115–27.

Bergkvist, L., Adami, H-O., Persson, I. *et al.* (1989) The risk of breast cancer after estrogen and estrogen-progestin replacement. *N Engl J Med* **321**: 293–7.

Bisson, R., Morandi, A. and Vecchnini, L. (1982) Synthetic salmon calcitonin treatment of choice in Sydeck's atrophy disease. *Minerva Ned* **63**: 1065–9.

Body, J.-J.B. and Heath III, H. (1983) Estimates of circulating monomeric calcitonin physiological studies in normal and thyroidectomized man. *J Clin Endocrinol Metab* **57**: 897–903.

Bouillon, R.A., Auwerx, J.H., Lissens, W.D. *et al.* (1987) Vitamin D status in the elderly. Seasonal substrate deficiency causes 1,25 dihydroxy-cholecalciferol deficiency. *Am J Clin Nutrition* **45**: 755–63.

Candona, J.M. and Pastur, E. (1997) Calcitonin vs Etidionate for treatment of postmenopausal osteoporosis: A meta-analysis of published clinical trials. *Osteoporosis Int* **7**: 165–74.

Civitelli, R., Gonnelli, S., Zaccei, F. *et al.* (1988) Bone turnover in postmenopausal osteoporosis. *J Clin Invest* **82**: 1268–74

Drinkwater, B.L., Bruemner, B., Chesnut III, C.H. (1990) Menstrual history as a determinant of current bone density in young athletes. *J Am Med Assoc* **263**: 545–8.

Eagan, A.B. (1989) The estrogen fix. No matter what your age or ailment, someday soon a doctor is going to suggest it. Ms. April pp. 38–43.

Ellerington, H.C., Holland, T.C. and Whitcroft, S.I. (1996) Intranasal salmon calcitonin for the prevention and treatment of postmenopausal osteoporosis. *Calcif Tissue Int* **59**: 675.

Ettinger, B., Genant, H.K. and Cann, C.E. (1987) Postmenopausal bone loss is prevented by treatment with low dosage estrogen with calcium. *Ann Intern Med* **106**: 40–5.

Eufemio, M.A. (1990) Advances in the therapy of osteoporosis. Steroid-induced osteoporosis. *Geriatr Med Today* **9**: 41–56.

Fiore, C.E., Castorina, F., Malatino, L.S. *et al.* (1983) Antalgic activity of calcitonin: effectiveness of the epidermal and subarachnoid routes in man. *Br J Clin Pharmacol Res* **3**: 257–60.

Gennari, C., Chierichetti, S.M., Bigazzi, S. *et al.* (1985) Comparative effects on bone mineral content of calcium and calcium plus salmon calcitonin given in two different regimens in postmenopausal osteoporosis. *Curr Ther Res* **38**: 455–64.

Graber, E.A. and Barber, H.R.K. (1975) The case for and against estrogen therapy. *Am J Nursing* **75**: 1766–70.

Graf, E., Holser, E., Chayen, R. *et al.* (1985) Cortisol and endorphin increase produced by calcitonin administration. *Isr J Med Sci* **21**: 483–4.

Gutteridge, D.H., Nicholson, C.C., Gruber, H.E. *et al.* (1984) A case of severe high-remodeling idiopathic osteoporosis effectively treated with calcitonin. In: *Osteroporosis*, (eds Christiansen, C., Arnaud, C.D. and Nordin, B.E.C.), Aalborg Stiftsbogtrykkeri, Copenhagen, pp. 531–3.

Heath III, H. and Sizemore, G.W. (1977) Plasma calcitonin in normal man. Differences between men and women. *J Clin Invest* **60**: 1135.

Hedlund, L.R. and Gallagher, J.C. (1989) Increased incidence of hip fracture in osteoporotic women treated with sodium fluoride. *J Bone Miner Res* **4**: 223–5.

Herzberg, L. and Bayless, E. (1980) Spinal-cord syndrome due to non-compressive Paget's disease of bone. A spinal artery steal phenomenon reversible with salmon calcitonin. *Lancet* **ii**: 13–15.

Hindley, A.C., Hill, E.B., Leyland, M.J. *et al.* (1982) A double-blind controlled trial of salmon calcitonin in pain due to malignancy. *Cancer Chemother Pharmacol* **9**: 71–4.

Johnston, C.C., Norton, J., Khairi, M.R.A. *et al.*

(1985) Heterogeneity of fracture syndromes in postmenopausal women. *J Clin Endocrinol Metab* **61**: 551–6.

Jones, K.P., Ravnikar, V.A., Tulchinsky, D. *et al.* (1990) Comparison of bone density in amenorrheic women due to athletics, weight loss, and premature menopause. *Obstet Gynecol* **66**: 5–8.

Joyce, J.M., Warren, D.L., Humphries, L.L. *et al.* (1990) Osteoporosis in women with eating disorders: comparison of physical parameters, exercise, and menstrual status with SPA and DPA evaluation. *J Nucl Med* **31**: 325–31.

Judd, H.L., Meldrum, D.R., Deftos, L.J. *et al.* (1983) Estrogen replacement therapy: indications and complications. *Ann Intern Med* **98**: 195–205.

Ludwig Breast Cancer Study Group (1988) Combination adjuvant chemotherapy for node-positive breast cancer. Inadequacy of a single perioperative cycle. *N Engl J Med* **319**: 677–83.

Luengo, M., Picado, C., Del Rio, L. *et al.* (1990) Treatment of steroid-induced osteopenia with calcitonin in corticosteroid-dependent asthma. *Am Rev Respir Dis* **142**: 104–7.

Lyritis, G.P., Tsakalakos, S., Magiasis, B *et al.* (1991) Analgesic effect of salmon calcitonin in osteoporotic vertebral fractures. Double-blind placebo-controlled study. *Calcif Tissue Int* **49**: 369–72.

MacIntyre, I., Whitehead, M.I., Banks, L.M. *et al.* (1988) Calcitonin for prevention of postmenopausal bone loss. *Lancet* **i**: 900–1.

Mamell, N., Meunier, P.J., Dusan, R., *et al.* (1988) Risk benefit ratio of sodium fluoride treatment in primary vertebral osteoporosis. *Lancet* **ii**: 361–5.

Mazess, R.B., Gallagher, J.C., Notelovitz, M. *et al.* (1989) Monitoring skeletal response to estrogen. *Am J Obstet Gynecol* **161**: 843–8.

Mazzuoli, G.F., Passeri, M., Gennari, C. *et al.* (1986) Effects of salmon calcitonin in postmenopausal osteoporosis: a controlled double-blind clinical study. *Calcif Tissue Int* **38**: 3–8.

Meunier, P.J., Delmas, P.D., Chaumet-Riffand, P.D. *et al.* (1991) Intranasal salmon calcitonin for prevention of postmenopausal bone loss. In: *Osteoporosis 1990*, (eds Christiansen, C. and Overgaard, K.), Osteopress, Copenhagen, pp. 1861–7.

Minaire, P., Meunier, P., Depassio, J. *et al.* (1984) Treatment of acute osteoporosis due to paraplegia with salmon calcitonin. *Horm Res* **20**: 88.

Montemurro, L., Schiraldi, G., Fraioli, P. *et al.* (1991) Prevention of corticosteroid-induced osteoporosis with salmon calcitonin in sarcoid patients. *Calcif Tissue Int* **49**: 71–6.

Nachtigall, L. and Heilman, J.R. (1986) Estrogen: the facts can change your life. Redbook September, pp. 17–22.

Nagant de Deuxchaisnes, C., (1983) Calcitonin in the treatment of Paget's disease. *Triangle* **22**: 103–28.

Nagant de Deuxchaisnes, C., Rombout-Lindemans, C., Huaux, J.P. *et al.* (1977) Roentgenologic evaluation of the efficacy of calcitonin in Paget's disease of bone. In: *Molecular Endocrinology*, (eds MacIntyre, I. and Szelke, M.), Elsevier/North Holland Biomedical Press, Amsterdam, pp. 213–33.

Overgaard K. (1994) Effect of intranasal salmon calcitonin therapy on bone mass and bone turnover in early postmenopausal women: a dose-response study. *Calcif Tissue Int* **55**: 82–6.

Overgaard K. and Christiansen, C. (1991) Long-term treatment of established osteoporosis with intranasal calcitonin. *Calcif Tissue Int* (suppl) **49**: S60–S63.

Overgaard, K. and Riis, B.J. (1994) Nasal salmon calcitonin in osteoporosis. *Calcif Tissue Int* **55**: 79–81.

Overgaard, K., Riis, B.J., Christiansen, C. *et al.* (1989a) Effect of calcitonin given intranasally on early postmenopausal bone loss. *Br Med J* **299**: 477–9.

Overgaard, K., Riis, B.J., Christiansen, C. *et al.* (1989b) Nasal calcitonin for treatment of established osteoporosis. *Clin Endrocinol* **30**: 435–42.

Overgaard, K., Hansen, M.A., Nelsen, V-A.H. *et al.* (1990) Discontinuous calcitonin treatment of established osteoporosis. Effects of withdrawal of treatment. *Am J Med* **102**: 319–24.

Overgaard, K. Hansen, N.H., Jensen, S.B. and Christiansen, C. (1992) Effect of salcalcitonin given intranasally on bone mass and fracture rates in osteoporosis. *Br Med J* **305**: 556–61.

Pacifici, R., Rupich, R., Griffin, M. *et al.* (1990) Dual energy radiography versus quantitative computer tomography for the diagnosis of osteoporosis. *J Clin Endocrinol Metab* **70**: 705–10.

Paul, T.L., Kerrigan, J., Kelly, A.M. *et al.* (1988) Long-term L-thyroxine therapy is associated with decreased hip bone density in premenopausal women. *J Am Med Assoc* **259**: 3137–41.

Quigley, M.M. and Hammond, C.B. (1979) Estrogen-replacement therapy – help or hazard? *N Engl J Med* **301**: 646–8.

Ravichandran, G. (1981) Spinal cord function in Paget's disease of the spine. *Paraplegia* **19**: 7–12.

Reginster, J.Y., Deroisy, R., Albert, A. *et al.* (1989) Relationship between whole plasma calcitonin levels, calcitonin secretory capacity and plasma levels of estrone in healthy women and post-menopausal osteoporosis. *J Clin Invest* **83**: 1073.

Rico, H., Hernandez, E.R., Diaz-Mediavilla, J. *et al.* (1990) Treatment of multiple myeloma with nasal spray calcitonin: a histomorphometric and biochemical study. *Bone Mineral* **8**: 231–7.

Rico, H., Hernandez, E.R., Revilla, M. *et al.* (1992) Salmon calcitonin reduces vertebral fracture rate in the postmenopausal crush fracture syndrome. *Bone Mineral* **16**: 131–8.

Riggs, B.L. and Melton III, L.J. (1983) Hetero-geneity of involutional osteoporosis: evidence for two osteoporosis syndromes. *Am J Med* **75**: 899–903.

Riggs, B.L., Hodgson, S.F. and O'Fallon, W.M. (1990) Effect of fluoride treatment on the fracture rate in postmenopausal women with osteoporosis. *N Engl J Med* **322**: 802–9.

Rivkees, S.A. and Crawford, J.D. (1988) The relationship of gonadal activity and chemotherapy-induced gonadal damage. *J Am Med Assoc* **259**: 2123–6.

Rosen, C.J., Chestnut, C.H., III and Mallinak, N.J.S. (1997) Predictive value of biochemical markers of bone turnover for bone mineral density in early postmenopausal women treated with hormone replacement or calcium supplementation. *J Clin Endocrinol Metab* **82**: 1904–10.

Samaa, M., Linthicum Jr, F.H., House, H.P. *et al.* (1986) Calcitonin as treatment in hearing loss in Paget's disease. *Am J Otol* **7**: 241–2.

Steingold, K.A., Judd, H.L., Nieberg, R.K. *et al.* (1986) Treatment of severe androgen excess due to ovarian hyperthecosis with a long-acting gonadotropin-releasing hormone agonist. *Am J Obstet Gynecol* **154**: 1241–8.

Steingold, K.A., de Ziegler, D., Cedars, M. *et al.* (1987) Clinical and hormonal effects of chronic gonadotropin-releasing hormone agonist treatment in polycystic ovarian disease. *J Clin Endocrinol Metab* **65**: 773–8.

Stock, J.L., Avioli, L.V., Baglink, D.J. *et al.* (1997) Calcitonin nasal spray reduces incidence of new vertebrae fracture in postmenopausal women. Three year interim results of study. *J Bone Miner Res* **12**: S149.

Szucs, J., Horvath, C., Kollin, E. *et al.* (1992) Three-year calcitonin combination therapy for post-menopausal osteoporosis with crush fractures of the spine. *Calcif Tissue Int* **50**: 7–10.

Thamsborg, G., Storm, T.L., Sykulski, R. *et al.* (1991) Effect of different doses of nasal salmon calcitonin on bone mass. *Calcif Tisue Int* **48**: 302.

Villareal, D.T., Civitelli, R., Avioli, L.V. *et al.* (1991) Subclinical vitamin D deficiency in post-menopausal women with decreased bone mass. *J Clin Endocrinol Metab* **72**: 628–34.

Warne, G.L., Fairley, K.F., Hobbs, J.B. *et al.* (1973) Cyclophosphamide-induced ovarian failure. *N Engl J Med* **289**: 1159–62.

Weinstein, M.C. (1980) Estrogen use in post-menopausal women – costs, risks, and benefits. *N Engl J Med* **303**: 308–16.

Wimalawansa, S.J. (1993) Long- and short-term side effects and safety of calcitonin in man: a prospective study. *Calcif Tissue Int* **52**: 90–3.

Whyte, M.P., Bergfeld, M.A., Murphy, W.A. *et al.* (1982) Postmenopausal osteoporosis. A heterogeneous disorder as assessed by histomorphometric analysis of iliac crest bone from untreated patients. *Am J Med* **72**: 193–202.

Woodhouse, N.J., Chalmers, A.H., Wells, I.P. *et al.* (1977) Paget's disease. Radiological changes occurring in untreated patients and those on salmon calcitonin therapy during two years' observation. *Br J Radiol* **50**: 699–705.

Zseli, J., Szucs, J., Steczek, K. *et al.* (1985) Decreased calcitonin reserve in accelerated post-menopausal osteoporosis. *Horm Metab Res* **17**: 696–7.

REQUIREMENTS FOR CALCIUM AND ITS USE IN THE MANAGEMENT OF OSTEOPOROSIS

11

J.A. Kanis

INTRODUCTION

There is a great deal of uncertainty concerning the requirements of calcium for skeletal health. Bone is the major reservoir for calcium, accounting for 99% of total body calcium. The skeleton contains about 25 g of elemental calcium at birth and this increases 40-fold by the time skeletal maturity is reached. Skeletal losses of calcium occur in the elderly and particularly in women in the years following the menopause. Indeed, women with hip fracture may have lost 50% of total body calcium. Indices of calcium metabolism have been available since the 1920s in the form of the metabolic balance and since the 1960s have been gradually replaced by densitometric techniques. Both measure calcium and because of the large shifts in calcium balance during life, this has led to the widespread view that calcium nutrition is of critical importance for the maintenance of skeletal health in the general population and particularly so in the osteoporotic population. Had these techniques measured phosphorus, magnesium or another bone constituent, our views on the role of calcium might have differed.

With respect to those involved in the world of calcium nutrition, they can be divided reasonably accurately into the evangelists and the nihilists. The evangelists will argue that:

- a higher than average dietary intake of calcium is important for building bone during growth. The term 'calciyummy' used to advertise cheese in the UK and the attempt to market high-calcium milk in the UK and cola in the US reinforce the view that mothers are negligent if they fail to appreciate the point;
- a higher than average intake of calcium is important to maintain skeletal mass at maturity. Thus, in women a high dietary intake during adult life is good insurance against the subsequent ravages of the menopause;
- a higher than average intake of calcium is important in women after the menopause because it prevents osteoporosis. Indeed, the evangelists view calcium as 'bone friendly', whereas other agents, including some bone-active drugs, are not (National Osteoporosis Society newsletter);
- a higher than average intake is important in all patients with osteoporosis since it decreases the risk of fractures. Indeed, it is no longer considered ethical not to provide calcium supplementation to the diet of patients with fractures (Ettinger *et al.*, 1987).

Osteoporosis. Edited by John C. Stevenson and Robert Lindsay. Published in 1998 by Chapman & Hall, London.
ISBN 0 412 48870 1

The nihilists, of course, argue the converse. What is of interest is that the same evidence is often cited to support both views. It is therefore the interpretation of the data which differs. This chapter reviews the reasons for these differences and the manner in which they arose. In so doing, it separates the considerations outlined above since the data and arguments relating to growth, for example, differ from those pertaining to the therapeutic use of calcium. The chapter draws heavily on earlier reviews by the author (Kanis and Passmore, 1989, 1990; Kanis, 1991, 1994) and the reader is referred elsewhere for views with a somewhat different perspective (Robinson, 1987; Barrett-Connor, 1989; Francis, 1989; Heaney, 1990; Nordin and Heaney, 1990; Anderson, 1990; National Osteoporosis Society, 1990; Schaafsma, 1992).

HISTORICAL PERSPECTIVE

We are all products of our heritage and it is of interest to examine the way in which concepts of the importance of calcium nutrition have arisen. Influential American textbooks in the 1920s encouraged the idea that calcium deficiency was common and that the ordinary dietary intake of calcium of the average American was 'a sorry spectacle' (Lusk, 1917). This conclusion arose from a paper by Tigerstedt (1911) who reported high dietary intakes of calcium in Finland. There was, however, no evidence provided that the Americans were disadvantaged in this respect. Biblical tradition would, however, have informed an American readership that milk was a desirable food (*Exodus* 3, 8).

Up until the 1950s influential textbooks perpetuated the view that the diet of both Americans and Europeans was 'more deficient in calcium than in other chemical elements' (Sherman, 1937). The conclusion was based, however, on more secure experimental observations (Sherman, 1920), which reported that the average daily requirement of young men was 450 mg and ranged from 270 to 829 mg. An analysis of diets in 225 typical Americans showed that one in six contained less than the indicated requirement of calcium. The requirement was calculated as the sum of the calcium balance and the dietary intake after abrupt changes in diet over a 3–8-day period. It was assumed, therefore, that in subjects with a negative balance for calcium, the addition of the apparent requirement of calcium to the diet would restore the balance. This implies that the intestinal absorption of the extra calcium would have been 100% – a notion which we now know to be false. This fallacy is illustrated by a significant relationship between dietary intake and 'requirements' for calcium calculated in this way (Kanis and Passmore, 1989) – the higher the calcium intake, the greater the apparent requirement, a view that even the evangelists might not consider reasonable.

By 1937 it was appreciated that not all the calcium in the diet was absorbed (Leitch, 1937; Kinsman *et al.*, 1939; Steggerda and Mitchell, 1946). This led to new approaches to determine the calcium requirements in man. The first was to examine the relationship between dietary intake and metabolic balance in populations. Mitchell (1939) found that men given a low-calcium diet lost calcium, whereas those with higher intakes did not. The intercept to a balance of zero was 9.7 mg of calcium/kg/day, which is equivalent to a daily requirement of 570 mg (range 245–760 mg), an advance on the figures of Sherman (1920).

A second approach was to study subjects on a low-calcium diet and to supplement the dietary calcium until balance was obtained (Leitch, 1937). This led to calculations of requirement based on the fractional absorption of calcium. Not surprisingly, the calculations increased the apparent requirement which in young adults were 662 mg daily (range 500–1000 mg; Outhouse *et al.*, 1941).

A third approach was to examine the relationship between dietary intake and total output (faecal and urinary) in subjects over a range of manipulated dietary intakes (Leitch, 1937). Women were always in negative balance below an intake of 135 mg daily and had an even chance of being in balance with an intake of 550 mg. By extrapolation, no women would be in negative balance with an intake of 1600 mg daily, yet another advance on the figures of Sherman.

All these studies therefore promoted the view that a high dietary intake of calcium was needed, but in many of these studies the dietary intake of calcium differed from that normally taken. It was therefore assumed that a decrease in calcium balance resulting from a decrease in dietary intake would be perpetuated indefinitely, a view which we now know to be wrong. The phenomenon of adaptation was appreciated as early as 1939 (Clark, 1926; Nichols and Nimalesuriya, 1939). It is ironic that even Sherman intuitively understood this when he stated that 'only those (balance) experiments in which there was a reasonably close approach to equilibrium of lime can be taken as indicating the lime requirement', but it had been forgotten by 1920. Nevertheless, the work of Sherman and his colleagues led American enthusiasts in the 1930s to advocate the drinking of a litre or more of milk daily to ensure an adequate intake of calcium.

Not surprisingly, in 1943 the United States Food and Nutrition Board set the allowance of calcium at 1000 mg (Food and Nutrition Board, 1943). Subsequent recommendations have hovered around this figure. The Consensus Conferences sponsored by the National Institutes of Health in 1984 and 1994 supported the dietary intake of calcium of 1000 mg for premenopausal women, but said that postmenopausal women who are not treated with oestrogen require about 1500 mg daily (National Institutes of Health, 1984, 1994). The recommendation was made largely on the basis of balance experiments.

Enthusiasm for calcium nutrition waned in the 1940s and 1950s when Albright proposed that osteoporosis was related to a defect in the formation of collagen matrix (Albright *et al.*, 1940), but a revival followed shortly afterwards (Whedon, 1959; Nordin, 1960; Harrison *et al.*, 1961), again based on balance studies, and since then has never gone away.

The flaws in interpreting early balance studies were appreciated as long ago as 1962 when the Food and Agricultural Organization and WHO Committee stated that high intakes of calcium were unnecessary and suggested a 'practical allowance' for adults of 400–500 mg daily (FAO, 1962). Several countries follow these recommendations whereas others follow the lead of or even outdo the United States (Truswell *et al.*, 1983).

We are left, therefore, with the recommendations of many authoritative bodies indicating a threefold difference in requirements between countries (Figure 11.1). The question arises whether these disparate views on calcium nutrition are based on a heritage littered with false assumptions or whether new evidence has emerged indicating the requirement for calcium to maintain skeletal health. An appreciation of adult bone biology is a useful starting point from which to address this issue.

BONE REMODELLING

In adults in whom longitudinal growth has ceased, much of the skeletal turnover (greater than 95%) is accounted for by remodelling of bone. The remodelling process comprises a series of discrete events well characterized morphologically but physiologically ill understood (Parfitt, 1983). The process is important for the self-repair of skeletal tissue and when remodelling is inhibited this gives rise to spontaneous fracture, presumably related to the inability of the skeleton to repair fatigue damage (Frost, 1960).

In the adult, bone comprises cortical (or compact) tissue and trabecular (or cancellous) bone. Approximately three-quarters of the skeleton is accounted for by cortical bone and the remainder by cancellous bone. Although

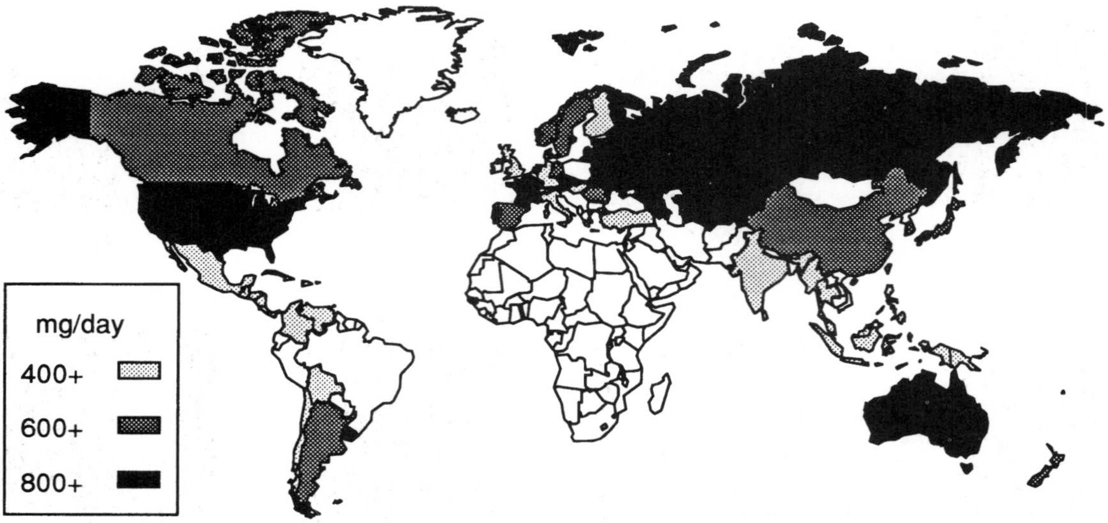

Figure 11.1 Recommended dietary allowances for calcium around the world.

cancellous bone accounts for a minority of skeletal mass, its surface-to-volume ratio is much higher than that of cortical bone. Since bone remodelling is a surface-based event, this means that the metabolic activity of cancellous bone is 10 times greater than that at cortical sites. The remodelling cascade (Figure 11.2) is a highly ordered sequence of cellular events comprising a resorption phase whereby old bone is removed, followed by the process of bone formation and mineralization. The phases of osteoclast activation and osteoclastic bone resorption result in the formation of a erosion (resorption) cavity. Mononuclear cells are found deep within the resorption bays and this is presumed to represent a later event in the resorption sequence (Baron *et al.*, 1983). These cells may be responsible for the signals that ultimately attract osteoblasts to the sites of previous resorption. The attraction of osteoblasts to sites of previous resorption is a phenomenon termed 'coupling' (Kanis, 1985). Coupling ensures that osteoblasts are attracted almost exclusively to sites of previous resorption. Osteoblasts thereafter synthesize an uncalcified osteoid matrix which undergoes mineralization several days later.

In the healthy adult who is neither gaining nor losing bone, the rate of bone resorption must equal the rate of new matrix formation and mineralization. Approximately 5 mmol of calcium is resorbed from bone daily and this is matched by an equal amount deposited during bone formation. Thus, the net flux of calcium from bone to the extracellular fluid attributable to bone remodelling is close to zero. At any one time approximately 10–15% of the bone surface is undergoing remodelling, the remaining surface being relatively quiescent.

It is important to recognize that accretion of calcium into bone occurs after matrix production and not before. Thus, the skeletal demands for calcium are governed by the rate of matrix synthesis rather than the other way round. If the skeletal demands for calcium are not met then hypocalcaemia and defective mineralization of bone will follow. Thus, low dietary intakes of calcium induce osteomalacia in mammals (Pettifor *et al.*, 1984) including man (Kooh *et al.*, 1977; Cundy *et al.* 1982). The question arises whether low dietary intakes of

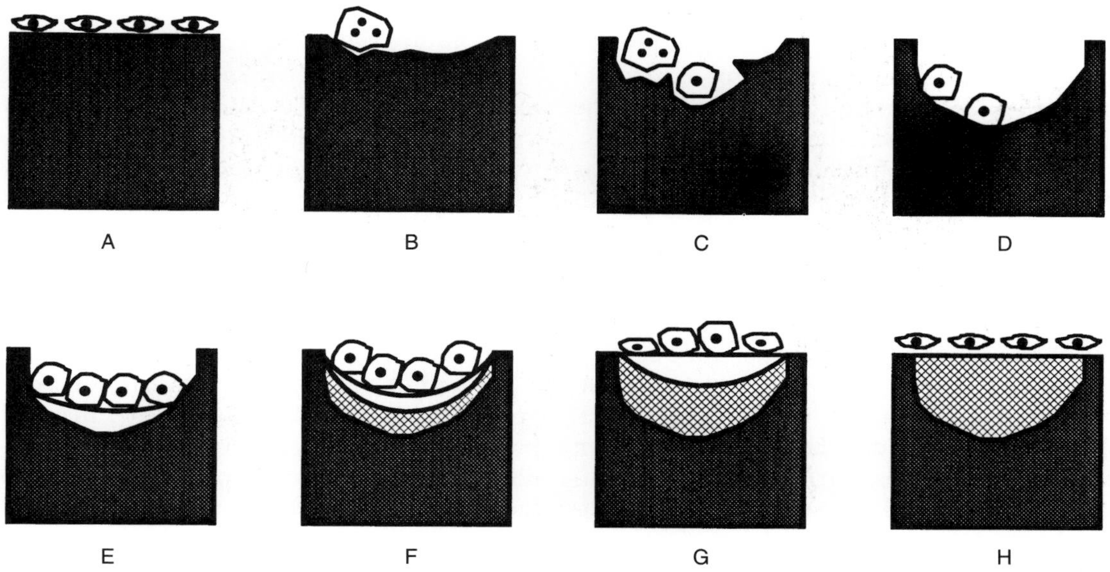

Figure 11.2 Steps in the remodelling sequence of cancellous bone. Early in the remodelling sequence osteoclasts are attracted to a quiescent bone surface (A) and excavate an erosion cavity (B, C). Mononuclear cells smooth off the erosion cavity (D) which is a subsequent site for the attraction of osteoblasts, which synthesize an osteoid matrix (E). Continuous new bone matrix synthesis (F) is followed by calcification (G) of the newly formed bone. When complete, lining cells once more overlie the trabecular surface (H).

calcium might decrease bone matrix synthesis in man. Most evidence suggests that this is not so since calcium supplementation decreases rather than increases the turnover of bone (Parfitt, 1980). This suggests that under normal conditions the skeletal requirements for calcium are governed by the rate of matrix synthesis rather than by the availability of calcium.

It is possible, nevertheless, that severe calcium deficiency might decrease the rate of matrix synthesis in man. In long-standing hypoparathyroidism, hypocalcaemia may result in osteomalacia (Nagant de Deuxchaisnes and Krane, 1978), but bone mass is not characteristically reduced. This is not, however, an adequate model of calcium deficiency since, although serum concentrations and intestinal absorption of calcium are low, so too is the rate of bone remodelling. In growing animals severe privation of dietary calcium does give rise to osteoporosis (Kalu and Masoro, 1990) but the relevance of these observations to the more modest variations of dietary intake in infancy, adolescence and young adulthood is not known.

BONE REMODELLING AND SKELETAL MASS

In health, as well as in a number of metabolic bone disorders, there is a close quantitative relationship between the amount of bone formed and that lost by bone resorption. For example, in Paget's disease, where bone remodelling may be augmented by as much as 10-fold, skeletal balance is usually close to zero, indicating that the high rates of bone resorption are accompanied by equally high rates of bone formation. In many metabolic bone disorders, including postmenopausal osteoporosis, accelerated rates of bone resorption are due to an increased activation rate of osteoclastic bone resorption, so that at any one time more bone remodelling units are extant on bone surfaces and a proportionately greater surface of bone is occupied by all the phases of bone remodelling.

An increase in the turnover of bone has several consequences. Since the process of bone remodelling implies a net deficit of bone (until resorption cavities are completely infilled), the skeletal volume missing at any one time will increase proportionately according to the number of functional bone-remodelling units (Figure 11.3). This skeletal deficit, termed the 'resorption space', is approximately 0.76% of total body calcium. From these considerations, Parfitt (1983) has calculated that a fivefold increase in bone turnover would produce a negative balance of 30 g or a decrease in total body bone volume of 3% under steady-state conditions.

A further consequence of increased skeletal remodelling relates to the turnover time of the skeleton. The amount of calcium normally removed by bone resorption is 250 mg daily from a total body calcium of 1 kg. Thus, for the whole skeleton the average turnover time is 11 years or 9% per annum. It is, however, much more rapid in cancellous bone than at cortical sites due to the higher surface activity of the former. If bone turnover is accelerated a proportionately greater amount of bone volume is occupied by young rather than old bone. In this regard, it is important to recognize that mineralization proceeds for many months after the completion of the bone-remodelling sequence. Thus, the proportion

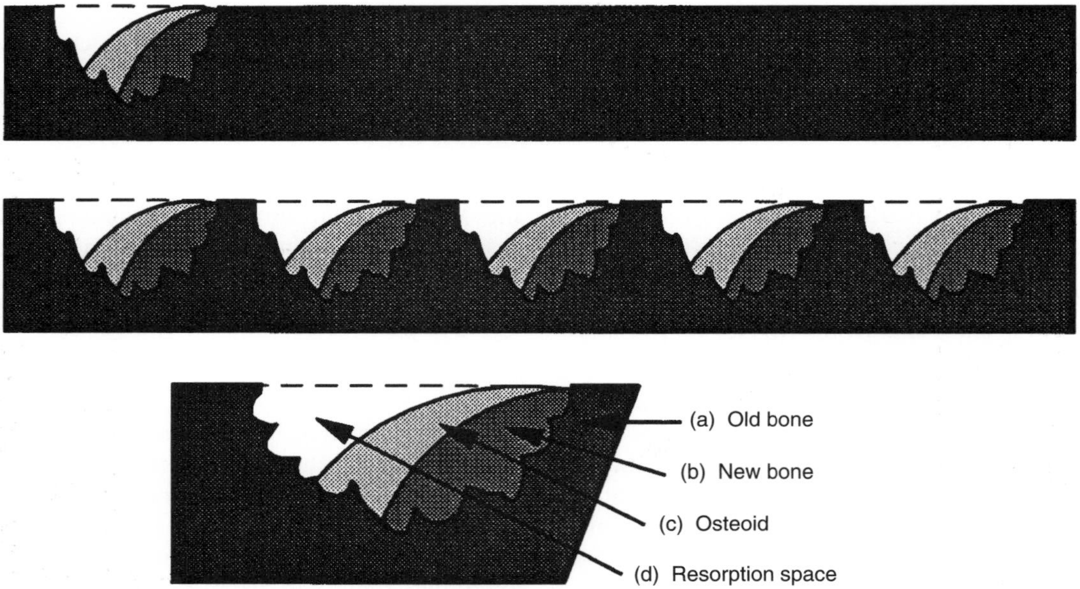

Figure 11.3 The effect of bone turnover on bone and calcium balance. The upper panel depicts normal bone-remodelling activity occurring on 15% of the trabecular surface. The resorption space (d) occupies 2% of the bone volume and a somewhat smaller amount is occupied by osteoid (1.5%) accounting for 3.5% of the bone volume. When bone turnover is increased fivefold (without affecting the balance between formation and resorption), the resorption space and osteoid space increase to 17.5% of bone volume. In addition, new bone formed at each site is not completely mineralized, increasing the mineral deficit so that trabecular density is increased by 20%.

of immature and incompletely mineralized bone will increase when turnover is increased and result in a decrease in bone mineral content.

A third consequence of increased remodelling is that the osteoid in the incompletely formed bone-remodelling units is not mineralized (see Figure 11.3). Thus, the calcium space exceeds the resorption space by a small but fixed proportion.

For these three reasons the mineral content of bone may be profoundly influenced by changes in bone turnover. In the cancellous bone of the ilium, a fivefold increase in turnover would decrease the actual bone volume by 20% and the mineral content by nearly double. This process is entirely reversible when bone turnover is decreased. The effects of changes in cortical bone turnover are less, but still significant so that a twofold increase in turnover at all skeletal sites would decrease bone mineral content by 1.5% (15 g) over the subsequent 2–3 years (Figure 11.4).

TRANSIENT AND STEADY STATES WITH RESPECT TO CALCIUM NUTRITION

In the healthy adult who is calcium deprived in the diet, the turnover of bone is increased due to an increase in the activation frequency of new bone-remodelling units. Conversely, when presented with high-calcium challenges, bone remodelling is decreased. A great deal of circumstantial evidence suggests that the mechanism for this relates to hormonal changes in calcium metabolism. Thus, during calcium depletion serum calcium tends to fall, which stimulates the secretion of parathyroid hormone and the synthesis of calcitriol. Parathyroid hormone

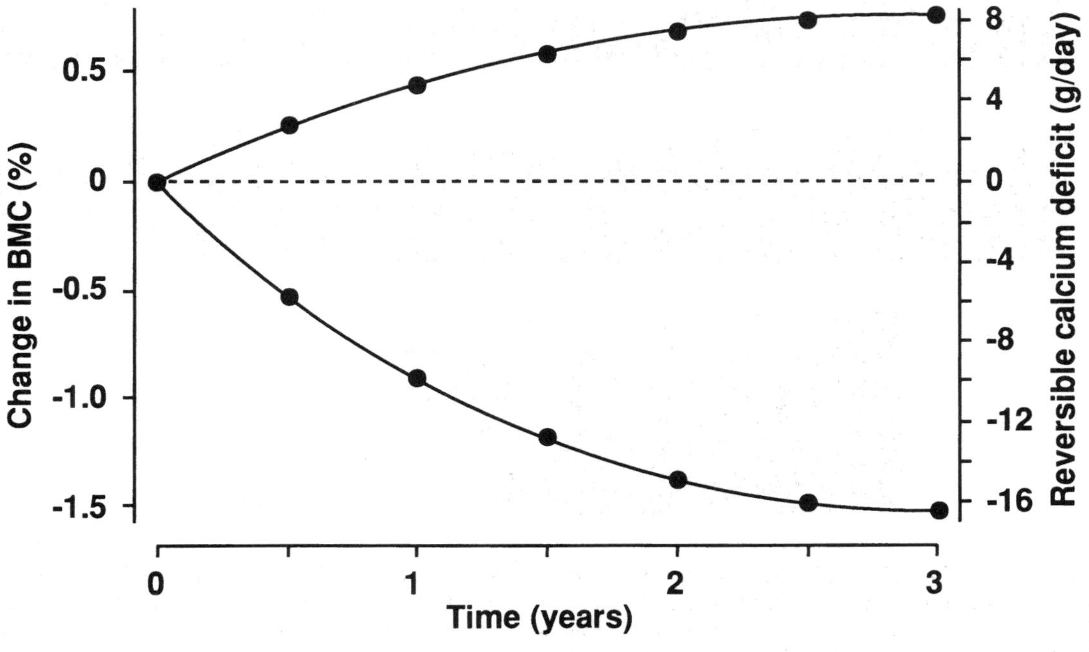

Figure 11.4 The anticipated effects of doubling or halving bone remodelling in a young healthy adult on bone mineral content and on reversible calcium deficit. The reversible skeletal deficit of calcium due to changes in bone remodelling is based on a total body calcium of 1000 g.

(PTH) may be the hormone responsible for the increased activation of bone remodelling. For the reasons outlined above, it would be expected that a substantial decrease in calcium intake would be associated with a finite but reversible deficit in bone mineral content. Conversely, an increased intake of calcium would increase the net intestinal absorption of calcium. The small rise in plasma calcium reduces secretion of PTH (and may increase that of calcitonin) (Nordin and Marshall, 1988) and thus the rate of bone turnover, giving rise to a small but finite increase in reversible bone mass. The reduction in PTH secretion would be expected to reduce the synthesis of calcitriol and offset to some extent the dietary calcium challenge.

For reasons related to the turnover time of bone (Parfitt, 1980; Kanis, 1984) these changes in bone mineral content may take several years to be complete. It would be expected, therefore, that the balance for calcium (intake minus total urinary, faecal and dermal excretion) would be negative for several years after a reduction in intake before the new equilibrium was attained (see Figure 11.4). Elegant studies undertaken by Malm (1958) in healthy prisoners given a low-calcium diet showed that calcium balance did indeed decrease. Over the ensuing years the balance for calcium became less negative. It is relevant to note that after a change in dietary calcium Malm's prisoners had not reached a new steady state of calcium balance, even after a year or more of follow-up (Figure 11.5; Kanis and Passmore, 1990). This clearly indicates that it may take several years for a new steady state to be achieved.

The question arises whether in health, particularly during growth, these adaptive mechanisms are adequate. A failure to adapt adequately to a low dietary calcium would decrease the availability of calcium for the mineralization of bone.

Some perspective of the problem can be gained by examining the amount of calcium that must be retained for normal skeletal growth (Figure 11.6). Peak requirements occur during the first month of life and during the adolescent growth spurt when up to 400 mg of calcium may be retained each day. At other times, retention is much lower, less than 100 mg daily and less than 20 mg after the age of 20 years. Minimum skeletal requirements for calcium are dictated by these factors, but actual requirements depend upon the amount in the diet, the efficiency of absorption and the obligatory losses in the urine, faeces and sweat. The efficiency with which the body must retain calcium to cope with skeletal demands throughout growth may be computed for any dietary load and may vary from 5% to 80%. Children and young adults are usually capable of such adaptation (Kanis and Passmore, 1989).

These considerations suggest that changes in calcium nutrition during growth or in young adult women are associated with changes in bone remodelling and a small but reversible change in bone mineral content is

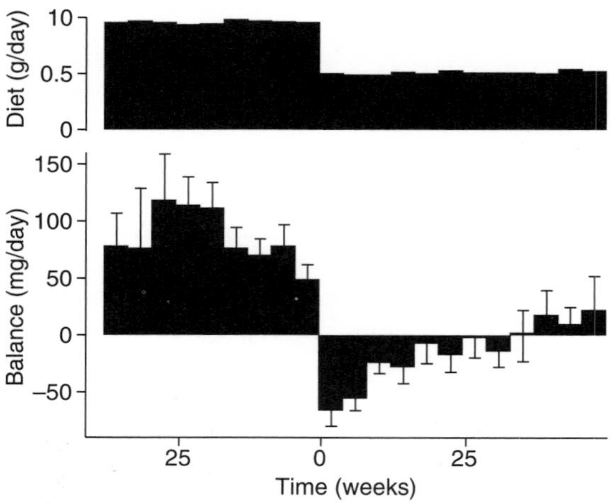

Figure 11.5 Mean (SEM) dietary calcium and calcium balance in healthy prisoners. Dietary calcium intake was decreased at time zero when calcium balance became negative. Note the slow attenuation of negative calcium balance thereafter. Data calculated from Malm (1958) from Kanis and Passmore (1989).

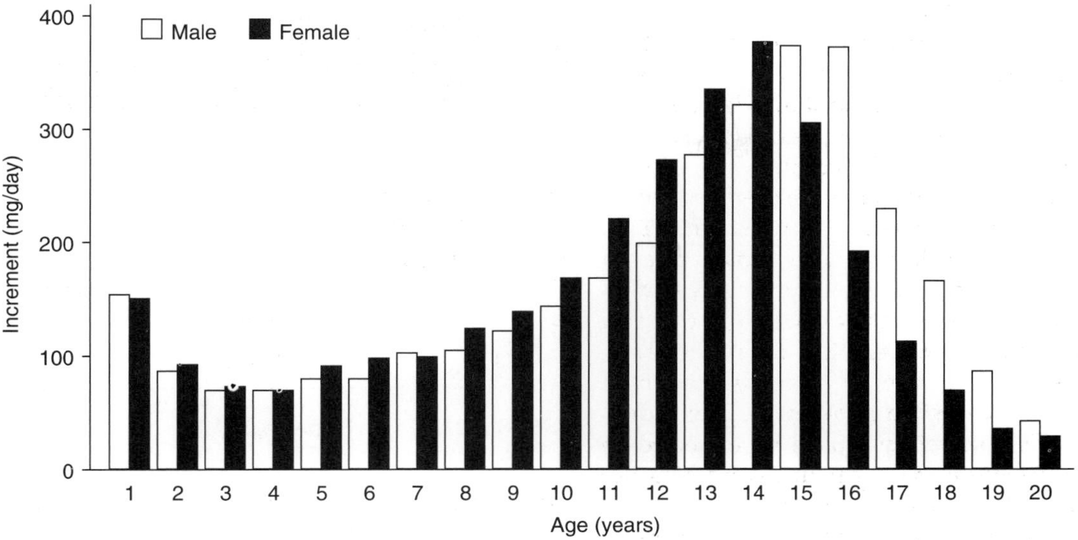

Figure 11.6 Estimated daily skeletal gains of calcium in men and women during growth. Data from Leitch (1937).

of no clinical significance. Where, then, is the evidence that the requirement of calcium in healthy adults is 10–50 times greater than the net skeletal gains of calcium at this age? The evidence for a high requirement and its computation comes from epidemiological and balance studies.

REQUIREMENTS FOR CALCIUM IN YOUNG HEALTHY WOMEN

A variety of epidemiological studies show an association between the lifetime intake of calcium and either bone density or the risk of fracture in women (Nordin, 1966; Kamiyama *et al.*, 1972; Matkovic *et al.*, 1979; Anderson and Tylavsky, 1984; Sandler *et al.*, 1985; Yano *et al.*, 1985; Holbrook *et al.*, 1988; Kanders *et al.*, 1988; Hansen *et al.*, 1991). On the other hand, it should be recognized that many studies show no such association over a range of dietary intakes (Smith and Frame, 1965; Smith and Rizek, 1966; Hegsted, 1967; Garn *et al.*, 1969; Donath *et al.*, 1975; Nilas *et al.*, 1984; Riggs *et al.*, 1987; Cooper *et al.*, 1988; Stevenson *et al.*, 1988, 1989; Wickham *et al.*, 1989; van Beresteijn *et al.*, 1990). Which are we to believe? Is it right to ignore that half of the data which fails to satisfy a particular hypothesis (Nordin and Heaney, 1990)?

We must be suspicious of both conclusions and examine the possible biases. A starting point is to ask what other nutritional differences there were between or within populations. This is not straightforward since most of the studies omit this aspect from their enquiry. It is perhaps ironic that the most cited and complete information available is that from Matkovic *et al.* (1979) showing a relationship between calcium intake, bone mass and fracture from two communities in Yugoslavia. One community had a substantially higher calcium intake, greater bone mass and fewer femoral fractures. Clearly shown in the paper but not commented on by the authors was the finding that where the calcium intake was higher, the energy intake was also higher (Table 11.1). It is of importance in this regard that the mean body weight in the two communities was identical.

Table 11.1 Nutritional and energy intake (mean ± SD) in women from two Yugoslavian communities (100 for each group). Note the significant increase in energy intake in women taking the higher calcium diets despite the similarity in body weight. Data computed from Matkovic *et al.* (1979)

	A *High dietary calcium*	*B* *Low dietary calcium*	*A/B*	*p<*
Calcium				
(mg/day)	876 ± 280	395 ± 276	2.22	0.001
Protein				
(g/day)	84.4 ± 19.5	56.9 ± 16.5	1.48	0.001
(kcal/day)	346 ± 80	233 ± 68	1.48	0.001
Fat				
(g/day)	92.6 ± 23.5	59.8 ± 21.2	1.55	0.001
(kcal/day)	861 ± 219	556 ± 197	1.55	0.001
Carbohydrate				
(g/day)	327 ± 71	345 ± 80	0.95	NS
(kcal/day)	1341 ± 291	1415 ± 328	0.95	NS
Body weight				
(kg)	68.8 ± 6.0	68.8 ± 6.0	1.00	NS
Total energy				
(kcal/day)	2548 ± 539	2204 ± 389	1.02	0.02
Waking energy expenditure				
(kcal/day)	2086 ± 539	1742 ± 389	1.20	0.02

Lower energy intake in populations with similar body weight indicates less physical activity and diminished activity is a well-recognized factor affecting skeletal mass (Chalmers and Ho, 1970; Smith and Raab, 1986; Cooper *et al.*, 1988). The data suggest that energy expenditure was 20% greater (assuming no difference in basal metabolic rate) between the communities in those patients with the higher dietary intakes for calcium. This increase in energy expenditure is equivalent to the activities of a blacksmith or a stone mason for one hour daily or to a daily three-mile walk.

A few studies have taken activity or energy expenditure into account and have shown a significant and independent relationship of calcium intake with bone density (Anderson and Tylavsky, 1984; Kanders *et al.*, 1988; Kelly *et al.*, 1990; Murphy *et al.*, 1994). Although these studies are necessarily limited by their cross-sectional nature, it is of interest that the differences in skeletal mass between high and low intakes of calcium are trivial and readily accounted for by differences in the reversible calcium space (Figure 11.7).

Studies between communities have not been very helpful. If calcium intake were important for peak bone density we would expect population studies to show differences in bone mass between communities with different intakes of calcium. Studies in the United States, Denmark, Central America and Switzerland show that this is not so (Smith and Frame, 1965; Smith and Rizek, 1966; Hegsted, 1967; Garn *et al.*, 1969; Donath *et al.*, 1975; Nilas *et al.*, 1984). Thus, the effect of genetic and environmental factors on bone mass may be greater than that of dietary calcium (Garn *et al.*, 1964; Nilsson and Westlin, 1971; Smith *et al.*, 1973; Elffors *et al.*, 1994).

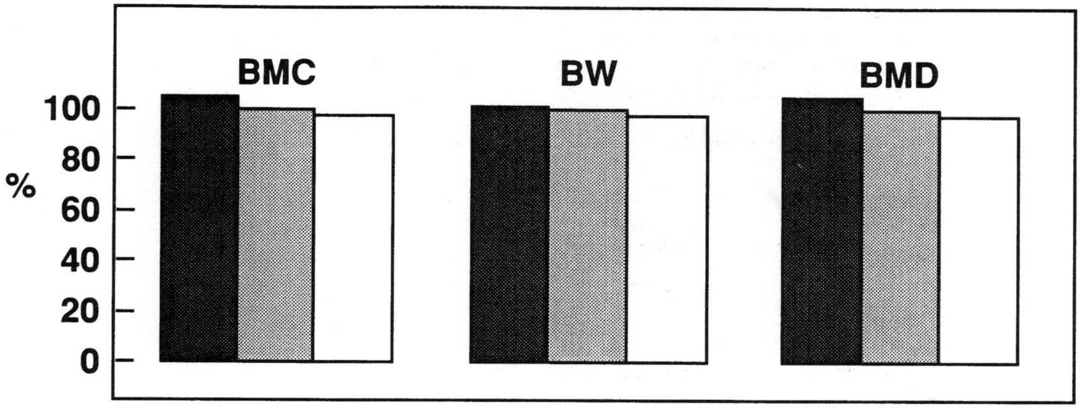

Figure 11.7 Bone mineral content (BMC), bone width (BW) and apparent mineral density (BMD) at the distal radius in elderly (shaded) women divided according to current intake of calcium. The dark bars refer to intakes of >800 mg daily and the open bars to an intake of <600 mg daily. Values were adjusted for age, energy, protein and phosphorus intake. Drawn from Anderson and Tylavsky (1984).

The problem with the epidemiological information is that even significant associations are not necessarily causal. Several epidemiological studies have shown an association between dietary intake of calcium and bone mass or density. So too is there an association between grey hair and a reduction in bone mass, but this should not necessarily be taken as evidence that dyeing the hair will beneficially affect the natural history of bone loss (Kanis and Passmore, 1990). The real problem lies in establishing the causality or otherwise of the relationships, which in turn depends in part on the plausibility of the association. This is weak in the case of advocating hair dye for the management of osteoporosis, but inconsistent in the case of calcium.

There are no prospective controlled studies to show whether an increase in calcium intake increases peak bone mass independently of energy intake, the resporption space or other nutritional factors. Two well-controlled studies report an effect of calcium supplements on bone density in adolescents given calcium or a placebo (Johnston *et al.*, 1992; Lloyd *et al.*, 1994), but the magnitude is small and consistent with a change in bone remodelling. Other studies reporting the effects of calcium supplementation in children are equivocal and have generally shown no effect on growth (Bausal *et al.*, 1964; Luyken *et al.*, 1967; Pettifor *et al.*, 1981). Short-term studies of calcium supplementation in school children have shown small and inconsistent changes that may have been related to changes in energy intake of their diets (Leighton and Clark, 1929; Ackroyd and Krishnan, 1938). Nor are there studies to show whether an increased calcium intake has any effect on skeletal consolidation or subsequent risk of fracture after longitudinal growth has ceased. These considerations suggest that global recommendations concernng the RDA for calcium in childhood and young adults should not be made on the basis of the presently available epidemiological evidence. We are left with studies of metabolic balance for any justification of the RDA.

The computation of the recommended dietary allowance in young healthy adults comes from the studies examining the relationship of skeletal or calcium balance to calcium intake. Many reputable investigators have shown that women on low-calcium diets are in negative calcium balance and conversely that women who consumed greater amounts were in positive balance (Whedon, 1959; Nordin, 1960, 1976; Harrison *et al.*, 1961; Heaney *et al.*, 1977a, b, 1978; Nordin *et al.*, 1987). These authors have argued on this basis that the availability of calcium in many women is inadequate to satisfy the skeletal demands for calcium and, furthermore, that osteoporosis is therefore due to calcium deficiency.

Heaney *et al.* (1977a, b) estimated calcium requirements in many healthy adult women from such balance studies. In addition to finding that women with the lower dietary intakes of calcium were in greater negative balance, they noted a positive correlation between calcium intake and balance (Figure 11.8). The intercept of the regression showed that the requirements in women before the menopause were in the order of 1 g and were even greater in postmenopausal women (Heaney *et al.* 1982; Heaney, 1982). Similar arguments have been put forward concerning the requirements in adolescents. The balance for calcium is greater the higher the dietary intake of calcium (Figure 11.9). In this study maximum balance occurred when the dietary intake exceeded 1 g daily (Matkovic, 1991), justifying the current US RDA for calcium in adolescence (1200 mg daily).

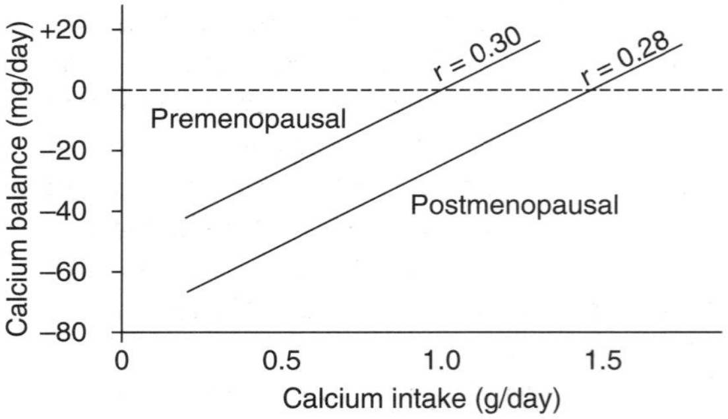

Figure 11.8 Relationship between external balance and dietary intake of calcium in 207 untreated premenopausal and 41 untreated postmenopausal women. Data provided from Heaney *et al.* (1978).

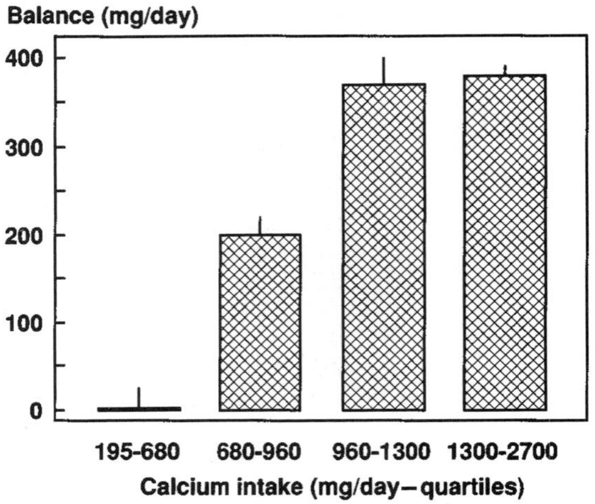

Figure 11.9 The relationship between calcium intake and balance for calcium in adolescents. Data drawn from Matkovic (1991).

The calculation of dietary requirements from balance studies in the way shown in Figures 11.8 and 11.9 is in part a statistical artefact and this type of evidence should no longer be put forward to promote the view that large dietary intakes of calcium are required to maintain skeletal health. By way of an example, some theoretical balance studies are presented in Table 11.2 (Kanis, 1990, 1991). Balance was computed in 40 cases where the dietary intake ranged from 100 to 1000 mg daily in increments of 100 mg. Balance for calcium was calculated from the difference between dietary intake and total excretion of calcium. The total excretion of calcium was randomly selected under double-blind conditions by four investigators. Thus, 10 randomly chosen dietary assessments were randomly matched to 10 estimates of calcium output by each investigator. There was a highly significant positive correlation between calcium intake and balance in all the 40 cases studied (Figure 11.10; $r = 0.63$; $p<0.001$). The mean requirement for calcium has been computed from where the linear regression describing this relationship inter-

Table 11.2 Calculated balance for calcium at 10 levels of dietary intake

Calcium intake (mg/day)	*Calcium balance (mg/day)*				
	A	*B*	*C*	*D*	*Mean ± SEM*
100	-30	-100	0	-90	-33 ± 20
200	0	-50	-40	-10	-25 ± 12
300	-40	-10	-60	+20	-23 ± 18
400	-20	-40	-60	-20	-35 ± 10
500	+20	-40	0	-30	-13 ± 14
600	-20	+50	+30	+40	25 ± 16
700	+60	+10	+50	+30	38 ± 11
800	+30	+30	+10	-10	15 ± 10
900	0	-10	+50	+40	20 ± 15
1000	0	+70	+20	+30	30 ± 15

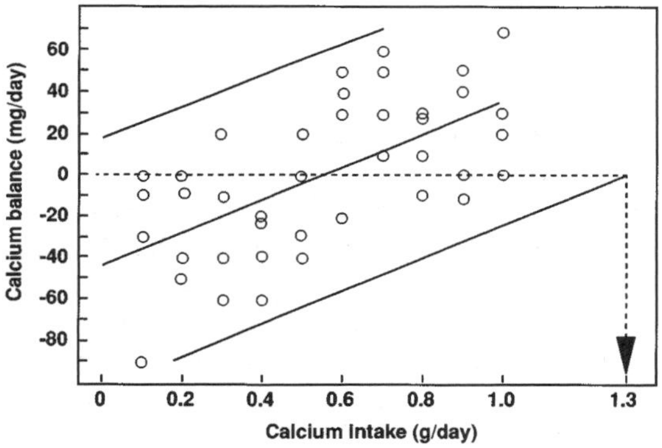

Figure 11.10 The relationship between calcium balance and calcium intake for 40 randomly chosen dietary intakes matched to random excretion values. The diagonal lines describe the mean relationship of the regression with 95% confidence intervals (Kanis, 1991).

cepts with zero balance. The calcium intake in this example at zero balance was 550 mg daily. The recommended dietary allowance computed from the 95% confidence estimates of this regression was 1300 mg daily.

The correlation between dietary intake and balance is an inevitable consequence of plotting two dependent variables (Cochran, 1939). The artefact arises because calcium intake is a measurement used in both sides of the equation (balance equals intake minus excretion). When dietary intake is high, a randomly chosen value for excretion is likely by chance to be lower and the balance positive. Conversely, when the intake is low, a randomly chosen value for excretion is likely to be higher and the balance for calcium negative. To treat intake and balance as independent is to introduce spurious correlations.

In practice, the situation is more complex since the dietary intake of calcium is not physiologically independent of its excretion. In examining the relationship between intake and excretion a non-linear function is expected where the slope is less steep at low levels of intake. Such relationships have not been adequately demonstrated, perhaps related to the poor precision and accuracy of the balance technique. These considerations suggest that the conclusions of studies computing requirements from balance cannot yet be interpreted.

If the epidemiological data, prospective or balance studies cannot provide information on the requirements for calcium, is there other information on which to base a recommendation? Several further arguments have been pursued.

The first is that the intake of calcium is habitually low in humans compared with that of many mammals, suggesting a daily dietary intake of 3–4 g might be phylogenetically appropriate (Mitchell, 1939; Heaney *et al.* 1977a; Heaney, 1990). Indeed, the point is pursued that the advent of organized agriculture decreased the habitual intake of calcium in man compared to our hunter-gatherer forefathers. The span of time since this change in lifestyle (12 000 years) is too brief to have permitted an evolutionary change. What we do not know is how our energy requirements have changed over this time and the intestinal absorption of calcium in our forefathers. Assuming a similar rate of bone remodelling, it seems plausible but difficult to prove that intestinal absorption of calcium was even lower due to their adaptation to a high-calcium diet.

A second argument relates to adaptation. Whereas it is now recognized that the phenomenon of adaptation to low-calcium diets does occur, the calcium protagonists have suggested that not all men are equal in their adaptive efficiency. There is some evidence for variations in the rate of adaptation (Malm, 1958), but not evidence to suggest that adaptation is ultimately incomplete in healthy women. Indeed, as reviewed subsequently, there is indirect evidence to suggest that adaptation even of postmenopausal women is efficient over a two-year period.

The lastest argument in a running debate has been that the losses of calcium in sweat have been underestimated (Charles *et al.*, 1983) and contribute significantly to obligatory losses of calcium in addition to those of the gut and urine (Nordin *et al.*, 1987; Peacock, 1991). Unfortunately, the argument is based indirectly on balance data where the missing calcium is assumed to be lost by sweat rather than by the inaccuracies of the technique. Moreover, the true obligatory losses in urine are not known: nor are those from the gut following adaptation to low-calcium diets. The calculation from such considerations (e.g. Peacock, 1991; Schaffsma, 1992) is therefore littered by assumptions which have not been tested.

The final argument raised by many is that it is wise to err on the side of exuberance when assessing requirements since calcium does no harm and may do good. This, in my view, is not only scientificaly hypocritical but also unwise. If we were to accept the premise that a gram of calcium was essential for skeletal health, we would have to admit that the vast majority of the world's population was calcium deficient and therefore at a disadvantage (Figure 11.11). This not only provokes anxiety but, if untrue, damages the credibility of nutritionists and the medical profession. Moreover, the resource implications for world health are enormous.

These considerations leave us with the uncomfortable conclusion that the RDA of young healthy women is unknown. Clearly, some calcium is required and the question of how much will continue to be asked. An honest answer would be that we do not yet know and that there is no good evidence to suggest that variations in dietary intake of calcium are prejudicial for skeletel health in young women who take a reasonably balanced diet.

SKELETAL METABOLISM AFTER THE MENOPAUSE

There is a great deal of evidence to indicate that osteoporosis is a disorder of bone remodelling. As previously discussed, the term 'coupling' describes the attraction of osteoblasts to sites of previous resorption. In osteoporosis the coupling process appears to be intact and the progressive decrease in bone mass is due to an imbalance between the amount of mineral and matrix removed and that subsequently incorporated into each erosion cavity. In postmenopausal osteoporosis and other types of osteoporosis, there is evidence to suggest that the imbalance between the amount of bone resorbed and

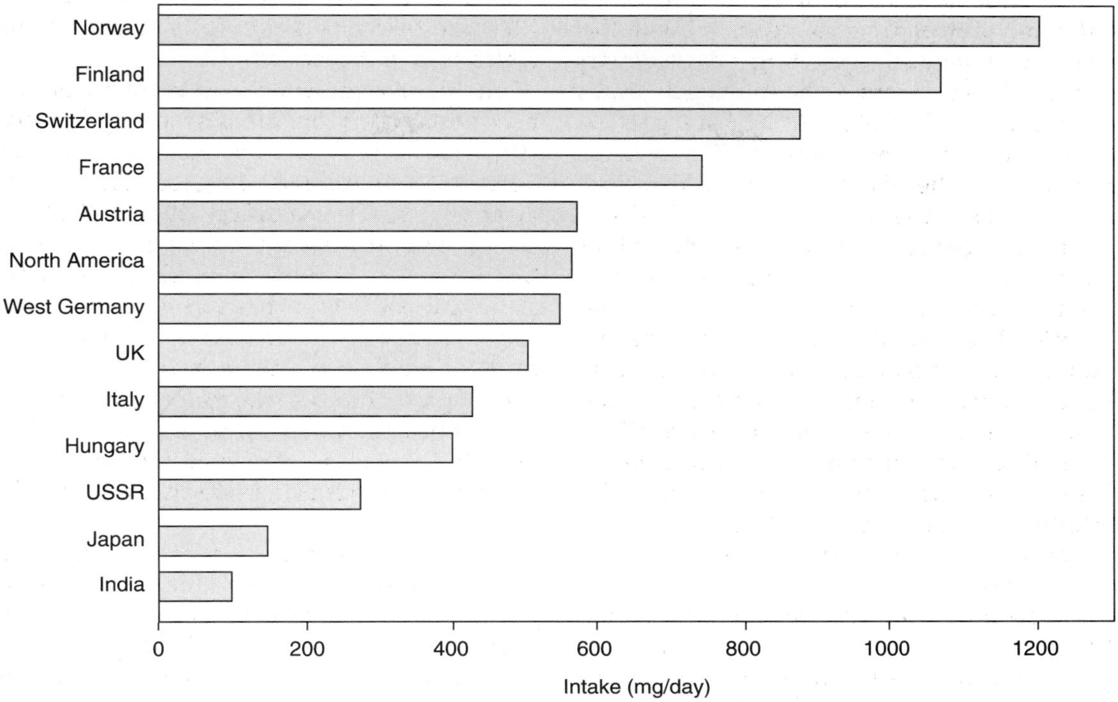

Figure 11.11 Calcium intake from milk and cheese in different countries.

that formed at each remodelling site is due to a decrease in the functional capacity of osteoblasts or a decrease in the recruitment of osteoblasts to previous resorption sites.

Irrespective of the mechanism, a finite deficit of bone is the end result of each remodelling sequence. If bone turnover is increased, the number of bone-remodelling units present at any one time also increases. If the imbalance at each site remains constant, the result of increasing bone turnover will be to amplify the rate of bone loss (Figure 11.12). There is now good evidence that oestrogen deficiency not only induces a focal imbalance at remodelling sites but also increases the remodelling rate of bone (Heaney *et al.*, 1978; Stepan *et al.*, 1987). In this way, bone loss is accelerated. The role of calcium in the treatment of established osteoporosis appears to be due to its ability to decrease bone turnover (Nordin and Need, 1989) and thereby decrease skeletal losses. It seems likely that this is related to the small increments in serum calcium and the resulting decrease in the activation of bone turnover in much the same way as seen in younger women.

It would be expected, then, that the inhibition of bone turnover would decrease the rate of bone loss but not prevent it entirely. The reason for this relates to the effect of calcium on bone remodelling. Thus, at each remodelling site a finite volume of bone is resorbed and in osteoporosis a somewhat lesser amount is formed. In terms of calcium transport, approximately 6 mmol of calcium is resorbed daily and 5 mmol put back by bone formation in the several million remodelling sites. This gives rise to a net deficit of 1 mmol of calcium per day (equivalent to bone loss of approximately 1% per annum). When bone

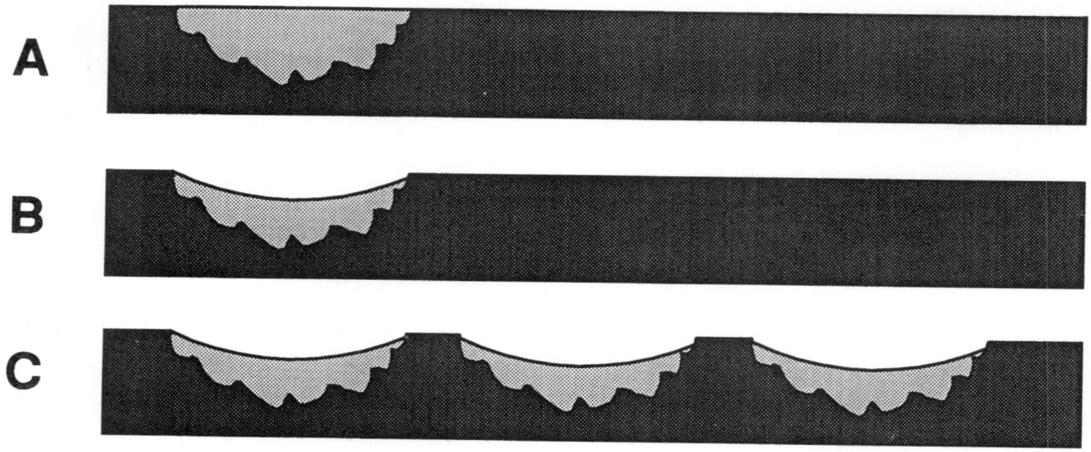

Figure 11.12 Schematic representation of a trabecular bone surface to illustrate the effect of balance and remodelling on the rate of bone loss. (A) The infilling of an erosion bay with an equal volume of new bone. In osteoporosis less bone is deposited in erosion cavities (B). If bone turnover is increased without altering this balance (C), the rate of cancellous bone loss will increase in proportion to the increment in bone turnover.

turnover alone is decreased the number of remodelling sites also decreases, but the imbalance between formation and resorption at each remodelling site persists. Thus, if bone turnover is decreased by 50%, bone loss would be reduced from 1% to 0.5% per annum.

A number of observations have shown that calcium supplements may be associated with the maintenance of or even an increase in skeletal mass, but this is modest (2–10% depending on the site measured) and ill sustained (Albanese *et al.*, 1975; Smith *et al.*, 1975, 1981; Horsman *et al.*, 1977; Recker *et al.*, 1977; Lamke *et al.*, 1978; Nordin *et al.*, 1980; Recker and Heaney, 1985). The reason for the transient increase in bone mass relates to the decreased activation of new remodelling sites. Early in treatment bone formation will continue at previously existing remodelling sites and bone mass will increase transiently to fill in the resorption space (Kanis, 1991). Since turnover is a slow process, the transient state may persist for up to three years and recent studies with the use of calcium supplements suggests that this is so (Stepán *et al.*, 1989) (Figure 11.13). Similar but more rapid effects are observed at cancellous bone sites (Figure 11.14).

The attainment of the new steady state after treatment with calcium is very similar to the adaptation of young adults to changes in dietary intake. The process is slow and takes several years to be complete. If adaptation were complete, it would be expected that intestinal absorption of calcium would decrease during the process and that the increment in absorbed calcium would decrease with time. This is precisely what is observed in prospective studies. Thus, after starting treatment with additional calcium, urine calcium excretion increases markedly in postmenopausal women (Nilas *et al.*, 1984). The effect is, however, attenuated with time and after two years reaches pretreatment values. This suggests that postmenopausal women are capable of adapting to increments in dietary intake (Kanis, 1990).

The difference in adaptation between pre- and postmenopausal women is that in the

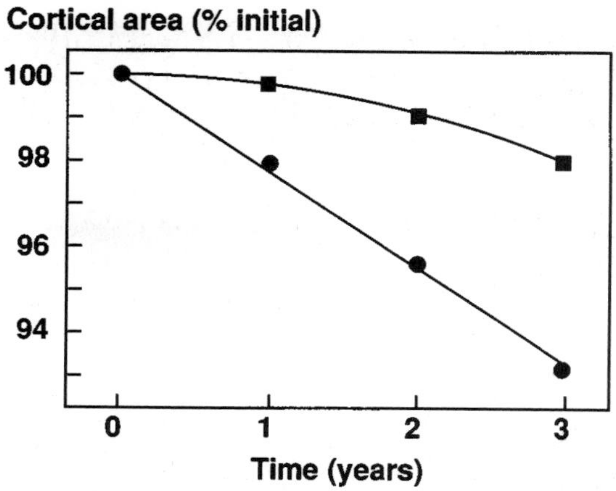

Figure 11.13 The effect of pharmacological doses of calcium (1.5 g daily) or placebo in women after a surgical menopause. This three-year placebo-controlled study indicates that calcium significantly delays the rate of bone loss. Data from Stepán *et al.* (1989).

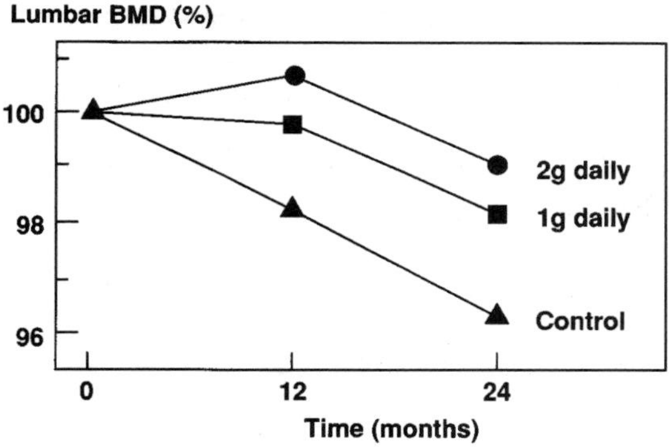

Figure 11.14 Effects of pharmacological intervention with two doses of calcium supplements on the rate of bone loss at the lumbar spine. Note the dose-dependent delay in the rate of loss. Data from Elders *et al.* (1991).

latter, bone loss persists, albeit it at a slower rate, since the balance of resorption and formation at remodelling sites remains unchanged. This imbalance, due to oestrogen deficiency, is not reversed by calcium. In contrast, bone loss is on average halted by oestrogen by correcting the imbalance and thereby preserving bone mass irrespective of the time that it is given after surgical castration or the menopause.

This and evidence reviewed elsewhere (Kanis and Passmore, 1989; Kanis, 1991, 1994) suggests that the use of calcium supplements is capable of decreasing the rate of bone loss in postmenopausal women.

IS OSTEOPOROSIS A CALCIUM-DEFICIENCY DISEASE?

Observations that pharmacological (even though phylogenetically appropriate) doses of calcium delay the rate of bone loss have been given as evidence that osteoporosis is indeed a calcium-defiency disorder (Nordin, 1960; Nordin and Morris, 1989; Nordin and Heaney, 1990). The elegant balance studies of Heaney indicate that intestinal absorption of calcium decreases after the menopause (Heaney *et al.*, 1977a, b, 1978). This is associated with low concentrations of calcitriol found by some but not all investigators (Gallagher *et al.*, 1973, 1979; Falch *et al.*, 1987). The argument depends critically upon whether reduced intestinal absorption of calcium is a cause or a conseqeunce of osteoporosis. Those favouring its causal role argue that oestrogens directly stimulate the production of calcitriol; deficiency at the menopause results in impaired production of calcitriol and malabsorption of calcium, thereby aggravating the osteoporosis. The converse view is that lack of oestrogens induce bone loss and infuse the extracellular fluid with calcium. This in turn induces the expected homoeostatic responses that offset the hypercalcaemic challenge of osteoporosis.

These opposing views are difficult to resolve from population studies. Population studies do not show differences in cortical bone loss between communities with very different intakes of calcium (Hegsted *et al.*, 1952; Garn *et al.*, 1969; Matkovic *et al.*, 1979). However, the decrement in calcium absorption appears to be similar over a wide range of dietary intakes and argues against calcium deficiency causing perimenopausal bone loss (Kanis and Passmore, 1989). Prospective studies would support this view (Falch *et al.*, 1987). These observations suggest that osteoporosis is not a disease due to calcium deficiency. Although skeletal calcium losses are clearly attenuated by the pharmacological manipulation of bone turnover, this argues that calcium deficiency causes osteoporosis only in the same sense that penicillin deficiency causes streptococcal infections. It is perhaps more appropriate to consider these as effective pharmacological interventions rather than causes of disease. The major cause of postmenopausal bone loss is oestrogen deficiency and a great deal of evidence suggests that the administration of oestrogens prevents this loss.

There are some useful analogies between the calcium losses of osteoporosis and the iron-deficiency anaemia that occurs with chronic gastrointestinal bleeding. Chronic bleeding clearly results in anaemia which is, in part, reversible by the administration of iron. In the same way, gonadal failure results in skeletal calcium losses. We should not, on this basis, argue that iron deficiency causes gastrointestinal bleeding. Nor can iron stop bleeding, even though it is well recognized that supplemental iron will improve anaemia. In the same way, calcium deficiency does not cause osteoporosis. Neither does it reverse the process, even though rates of bone loss can be attenuated.

For all these reasons, there is clearly potential for calcium supplementation of the postmenopausal woman who can be shown to be at risk of osteoporosis. The rationale depends upon the strength of the assumption that a decrease in the rate of bone loss in the elderly at risk would decrease the risk of osteoporotic fracture.

EFFECTS OF CALCIUM IN OSTEOPOROSIS

Bone loss continues throughout later life, but the amount of bone lost falls with advancing years (Garn *et al.*, 1969; Kanis and Adami, 1994). The question arises whether calcium intake affects the rate of bone loss in women well past the menopause and who have undergone fracture. Many studies of calcium requirement have been undertaken in the elderly using balance techniques (Roberts *et al.*, 1948; Ohlson *et al.*, 1952; Whedon, 1959; Harrison *et al.*, 1961; Nordin, 1962). As expected, none showed a mean of apparent requirement of less than 800 mg, but none may be interpreted with confidence. Other surveys of elderly people have shown that patients with osteoporosis took less calcium in their diets than those without osteoporosis (Nordin, 1960, 1962; Riggs *et al.*, 1967; Hruxthal and Vose, 1969). One obvious interpretation would be that if such patients had taken more calcium they would have been spared their osteoporosis. The alternative view, that patients with osteoporosis were smaller or took less exercise and so selected diets of lower energy and calcium content, seems not to have been considered.

More persuasive evidence comes from controlled prospective studies which have examined the effect of calcium on the rate of bone loss in osteoporotic patients (Smith *et al.*, 1975; Lamke *et al.*, 1978; Nordin *et al.*, 1980). These studies in osteoporotic patients are similar to the findings in postmenopausal women without osteoporosis and show that the administration of pharmacological amounts of calcium delays the rate of bone loss. The evidence for this has recently been reviewed (Kanis, 1991) and several more recent publications support this view (e.g. Dawson-Hughes *et al.*, 1990; Dawson-Hughes, 1991; Elders *et al.*, 1991).

The ultimate arbiter of the efficacy of calcium is the study of fracture rates. Until recently there were very few adequate studies on fracture in women with osteoporosis and several clinical and epidemiological studies claiming an effect of calcium were subject to other interpretations (Kanis, 1984). Individuals who elect to take high-calcium diets differ significantly from non-calcium-taking counterparts in terms of their general health, education, physical activity and other possible confounding factors. Such studies of dietary calcium should be distinguished from those that examine the pharmacological use of calcium.

Several studies have reported the beneficial effects of calcium treatment on the frequency of fracture (Nordin *et al.*, 1980; Riggs *et al.*, 1982), but in both the design of the trial was flawed (Kanis, 1984). Only recently have the effects of calcium been studied using adequate trial methodology (Recker *et al.*, 1994). This community-based study showed that those women with prevalent vertebral fractures who took calcium (600 mg daily) sustained 45% less vertebral fractures than those given placebo. Other recent studies show comparable effects (Chevalley *et al.*, 1994; Reid *et al.*, 1995). Attempts to increase the intestinal availability of calcium with derivatives of vitamin D have not shown a consistently beneficial effect on the frequency of fractures (Kanis, 1984; Ott and Chesnut, 1987, 1989). Two recent studies have shown an effect of vitamin D on vertebral fracture frequency (Orimo *et al.*, 1987; Tilyard *et al.*, 1992).

We have reported that the risk of hip fractures decreased in women taking pharmacological amounts of calcium for osteoporosis (Kanis *et al.*, 1992). The data were derived from a retrospective epidemiological survey, but the effect persisted even when adjusting for potential confounding factors (Figure 11.15). Of particular interest is the observation that calcium supplements were taken on average at the age of 70 years whereas the average age of hip fractures in our study was 75 years. Thus treatment, even late in the natural history of bone loss, may have significant clinical dividends.

Recently, a controlled prospective study of the use of calcium in the institutionalized elderly has shown that calcium and vitamin D significantly decrease the frequency of hip fracture in women over the age of 75 years (Chapuy *et al.*, 1992). Over an 18-month follow-up of more than 3000 women there was a significant decrease in both femoral and other non-vertebral fractures (Table 11.3). This finding adds credibility to our retrospective studies and earlier but less well-controlled studies supporting an effect of calcium on fracture frequency but may not be applicable to the general population. It is, however, consistent with the view that

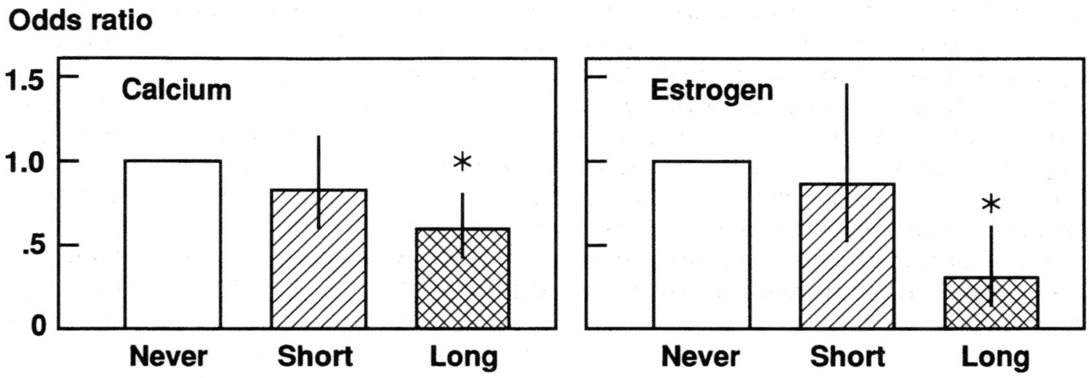

Figure 11.15 Relative risk of hip fracture in elderly women given calcium supplements or hormone replacement treatment. Both interventions show a significant duration-dependent effect but the effects of calcium are less complete (Kanis *et al.*, 1992).

Table 11.3 Effects of calcium with vitamin D or placebo on the occurrence of extravertebral fractures in 3270 women (Chapuy *et al.*, 1992). There was a significant decrease in femoral and other (non-vertebral) fractures ($p < 0.05$ and < 0.02 respectively)

	Treatment		*Placebo*	
Interval and follow-up (months)	*All fractures*	*Hip fractures*	*All fractures*	*Hip fractures*
0–6	55	30	76	36
6–12	52	24	62	30
12–18	44	19	66	37
0–18	151	73	204	103

treatment, even relatively late in the natural history of osteoporotic bone loss, significantly reduces the risk of hip fracture.

There is an obvious disparity between ecological studies and case control or intervention studies examining the effects of calcium on fracture rate. From a worldwide perspective there is a direct rather than inverse relation between calcium intake and the frequency of hip fracture (Kanis and Passmore, 1989). Such observations should not be used to argue that calcium causes hip fracture, but only that variations in calcium intake around the world cannot explain the differences in risk between the communities. For the same reasons, findings derived from other ecological studies suggesting that a high intake of animal protein causes hip fractures (Abelow *et al.*, 1992) or that fluoride causes or protects against hip fracture (Melton, 1990) should be regarded as hypotheses. Nevertheless, the observations do suggest that different patterns of calcium nutrition around the world cannot explain the variations in risk between populations, but that treatment with calcium in osteoporotic women within communities can clearly affect the rate of bone loss and decreases the risk of osteoporotic fractures.

WHO AND HOW TO TREAT

A wide variety of calcium preparations is available. Prescription products available in the United Kingdom are listed in Table 11.4. Many non-proprietary forms are also available, but the calcium content is small, so that more than 10 tablets need to be taken daily in order to provide a dose of 1000 mg. There are small differences in the bioavailability of calcium between these prescription products, but they are unlikely to be of therapeutic significance. The same is not true of some over-the counter brands where the availability of calcium may be markedly reduced. A similar situation applies to some foodstufs where the availability of calcium, for example from green vegetables, appears to be significantly less than that from dairy products (Weaver *et al.*, 1991). Apart from this caveat, there is no reason to believe that the consumption of calcium, particularly in the form of dairy products, would not have the same ultimate effect, though this is yet to be formally demonstrated.

The major problem which arises is whom to treat. Many prospective studies have now shown a clear relationship between bone mineral density and the future risk of fracture (Ross *et al.*, 1987; Hui *et al.*, 1988; Wasnich *et al.*, 1989; Cummings *et al.*, 1990; Nordin *et al.*, 1990; Black *et al.*, 1991). The sensitivity and specificity of bone mineral density measurements is similar to that of blood pressure for cerebrovascular disease, and suggests that the measurement of bone density might be a useful test to enable calcium supplements to be targeted to those most at risk. The role of

Table 11.4 Proprietary preparations of calcium available in the UK

Name	*Calcium salt*	*Calcium content mg*	*Formulation*	*Daily dose*[a]	*Monthly cost (£)*[b]
Cacit	Carbonate	500	Effervescent tablet	2	15.50
Calcichew	Carbonate	500	Chewable tablet	2	6.75
Calcichew-D_3[c]	Carbonate	500	Chewable tablet	2	8.40
Calcidrink	Carbonate	1000	Sachet of granules	1	8.70
Calcium Sandoz	Glubionate + lactobionate	324	Syrup 15 ml	3	6.67
Citrical	Carbonate	500	Sachet of granules	2	16.00
Ossopan 800	Hydroxyapatite	176	Tablets	6	37.26
Ossopan granules	Hydroxyapatite	712	Sachet of granules	2[d]	39.64
Sandocal 400	Carbonate + lactate gluconate	400	Effervescent tablet	3[e]	6.63
Sandocal 1000	Carbonate and lactate gluconate	1000	Effervescent tablet	1	6.63
Titrilac	Carbonate	190	Tablet	5	1.86

[a] The daily dose is that to provide approximately 1 g of elemental calcium (25 mmol) daily
[b] May 1992
[c] Contains 5 μg (200 IU) vitamin D_3 per tablet
[d] 1424 mg
[e] 1200 mg

bone density measurements in the assessment of fracture risk is as controversial as the RDA for calcium (Freemantle, 1992; Stevenson *et al.*, 1992), but many believe that bone density measurements will form a component of directing treatment at least for non-hormonal interventions (Kanis *et al.*, 1994). In the meantime, the risk of fracture is certainly increased markedly following a first osteoporotic fracture (Ross *et al.*, 1991). In such women it appears to be appropriate to offer an intervention and calcium is certainly a potential candidate.

In 1986 approximately $166 million was spent in the United States on calcium supplements (Kolata, 1986). In the UK prescriptions for calcium more than doubled between 1985 and 1989 (Figure 11.16) and clearly there is a need to target these rising costs to an appropriate segment of the community.

The question arises of how calcium is placed within the ever-increasing therapeutic armamentarium available to manage patients with established osteoporosis. The effects of calcium are certainly less complete than those of oestrogens or other gonadal steroids, but many women, particularly those well after the menopause, are reluctant to accept the

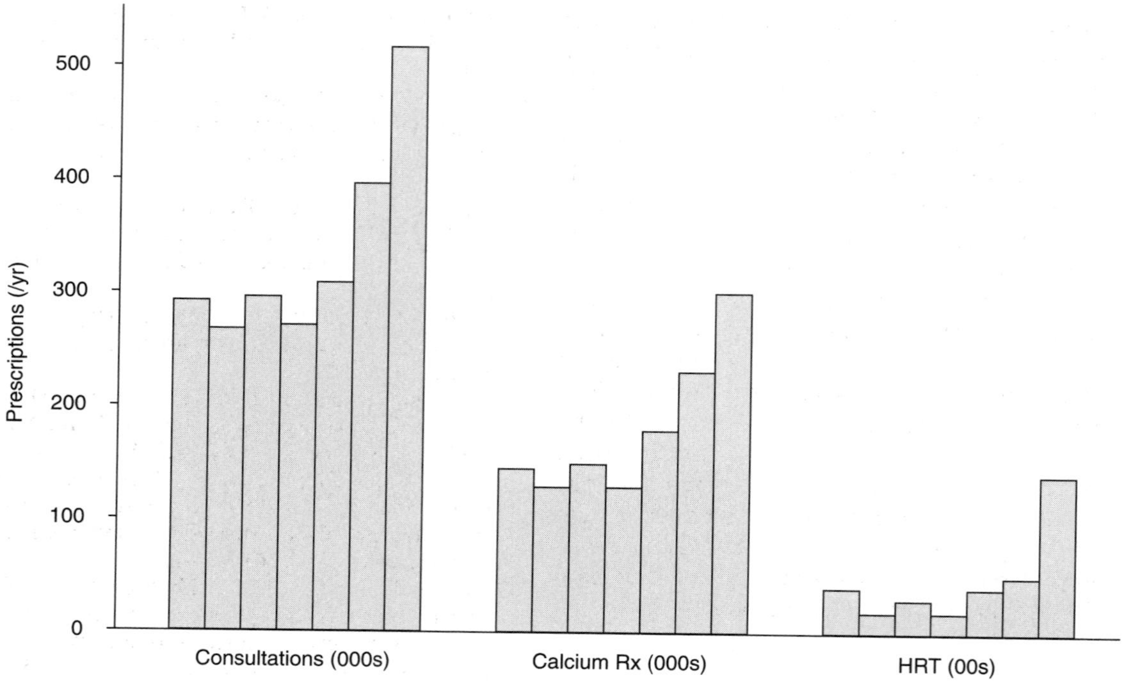

Figure 11.16 Yearly numbers of consultations and prescriptions of calcium and hormone replacement treatment (HRT) in the UK for osteoporosis between 1983 (left-hand bars) and 1989 (right-hand bars).

long-term use of HRT. There is thus a clear place for other interventions in the management of osteoporosis. Other interventions also have more complete effects than calcium, at least on bone density. These include the calcitonins, the bisphosphonates and the anabolic steroids. The effects of some of these agents on fracture frequency are less secure and must await the outcome of well-designed prospective studies.

CONCLUSION

There is no doubt that humans are capable of adapting to large changes in the dietary intake of calcium. This adaptation may take many years to be complete, but occurs in healthy adults and in postmenopausal women. In both, a change in calcium nutrition induces transient changes in bone turnover until a new steady state comes about several years later. Whereas acute changes in dietary intake of calcium can alter calcium balance, the steady-state effect of altered calcium intake can only be determined from long-term studies.

There are still no adequately controlled studies to show whether an increase in calcium intake increases bone mass in the young over and above that expected from changes in remodelling independently of energy intake. Nor are there studies to show whether an increased calcium intake has an effect on skeletal consolidation or subsequent fracture risk after longitudinal growth has ceased. For this reason, recommendations concerning the dietary allowance for calcium in young healthy women depend largely upon the extrapolation of data obtained in studies of metabolic balance. The interpretation of such studies is flawed. Thus, the view that the amount of calcium taken in our diet critically affects skeletal capital is an hypothesis which needs to be tested formally.

In contrast, skeletal calcium losses after the menopause are attentuated by pharmacological manipulation of bone turnover with high dietary intakes of calcium. Indeed, there are well-controlled prospective studies which indicate that pharmacological doses of calcium delay the rate of bone loss in women after surgical castration, in the postmenopausal state and in established osteoporosis. The probable mechanism for this relates to the effects of calcium in suppressing bone turnover. It might be expected that a decrease in the rate of bone loss would decrease the risk of osteoporotic fracture. A variety of epidemiological data and prospective studies indicate that this is so, particularly in the elderly.

REFERENCES

Abelow, B.J., Holford, T.R. and Insogna, K.L. (1992) Cross-sectional associations between dietary animal protein and hip fracture. A hypothesis. *Calcif Tissue Int* **50**: 14–18.

Ackroyd, W.R. and Krishnan, B.G. (1938) Effect of calcium lactate on children in a nursery school. *Lancet* **ii**: 153–5.

Albanese, A.A., Edelson, A.H., Lorenze, E.J., Woodhull, M.L. and Wein, E.H. (1975) Problems of health in the elderly: ten year study. *NY State J Med* **75**: 326–36.

Albright, F., Bloomberg, E. and Smith, P.H. (1940) Postmenopausal osteoporosis. *Trans Assoc Am Physicians* **55**: 298–305.

Anderson, J.J.B. (1990) Dietary calcium and bone mass through the life cycle. *Nutrition Today* **25**: 9–14.

Anderson, J.J.B. and Tylavsky, F.A. (1984) Diet and osteopenia in elderly caucasian women. In: *Osteoporosis*, (eds Christiansen, C., Arnaud, C.D., Nordin, B.E.C. *et al.*), Glostrup Hospital, Copenhagen, pp. 299–303.

Baron, R., Vignery, A. and Horowitz, M. (1983) Lymphocytes, macrophages and the regulation of bone remodelling. In: *Bone and Mineral Research Annual*, (ed. Peck, W.A.), Elsevier, Amsterdam, pp. 175–184.

Barrett-Connor, E. (1989) The RDA for calcium in the elderly: too little too late. *Calcif Tissue Int* **44**: 303–7.

Bausal, P., Rao, R., Venkatachalam, P. and Goplan, G. (1964) Effect of calcium supplementation on children in a rural community. *Indian J Med* Res **52**: 219–23.

Black, D.M., Cummings, D.M., Genant, H.K. *et al.* (1991) Axial bone mineral density predicts fractures in older women. *J Bone Miner Res* **6** (Suppl 1): S136.

Chalmers, J. and Ho, K.C. (1970) Geographical variations in senile osteoporosis. *J Bone Joint Surg* **52B**: 667–75.

Chapuy, M.C., Arlot, M.E., Dubeof, F. *et al.* (1992) Vitamin D_3 and calcium to prevent hip fractures in elderly women. *N Engl J Med* **327**: 1637–42.

Charles, P., Taagehoj Jensen, F., Mosekilde, L. and Hvid Hansen, H. (1983) Calcium metabolism evaluated by ^{47}Ca kinetics: estimation of dermal calcium loss. *Clin Sci* **65**: 415–22.

Chevalley, T., Rizzoli, R. and Nydegger, V. (1994) Effects of calcium supplements on femoral bone density and vertebral fracture rate in vitamin D replete elderly patients. *Osteoporosis Int* **4**: 245–52.

Clark, G.W. (1926) Studies in the mineral metabolism in adult man. *University of California Publications in Physiology* **5**: 195–287.

Cochran, W.G. (1939) Long term agricultural experiments. *J Roy Statist Soc* **6** (Suppl): 104.

Cooper, C., Barker, D.J.P. and Wickham, C. (1988) Physical activity, muscle strength and calcium intake in fracture of the proximal femur in Britain. *Br Med J* **297**: 1443–5.

Cummings, S.R., Black, D.M., Nevitt, M.C. *et al.* (1990) Appendicular bone density and age predict hip fracture in women. *J Am Med Assoc* **263**, 665–8.

Cundy, T.C., Kanis, J.A., Heynen, G. *et al.* (1982) Failure to heal vitamin D-deficient rickets and suppress secondary hyperthyroidism with conventional doses of 1,25-dihydroxyvitamin D_3. *Br Med J* **284**: 883–5.

Dawson-Hughes, B. (1991) Effects of calcium intake on calcium retention and bone density in postmenopausal women. In: *Nutritional Aspects of Osteoporosis*, (eds Burkhardt, P. and Heaney, R.P.), Serono Symposium Publications, Raven Press, New York, pp. 331–45.

Dawson-Hughes, B., Dallal, G.E., Krall, E.A. *et al.* (1990) A controlled trial of the effect of calcium supplementation on bone density in postmenopausal women. *N Engl J Med* **323**: 878–83.

Donath, A., Indermuhle, P. and Baud, R. (1975) Influence of the national calcium and fluoride supply and of a calcium supplementation on bone mineral content of health population in Switzerland. Proceedings of an International Conference on Bone Mineral Measurements, Department of Health, Education and Welfare, London.

Elders, P.J.M., Netelenbos, J.C., Lips, P. *et al.* (1991) Calcium supplementation reduces vertebral bone loss in perimenopausal women: a controlled trial in 248 women between 46 and 55 years of age. *J Clin Endocrinol Metab* **73**: 533–40.

Elffors, L., Allander, E., Kanis, J.A. *et al.* (1994) The variable incidence of hip fracture in Southern Europe. The MEDOS Study. *Osteoporosis Int* **4**: 253–63.

Ettinger, B., Genant, H.K. and Cann, C.E. (1987) Postmenopausal bone loss is prevented by treatment with low-dose estrogen with calcium. *Ann Intern Med* **106**: 40–5.

Falch, J.A., Odeggard, O.R., Finnanger, A.M. and Matheson, I. (1987) Postmenopausal osteoporosis: no effect of three years treatment with 1,25-dihydroxycholecaliciferol. *Acta Med Scand* **221**: 199–204.

Food and Agricultural Organization and World Health Organization (1962) Calcium Requirements, WHO Technical Report Services No 230, WHO, Geneva.

Food and Nutrition Board (1943) Recommended Dietary Allowances, National Research Council Reprint and Circular Series No 115.

Francis, R.M. (1989) Calcium's role in preventing and treating osteoporosis. *Geriat Med* **19**: 24–6.

Freemantle, N. (1992) Screening for osteoporosis to prevent fractures. In: *Effective Health Care No 1*, School of Public Health, Leeds.

Frost, H.M. (1960) Presence of microscopic cracks *in vivo* in bone. *Henry Ford Hosp Bull* **8**: 25–35.

Gallacher, J.C., Aaron, J., Horsman, A. *et al.* (1973) The crush fracture syndrome in postmenopausal women. *Clin Endocrinol Metab* **2**: 293–315.

Gallacher, J.C., Riggs, B.L., Eisman, J. *et al.* (1979) Intestinal calcium absorption and serum vitamin D metabolites in normal subjects and osteoporosis patients: effect of age and dietary calcium. *J Clin Invest* **64**: 729–36.

Garn, S.M., Pao, E.M. and Rihl, M.E. (1964) Compact bone in Chinese and Japanese. *Science* **143**: 1439–40.

Garn, S.M., Rohmann, C.G., Wagner, B., Davila, G.H. and Ascoli, W. (1969) Population similarities in the onset and rate of adult endosteal bone loss. *Clin Orthop* **65**: 51–60.

Hansen, M.A., Overgaard, K., Riis, B.J. and Christiansen, C. (1991) Potential risk factors for development of postmenopausal osteoporosis examined over a 12 year period. *Osteoporosis Int* **1**: 95–102.

Harrison, M., Fraser, R. and Mullan, B. (1961) Calcium metabolism in osteoporosis. *Lancet* **i**: 1015–19.

Heaney, R.P. (1982) Calcium intake, requirement and bone mass in the elderly. *J Lab Clin Med* **100**: 309–12.

Heaney, R.P. (1990) Calcium. In: *Progress in Basic and Clinical Pharmacology*, (ed. Kanis, J.A.), Karger; Basel, pp. 28–54.

Heaney, R.P., Recker, R.R. and Saville, P.D. (1977a) Calcium balance and calcium requirement in middle aged women. *Am J Clin Nutrition* **30**: 1603–11.

Heaney, R.P., Recker, R.R. and Saville, P.D. (1977b) Menopausal changes in calcium balance performance. *J Lab Clin Med* **92**: 953–63.

Heaney, R.P., Recker, R.R. and Saville, P.D. (1978) Menopausal changes in bone remodelling. *J Lab Clin Med* **92**: 964–70.

Heaney, R.P., Gallacher, J.C., Johnston Jr, C.C. *et al.* (1982) Calcium nutrition and bone health in the elderly. *Am J Clin Nutrition* **36**: 986–1013.

Hegsted, D.M. (1967) Mineral intake and bone loss. *Federation Proceedings* **26**: 1747–1754.

Hegsted, J.M., Moscosco, I., Collazos, C.H.C. (1952) Study of minimum calcium requirements by adult man. *J Nutr* **46**: 181–201.

Holbrook, T.L., Barrett-Connor, E. and Wingard, D.L. (1988) Dietary calcium intake and risk of hip fracture: 14 year prospective population study. *Lancet*, **ii**: 1046–9.

Horsman, A., Gallacher, J.C., Simpson, M., Nordin, B.E.C. (1977) Prospective trial of oestrogen and calcium in postmenopausal women. *Br Med J*, **ii**: 789–92.

Hruxthal, L.M. and Vose, G.P. (1969) The relationship of dietary calcium intake to radiographic bone density in normal and osteoporotic persons. *Calcif Tissue Res*, **4**: 245–56.

Hui, S.L., Slemenda, C.S., Johnston, C.C. (1988) Age and bone mass as predictors of fracture in a prospective study. *J Clin Invest* **81**: 1804–9.

Johnston, C.O., Miller, J.Z., Slemenda, C.W. *et al.* (1992) Calcium supplementation and increases in bone mineral density in children. *N Engl J Med* **327**: 82–7.

Kalu, D.N. and Masoro, E.J. (1990) Undernutrition as a modulator of general and bone aging in the rat. In: *Nutrition and Bone Development*, (ed. Simmons, D.J.), Oxford University Press, Oxford, pp. 93–113.

Kamiyama, S., Kobayashi, S., Abe, S. *et al.* (1972) Osteoporosis prevalence and nutritional intake among the people in farm, fishing and urban districts. *Tohoku J Exp Med* **107**: 387–94.

Kanders, B., Dempster, D.W. and Lindsay, R. (1988) Interaction of calcium nutrition and physical activity on bone mass in young women. *J Bone Miner Res* **3**: 145–9.

Kanis, J.A. (1984) Treatment of osteoporotic fracture. *Lancet*, **i**: 27–33.

Kanis, J.A. (1985) Osteoporosis. In: *The Chemistry and Biology of Mineralised Tissues*, (ed. Butler, W.T.), EBSCO Media, Birmingham, Alabama, pp. 398–407.

Kanis, J.A. (1990) The nutritional requirements for calcium derived from balance studies: fact or artefact? In: *Osteoporosis 1990*, (eds Christiansen, C. and Overgaard, K.), Osteopress, Copenhagen, pp. 341–2.

Kanis, J.A. (1991) Requirements of calcium for optimal skeletal health. *Calcif Tissue Int* **49** (Suppl), S33–41.

Kanis, J.A. (1994) Calcium nutrition and its implications for osteoporosis. *Eur J Clin Nutrition* **48**: 757–67, 833–41.

Kanis, J.A. and Adami, S. (1994) Bone loss in the elderly. *Osteoporosis Int* 4 (Suppl 1), 56–65.

Kanis, J.A. and Passmore, R. (1989) Calcium supplementation of the diet. *Br Med J* **298**, 137–40, 205–8, 673–4.

Kanis, J.A. and Passmore, R. (1990) Calcium supplementation of the diet. *Br Med J* **300**, 1523.

Kanis, J.A., Johnell, O., Gullberg, B. *et al.* (1992) Evidence for the efficacy of drugs affecting bone metabolism in the prevention of hip fracture. *Br Med J* **305**, 1124–8.

Kanis, J.A. and the WHO Study Group (1994) Assessment of fracture risk and its application to screening for postmenopausal osteoporosis. *Osteoporosis Int* **4**: 368–81.

Kelly, P.J., Pocock, N.a., Sambrook, P.N. and Eisman, J.A. (1990) Dietary calcium, sex hormones and bone mineral density in man. *Br Med J* **300**, 1361–4.

Kinsman, G.D., Sheldon, R., Jensen, M. *et al.* (1939) The utilization of calcium of milk by preschool children. *J Nutrition* **17**, 429–41.

Kolata, G. (1986) How important is dietary calcium in preventing osteoporosis? *Science* **233**: 519–20.

Kooh, S.W., Fraser, D., Reilly, B.J. *et al.* (1977) Rickets due to calcium deficiency. *N Engl J Med* **297**, 1264–6.

Lamke, B., Sjoberg, H.E. and Sylven, M. (1978) Bone mineral content in women with Colles' fracture: effect of calcium supplementation. *Acta Orthop Scand* **49**, 143–9.

Leighton, G. and Clark, M.L. (1929) Milk consumption and the growth of school children. *Lancet* **i**: 40–3.

Leitch, I. (1937) The determination of the calcium requirements of man. *Nutrition Abstr Rev* **6**, 553–78.

Lloyd, T., Chrischilli, V. and Rollings, N. (1994) Bone acquisition in adolescent girls: the effect of starting calcium supplements at age 12 or 14. In: *Current Research in Osteoporosis and Bone Mineral Measurements III*, (eds Ring, E.J.F., Elvins, D.M., and Bhalla, A.K.), British Institute of Radiology, London, pp. 82–3.

Lusk, G. (1917) *The Science of Nutrition*, 3rd edn. W.B. Saunders, Philadelphia.

Luyken, R., Luyken-Koning, F.W.M., Cambridge, T.H., Dohle, T. and Rosh, R. (1967) Studies on the physiology of nutrition in Surinam. X. Protein metabolism and influence of extra calcium on the growth of and calcium metabolism in boarding school children. *Am J Clin Nutrition* **20**: 34–42.

Malm, O.J. (1958) Calcium requirement and adaptation in adult men. *Scand J Clin Lab Invest* **10** (Suppl 36).

Matkovic, V. (1991) Calcium metabolism and calcium requirements during skeletal modelling and consolidation. *Am J Clin Nutrition 54*, 245–60.

Matkovic, V., Kostial, K., Simonovic, I. *et al.* (1979) Bone status and fracture rates in two regions of Yugoslavia. *Am J Clin Nutrition*, **32**, 540–9.

Melton III, L.J. (1990) Fluoride in the prevention of osteoporosis and fractures. *J Bone Miner Res* **5** (Suppl 1): s163–7.

Mitchell, H.H. (1939) The dietary requirements of calcium and its significance. In: *Actualites Scientifiques et Industrielles 18*, (ed. Mitchell, H.H.), Hermann and Company, Paris.

Murphy, S., Khaw, K-T., May, H. and Compston, J.E. (1994) Milk consumption and bone mineral density in middle aged and elderly women. *Br Med J* **308**, 933–41.

Nagant de Deuxchaisnes, C. and Krane, S.M.

(1978) Hypoparathyroidism. In: *Metabolic Bone Disease*, (eds Avioli, L.V. and Krane, S.M.), Academic Press, New York, pp. 218–445.

National Institutes of Health (1984) Osteoporosis: consensus conference. *J Am Med Assoc* **252**: 799–802.

National Institutes of Health (1994) Optimal calcium intake: NIH Consensus Statement. *Nutrition* **12:** 1–31.

National Osteoporosis Society (1990). Calcium. In: *Recommended Daily Allowances*, NOS, Bath.

Nichols, L. and Nimalesuriya, A. (1939) Adaptation to a low calcium intake in reference to the calcium requirements of a tropical population. *J Nutrition* **18**, 563–77.

Nilas, L., Christiansen, C. and Rodbro, P. (1984) Calcium supplementation and postmenopausal bone loss. *Br Med J* **289**: 1103–6.

Nilsson, B.E. and Westlin, N.E. (1971) Bone density in athletes. *Clin Orthop* **77**, 179–82.

Nordin, B.E.C. (1960) Osteoporosis and calcium deficiency. *Proc Nutrition Soc* **19**, 129–37.

Nordin, B.E.C. (1962) Calcium balance and calcium requirement in spinal osteoporosis. *Am J Clin Nutrition* **10**: 384–90.

Nordin, B.E.C. (1966) International patterns of osteoporosis. *Clin Orthop* **45**: 17–30.

Nordin, B.E.C. (1976) Nutritional considerations. In: *Calcium, Phosphate and Magnesium Metabolism*, (ed. Nordin, B.E.C.), Churchill Livingston, Edinburgh, pp. 1–35.

Nordin, B.E.C. and Heaney, R.P. (1990) Calcium supplementation of the diet: justified by the present evidence. *Br Med J* **300**: 1056–9.

Nordin, B.E.C. and Marshall, D.H. (1988) Dietary requirements for calcium. In: *Calcium in Human Biology*, (ed. Nordin, B.E.C.), Springer, Berlin, pp. 447–71.

Nordin, B.E.C. and Morris, H.A. (1989) The calcium deficiency model for osteoporosis. *Nutrition Rev* **47**: 65–72.

Nordin, B.E.C. and Need, A.G. (1989) The rationale for calcium therapy in the prevention and treatment of osteoporosis. *Triangle* **28** (Suppl 1): 49–56.

Nordin, B.E.C., Horsman, A., Crilly, R.G., Marshall, D.H. and Simpson, M. (1980) Treatment of spinal osteoporosis in postmenopausal women. *Br Med J* **280**: 451–4.

Nordin, B.E.C., Polley, K.Y., Need, A.G., Morris, H.A. and Marshall, D. (1987) The problem of calcium requirement. *Am J Clin Nutrition* **45**: 1295–304.

Nordin, B.E.C., Need, A.G., Chatterton, B.E. Horowitz, M. and Cleghorn, D.B. (1990) Bone density screening for osteoporosis. *Lancet* **336**: 1327–8.

Ohlson, M.A., Brewer, W.D., Jackson, L. *et al.* (1952) Intakes and retention of nitrogen, calcium and phosphorus by 136 women between ages 30 and 85 years. *Federation Proc* **11:** 775–83.

Orimo, H., Shiraki, M., Hayashi, T. and Nakamura, T. (1987) Reduced occurrence of vertebral crush fractures in senile osteoporosis treated with 1α(OH)-vitamin D_3. *Bone Mineral* **3**: 47–52.

Ott, S.M. and Chesnut, C.H. (1987) Calcitriol treatment in patients with postmenopausal osteoporosis. In: *Osteoporosis*, (eds Christiansen, C., Johansen, J.S. and Riis, B.J.) Osteopress ApS, Copenhagen, pp. 884–9.

Ott, S.M. and Chesnut, C.H. (1989) Calcitriol treatment is not effective in postmenopausal osteoporosis. *Ann Intern Med* **110**: 267–74.

Outhouse, J., Breiter, H., Rutherford, E. *et al.* (1941) The calcium requirement of man: balance studies on seven adults. *J Nutrition* **21**: 566–75.

Parfitt, A.M. (1980) Morphological basis of bone mineral measurements: transient and steady state effects of treatment in osteoporosis. *Mineral Electrolyte Metab* **4**, 273–87.

Parfitt, A.M. (1983) The physiologic and clinical significance of bone histomorphometric data. In: *Bone Histomorphometry Techniques*, (ed. Recker, R.), CRC Press, Boca Raton, pp. 143–223.

Peacock, M. (1991) Estimates for requirement of calcium in growth and development. In: *Nutritional Aspects of Osteoporosis*, (eds Burkhardt, P. and Heaney, R.P.), Serono Symposium Publications, Raven Press, New York, pp. 49–65.

Pettifor, J.M., Ross, P., Moodley, G. and Shuenyane, E. (1981) The effect of dietary calcium supplementation on serum calcium, phosphorus and alkaline phosphatase concentrations in a rural black population. *Am J Clin Nutrition* **34**, 2187–91.

Pettifor, J.M., Marie, P.J., Sly, M.R. *et al.* (1984) The effect of differing dietary calcium and phosphorus contents on mineral metabolism and bone histomorphometry in young vitamin D-replete baboons. *Calcif Tissue Int* **36**, 668–76.

Recker, R.R. and Heaney, R.D. (1985) The effect of milk supplements on calcium metabolism, bone metabolism and calcium balance. *Am J Clin Nutrition* **41**, 254–63.

Recker, R.R., Saville, P.D. and Heaney, R.P. (1977) Effect of estrogens and calcium carbonate on bone loss in postmenopausal women. *Ann Intern Med* **87**, 649–55.

Recker, R.R., Kimmel, D.B., Hinders, S. and Davies, K.M. (1994) Antifracture efficacy of calcium in elderly women. *J Bone Miner Res* **9** (Suppl 1): S154.

Reid, I.R., Evans, R.W., Gamble, G.D. and Sharpe, S.J. (1995) Long-term effects of calcium supplementation on bone loss and fractures in postmenopausal women. A randomised controlled trial. *Am J Med* **98**, 331–5.

Riggs, B.L., (1986) Involutional osteoporosis. *N Engl J Med* **314**: 1676–86.

Riggs, B.L., Kelly, P.J., Kinney, V.R., Scholz, D.A. and Bianco, A.J. (1967) Calcium deficiency in osteoporosis: observations in one hundred sixty-six patients and critical review of the literaure. *J Bone Joint Surg* (Am) **49**, 915–24.

Riggs, B.L., Seeman, E., Hodgson, S.F., Taves, D.R. and O'Fallon, W.M. (1982) Effect of the fluoride/calcium regimen on vertebral fracture occurrence in postmenopausal osteoporosis. Comparison with conventional therapy. *N Engl J Med* **306**, 446–50.

Riggs, B.L., Wahner, H.W., Melton III, L.J. *et al.* (1987) Dietary calcium intake and rates of bone loss in women. *J Clin Invest* **80**: 979–82.

Roberts, P.H., Kerr, C.H. and Ohlson, M.A. (1948) Nutritional status of older women. *J Am Diet Assoc* **24**: 292–9.

Robinson, C.J. (1987) The importance of calcium intake in preventing osteoporosis. *Int Med* **12** (Suppl), 28–9.

Ross, P.D., Wasnich, R.D., MacLean, C.J. and Vogel, J.M. (1987) Prediction of individual lifetime fracture expectancy using bone mineral measurements. In: *Osteoporosis*, (eds Christiansen, C., Johansen, and J.S., Riis, B.J.), Osteopress, Copenhagen, pp. 288–93.

Ross, P.D., Davis, J.W., Epstein, R.S. and Wasnich, R.D. (1991) Pre-existing fractures and bone mass predict vertebral fracture incidence in women. *Ann Intern Med* **114**: 919–23.

Sandler, R.B., Slemendra, C.W. and LaPorte, R.E. (1985) Postmenopausal bone density and milk consumption in childhood and adolescence. *Am J Clin Nutrition* **42**, 270–4.

Schaafsma, G. (1992) The scientific basis of recommended dietary allowances for calcium. *J Intern Med* **231**, 187–94.

Sherman, H.C. (1920) Calcium requirements of maintenance in man. *J Biol Chem* **44**, 21–7.

Sherman, H.C. (1937) *Chemistry of Food and Nutrition*, 5th edn. Macmillan, New York.

Smith, D.A., Anderson, J.J.B., Aitken, J.M. and Shimmins, J. (1975) The effects of calcium supplements of the diet on bone mass measurements. In: *Calcium Metabolism, Bone and Metabolic Bone Disease*, (eds Kuhlencordt, F. and Kruse, H.P.), Springer, Berlin, pp. 278–82.

Smith, D.M., Nance, W.E., Kang, K.W., Christian, J.C. and Johnston, C.C. (1973) Genetic factors in determining bone mass. *J Clin Invest* **52**: 2800–8.

Smith, E.L. and Raab, D.M. (1986) Osteoporosis and physical activity. *Acta Med Scand* **711** (Suppl), 149–56.

Smith, E.L., Reddan, W. and Smith, P.E. (1981) Physical activity and calcium modalities for bone mineral increase in aged women. *Med Sci Sports Exerc* **13**, 60–4.

Smith, R.W. and Frame, B. (1965) Concurrent axial and appendicular osteoporosis. Its relation to calcium consumption. *N Engl J Med* **273**, 73–8.

Smith, R.W. and Rizek, J. (1966) Epidemiological studies of osteoporosis in women of Puerto Rico and Southwest Michigan with special reference to age, race, nationality and other associated findings. *Clin Orthop* **45**, 31–48.

Steggerda, F.R. and Mitchell, H.H. (1946) Variability in the calcium metabolism and calcium requirements of adult human subjects. *J Nutrition* **31**, 407–22.

Stepán, J.J., Pospichal, J., Presl, J. and Pacovsky, V. (1987) Bone loss and biochemical indices of bone remodelling in surgically induced postmenopausal women. *Bone* **8**: 279–84.

Stepán, J.J., Pospichal, J., Presl, J. and Pacovsky, V. (1989) Hydroxyapatite compound in surgically induced postmenopausal women. *Bone* **10**: 179–85.

Stevenson, J.C., Whitehead, M.I., Padwick, M. *et al.* (1988) Dietary intake of calcium and postmenopausal bone loss. *Br Med J* **297**: 15–17.

Stevenson, J.C., Lees, B., Cust, M.P. and Ganger, K.F. (1989) Determinants of bone density in normal women: risk factors for future osteoporosis. *Br Med J* **298**: 924–8.

Stevenson, J.C., Kanis, J.A. and Christiansen, C. (1992) Bone density measurement. *Lancet* **339**: 370–1.

Tigerstedt, R. (1911) Zur Kenntnis der Aschebestandteile in der frei gewahlten Kost des

Menschen. *Skandinavisches Archiv fur Physiologie* **24**, 97–112.

Tilyard, N.W., Spears, G.F.S., Thomson, J. and Dovey, S. (1992) Treatment of postmenopausal osteoporosis with calcitriol or calcium. *N Engl J Med* **326**: 357–62.

Truswell, A.S., Irwin, T., Beaton, G.H. *et al.* (1983) Recommended dietary intake around the world. *Nutrition Abstr Rev* **53**: 939–1015.

Van Beresteijn, E.C.H., van t'Hof, M.A., de Waard, H., Raymakers, J.A. and Duursma, S.A. (1990) Relation of axial bone mass to habitual calcium intake and to cortical bone loss in healthy early postmenopausal women. *Bone* **11**: 7–13.

Wasnich, R.D., Ross, P.D., Davis, J.W. and Vogel, J.M. (1989) A comparison of single and multisite BMC measurements for assessment of spine fracture probability. *J Nucl Med* **30**: 1166–71.

Weaver, C.M., Martin, R.H. and Heaney, R.P. (1991) Calcium absorption from foods. In: *Nutritional Aspects of Osteoporosis*, (eds Burkhardt, P. and Heaney, R.P.), Serono Symposium Publications, Raven Press, New York, pp. 133–9.

Whedon, G.D. (1959) Effects of high calcium intakes on bone, blood, and soft tissue; relationship of calcium intake to balance in osteoporosis. *Federation Proc* **18**: 1112–18.

Wickham, C.A.C., Walsh, K., Cooper, C. *et al.* (1989) Dietary calcium, physical activity and risk of hip fracture: a prospective study. *Br Med J* **299**: 889–92.

Yano, K., Heilbrun, L.K., Wasnich, R.D., Hankin, J. and Vogel, J.M. (1985) The relationship between diet and bone mineral content of multiple skeletal sites in elderly Japanese-American men and women living in Hawaii. *Am J Clin Nutrition* **42**: 877–88.

VITAMIN D TREATMENT IN OSTEOPOROSIS AND OSTEOMALACIA

12

J.C. Gallagher

INTRODUCTION

Vitamin D has a long history of use in the treatment of osteoporosis after early studies found that it increased calcium absorption, but few trials of vitamin D have actually been carried out in osteoporotics. In fact, much more information has been collected on the effects of vitamin D metabolites or analogs in the treatment of osteoporosis. Before discussing the therapeutic effects of vitamin D, it may be helpful to review the metabolism of vitamin D and its interaction with calcium absorption.

VITAMIN D METABOLISM

It is now recognized that vitamin D is both a hormone and a vitamin (DeLuca, 1988). The prohormone vitamin D_3 is produced in skin through the effect of ultraviolet light (UV-B) and transported to the liver where it is hydroxylated to 25-hydroxyvitamin D_3 (25-OHD_3), which in turn is hydroxylated in the kidney to form 1,25-dihydroxyvitamin D_3 (1,25$(OH)_2D_3$), the hormonally active form. Its production in the kidney is closely regulated by parathyroid hormone and serum phosphate. 1,25$(OH)_2D$ functions like a steroid hormone by binding to specific receptors and initiating gene transcription of different proteins (Baker *et al.*, 1988). It has a number of specific actions on mineral metabolism and on the hematopoietic system and less well-defined effects on many other tissues in the body. Some of the specific actions relating to mineral metabolism are its binding to specific receptors in the intestine and generation of calcium-binding proteins which increase calcium absorption (Desplan *et al.*, 1983). 1,25$(OH)_2D$ binds to specific receptors in bone cells and stimulates osteoblasts to make osteocalcin, specific protein involved in bone mineralization (Lian *et al.*, 1989) and it is involved in the differentiation of stem cells in the marrow, increasing the formation of osteoclasts which are involved in bone resorption (Roodman *et al.*, 1985). 1,25$(OH)_2D$ is involved in the differentiation of cells in the hematopoietic system (Tanaka *et al.*, 1982) in T and B cell lymphocyte function (Manolagas *et al.*, 1985) and in inhibiting proliferation of cancer cells (Colston *et al.*, 1981) or epidermal cells, as occurs in psoriasis (Smith *et al.*, 1986). If all of the 1,25$(OH)_2D$ could be supplied through the action of UV light, then vitamin D could be classified as a hormone but, as will be apparent from the discussion later on, one cannot live by UV light alone, especially in northern areas of the world, and so there is a need for dietary intake of vitamin D, thus fulfilling the definition of a vitamin.

Osteoporosis. Edited by John C. Stevenson and Robert Lindsay. Published in 1998 by Chapman & Hall, London. ISBN 0 412 48870 1

Vitamin D_3 (cholecalciferol) is produced in skin when ultraviolet (UV-B) light converts 7-dehydrocholesterol (provitamin D_3) to pre-vitamin D_3 and then vitamin D_3 in the epidermis (Holick *et al.*, 1980). The skin production of vitamin D varies with the season (Webb *et al.*, 1988), the time of the day when UV light is effective on skin synthesis (Webb *et al.*, 1988) amount of skin pigmentation (Clemens *et al.*, 1982a), clothing, sunscreen applications (Matsuoka *et al.*, 1987) and aging (Maclaughlin and Holick, 1985; Holick *et al.*, 1989). Vitamin D_3 formed in skin has a short half-life of about 24 hours and because it is markedly influenced by the factors mentioned above (Clemens *et al.*, 1982b), serum vitamin D is not the best measurement of vitamin D status. The other main source of vitamin D is the diet. Either vitamin D_2 (ergocalciferol) or D_3 (cholecalciferol) can be ingested in the diet. The major dietary sources of vitamin D are fish (sardines, salmon, cod), liver and egg yolk. In the USA and in Scandinavia, dairy products are supplemented with vitamin D and each quart of milk is fortified with 400 IU of either vitamin D_2 or D_3, but in other countries milk is not usually supplemented. For this reason the dietary intake of vitamin D in supplemented countries should be higher than in most other countries.

Vitamin D derived from skin or diet is transported to the liver and converted to 25-OHD. Because 25-OHD has a much longer half-life of 3–4 weeks, the serum levels remain fairly constant and serum 25-OHD is the measurement of choice when assessing the nutritional status of the individual (Davie *et al.*, 1982). Usually in younger subjects, serum 25-OHD level ranges from 10 to 50 ng/ml but it depends on the time of the year when the sample is taken. 25-OHD probably is not physiologically active at these normal concentrations, but is converted in the kidney to the active metabolite $1,25(OH)_2D$. Usually serum $1,25(OH)_2D$ level averages 35 pg/ml but it ranges from 25 to 50 pg/ml (Hollis, 1986). Serum $1,25(OH)_2D$ is stable throughout the year and is not affected by vitamin D deficiency until the serum 25-OHD level decreases to less than 10 ng/ml (Bouillon *et al.*, 1987; Lips *et al.*, 1987).

CALCIUM ABSORPTION: EFFECTS OF DIETARY CALCIUM, $1,25(OH)_2D$ AND AGE

One of the major target organs for $1,25(OH)_2D$ is the intestine where it binds to a specific receptor and initiates gene transcription of calbindin-D, a calcium-binding protein correlated closely with stimulation of calcium absorption. When calcium intake is low, there is an increase of parathyroid hormone (PTH) secretion which stimulates increases in the renal production of $1,25(OH)_2D$ and calcium absorption (Gallagher *et al.*, 1979). When calcium intake is high, serum PTH and $1,25(OH)_2D_3$ production are both suppressed, leading to a decrease in calcium absorption. Typically, on a low-calcium diet the amount of calcium absorbed is about 40% whereas on a high-calcium intake this decreases to about 10%. This variation in calcium absorption on low- and high-level calcium intakes is a physiologic process known as adaptation which is hormonally controlled by PTH and $1,25(OH)_2D$ (Figure 12.1). Calcium absorption decreases with aging in normal people (Alevizaki *et al.*, 1965; Avioli *et al.*, 1965; Bullamore *et al.*, 1970; Gallagher *et al.*, 1979).

A variety of techniques have been used to demonstrate the decrease in calcium absorption, the most common method being radiocalcium absorption tests. When calcium absorption is measured with a small carrier load such as 20 mg, the results show that calcium absorption remains normal until age 65 and then decreases with each decade (Bullamore *et al.*, 1970). When larger amounts of calcium are used in the absorption test, such as 250 mg, the decrease in calcium absorption appears to be linear from age 40.

Measurement of calcium absorption using a

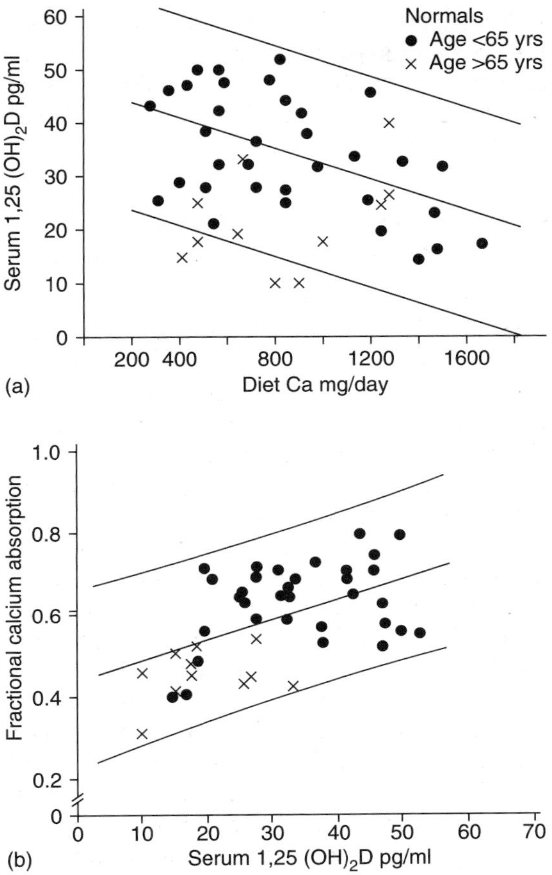

Figure 12.1 (a) Relationship between calcium intake and dietary calcium intake in normal women. Elderly women have a lower serum $1,25(OH)_2D$ relative to the calcium intake. (b) Relationship between calcium absorption and serum $1,25(OH)_2D_3$ in normal women. Solid lines represent mean ± 95% confidence limits.

metabolic balance technique shows a decrease in calcium absorption from about age 60 (Nordin *et al.*, 1976), but one study of absorption of calcium 44 from meals showed no change with age (Eastell *et al.*, 1991). It is likely that these different results provide information on different aspects of calcium absorption (Reeve *et al.*, 1980). Using an intestinal lavage technique, Sheikh *et al.* (1988) found that with a low-calcium meal (120 mg), all of the calcium transport was mediated by an active transport process, but with a larger (300 mg) calcium load both active and passive transport systems were involved.

A number of different studies have looked at the effect of age on serum $1,25(OH)_2D$, but the results have not always been in agreement, some studies reporting decreased levels with aging (Gallagher *et al.*, 1979; Manolagas *et al.*, 1983; Fujisawa *et al.*, 1984; Peacock and Hordon, 1989; Quesada *et al.*, 1992) and others reporting normal levels up to age 65 and then a decline (Epstein *et al.*, 1986; Eastell *et al.*, 1991). What seems to be the most important factor determining production of $1,25(OH)_2D_3$ with aging is the degree of renal function (Francis *et al.*, 1984a). Serum $1,25(OH)_2D$ levels are reduced in subjects with decreased renal function (Francis *et al.*, 1984a), are very low in patients with end-stage chronic renal failure and are undetectable in anephric patients (Reinhardt *et al.*, 1984). The aging kidney shows a reduced response to stimulation with parathyroid hormone (Tsai *et al.*, 1984; Kinyamu *et al.*, 1996) and this may account for lower serum $1,25(OH)_2D$ in the elderly. However, without the development of age-related secondary hyperparathyroidism (Gallagher *et al.*, 1980), it is possible that serum $1,25(OH)_2D$ would be even lower. Some elderly subjects, however, have been found to have malabsorption of calcium with normal levels of serum $1,25(OH)_2D$ (Gallagher *et al.*, 1979; Francis *et al.*, 1984b). This finding could be explained by a decline in the vitamin D receptor concentration in the intestine with age, as reported by one group (Ebeling *et al.*, 1992) but not confirmed by others (Kinyamu *et al.*, 1995) or by some other impairment of the calcium transport system.

CALCIUM ABSORPTION IN OSTEOPOROTICS

Patients with osteoporosis usually exhibit a more severe decrease in calcium absorption than age-matched controls. A number of studies have shown that 50–70% of patients with type I postmenopausal osteoporosis with vertebral fractures have marked impairment of calcium absorption (Caniggia *et al.*, 1963; Gallagher *et al.*, 1973, 1979; Nordin *et al.*, 1980; Francis *et al.*, 1984a). Many of these patients have reduced levels of serum $1,25(OH)_2D$ (Gallagher *et al.*, 1979; Lawoyin *et al.*, 1980; Lund *et al.*, 1982; Caniggia *et al.*, 1984; Aloia *et al.*, 1985), but some have normal levels with malabsorption of calcium (Gallagher *et al.*, 1979; Francis *et al.*, 1984b; Eastell *et al.*, 1991; Ebeling *et al.*, 1992). It has been hypothesized that the cause of low serum $1,25(OH)_2D$ and malabsorption of calcium in patients with type I postmenopausal osteoporosis is due to lower PTH levels caused by increased bone resorption and a slightly higher serum calcium (Riggs and Melton, 1986). In those patients with malabsorption and a normal serum $1,25(OH)_2D$, the primary defect must be in the non-D-mediated control of calcium transport in the gut. This 'resistance' in the gut of younger women with vertebral osteoporosis may be similar to that described above in some elderly people aged 75+. In one study, osteoporotics with low calcium absorption were matched to controls with similar absorption and treated with oral synthetic 25-OHD_3. Although the increase in serum $1,25(OH)_2D_3$ after 25-OHD_3 administration was similar in both groups, calcium absorption increased more in controls than osteoporotics (Francis *et al.*, 1984b). However, treatment with oral $1,25(OH)_2D_3$ always normalizes absorption (Gallagher *et al.*, 1982), perhaps because oral administration has a first-pass effect on the gut.

VITAMIN D DEFICIENCY

Vitamin D deficiency develops when serum 25-OHD falls below the normal range of 37.5 nmol/l (15 ng/ml). During the initial stage of vitamin D deficiency, mild hypocalcemia leads to secondary hyperparathyroidism. As the degree of osteomalacia progresses, there is an increase in the amount of bone that is unmineralized. Eventually, with severe vitamin D deficiency, the amount of unmineralized bone surface may be as much as 80–90% of the total surface (normal is less than 25%). It is not clear what level of serum 25-OHD is associated with histological evidence of osteomalacia but it is probably less than 25 nmol/l (10 ng/ml) and decreased mineralization of bone becomes more severe with decreasing levels of serum 25-OHD.

SEASONAL CHANGES IN SERUM 25-OHD

Several studies in Europe, North America and Japan in all age groups have shown lower levels of serum 25-OHD in late winter and early spring and higher values in late summer and autumn (Lester *et al.*, 1977; Somerville *et al.*, 1977; Lawson *et al.*, 1979; Stryd *et al.*, 1979; Poskitt *et al.*, 1979; Devgun *et al.*, 1981; Omdahl *et al.*, 1982; Kobayashi *et al.*, 1983; Dattani *et al.*, 1984; Corless *et al.*, 1985; McKenna *et al.*, 1985; Davies *et al.*, 1986; Sowers *et al.*, 1986; Gibson *et al.*, 1986; Chapuy *et al.*, 1987; Bouillon *et al.*, 1987; Lips *et al.*, 1987, 1988; Egsmose, 1987; Toss *et al.*, 1988; Delvin *et al.*, 1988; Krall *et al.*, 1989; Aksnes *et al.*, 1989; Himmelstein *et al.*, 1990; Webb *et al.*, 1990; Sherman *et al.*, 1990; Honkanen *et al.*, 1990; Quesada *et al.*, 1992). In younger people aged 30–60 years living in the USA, serum 25-OHD increased from 32 to 77 nmol/l (13 to 31 ng/ml) between winter and summer (Stryd *et al.*, 1979). In a study of gardeners in Scotland serum 25-OHD increased seasonally from 42 to 82 nmol/l (17 to 33 ng/ml) (Devgun *et al.*, 1981). In Japan, young subjects increased seasonally from 40 to 70 nmol/l (16 to 28 ng/ml) (Kobayashi *et al.*, 1983). In Belgium a study of young volunteers showed seasonal increases in serum 25-OHD from 52 to 67 nmol/l (21 to 27 ng/ml) (Bouillon *et al.*, 1987). Although serum 25-OHD for young subjects is often quoted as 50 to 125 nmol/l (20–50 ng/ml), this range probably reflects the time of the year that blood was collected. These studies in younger people show that serum 25-OHD is consistently lower in winter/spring than in the summer/autumn, with average serum 25-OHD increasing seasonally from 42 to 72 nmol/l (17 to 29 ng/ml).

In the elderly, serum 25-OHD shows a smaller seasonal increase than in younger people (Lester *et al.*, 1977; Somerville *et al.*, 1977; Lawson *et al.*, 1979; Stryd *et al.*, 1979; Poskitt *et al.*, 1979; Devgun *et al.*, 1981 Omdahl *et al.*, 1982; Kobayashi *et al.*, 1983; Dattani *et al.*, 1984; Corless *et al.*, 1985; McKenna *et al.*, 1985; Davies *et al.*, 1986; Sowers *et al.*, 1986; Gibson *et al.*, 1986; Chapuy *et al.*, 1987; Bouillon *et al.*, 1987; Lips *et al.*, 1987, 1988; Egsmose *et al.*, 1987; Toss *et al.*, 1988; Delvin *et al.*, 1988; Krall *et al.*, 1989; Aksnes *et al.*, 1989; Himmelstein *et al.*, 1990; Webb *et al.*, 1990; Sherman *et al.*, 1990; Honkanen *et al.*, 1990) (Figure 12.2). In the studies cited above, the average serum 25-OHD level increased from 20 nmol/l in winter/spring to 32 nmol/l in summer (8 to 12 ng/ml), although the seasonal change may be underestimated if blood testing is not done at the peak. In a study of several hundred elderly people in England, Dattani *et al.* (1984) found a larger seasonal increase from 25 to 47 nmol/l (10 to 19 ng/ml). They also showed a larger seasonal change in serum 25-OHD in 65-year-old men and women compared to 90-year-old subjects. Elderly subjects who are not functionally independent and live in long-term care facilities may have even lower serum 25-OHD values, ranging from 8 to 22 nmol/l (4 to 8 ng/ml) (Devgun *et al.*, 1981; Corless *et al.*, 1985; McKenna *et al.*, 1985; Davies *et al.*, 1986; Bouillon *et al.*, 1987; Lips *et al.*, 1987, 1988; Chapuy *et al.*, 1987).

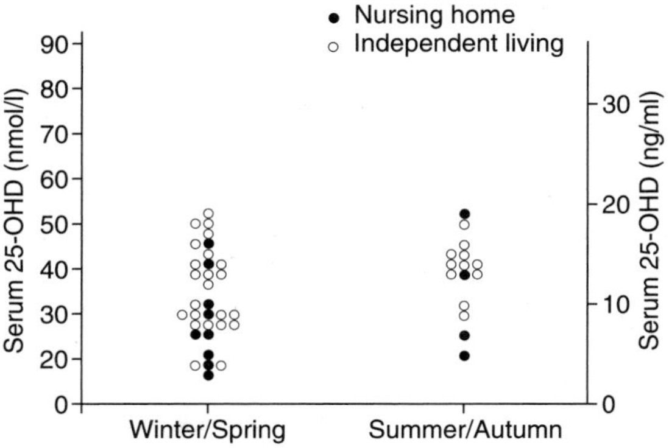

Figure 12.2 Seasonal changes in serum 25-OHD in elderly male and female subjects, some living independently at home and others in a nursing home.

There are a number of different reasons for the seasonal change in vitamin D. In countries in the northern latitudes ultraviolet light is ineffective in producing vitamin D in winter because the angle of the sun is too low (<35°) to allow effective UV activation of skin synthesis of 7-dihydrocholesterol and, as shown in Figure 12.3, UV-B light will only be effective for seven months of the year. Skin synthesis of vitamin D is reduced in the aging and less vitamin D is formed in the skin of the elderly compared to younger people after exposure to the same dose of UV light (Holick *et al.*, 1989). Also, elderly people have less exposure to the sun because they stay indoors more and clothing usually covers most of the skin when they go outside. When these factors are taken into account, it is likely that diet is the main contributor to a serum 25-OHD value of 15 nmol/l (6 ng/ml) in the elderly. In summer, if ultraviolet light increases the level of serum 25-OHD on average by another 9 ng/ml (Dattani *et al.*, 1984), then dietary vitamin D provides about 40% and UV exposure about 60% to the serum 25-OHD level. Interestingly, in a study of 32 adults who received 250 IU/day of vitamin D_2 through parenteral nutrition, Glenville Jones and colleagues (1979) calculated that D_2 contributed 25 nmol/l (10 ng/ml, i.e. 53%) to a total serum 25-OHD of 48 nmol/l (19 ng/ml) and skin synthesis produced 22 nmol/l (9 ng/ml, i.e. 47%). The amount of D_3 synthesized in skin was equivalent to a daily

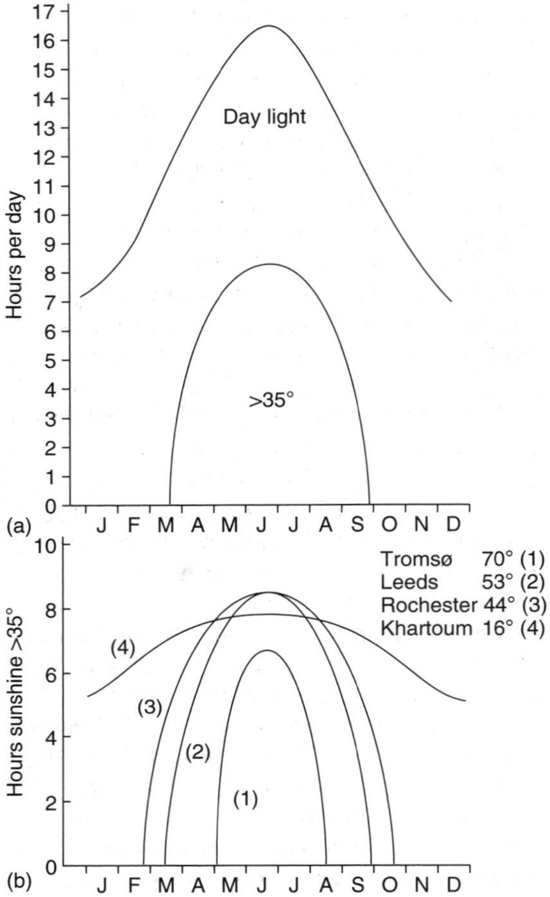

Figure 12.3 (a) Comparison of the hours of ultraviolet light available for skin synthesis of vitamin D (angle of sun >35° from horizontal) compared to hours of sunlight. (b) Available UV-B light for different cities: Tromso (Norway), Leeds (England), Rochester (Minnesota, USA) and Khartoum (Sudan).

dietary vitamin D intake of 177 IU in winter and 238 IU in summer.

A number of studies have demonstrated correlations between the dietary intake of vitamin D and serum 25-OHD (Lester *et al.*, 1977; Davies *et al.*, 1986; Sowers *et al.*, 1986; Gibson *et al.*, 1986; Lips *et al.*, 1987; Asknes *et al.*, 1989; Webb *et al.*, 1990). These results suggest that a daily dietary intake of 250 IU of vitamin D_2 is not enough to maintain a satisfactory 25-OHD level unless there is adequate exposure to UV light. It is difficult to say what a normal level of serum 25-OHD should be, but an estimate is 75–100 nmol/l (30–40 ng/ml).

EFFECT OF VITAMIN D SUPPLEMENTATION ON SERUM 25-HYDROXYVITAMIN D AND PARATHYROID HORMONE

Without bone histology it is not clear what exact level of serum 25-OHD is associated with vitamin D deficiency, although secondary hyperparathyroidism may provide some indication. However, a single measurement of PTH is not helpful clinically since the value in elderly subjects is often higher compared to younger people, especially if they have impaired renal function or malabsorption of calcium. Neither is a decrease in serum PTH following administration of vitamin D enough to support a diagnosis of vitamin D deficiency because of the direct effect of $1,25(OH)_2D$ on the parathyroid gland.

There have been several studies of the effects of vitamin D supplementation on serum 25-OHD in the elderly (Figure 12.4). Lips *et al.* (1988) completed a randomized study of vitamin D_3 400 IU in Dutch subjects,

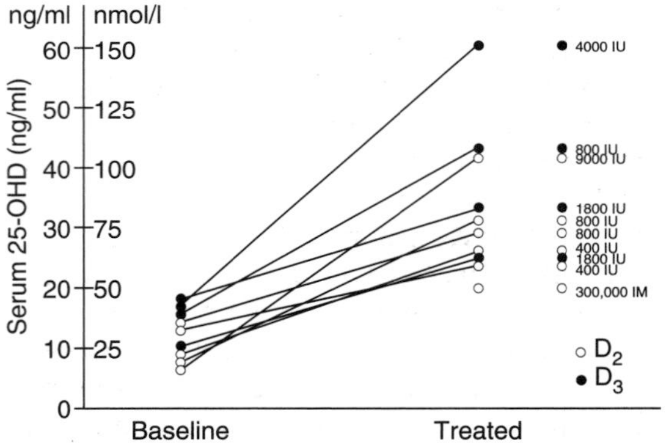

Figure 12.4 Effect of vitamin D_2 or D_3 on serum 25-OHD in elderly subjects.

age 84 years, from a nursing home and an old people's home. In the control group baseline serum 25-OHD was 22 nmol/l (9 ng/ml) and remained unchanged over one year. In the treated group serum 25-OHD increased from 22 to 40 nmol/l (9 to 16 ng/ml) and serum PTH was reduced by 15%. In two studies from France by Chapuy *et al.* (1987, 1992), administration of vitamin D_3 800 IU daily increased serum 24-OHD from 40 nmol/l (16 ng/ml) to 105 pmol/l (42 ng/ml) and serum PTH decreased by 48% after 18 months of treatment.

Taken together, these large studies support the concept that a value of serum 25-OHD below 40 nmol/l (16 ng/ml) leads to secondary hyperparathyroidism, increased bone resorption and fractures. This stage could be termed 'hypovitaminosis D', which may develop into more severe vitamin D deficiency associated with histological findings of osteomalacia. Since bone biopsies were not performed in these studies, it is uncertain whether these women had osteomalacia. In a study of hip fracture patients in England, bone histomorphometry showed increases in the percentage of osteoid surfaces and decreases in the percentage calcification front during early spring, but not in summer (Aaron *et al.*, 1974; Gallagher, 1976). Although serum 25-OHD was not measured in that study, later measurements of serum 25-OHD from another group of hip fracture patients in the same town showed very low levels (12.5 nmol/l [5 ng/ml]) (Hordon and Peacock, 1987). Hip fracture patients in Holland have also been shown to have very low serum 25-OHD levels of 20 nmol/l (8 ng/ml) (Lips *et al.*, 1987) and seasonal PTH increases in hip fracture patients have been found during the late winter and spring (Aaron *et al.*, 1974).

In a study from Denmark, 94 geriatric hospital inpatients aged 81 were found to have serum 25-OHD levels of 35 nmol/l (14 ng/ml) if mobile and 17 nmol/l (7 ng/ml) if bedridden (Egsmose *et al.*, 1987); 50% of the patients had values less than 12 nmol/l (5 ng/ml). Those supplemented with vitamin D had higher serum 25-OHD levels of 30 nmol/l (11.9 ng/ml) versus 17 nmol/l (7.0 ng/ml) if not supplemented. Another study from Finland showed that serum 25-OHD levels were 25 nmol/l (10 ng/ml) in institutionalized elderly subjects and 37.5 nmol/l (15 ng/ml) in independent living subjects (Honkanen *et al.*, 1990). After 11 weeks of treatment with 1800 IU of vitamin D_3, levels increased in the treated patients from 42 to 77 nmol/l (17 to 31 ng/ml) in those living at home and from 25 to 65 nmol/l (10 to 26 ng/ml) in the inpatients. Elderly subjects in Norway, aged 84 years, treated with vitamin D_2 400 IU/day had an increase in serum 25-OHD from 35 to 65 nmol/l (14 to 26 ng/ml) (Asknes *et al.*, 1989) and in France, 75-year-old inpatients given vitamin D_2 800 IU daily, showed levels increased from 22 to 60 nmol/l (9 to 24 ng/ml) (Chapuy *et al.*, 1987). In a study from England, 302 subjects (average age 82 years) given vitamin D_2 9000 IU daily demonstrated increased serum 25 hydroxyvitamin D from 17 to 106 nmol/l (7 to 42 ng/ml) after nine months of treatment (Corless *et al.*, 1985).

There is insufficient information in the literature to determine whether one should use vitamin D_2 or D_3 in normal elderly subjects, although there may be differences in D_2 and D_3 metabolism in humans. Tjellesen *et al.* (1985) found a marked increase in total serum 25-OHD after administration of vitamin D_3 to epileptics on tegretol but no change on vitamin D_2.

Oral administration of 25-hydroxyvitamin D3 has been used to increase serum 25-OHD levels. Bouillon *et al.* (1987) gave 10 μg/day after a loading dose of 200 μg and serum 25-hydroxyvitamin D increased from 42 to 89 nmol/l (17 to 36 ng/ml) in vitamin D-replete subjects and from 12 to 35 nmol/l (5 to 14 ng/ml) in deficient subjects. Francis *et al.* (1984b) treated elderly subjects with 40 μg for seven days and serum 25-OHD increased from about 12 to 50 nmol/l (5 to 20 ng/ml).

In view of the fact that seasonal vitamin D is in short supply in northern Europe, an RDA for vitamin D of 200 IU for elderly subjects appears insufficient. The fact that supplementation with vitamin D 400 IU per day increases serum 25-OHD to normal 60 nmol/l (24 ng/ml) and decreases serum parathyroid hormone in normal elderly people (Lips *et al.*, 1988) suggests that at least 500 IU (i.e. 400 IU from the supplement plus an average dietary intake 100 IU) per day provides minimally adequate 25-OHD levels. On vitamin D_3 800 IU daily, the average serum 25-OHD level increased to 42 ng/ml (Jones *et al.*, 1979). If dietary vitamin D is assumed to be 100 IU then these subjects received about 900 IU/day. The level of 42 ng/ml is higher than the average serum 25-OHD found in younger subjects of 80 nmol/l (32 ng/ml) in the USA and 25 ng/ml in northern Europe, so that a daily intake of 800 IU of vitamin D_3 may be higher than is necessary. The results suggest that a vitamin D supplement of 400 IU daily in addition to the diet may be enough to produce a normal serum 25-OHD level. On this basis, vitamin D supplementation of 40 IU in elderly subjects in Europe is sufficient to avoid vitamin D deficiency and is a more appropriate RDA than 200 IU daily, especially for elderly subjects at high risk.

VITAMIN D_2 OR D_3 TREATMENT IN TYPE I POSTMENOPAUSAL OSTEOPOROSIS

In a one-year study of bone histomorphometry in 18 osteoporotics in the USA (Riggs *et al.*, 1976) a group treated with 2.5 g calcium + vitamin D_2 400 IU daily were compared to a group receiving 1.5–2 g of calcium daily and 50 000 units of vitamin D_2 twice weekly (average 14 000 IU/day). In both groups, there was a significant decrease in bone resorption on the 3–4-month bone biopsies and a significant reduction in resorption and formation only in the group treated with the larger dose of vitamin D at the end of one year. Because serum PTH levels decreased significantly in both groups, it was suggested that the main effect of calcium and vitamin D therapy was to reduce bone turnover by reducing PTH secretion. This reduction in bone turnover could have been a transient effect, since it seems to occur with other antiresorptive therapies. In osteoporotics treated with varying doses of vitamin D, calcium absorption did not increase to normal in every patient given 1000 IU or 10 000 IU/day (Figure 12.5). Many required 10 000–40 000 IU/day to normalize absorption.

Longitudinal studies of the effect of vitamin D_2 on metacarpal cortical bone loss in English patients with type I postmenopausal osteoporosis showed that vitamin D_2 doses less than 10 000 IU/day were ineffective in preventing metacarpal cortical bone loss whereas doses of 20 000 IU/day prevented metacarpal bone loss (Nordin *et al.*, 1975). Further analysis showed that bone loss was only prevented in those patients in whom calcium absorption increased after vitamin D therapy. The fact that larger doses of vitamin D_2 were needed to increase calcium

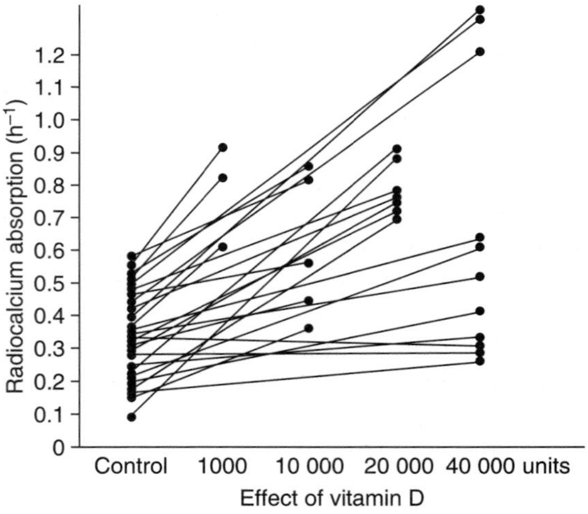

Figure 12.5 Dose response of vitamin D_2 on calcium absorption in postmenopausal osteoporosis (type I). 1 IU = 40 μg.

absorption supports the concept that there is a 'resistance' in the gut in osteoporotics. There have been no controlled studies of the effect of vitamin D_2 or D_3 on fracture incidence in patients with type I postmenopausal osteoporosis.

VITAMIN D_2 OR D_3 TREATMENT IN TYPE II SENILE OSTEOPOROSIS

Metacarpal bone loss was also measured in a study of 137 normal ambulatory elderly women aged 65–74 years, given either vitamin D_2 15 000 IU once a week (average 2100 IU/day) or placebo (Nordin *et al.*, 1985). Serum 25-hydroxyvitamin D increased in the treated group from 20 to 60 nmol/l (8 to 24 ng/ml). There was a small but significant increase in bone mass in the D-treated group and a decrease in the placebo group.

There have recently been two studies of the effect of vitamin D on fracture incidence in elderly patients with type II senile osteoporosis, but it is likely that many of the patients had vitamin D deficiency. One was a four-year randomized trial of 799 subjects in Finland, 480 outpatients living at home and 320 living in an old people's home (Heikinheimo *et al.*, 1992). Patients were at least 75 years old and many were over 85. They were randomized to treatment with an annual injection of vitamin D_2, 150 000 IU in the first year of the trial increased to 300 000 IU in subsequent years; the control group received no treatment. There was no difference in fracture incidence in male subjects between the treated and control groups. However, in females, there was a statistical decrease in fracture incidence in the vitamin D_2-treated group compared to the control group (18% versus 25% respectively), but the decrease occurred mainly in upper limb fractures and not in hip fractures.

In the second study, from France, 3270 ambulatory women, mean age 84 years, were randomized to treatment with calcium 1.2 g daily plus vitamin D_3 800 IU daily compared to placebo (Jones *et al.*, 1979). After a period of 18 months treatment, fractures occurred in 9.9% of the treated group compared to 15.1% in controls. There was a significant reduction in hip fracture incidence, occurring in 2.4% of the treated group compared to 4.2% in the control group. The results from the first 1.5 years of the study support the efficacy of vitamin D_2 or D_3 therapy in the prevention of bone loss and fractures in elderly people with vitamin D deficiency. In a recent update of the same study, the hip fracture incidence between 18 months and three years was the same as that of the control group (Meunier *et al.*, 1995).

So, the question of the long-term efficacy of this treatment in preventing fractures is questionable. Whether vitamin D_2 or D_3 has an important role in preventing bone loss and fractures in elderly subjects after vitamin D deficiency has been corrected is unproven. Biochemical measurements in subgroups showed that the mean serum 25-OHD increased after one year on treatment from 40 to 100 nmol/l (16 to 40 ng/ml) but remained similar in the control group at 32 to 27 nmol/l (13 to 11 ng/ml) and serum PTH decreased by 44% in the treated group. These low values, together with the elevated serum PTH, suggest that many of these patients had significant vitamin D deficiency with secondary hyperparathyroidism. The only ways that vitamin D could have reduced the fracture rate in this study would be by preventing falls or by reducing the number of stress fractures in the femoral neck that lead to spontaneous fractures. Other studies have shown that subjects who suffer hip fracture have a slower gait and fall more frequently (Seeley *et al.*, 1992). On the other hand, a double-blind randomized study of vitamin D_2 9000 IU daily in elderly English subjects showed no improvement in activities of daily living (ADL) or in tests of mental function after nine months of treatment (Corless *et al.*, 1985).

METABOLITES OR ANALOGS OF VITAMIN D IN OSTEOPOROSIS TREATMENT

DIHYDROTACHYSTEROL (DHT_2, DHT_3)

Dihydrotachysterol is a modified form of vitamin D_2 or D_3. Its chemical structure is similar to that of $1{,}25(OH)_2D$ except that it lacks the 25 hydroxyl group, which is attached once DHT passes through the liver. Because of its structural similarity to $1{,}25(OH)_2D$ it is active in anephric patients, but it is not as potent as 1α-OHD_3 or $1{,}25(OH)_2D_3$. It is about 1/400 as active as vitamin D in the antirachitic assay but when given in large doses, it is more potent than vitamin D in mobilizing calcium. Although DHT has been used in the past to treat renal osteodystrophy and hypoparathyroidism, its role in therapy is limited now that 1α-OHD_3 and $1{,}25(OH)_2D_3$ are available.

25-HYDROXYVITAMIN D_3 (25-OHD_3)

Synthetic 25-hydroxyvitamin D_3 has had limited evaluation in osteoporosis. In a study of osteoporotics given 50 μg of 25-OHD_3 for one year, calcium absorption increased in only half of the patients and remained low in the others. There was no increase in serum $1{,}25(OH)_2D$ and it is possible that those who did not increase absorption may have had impaired 1α-hydroxylase activity in the kidney (Zerwekh *et al.*, 1983). On the other hand, in another study, a group of osteoporotics matched for absorption with controls were given 40 μg daily of 25-OHD_3. Both groups showed a similar increase in serum $1{,}25(OH)_2D$ but osteoporotics had a smaller increase in calcium absorption than controls, suggesting that there could be resistance to $1{,}25(OH)_2D$ at the gut level (Francis *et al.*, 1984b). Another group of elderly women were given 25-OHD ranging in dose from 5 to 120 μg daily. Calcium absorption did not increase on 5–10 μg but showed increasing response with further increase in 25-OHD dose. Twenty micrograms produced a more physiologic increase in serum 25-OHD to 62 nmol/l (25 ng/ml) whereas 40 μg increased serum 25-OHD to 100 nmol/l (40 ng/ml) (Francis *et al.*, 1983).

Orwoll *et al.* (1989) compared the effects of 25-OHD_3 40 μg daily plus 1200 mg of calcium with 1200 mg calcium alone on bone histomorphometry and radial density in women over a period of two years. Many subjects had low levels of serum 25-OHD at baseline compatible with vitamin D deficiency. On treatment, serum 25-OHD increased into the supranormal range of 225 nmol/l (90 ng/ml), but serum $1{,}25(OH)_2D_3$ was unchanged. There was no difference in radial density between the two treated groups. The authors concluded that 25-OHD_3 may not be a suitable agent for the treatment of osteoporosis since it failed to increase serum $1{,}25(OH)_2D$ levels, but a lack of change in serum $1{,}25(OH)_2D_3$ is not unexpected because production of $1{,}25(OH)_2D$, which is a hormone, is tightly regulated.

24,25-DIHYDROXYVITAMIN D_3

Initial studies with this metabolite in osteoporosis using 2 μg daily showed an increase in calcium absorption and calcium balance after two weeks of treatment, but a return to baseline values after six months of treatment (Reeve *et al.*, 1982). In a study of early postmenopausal bone loss, women aged 50 were given either 10 μg daily of $24{,}25(OH)_2D_3$ or placebo for two years; no difference in bone density of the spine or radius was seen between the two groups (Riis *et al.*, 1986). In a three-year study of 131 osteoporotic patients, two doses of $24{,}25(OH)_2D_3$, 10 or 40 ug daily, were compared to a combination of 1α-OHD_3 plus $24{,}25(OH)_2D_3$ 10 μg daily or a placebo (Menczel *et al.*, 1991). There was a significant increase of 2.6%/year in radial density on 40 μg/day of $24{,}25(OH)_2D_3$ and a decrease of –2.6%/year in the placebo group.

This is the only positive study reported on this metabolite, but the dose used was much larger than that used previously. Further studies, perhaps with larger doses, are needed to answer fully the question of 24,25$(OH)_2$D efficacy in osteoporosis.

1α-HYDROXYVITAMIN D_3 (1α-OHD_3)

The first vitamin D analog to be used in the treatment of osteoporosis was 1α-hydroxy D_3 (1α-OHD_3). This compound was easier to synthesize than the natural metabolite 1,25$(OH)_2D_3$ and so became readily available. 1α-OHD_3 is absorbed intact through the intestine and then converted in the liver to 1,25$(OH)_2D_3$. Metabolic balance studies were performed with 1α-OHD_3 1–2 μg daily in patients with type I postmenopausal osteoporosis. Calcium balance studies showed that calcium absorption was not always normalized on 1 μg but always increased to normal on 2 μg/day (Marshall *et al.*, 1977). Urinary calcium excretion increased more on the larger dose and calcium balance improved on those patients given 2 μg/day, but was still slightly negative. When estrogen was combined with 1α-OHD_3, calcium balance improved and became positive in most of the patients on 2 μg and became positive in some of the patients on the 1 μg dose (Crilly *et al.*, 1980).

Krolner *et al.* (1980) gave 1α-OHD_3 0.5–1.0 μg daily to 21 osteoporotics in Denmark and found an increase of 5.5% in lumbar spine density after two years of treatment. In a Swedish study, 25 osteoporotics were treated for two years with 1α-OHD_3 1 μg/day plus calcium supplement and showed an increase in radial density (Lindholm *et al.*, 1981). In another study from Denmark, 22 osteoporotic patients were treated with 1α-OHD_3 1 μg/day and followed for five years. Spine density increased by 1% at two years and by 5% after five years of treatment. In these patients there was a significant increase in radial density during the first 24 months and then a return to baseline by the end of five years (Lund *et al.*, 1985).

In osteoporotic patients in Japan, 1α-OHD_3 has been used extensively. Shiraki *et al.* (1985) compared the effect of 1α-OHD_3 and 1,25$(OH)_2D_3$ in osteoporotics. Radial density increased or remained stable in the treated groups but decreased in the control group and patients on 1α-OHD_3 showed a slightly higher increase in radial density compared to patients on 1,25$(OH)_2D_3$. In a study from Belgium by Geusens and Dequeker (1986), 34 patients with osteoporosis were randomized to treatment with anabolic steroids or 1α-OHD_3 or to a calcium infusion treatment group. Patients on anabolic steroids and 1α-OHD_3 showed an increase in radial density compared to a decrease in the calcium-treated group; however, measurements on the metacarpal cortex were different and showed a decrease on 1α-OHD_3 or calcium and an increase on nandrolone.

In the most recent study from Japan 80 osteoporotic patients were randomly assigned to receive 1α-OHD_3 1 μg/day or placebo (Orimo, 1993). Measurement of spine density at the end of one year showed an increase of 0.65% in the treated group compared to a decrease of –1.14% in the placebo group. There were no significant differences in femoral neck density between the two groups, but trochanteric density increased by 4.2% in the treated group and decreased by 2.3% on placebo.

There have been two studies of the effect of 1α-OHD_3 on vertebral fracture rates in patients with osteoporosis. In a study from Japan, 86 patients with osteoporosis were treated with either 1α-OHD_3 1 μg/day, 1α-OHD_3 plus calcium or calcium 1000 mg/day (Orimo *et al.*, 1987). After one year, the vertebral fracture rate was 35% lower in the group given 1α-OHD_3 (330/1000 patient-years compared to 950/1000 patient-years in the control group) and was reduced by 85% to 150/1000 patient-years in the group treated with 1α-OHD_3 plus calcium. The better reduction in fracture incidence in the group given 1α-OHD_3 plus calcium can probably be explained by the very low calcium intake in Japan and 1α-OHD_3 needs a minimum dietary calcium for full effectiveness. In another study from Japan, 666 women were randomly assigned to 1α-OHD_3 1 μg/day or to a control group (Hayashi *et al.*, 1992). The vertebral fracture rate of 411/1000 patient-years in the 1α-OHD_3-treated group was significantly lower than that in the control group of 759/1000 patient-years. In summary, in both studies, the vertebral fracture rate was reduced by at least 50% in patients treated with 1α-OHD_3.

1α-HYDROXYVITAMIN D_2 (1α-OHD_2)

Preliminary work with 1α-OHD_2 treatment of type II osteoporosis has just started. In a dose-ranging study, 1α-OHD_2 was found to be well tolerated at doses of 3–5 μg daily (Gallagher *et al.*, 1994). At doses of 5 μg daily, hypercalciuria occurred in a significant proportion of patients, but hypercalcemia was uncommon and the average daily dose which maintained normal serum and urine calcium was 3.8 μg. Clinical trials of 1α-OHD_2 in osteoporosis are now in progress.

SYNTHETIC 1,25-DIHYDROXYVITAMIN D_3 (1,25$(OH)_2D_3$, ROCALTROL)

Since the discovery in the early 1970s that 1,25$(OH)_2D_3$ was the active metabolite responsible for the physiologic actions of vitamin D, there has been interest in the use of this agent for reversing malabsorption and improving calcium balance in patients with osteoporosis. The first metabolic study carried out in 1982 measured the effect of synthetic 1,25-dihydroxyvitamin D_3 or placebo on 0.5 μg daily on calcium balance, bone turnover and bone histomorphometry in type I postmenopausal osteoporotics (Aloia *et al.*, 1985). Calcium absorption increased on 1,25$(OH)_2D_3$ in every patient and calcium balance, which was initially negative, became positive. Radiocalcium kinetic studies and bone histomorphometry measurements of bone turnover showed a decrease in bone formation and resorption rate at six months, but an increase in bone turnover after two years.

In a separate study (Gallagher and Recker, 1985), 1,25$(OH)_2D_3$ was given at a high dose of 2 μg daily for six months and bone histomorphometry performed after six weeks and six months showed a significant increase in the bone formation rate (Figure 12.6). After 1,25$(OH)_2D_3$ was discontinued and patients were placed on calcium supplements for six months, subsequent biopsies showed a decrease in the bone formation rate (Figure 12.6). The effect of 1,25$(OH)_2D_3$ on the bone formation rate is in marked contrast to that of calcium supplements and suggests that 1,25$(OH)_2D_3$ has a direct effect on bone cells independent of its effect in increasing calcium and phosphate transport into bone.

In a study from Denmark patients with osteoporosis were randomly assigned to

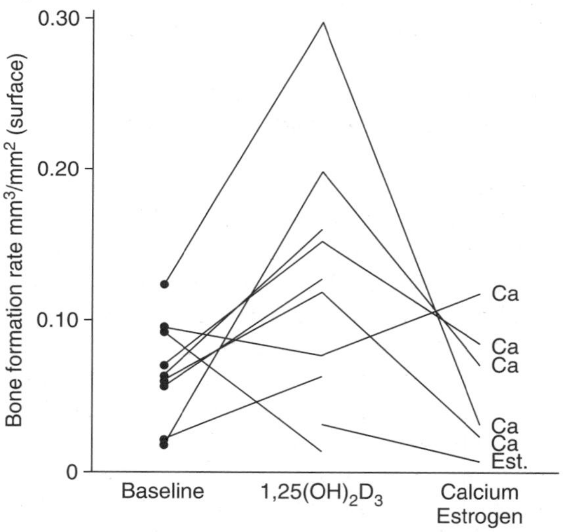

Figure 12.6 Comparison of the effect of synthetic 1,25$(OH)_2D_3$, 2 μg daily, with that of calcium supplements 1500 mg/day, on bone formation measured by histomorphometry. Adapted from Hayashi *et al.* (1992).

treatment with either estrogen alone or estrogen plus 1,25(OH)$_2$D$_3$ 0.5 µg/day and followed for two years. There was an increase in radial density on the combined therapy compared to a decrease of 1% in the group treated with estrogen (Lund *et al.*, 1984). In a study of osteoporosis in patients in Italy, a high dose of 1,25(OH)$_2$D$_3$ 1 µg daily was administered only to patients with decreased calcium absorption. After three years of treatment, calcium absorption was normalized and there were increases in radial density and total body calcium (Caniggia *et al.*, 1990, 1993).

In three similar double-blind randomized studies carried out in the USA by Aloia *et al.* (1988), Gallagher and Goldgar (1990) and Ott and Chesnut (1989), 1,25(OH)$_2$D$_3$ was administered to patients with type I postmenopausal osteoporosis. Both treated and control groups were also given vitamin D$_3$ 400 IU/day. In these studies the dose of 1,25(OH)$_2$D$_3$ was titrated upwards to the point of toxicity (hypercalciuria or hypercalcemia) and then maintained just below the dose that produced toxicity. In the study by Aloia *et al.*, the final dose of 1,25(OH)$_2$D$_3$ averaged 0.8 µg daily and in the study by Gallagher and Goldgar, the final dose averaged 0.62 µg daily. In both of these studies there were significant increases in bone mineral density of the spine and total body calcium. In the third study, by Ott and Chesnut, the average maintenance dose of 1,25(OH)$_2$D 0.43 µg/day was lower and no significant difference was seen in total body calcium or spine density between the treated and control group. In a subsequent analysis, Ott and Chesnut (1990) showed that the changes in spine density and total body calcium in the treated group were dose related and that patients given higher doses of 1,25(OH)$_2$D$_3$ (>0.5 µg/day) showed increases in spine density. This reanalysis supports the other studies in which higher doses of 1,25(OH)$_2$D$_3$ (0.8 and 0.67 µg daily) were effective.

There have been a small number of other types of studies which showed no efficacy. A study of women with Colles fractures with or without vertebral fractures showed similar decreases in radial density in the groups given either 1,25(OH)$_2$D$_3$ 0.5 µg daily or placebo (Falch *et al.*, 1987). In a study of normal 70-year-old patients without fractures, in whom the average treatment dose of 1,25(OH)$_2$D$_3$ was only 0.39 µg daily, Jensen *et al.* (1982) found a decrease in ultradistal radial density on 1,25(OH)$_2$D$_3$ similar to that in the control group and an increase in an estrogen-treated group. A small study of 14 elderly women without fractures looked at the effect of 1,25(OH)$_2$D$_3$, average dose 0.4 µg daily, on vertebral height (Jensen *et al.*, 1985). The cumulative anterior vertebral height was calculated for all vertebrae from T6 to L5 at baseline; at one year of treatment, the 1,25(OH)$_2$D$_3$-treated group showed a mean decrease of 1 mm and the placebo group had a mean decrease of 0.12 mm. These changes are so small that it is doubtful whether they have any meaningful clinical significance.

There have been two randomized studies of vertebral fracture rates in patients with type I postmenopausal osteoporosis and vertebral fractures. In these trials in the USA, osteoporotic patients were randomized double blind to either 1,25(OH)$_2$D$_3$ 0.5–0.75 µg daily or placebo for a period of one year (Gallagher *et al.*, 1989). After one year there was a significant reduction (~50%) in the vertebral fracture rate. At the end of the first year, all patients were crossed over to active treatment and in the second and third years there was a further 25% reduction in the number of fractures. In a large study of vertebral fracture rates in type I osteoporotics by Tilyard and colleagues (1992), approximately 600 patients were randomized to either 1,25(OH)$_2$D$_3$ 0.5 µg daily or calcium 1000 mg/day. The patients in the 1,25(OH)$_2$D$_3$-treated group had a significant reduction in vertebral fracture rate in the second and third years of study. By the end of the third year only 9% of the patients on 1,25(OH)$_2$D$_3$ had suffered vertebral fracture compared to 32% on calcium, a reduction in fractures of 72%. The decrease in fracture incidence was more marked in patients who had malabsorption of calcium.

In the ulimate analysis, a decrease in vertebral fracture rate is probably the most important measure of drug efficacy. It should be pointed out, however, that in these studies a vertebral fracture has been defined as a 15% reduction in anterior vertebral height and represents a change in the degree of wedging or compression of the vertebrae rather than a clinical fracture event.

The overall results summarized above support the efficacy of $1,25(OH)_2D_3$ and 1α-OHD_3 in the treatment of osteoporotic patients and the negative studies can be explained on the basis that the dose of $1,25(OH)_2D_3$ used was too low for efficacy (<0.5 μg daily). $1,25(OH)_2D_3$ therapy has also been shown to prevent steroid-induced osteoporosis. In contrast, calcium supplements were ineffective. In a three-year double-blind study of steroid osteoporosis, vitamin D 50 000 IU weekly plus a calcium supplement of 1000 mg/day failed to prevent bone loss (Sambrook *et al.*, 1993). Thus, $1,25(OH)_2D_3$ therapy offers superior efficacy in steroid osteoporosis (Adachi *et al.*, 1996). The therapeutic window for $1,25(OH)_2D_3$ is narrower than for 1α-OHD_3 and whereas $1,25(OH)_2D_3$ 0.4 μg daily does not always increase calcium absorption, a dose of 0.5 μg daily is usually effective and a dose greater than 0.75 μg daily causes hypercalciuria in a third of patients unless the calcium intake is maintained between 600 and 800 mg/day (Riggs and Nelson, 1985). For 1α-OHD_3, the therapeutic window is between 0.5 and 2 μg/day on a normal calcium intake.

SAFETY OF VITAMIN D ADMINISTRATION IN OSTEOPOROSIS

Vitamin D poisoning or intoxication usually refers to hypercalcemia and has most often been associated with the use of high doses (50 000–200 000 IU/day) of vitamin D_2 or D_3 (Davies and Adams, 1978), usually for treatment of hypoparathyroidism. These doses should not be used in the treatment of osteoporosis. In a recent study in France of several hundred women treated with vitamin D_3 800 IU and 1.25 g elemental calcium, there were no cases of hypercalcemia after 18 months of treatment (Jones *et al.*, 1979). Hypercalcemia did not occur in 32 elderly women in England given 9000 IU/day of vitamin D_2, in 23 women given vitamin D_2 35 000 IU/day plus 300 mg elemental calcium (Buring *et al.*, 1974) or in 60 women given 15 000 IU vitamin D_2 weekly (Nordin *et al.*, 1985). Four cases of hypercalciuria but none of hypercalcemia occurred in four women given 50 000 IU vitamin D_2 twice weekly plus 2–2.5 g of elemental calcium (Riggs *et al.*, 1976).

Administration of 25-OHD_3 50 μg/day to 15 women for one year produced a mean serum 25-OHD level of 225 nmol/l (90 ng/ml) and no cases of hypercalcemia or hypercalciuria (Francis *et al.*, 1983). Another 14 women given 25-OHD_3 40 μg/day for two years had a mean (±SD) serum 25-OHD of 270 to 225 ± 87 nmol/l (108 to 90 ± 35 ng/ml) and no reported cases of hypercalcemia or hypercalciuria (Orwoll *et al.*, 1989). Hypercalcemia was reported in several American subjects who consumed milk which had been oversupplemented with vitamin D_3 with as much as 230 000 IU per quart (Jacobus *et al.*, 1992). Serum 25-OHD levels in these patients ranged from 424 to 1660 nmol/l (170 to 664 ng/ml).

These results suggest that hypercalcemia occurs after the serum 25-OHD level exceeds 424 nmol/l or 170 ng/ml. As noted earlier (Figure 12.4), on vitamin D_3 4000 IU/day the mean serum 25-OHD was 150 nmol/l (60 ng/ml). Based on the serum 25-OHD values, it is unlikely that small doses of vitamin D (<1000 IU/day) lead to vitamin D toxicity because the increase in serum 25-OHD is relatively small.

The analogs and metabolites of vitamin D are much more potent in producing hypercalcemia and hypercalciuria because there is no negative feedback control for 1,25$(OH)_2D$. In 213 elderly women given 1,25$(OH)_2D_3$ 0.25 μg twice daily (Tilyard *et al.*, 1992), hypercalcemia occurred in 0.5% over a period of three years (hypercalciuria was not monitored). In a two-year study of patients given 1,25$(OH)_2D_3$ 0.75 μg daily, calcium absorption was above normal and mild hypercalcemia and hypercalciuria occurred in 30% of the group (Riggs and Nelson, 1985). In a dose titration study hypercalcemia and hypercalciuria occurred in most patients given 1,25$(OH)_2D_3$ in doses of 1–2 μg daily; however, this problem was dependent on the calcium intake and did not occur if the calcium intake was less than 600 mg/day (Gallagher, 1990). On a dose of 1 μg of 1α-OHD_3 in 7000 Japanese women, hypercalcemia occurred in only 0.4% of the patients (Orimo and Shiraki, 1990).

Because of the potential for producing hypercalcemia and hypercalciuria these potent forms of vitamin D could affect renal function after long-term use. With the exception of patients with hypophosphatemic rickets, long-term follow-up has shown no deterioration in creatinine clearance, no increased incidence of renal stones nor nephrocalcinosis (Buring *et al.*, 1974; Tilyard *et al.*, 1992).

ACKNOWLEDGEMENTS

Supported by NIH grants U01-AG10373 and R01-AG10358.

REFERENCES

Aaron, J.E., Gallagher, J.C., Anderson, J. *et al.* (1974) Frequency of osteomalacia and osteoporosis in fractures of the proximal femur. *Lancet* **i**: 229–33.

Adachi, J.D., Bensen, W.G., Bianchi, F. *et al.* (1996) Vitamin D and calcium in the prevention of corticosteroid induced osteoporosis. A 3 year follow up. *J Rheumatol* **23**: 995–1000.

Aksnes, L., Rodland, O., Odegaard, O.R., Baake, K.J. and Aarskog, D. (1989) Serum levels of vitamin D metabolites in the elderly. *Acta Endocrinol* **121**: 27–33.

Alevizaki, C.C., Ikkos, D.G. and Singhelakis, P. (1965) Progressive decrease of true intestinal calcium absorption with age in normal man. *J Nucl Med* **14**: 760–2.

Aloia, J.F., Cohn, S.H., Vaswani, A. *et al.* (1985) Risk factors for postmenopausal osteoporosis. *Am J Med* **78**: 95–100.

Aloia, J.F., Vaswani, A., Yeh, J.K. *et al.* (1988) Calcitriol in the treatment of postmenopausal osteoporosis. *Am J Med* **84**: 401–8.

Avioli, L.V., McDonald, J.E. and Lee, S.W. (1965) The influence of age on the intestinal absorption of ^{47}Ca in women and its relation to ^{47}Ca absorption in postmenopausal osteoporosis. *J Clin Invest* **44**: 1960–7.

Baker, A.R., McDonnell, D.P., Hughes, M.R. *et al.* (1988) Cloning and expression of full-length cDNA encoding human vitamin D receptor. *Proc Natl Acad Sci USA* **85**: 3294–8.

Bouillon, R.A., Auwerx, J.H., Lissens, W.D. and Pelemans, W.K. (1987) Vitamin D status in the elderly: seasonal substrate deficiency causes 1,25 dihydroxy-cholecalciferol deficiency. *Am J Clin Nutrition* **45**: 755–63.

Bullamore, J.R., Gallagher, J.C., Wilkinson, R., Nordin, B.E.C. and Marshall, D.H. (1970) Effect of age on calcium absorption. *Lancet* **ii**: 535–7.

Buring, K., Hulth, A.G., Nilsson, B.E., Westlin, N.E. and Wiklund, P.E. (1974) Treatment of osteoporosis with vitamin D. *Acta Med Scand* **195**: 471–2.

Caniggia, A., Gennari, C., Vianchi, V. and Guideri, R. (1963) Intestinal absorption of Ca in senile osteoporosis. *Acta Med Scand* **173**: 613.

Caniggia, A., Nuti, R., Lore, F. *et al.* (1990) Long-term treatment with calcitriol in post-menopausal osteoporosis. *Metabolism* **39**: 43–9.

Caniggia, A., Nuti, R., Lore, F. *et al.* (1993) Total body absorptiometry in post menopausal osteoporotic patients treated with 1α-hydroxylated vitamin D metabolites. *Osteoporosis Int* **3**: 181–5.

Caniggia, A., Nuti, R., Lorie, F. and Vattimo, A. (1984) The hormonal form of vitamin D in the pathophysiology and therapy of post-menopausal osteoporosis. *J Endocrinol Invest* **7**: 373–8.

Chapuy, M.C., Arlot, M.E., Duboeuf, F. *et al.* (1992) Vitamin D_3 and calcium to prevent hip fractures in elderly women. *N Engl J Med* **327**: 1637–42.

Chapuy, M.C., Chapuy, P. and Meunier, P.J. (1987) Calcium and vitamin D_2 supplements: effects on calcium metabolism in elderly people. *Am J Clin Nutrition* **46**: 324–8.

Clemens, T.L., Adams, J.S. and Holick, M.F. (1982b) Measurement of circulating vitamin D in man. *Clin Chim Acta* **121**: 301–8.

Clemens, T.L., Henderson, S.L., Adams, J.S. and Holick, M.F. (1982a) Increased skin pigment reduces the capacity of skin to synthesize vitamin D_3. *Lancet* **i**: 74–6.

Colston, K., Colston, M.J. and Feldman, D. (1981) 1,25 dihydroxyvitamin D, and malignant melanoma: the presence of receptors and inhibition of cell growth in culture. *Endocrinology* **108**: 1083–6.

Corless, D., Dawson, E., Fraser, F. *et al.* (1985) Do vitamin D supplements improve the physical capabilities of elderly hospital patients? *Age Ageing* **14**: 76–84.

Crilly, R.G., Marshall, D.H., Horsman, A. and Nordin, B.E.C. (1980) 1 alpha hydroxy D_3 with and without oestrogen in the treatment of osteoporosis. In: *Osteoporosis: Recent Advances in Pathogenesis and Treatment*, (eds DeLuca, H.F., Frost, H.M., Jee, W.S.S. and Johnston Jr, C.C.), University Park Press, Baltimore.

Dattani, T., Exton-Smith, A.N. and Stephen, J.M.L. (1984) Vitamin D status of the elderly in relation to age and exposure to sunlight. *Hum Nutrition* **38C**: 131–7.

Davie, M.W.J., Lawson, D.E.M., Emberson, C. *et al.* (1982) Vitamin D from skin: contribution to vitamin D status compared with oral vitamin D in normal and anticonvulsant treated subjects. *Clin Sci* **63**: 461–72.

Davies, M. and Adams, P.H. (1978) The continuing risk of vitamin-D intoxication. *Lancet* **ii**: 621–3.

Davies, M., Mawer, E.G., Hann, J.T. and Taylor, J.L. (1986) Seasonal changes in the biochemical indices of vitamin deficiency in the elderly: a comparison of people in residential homes, long-stay wards and attending a day hospital. *Age Ageing* **15**: 77–83.

DeLuca, H.F. (1988) The vitamin D story: a collaborative effort of basic science and clinical medicine. *FASEB J* **2**: 224–36.

Delvin, E.E., Imbach, A. and Copti, M. (1988) Vitamin D nutritional status and related biochemical indices in an autonomous elderly population. *Am J Clin Nutrition* **48**: 373–8.

Desplan, C., Thomasset, M. and Moukhtar, M. (1983) Synthesis, molecular cloning, and restriction analysis of DNA complementary to vitamin D-dependent calcium binding protein mRNA from rat duodenum. *J Biol Chem* **258**: 2762–5.

Devgun, M.S., Paterson, C.R., Johnson, B.E. and Cohen, C. (1981) Vitamin D nutrition in relation to season and occupation. *Am J Clin Nutrition* **34**: 1501–4.

Eastell, R., Yergey, A.L., Vierira, N.E. *et al.* (1991) Interrelationship among vitamin D metabolism, true calcium absorption, parathyroid function, and age in women: evidence of an age-related intestinal resistance to 1,25 dihydroxyvitamin D action. *J Bone Miner Res* **6**(2): 125–32.

Ebeling, P.R., Sandgren, M.E., DiMagno, E.P. *et al.* (1992) Evidence of an age-related decrease in intestinal responsiveness to vitamin D: Relationship between serum 1,25 dihydroxyvitamin D_3 and intestinal vitamin D receptor concentrations in normal women. *J Clin Endocrinol Metab* **75**(1): 176–82.

Egsmose, C., Lund, B., McNair, P. *et al.* (1987) Low serum levels of 25 hydroxyvitamin D and 1,25 dihydroxyvitamin D in institutionalized old people: influence of solar exposure and vitamin D supplementation. *Age Ageing* **16**: 35–40.

Epstein, S., Bryce, G., Hinman, J.W. *et al.* (1986) The influence of age on bone mineral regulating hormones. *Bone* **7**: 421–5.

Falch, J.A., Odegaard, O.R., Finnanger, A.M. and Matheson, I. (1987) Postmenopausal osteoporosis: no effect of three years treatment with 1,25 dihydroxycholecalciferol. *Acta Med Scand* **221**: 199–204.

Francis, R.M., Peacock, M. and Barkworth, S.A. (1984a) Renal impairment and its effect on calcium metabolism in elderly women. *Age Ageing* **13**: 14–20.

Francis, R.M., Peacock, M., Storer, J.H. *et al.* (1983) Calcium malabsorption in the elderly: the effects of treatment with oral 25-hydroxyvitamin D_2. *Eur J Clin Invest* **13**: 391–6.

Francis, R.M., Peacock, M., Taylor, G.A., Storer, J.H. and Nordin, B.E.C. (1984b) Calcium malabsorption in elderly women with vertebral fractures: evidence for resistance to the action of vitamin D metabolites on the bowel. *Clin Sci* **66**: 103–7.

Fujisawa, Y., Kida, K. and Matsuda, H. (1984) Role of change in vitamin D metabolism with age in calcium and phosphorus metabolism in normal human subjects. *J Clin Endocrinol Metab* **59**: 719–26.

Gallagher, J.C. (1976) The pathogenesis of fracture of the proximal femur: histological, biochemical and radiological results. MD thesis, University of Manchester.

Gallagher, J.C. (1990) Metabolic effects of synthetic calcitriol (rocaltriol) in the treatment of post-menopausal osteoporosis. *Metabolism* **39**(S1): 27–9.

Gallagher, J.C., Aaron, J., Horsman, A. *et al.* (1973) The crush fracture syndrome in postmenopausal women. *Clin Endocrinol Metab* **2**: 293–315.

Gallagher, J.C., Bishop, C.W., Knutson, J.C., Mazess, R.B. and DeLuca, H.F. (1994) Effect of increasing doses of 1a hydroxyvitamin D_2 on calcium homeostatis in postmenopausal osteopenic women. *J Bone Miner Res* **9**(5): 607–14.

Gallagher, J.C. and Goldgar, D. (1990) Treatment of postmenopausal osteoporosis with high doses of synthetic calcitriol. A randomized controlled study. *Ann Intern Med* **113**: 649–55.

Gallagher, J.C., Jerpbak, C.M., Jee, W.S.S. *et al.* (1982) 1,25 dihydroxyvitamin D_3: short- and long-term effects on bone and calcium metabolism in patients with postmenopausal osteoporosis. *Proc Natl Acad Sci USA* **79**: 3325–9.

Gallagher, J.C. and Recker, R.R. (1985) A comparison of the effects of calcitriol or calcium supplements. In: *Vitamin D: A Chemical, Biochemical and Clinical Update*, (eds Norman, A.W., Schaefer, K., Grigoleit, H.G. and Herrath, D.V.), Walter de Gruyter, Berlin, pp. 971–5.

Gallagher, J.C., Riggs, B.L., Eisman, J. *et al.* (1979) Intestinal calcium absorption and serum vitamin D metabolites in normal subjects and osteoporotic patients. *J Clin Invest* **64**: 729–36.

Gallagher, J.C., Riggs, B.L., Jerpbak, C. and Arnaud, C.D. (1980) The effect of age on serum immunoreactive parathyroid hormone in normal and osteoporotic women. *J Lab Clin Med* **95**: 373–85.

Gallagher, J.C., Riggs, B.L., Recker, R.R. and Goldgar, D. (1989) The effect of calcitriol on patients with postmenopausal osteoporosis with special reference to fracture frequency. *Proc Soc Exp Biol Med* **191:** 287–92.

Geusens, P. and Dequeker, J. (1986) Long-term effect of nandrolone decanoate, 1 alpha-hydroxy-vitamin D_3 or intermittent calcium infusion therapy on bone mineral content, bone remodeling and fracture rate in symptomatic osteoporosis: a double-blind controlled study. *Bone Mineral* **1**: 347–57.

Gibson, R.S., Draper, H.H., McGirr, L.G., Nizan, P. and Martinez, O.B. (1986) The vitamin D status of a cohort of postmenopausal non institutionalized Canadian women. *Nutrition Res* **6**: 1179–87.

Hayashi, Y., Fugita, T. and Inoue, T. (1992) Decrease of vertebral fracture in osteoporotics by administration of 1a hydroxy-vitamin D_3. *IBBM* **10**(2): 184–8.

Heikinheimo, R.J., Inkovaara, J.A., Harju, E.J. *et al.* (1992) Annual injection of vitamin D and fractures of aged bones. *Calcif Tissue Int* **51**: 105–10.

Himmelstein, S., Clemens, T.L., Rubin, A. and Lindsay, R. (1990) Vitamin D supplementation in elderly nursing home residents increases 25(OH)D but not $1,25(OH)_2D$. *Am J Clin Nutrition* **52**: 701–6.

Holick, M.R., Matsuoka, L.Y. and Wortsman, J. (1989) Age, vitamin D, and solar ultraviolet radiation. *Lancet* **ii**, 1104–5.

Holick, M.F., Maclaughlin, J.A., Clark, M.B. *et al.* (1980) Photosynthesis of previtamin D in human skin and the physiologic consequences. *Science* **210**: 203–5.

Hollis, B.W. (1986) Assay of circulating 1,25 dihydroxyvitamin D involving a novel single-cartridge extraction and purification procedure. *Clin Chem* **32**: 2060–3.

Honkanen, R., Alhava, E., Parviainen, M., Talasniemi, S. and Monkkonen, R. (1990) The necessity and safety of calcium and vitamin D in the elderly. *J Am Geriatr Soc* **38**: 862–6.

Hordon, L.D. and Peacock, M. (1987) Vitamin D metabolism in women with femoral neck fracture. *Bone Miner* **2**: 413–26.

Jacobus, C.H., Holick, M.F., Shao, Q. *et al.* (1992) Hypervitaminosis D associated with drinking milk. *N Engl J Med* **326**: 1173–7.

Jensen, G.F., Christiansen, C. and Transbol, I. (1982) Treatment of postmenopausal osteoporosis. A controlled therapeutic trial comparing oestrogen/gestagen, 1,25 dihydroxyvitamin D_3 and calcium. *Clin Endocrinol Oxf* **16**: 515–24.

Jensen, G.F., Meinecke, B., Boesen, J. and Transbol, I. (1985) Does $1,25(OH)_2D_3$ accelerate spinal bone loss? A controlled therapeutic trial in 70-year-old women. *Clin Orthop* 215–21.

Jones, G., Byrnes, B., Duthie, D. *et al.* (1979) Contribution of skin vitamin D_3 synthesis in patients receiving total parenteral nutrition. In: *Vitamin D, Basic Research and its Clinical Application*, (eds Norman, A.W., Schaefer, K. and Grigoleit, H.G.), Gruyter, Berlin.

Kinyamu, H.K., Gallagher, J.C., DeLuca, H.F. *et al.* (1995) Relationship between intestinal vitamin D receptor, VDR genotypes, calcium absorption, and serum 1,25 dihydroxyvitamin D in normal women. *J Bone Miner Res* **10**(S1): 94.

Kinyamu, H.K., Gallagher, J.C., Petranick, K.M. and Ryschon, K.L. (1996) Effect of parathyroid hormone [hPTH(134)] infusion on serum 1,25 dihydroxyvitamin D and parathyroid hormone in normal women. *J Bone Miner Res* **11**(10): 1400–50.

Kobayashi, T., Okano, T., Shida, S. *et al.* (1983) Variation of 25-hydroxyvitamin D_3 and 25-hydroxyvitamin D_2 levels in human plasma obtained from 758 Japanese healthy subjects. *J Nutrition Sci Vitaminol* **29**(3): 271–81.

Krall, E.A., Sahyoun, N., Tannenbaum, S., Dallai, G.E. and Dawson Hughes, B. (1989) Effect of vitamin D intake on seasonal variations in parathyroid hormone secretion in post-menopausal women. *N Engl J Med* **321**: 1777–83.

Krolner, B., Nielsen, S.P., Lund, B. *et al.* (1980) Lumbar spine bone mineral content in post menopausal osteoporosis. *Calcif Tissue Int* **31S**: 77A.

Lawoyin, S., Zerwekh, J.E., Glass, K. and Pak, C.Y.C. (1980) Ability of 25-hydroxyvitamin D_3 therapy to augment serum 1,25- and 24,25-dihydroxyvitamin D in postmenopausal osteoporosis. *J Clin Endocrinol Metab* **50**: 593–6.

Lawson, D.E.M., Paul, A.A., Black, A.E. *et al.* (1979) Relative contributions of diet and sunlight to vitamin D state in the elderly. *Br Med J* **2**: 303–5.

Lester, E., Skinner, R.K. and Wills, M.R. (1977) Seasonal variation in serum-25-hydroxyvitamin-D in the elderly in Britain. *Lancet* **i**: 979–80.

Lian, J.B., Stewart, C., Puchacz, E. *et al.* (1989) Structure of the rat osteocalcin gene and regulation of vitamin D-dependent expression. *Proc Natl Acad Sci USA* **86**: 1143–7.

Lindholm, T.S., Nilsson, O.S., Kyhle, B.R. *et al.* (1981) Failures and complications in treatment of osteoporotic patients treated with 1 dihydroxyvitamin D_3 supplemented by calcium. In: *Osteoporosis*, (eds Christiansen, C., Arnaud, C.D., Nordin, B.E.C. *et al.*), Aalborg Stiftsbogtrykkeri, Glostrup, pp. 351–7.

Lips, P., van Ginkel, F.C., Jongen, M.J.M. (1987) Determinants of vitamin D status in patients with hip fracture and in elderly control subjects. *Am J Clin Nutrition* **46**: 1005–10.

Lips, P., Wiersinga, A., van Ginkel, F.C. *et al.* (1988) The effect of vitamin D supplementation on vitamin D status and parathyroid function in elderly subjects. *J Clin Endocrinol Metab* **67**: 644–50.

Lund, B., Holm, P., Egsmose, C. *et al.* (1984) A controlled double-blind study comparing the effect of estrogen with estrogen and 1,25 dihydroxyvitamin D_3 in postmenopausal osteoporosis. In: *Osteoporosis*, (eds Christiansen, C., Arnaud, C.D., Nordin, B.E.C. *et al.*), Aalborg Stiftsbogtrykkeri, Glostrup, pp. 763–76.

Lund, B., Sorensen, O.H., Anderson, R.B. *et al.* (1985) Long-term treatment of senile osteopenia with 1 alphahydroxycholecalciferol. In: *Vitamin D. A Chemical, Biochemical and Clinical Update*, (eds Norman, A.W., Schaefer, K., Grigoleit, H.G. and Herrath, D.V.), Walter de Gruyter, Berlin, pp. 1039–40.

Lund, B., Sorensen, O.H., Lund, B. and Agner, E. (1982) Serum 1,25 dihydroxyvitamin D in normal subjects and in patients with post-menopausal osteopenia. Influence of age, renal function and oestrogen therapy. *Horm Metab Res* **14**: 271–4.

McKenna, M.J., Freaney, R., Meade, A. and Muldowney, F.P. (1985) Hypovitaminosis D and elevated serum alkaline phosphatase in elderly Irish people. *Am J Clin Nutrition* **41**(1): 101–9.

Maclaughlin, J. and Holick, M.F. (1985) Aging decreases the capacity of human skin to produce vitamin D. *J Clin Invest* **76**: 1536–8.

Manolagas, S.C., Culler, F.L., Howard, J.E., Brickman, A.S. and Deftos, L.J. (1983) The cytoreceptor assay for 1,25-dihydroxyvitamin D and its application to human studies. *J Clin Endocrinol Metab* **56**: 751–60.

Manolagas, S.C., Provvedini, D.M. and Tsoukas, C.D. (1985) Interactions of 1,25-dihydroxyvitamin D_3 and the immune system. *Mol Cell Endocrinol* **43**: 113–22.

Marshall, D.H., Gallagher, J.C., Guha, P. *et al.* (1977) The effect of 1 alphahydroxycholecalciferol and hormone therapy on the calcium balance of post-menopausal osteoporosis. *Calcif Tissue Res* **225**: 78–84.

Matsuoka, L.Y., Ide, L., Wortsman, J., Maclaughlin, J. and Holick, M.F. (1987) Sunscreens suppress cutaneous vitamin D_3 synthesis. *J Clin Endocrinol Metab* **64**: 1165–8.

Menczel, J., Foldes, J., Steinberg, R. *et al.* (1991) The role of $24,25(OH)_2D_3$ in the treatment of osteoporosis. Eighth Workshop on Vitamin D, (eds Norman, A.W., Bouillon, R. and Thomasset, M.), Walter de Gruyter, Berlin.

Meunier, P.J., Chapuy, M.C., Arlot, M.E., Delmas, P.D. and Duboeuf, F. (1995) Can we stop bone loss and prevent hip fractures in the elderly? *Osteoporosis Int* **4**(S1): S71–S76.

Nordin, B.E.C., Horsman, A. and Gallagher, J.C. (1975) Effect of various therapies on bone loss in women. In: *Calcium Metabolism, Bone and Metabolic Bone Disease*, (eds Kuhlencordt, F. and Kruse, H.P.), Springer Verlag, New York, pp. 233–42.

Nordin, B.E.C., Wilkinson, R., Marshall, D.H. *et al.* (1976) Calcium absorption in the elderly. *Calcif Tissue Res* **21S**: 442–51.

Nordin, C., Baker, M.R., Horsman, A. and Peacock, M. (1985) A prospective trial of the effect of vitamin D supplementation on metacarpal bone loss in elderly women. *Am J Clin Nutrition* **42**: 470–4.

Omdahl, J.L., Garry, P.J., Hunsaker, L.A., Hunt, W.C. and Goodwin, J.S. (1982) Nutritional status in a healthy elderly population: vitamin D. *Am J Clin Nutrition* **36**: 1225–33.

Orimo, H. (1993) Alfacalcidol in the treatment of established osteoporosis. Fourth International Symposium on Osteoporosis, (eds Christiansen, C. and Riis, B.), Handelstrykkeriet, Aalborg.

Orimo, H., Shiraki, M., Hayashi, T. and Nakamura, T. (1987) Reduced occurrence of vertebral crush fractures in senile osteoporosis treated with 1 alpha(OH)-vitamin D_3. *Bone Mineral* **3**, 47–52.

Orimo, H. and Shiraki, M. (1990) Long term use of 1a(OH)D3 in involutional osteoporosis. In: *Osteoporosis: Physiological Basis, Assessment, and Treatment*, (eds DeLuca, H.F. and Mazess, R.), Elsevier, New York, pp. 223–9.

Orwoll, E.S., McClung, M.R., Oviatt, S.K., Recker, R.R. and Weigel, R.M. (1989) Histomorphometric effects of calcium or calcium plus 25-hydroxyvitamin D_3 therapy in senile osteoporosis. *J Bone Miner Res* **4**(1): 81–8.

Ott, S.M. and Chesnut, C.H. (1989) Calcitriol treatment is not effective in postmenopausal osteoporosis: see comments. *Ann Intern Med* **110**: 267–74.

Ott, S. and Chesnut, C. (1990) Tolerance to doses of calcitriol is associated with improved bone density in women with postmenopausal osteoporosis. *J Bone Miner Res* **5**(S2): 746.

Peacock, M. and Hordon, L. (1989) Femoral fracture: the role of vitamin D. In: *Clinical Disorders of Bone and Mineral Metabolism*, (eds Kleerekoper, M. and Krane, S.M.), Mary Ann Liebert, New York, pp. 265–71.

Poskitt, E.M.E., Cole, T.J. and Lawson, D.E.M. (1979) Diet, sunlight, and 25-hydroxy vitamin D in healthy children and adults. *Br Med J* **1**: 221–3.

Quesada, J.M., Coopmans, W., Ruiz, B. *et al.* (1992) Influence of vitamin D on parathyroid function in the elderly. *J Clin Endocrinol Metab* **75**: 494–501.

Reeve, J., Bijvoet, O.L.M., Neer, R.M. *et al.* (1980) A comparison between the balance method and radiotracer methods for measuring calcium absorption in treated and untreated patients with osteoporosis. *Metab Bone Dis Rel Res* **2**: 233–8.

Reeve, J., Tellez, M., Green, J.R. *et al.* (1982) Long-term treatment of osteoporosis with 24,25 dihydroxycholecalciferol. *Acta Endocrinol* **101**: 636–40.

Reinhardt, T.A., Horst, R.L., Orf, J.W. and Hollis, B.W. (1984) A microassay of 1,25-dihydroxyvitamin D not requiring high performance liquid chromatography: application to clinical studies. *J Clin Endocrinol Metab* **58**(1): 91–8.

Riggs, B.L., Jowsey, J., Kelly, P.G., Hoffman, D.L. and Arnaud, C.D. (1976) Effects of oral therapy with calcium and vitamin D in primary osteoporosis. *J Clin Endocrinol Metab* **42**: 1139–44.

Riggs, B.L. and Melton III, L.J. (1986) Involutional osteoporosis. *N Engl J Med* **314**: 1676–86.

Riggs, B.L. and Nelson, K. (1985) Effect of long term treatment with calcitriol on calcium absorption and mineral metabolism in postmenopausal osteoporosis. *J Clin Endocrinol Metab* **61**: 457–61.

Riis, B.J., Thomsen, K. and Christiansen, C. (1986) Does $24R,25(OH)_2$ vitamin D_3 prevent postmenopausal bone loss? *Calcif Tissue Int* **39**: 128–32.

Roodman, G.D., Ibbotson, K.J., MacDonald, B.R., Kuehl, T.J. and Mundy, G.R. (1985) $1,25(OH)_2$ vitamin D_3 causes formation of multinucleated cells with osteoclast characteristics in cultures of primate marrow. *Proc Natl Acad Sci USA* **82**: 8213–17.

Sambrook, P., Birmingham, J. and Kelly, P. (1993) Prevention of corticosteroid osteoporosis. *N Engl J Med* **328**: 1747–52.

Seeley, D.G., Kelsey, J., Nevitt, M.C., Tao, J.L. and Cummings, S.R. (1992) Predictors of ankle and foot fractures in elderly women. *Bone Miner Res* **7**(S1): 137.

Sheikh, M.S., Ramirez, A., Emmett, M. *et al.* (1988) Role of vitamin D-dependent and vitamin D-independent mechanisms in absorption of food calcium. *J Clin Invest* **81**: 126–32.

Sherman, S., Hollis, B.W. and Tobin, J.D. (1990) Vitamin D status and related parameters in a healthy population: the effects of age, sex, and season. *J Clin Endocrinol Metab* **71**: 405–13.

Shiraki, M., Orimo, H., Ito, H. *et al.* (1985) Long-term treatment of postmenopausal osteoporosis with active vitamin D_3, alpha-hydroxycholecalciferol (1 alpha OHD_3) and 1,24 dihydroxy-cholecalciferol (1,24$(OH)_2D_3$). *Endocrinol Jpn* **32**: 305–15.

Smith, E.L., Walworth, N.C. and Holick, M.F. (1986) Effect of 1,25 dihydroxyvitamin D on the morphologic and biochemical differentiation of cultured human epidermal keratinocytes grown in serum-free conditions. *J Invest Dermatol* **86**: 709–14.

Somerville, P.J., Lien, J.W.K. and Kaye, M. (1977) The calcium and vitamin D status in an elderly female population and their response to administered supplemental vitamin D_3. *J Geront* **32**(6): 659–63.

Sowers, M.F.R., Wallace, R.B., Hollis, B.W. and Lemke, J.H. (1986) Parameters related to 25-OH-D levels in a population based study of women. *Am J Clin Nutrition* **43**: 621–8.

Stryd, P., Gilbertson, T.J. and Brunden, M.N. (1979) A seasonal variation study of 25-hydroxyvitamin D_3 serum levels in normal humans. *J Clin Endocrinol Metab* **48**: 771–5.

Tanaka, H., Abe, E., Miyaura, C. *et al.* (1982) 1,25 dihydroxycholecalciferol and hyman myeloid leukemia cell line (HL-60): the presence of cytosol receptor and induction of differentiation. *Biochem J* **204**: 713–19.

Tilyard, M.W., Spears, G.F.S., Thomson, J. and Dovey, S. (1992) Treatment of postmenopausal osteoporosis with calcitriol or calcium. *N Engl J Med* **326**: 357–62.

Tjellesen, L., Christiansen, C., Rodbro, P. and Hummer, L. (1985) Different metabolism of vitamin D_2 and vitamin D_3 in epileptic patients on carbamazepine. *Acta Neurol Scand* **1**: 385–9.

Toss, G., Almqvist, S., Larson, L. and Zetterqvist, H. (1988) Vitamin D deficiency in welfare institutions for the aged. *Acta Med Scand* **208**: 87–9.

Tsai, K-S., Heath III, H., Kumar, R. and Riggs, B.L. (1984) Impaired vitamin D metabolism with aging in women. Possible role in pathogenesis of senile osteoporosis. *J Clin Invest* **73**: 1668–72.

Webb, A.R., Kline, L. and Holick, M.F. (1988) Influence of season and latitude on the cutaneous synthesis of vitamin D_3: exposure to winter sunlight in Boston and Edmonton will not promote vitamin D_3 synthesis in human skin. *J Clin Endocrinol Metab* **67**: 373–8.

Webb, A.R., Pilbeam, C., Hanafin, N. and Holick, M.F. (1990) An evaluation of the relative contributions of exposure to sunlight and of diet to the circulating concentrations of 25-hydroxyvitamin D in an elderly nursing home population in Boston. *Am J Clin Nutrition* **51**: 1075–81.

Wiklund, P.E. (1974) Treatment of osteoporosis with vitamin D. *Acta Med Scand* **195**: 471–2.

Zerwekh, J., Sakhaee, K., Glass, K. and Pak, C.Y.C. (1983) Long term 25 hydroxyvitamin D_3 therapy in postmenopausal osteoporosis: demonstration of responsive and nonresponsive subgroups. *J Clin Endocrinol Metab* **56**: 410–13.

ANABOLIC STEROIDS 13

C. Christiansen

INTRODUCTION

Anabolic steroids were introduced into therapeutic medicine late in the 1950s. At that time they were thought to be suitable for the treatment of a vast number of indications (Kockakian, 1976). Some of these, e.g. muscular dystrophies and diabetic retinopathy, were never sufficiently supported by convincing data and were therefore dropped by most therapists in the course of time. The validity of others, such as stunted growth, mammary carcinoma, certain anemias, deficiency states and catabolic conditions as well as some organic diseases, has been established in clinical pharmacological investigations; as a consequence these indications are widely accepted (Kopera, 1985). A few indications, however, including osteoporosis, survived more on account of positive subjective impressions than on clearcut reproducible results obtained in clinical trials, so that many physicians hesitate to regard them as true indications for anabolic steroids. It is therefore understandable that some of those involved in the treatment of osteoporosis might not be very familiar with anabolic steroids.

Anabolic steroids are chemically related to natural androgens. They are distinguished from the latter by a powerful protein anabolic effect in doses which produce little androgenic effect. A complete separation of both activities is not possible as they differ only with respect to their location and not in essence: anabolic activity is indicated when extragenital stimulation of protein synthesis is produced whereas androgenic activity is defined as the anabolic effect in the area of sex organs.

THE EFFECT ON THE HUMAN BONE CELL

The mechanism by which androgens exert their effect on bone cells is not known but the action of androgens on other target tissues has been thought to be mediated by growth factors (Ishii and Shooter, 1975; Gresik and Barka, 1983). Kasperk *et al.* (1990) have previously reported that in bone cells androgens stimulate cell proliferation and differentiation *in vitro* and dihydroxytestosterone increases TGFβ production and increases IgF-II receptors in human bone cells. These studies were intended to examine the action of the testosterone analog nandrolone – a compound which has been shown to increase bone mass in osteoporotic patients (Geusens and Dequeker, 1986; Gennari *et al.*, 1989) – to determine its mechanism of action on osteoblastic cells. Nandrolone was tested on various human bone cell parameters *in vitro*. As with the action of dihydroxytestosterone, nandrolone increased both cell proliferation and differentiation of human bone cells. In summary, these studies have shown that

Osteoporosis. Edited by John C. Stevenson and Robert Lindsay. Published in 1998 by Chapman & Hall, London.
ISBN 0 412 48870 1

nandrolone can increase bone cell proliferation and ALP in a dose-dependent manner. Furthermore, the effects on bone cell proliferation may be mediated in part by IgF-II because nandrolone increased IgF-II receptor number and the maximum mitogenic action of IgF-II. In conclusion, nandrolone has the unique ability to increase both proliferation and differentation of bone cells; this could explain the positive clinical bone responses to nandrolone at least in part.

THE EFFECTS ON THE OVARIECTOMIZED RAT

In experimental animals osteoporosis does not develop spontaneously, as in man, but can readily be induced, for example in rats or dogs (Saville, 1969; Hodgkinson *et al.*, 1978; Wronski *et al.*, 1985; Malluche *et al.*, 1986; Turner *et al.*, 1987). In particular, the ovariectomized rat is frequently used as an animal model for early postmenopausal bone loss. In this model significant reduction in trabecular bone mass in the distal metaphysis of the long bones becomes manifest by 2–4 weeks after ovariectomy. The reduction in bone mass is due to a greater increase in bone resorption than in bone formation. The latter finding indicates that in this respect the etiology of bone loss in the rat model closely resembles that of bone loss in early postmenopausal women. The model has, however, been criticized because the skeleton of the rat grows continuously and regulation of calcium metabolism in the ovariectomized rat and early postmenopausal women is not identical. Therefore the use of elderly rats (>12 months old) is recommended (Kalu *et al.*, 1989).

Recent studies have indicated that trabecular bone loss in ovariectomized rats can be inhibited not only with estrogen, but also with other naturally occurring steroids such as androstenedione and progesterone (Turner *et al.*, 1989a,b).

Synthetic steroids also affect the bone mass of ovariectomized rats. Schot and Schuurs (1987) have demonstrated that the anabolic steroid nandrolone decanoate significantly stimulates longitudinal and periosteal bone formation. Since this steroid has been shown to increase bone mass in postmenopausal women with established osteoporosis (Dequeker and Geusens, 1985; Need *et al.*, 1987; Gennari *et al.*, 1989), Schot and Schuurs performed two studies in ovariectomized rats to investigate further the effect of nandrolone decanoate on trabecular and cortical bone mass (Schot *et al.*, 1989).

EFFECTS ON TRABECULAR BONE MASS

Histomorphometrical analysis of trabecular bone volume (TBV) of the metaphyseal bone of the distal femur showed that ovariectomy causes a significant decrease of TBV. Treatment with 2 mg nandrolone decanoate for eight weeks resulted in a TBV significantly higher than in the ovariectomized rats, but significantly lower than in the intact rats; 0.5 and 1 mg of nandrolone decanoate had no significant effects on TBV. Measurement of plasma levels of osteocalcin revealed that bone-remodeling activity was significantly increased by ovariectomy and reduced by nandrolone decanoate.

EFFECTS ON CORTICAL BONE MASS

The effects of ovariectomy and nandrolone decanoate treatment on various bone parameters of the femur were studied. Dry weight and femur length were significantly stimulated by 1 and 2.5 mg nandrolone decanoate. In the intact animals no change in the density of the metaphysis and the mid-diaphysis of the femur was found during the experiment. Nandrolone decanoate prevented ovariectomy-induced decrease in bone density in both the metaphysis and the diaphysis. The values even exceeded those of the two intact groups. Ovariectomy caused an increase in plasma levels of osteocalcin, whilst nandrolone decanoate treatment caused a dose-dependent reduction of this parameter.

From the above-mentioned studies, it was concluded that nandrolone decanoate reverses bone loss in both young and old ovariectomized rats, probably due to correction of unbalanced bone turnover.

THE EFFECTS OF ANABOLIC STEROIDS IN MAN

Many anabolic steroids have been used in man. Those most commonly used in osteoporosis are stanozolol and nandrolone but they are not universally available. Stanozolol is given by mouth and nandrolone by intramuscular injection of the decanoate. Other agents tested in osteoporosis are danazol, oxymethalone, oxandrolone and methandrostenolone. Differences in the effects of anabolic agents probably lie more in their side effects than in their activity on bone, which is reviewed briefly below.

BIOCHEMICAL EFFECTS

The biochemical changes induced by anabolic steroids in postmenopausal women include an early and marked decrease in the fasting urinary excretion of calcium which is widely interpreted to indicate a decrease in the net release of calcium from bone (Chesnut *et al.*, 1983; Need *et al.*, 1987; Benéton *et al.*, 1991). Since the fasting urinary excretion of calcium is expressed as a fraction of creatinine excretion, the question arises whether the changes are attributable to effects on calcium or creatinine metabolism or both. In a study of stanozolol (Benéton *et al.*, 1991) there were significant increases in serum and urinary creatinine which rose by 23%, presumably due to an increase in creatinine production. The increase in creatinine output, however, accounts for only a third of the decrease in the calcium–creatinine ration. It thus seems likely that the changes in the fasting urinary excretion of calcium are due mainly to a decrease in the net efflux of calcium from bone to the extracellullar fluid. These observations suggest that anabolic steroids stimulate bone formation, decrease bone resorption or both.

The indirect indices of skeletal turnover, such as total alkaline phosphatase and hydroxyproline excretion, do not change markedly and therefore do not help to determine the mechanism of this effect. The lack of effect on alkaline phosphatase might be due to the lack of specificity of the measurement, since an increase in the skeletal-derived fraction has been reported.

The effect in elderly postmenopausal women of nandrolone decanoate and estrogen-progestogen therapy on serum concentration of procollagen type III amino terminal propeptide (PIIINP), a measure of collagen synthesis (type III collagen is present in loose and dense connective tissues throughout the body), and serum type I procollagen carboxy terminal propeptide (PICP), a measure of bone formation (type I collagen is almost only found in bone), was studied in double-blind trials. The biochemical parameters were measured every three months during the 12-month study period (Hassager *et al.*, 1990, 1991).

Anabolic steroid therapy resulted in a more than 50% increase in PIIINP. In the estrogen-progestogen group, PIIINP increased too, but to a lesser extent (Figure 13.1). This study thus demonstrated that nandrolone decanoate increases the collagen type III synthesis significantly. PICP decreased by about 30% in the group treated with estrogen-progestogen whereas this marker of bone formation was hardly affected by nandrolone decanoate (Figure 13.2).

More recently, marked changes in carboxy terminal pyridinoline crosslinked telopeptide of type I collagen in serum have been demonstrated in response to nandrolone decanoate therapy in postmenopausal osteoporosis (Hassager *et al.*, 1994).

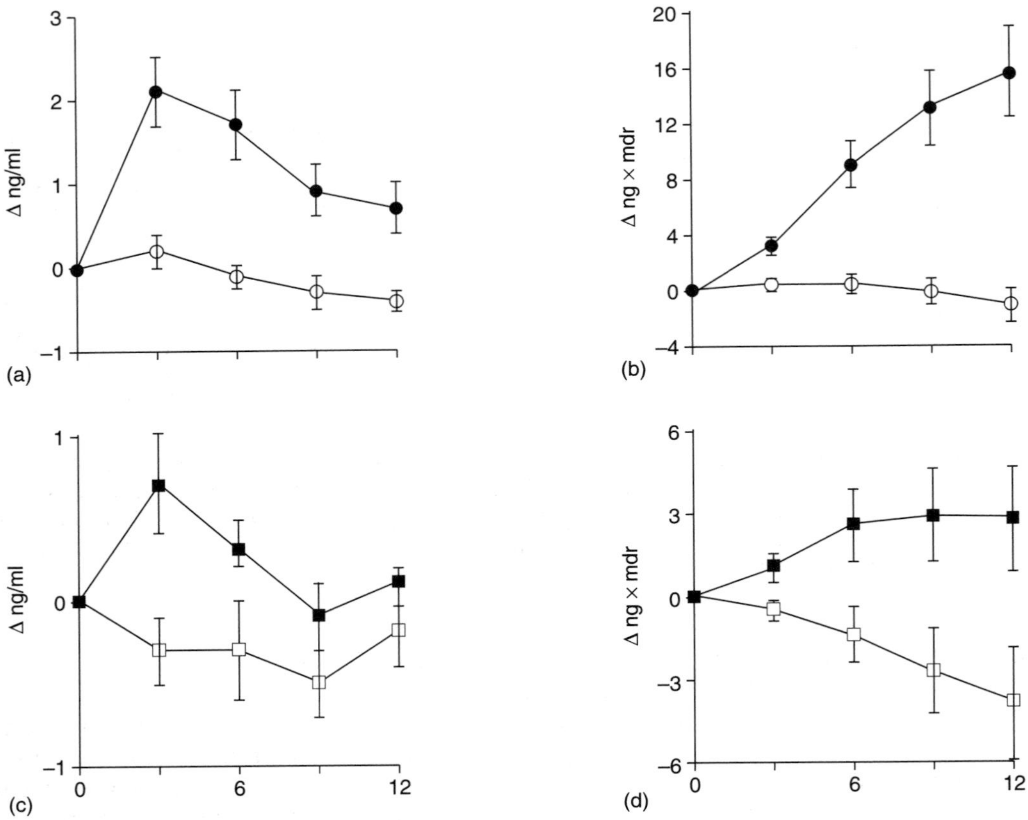

Figure 13.1 Change in serum PIIINP and cumulative change in serum PIIINP. (a and b) During treatment with nandrolone decanoate (●), active (n = 19); (○), placebo (n = 17). (c and d) During estrogen-progestogen substitution therapy (■), active (n = 16); (□), placebo (n = 15). Values are given as difference from the initial values as mean ± SEM. Significance of difference from placebo; *$p < 0.05$; **$p < 0.01$; ***$p < 0.001$. Reproduced with permission from Hassager *et al.* (1990).

EFFECTS ON BONE MASS

The effects of anabolic steroids on bone mass are generally consistent with a preferential effect of these agents at cortical bone sites. Treatment with methandrostenolone or with stanozolol increases total body calcium as measured by neutron-activation analysis (Chesnut *et al.*, 1977, 1983). Total body calcium increased progressively over a treatment period of 29 months. The increment on bone mass over the first year of treatment was similar to that over the second year, which is unlike the effects of inhibitors of bone resorption (e.g. calcitonin, bisphosphonate, calcium, etc.) but more in keeping with the effects of anabolic regimens such as fluoride. Longer term studies would be required, however, to document whether steady-state conditions had been achieved.

The effects of anabolic steroids on regional skeletal sites vary according to the site and technique used. At the metacarpal, nandrolone prevents cortical bone loss (Geusens *et al.*, 1986) consistent with a

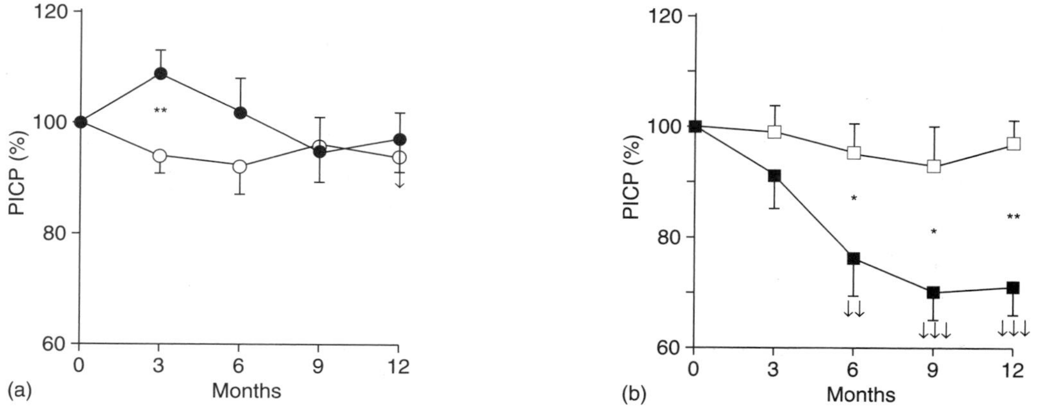

Figure 13.2 Changes in PICP during (a) treatment with nandrolone decanoate therapy (●, active; ○, placebo) and (b) during estrogen-progestogen substitutional therapy (■, active; □, placebo). Values are given as a percentage of the initial values as mean ± SEM. Significance of difference from initial values (↓,↓↓,↓↓↓) or difference from initial values from placebo (*,**,***) for $p < 0.05$; $p < 0.01$; and $p < 0.001$, respectively. Reproduced with permission from Hassager *et al.* (1991).

protective effect on endocortical loss at this site. The same authors showed an increase in forearm bone mineral content (at a cortical site) but the increment in the first year was greater than in the second year of treatment. The width of the bone did not increase (Need *et al.*, 1989). This might suggest that an early response is due to increased cortical density and that the long-term response is due to a progressive increase in cortical width at the endocortical site, as suggested by the histological findings.

Many studies of nandrolone have shown increases in bone mass over periods of 1–2 years of absorptiometric techniques at different sites, including a component of cancellous bone. These need to be interpreted cautiously because of the effects of anabolic steroids on other components of body composition (Hassager *et al.*, 1989). Anabolic steroids decrease the ratio of fat to lean body mass and this introduces errors into the methodology. Thus the apparent increments in bone mineral density are due in part to these effects (Figure 13.3).

EFFECTS OF FRACTURE

There have been no prospective randomized studies to determine whether anabolic steroids reduce fracture frequency. Two studies examining the effects of stanozolol or nandrolone on bone mass report fewer vertebral fractures compared with the control arm of the study (Chesnut *et al.*, 1983; Geusens *et al.*, 1986). A retrospective case control study (the MEDOS study) has shown that the use of anabolic steroids in women was associated with a marked (RR = 0.60) but not significant decrease in the relative risk of hip fracture (Kanis *et al.*, 1992). Analysis of these data for Italy, the country with the greatest use, showed a marked and significant reduction in the risk of hip fracture (RR = 0.20; $p = 0.008$). In this study, users of anabolic steroids were more likely to have taken estrogen following hysterectomy, have a higher degree of physical activity and have a poorer mental score. Adjustment for these factors did not alter the significance of these findings (RR = 0.07; 95% CI 0.01–0.55). A further problem in the interpretation of these data is that controls

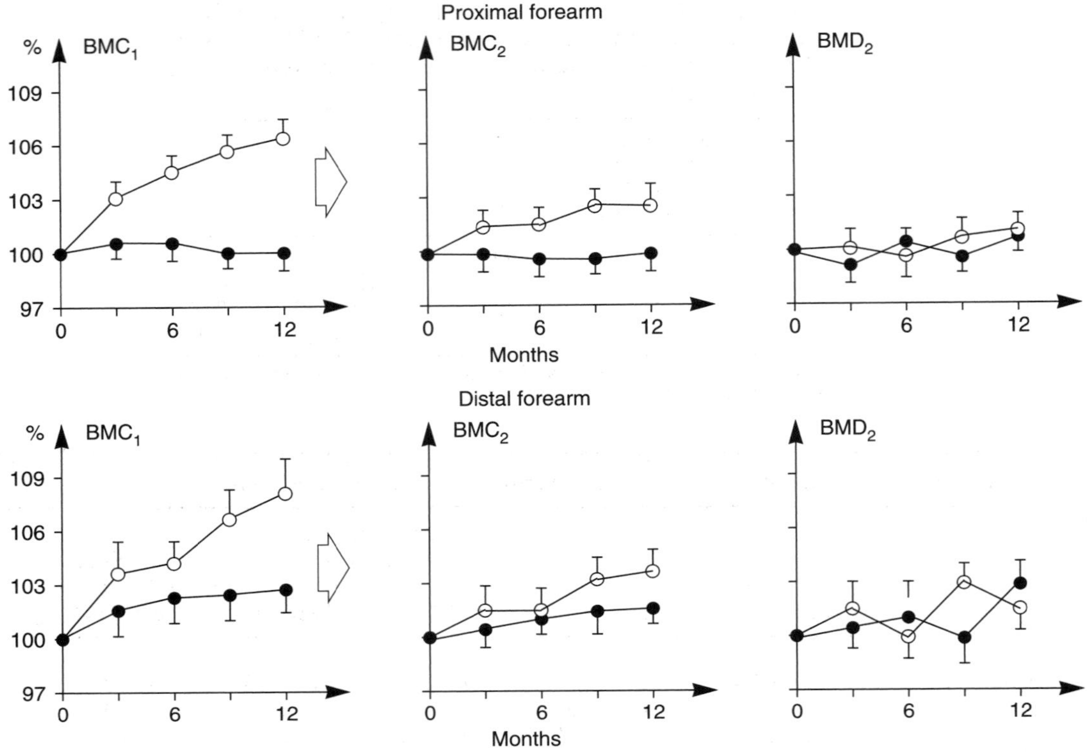

Figure 13.3 Forearm bone mass during treatment with nandrolone decanoate (○) or placebo (●). BMC_1 = uncorrected bone mineral content; BMC_2 = fat-corrected bone mineral content; BMD_2 = fat-corrected bone mineral density. Proximal and distal refer to two different measurement sites. Values are given in percent of initial values as mean ± 1 SEM. Reproduced with permission from Hassager *et al.* (1989).

exposed to anabolic steroids are commonly also treated with other agents. In Italy, the use of cacitonin is significantly higher among takers of anabolic steroids than those not taking anabolic steroids. The relative contribution of calcitonin to the effects of anabolic steroids was, however, independent by multivariate analysis (Table 13.1), suggesting that a protective effect of anabolic steroids was unlikely to be due to the concurrent use of calcitonin.

EFFECTS ON BODY COMPOSITION

Since muscle mass correlates with bone mass (Kenyon *et al.*, 1940) and anabolic steroids have been shown to create a positive nitrogen balance (Johansen *et al.*, 1989), the observed increase in bone mass during such therapy might be secondary to an increase in muscle mass.

In a double-blind study, nandrolone decanoate resulted in major quantitative changes in various soft tissue compartments in postmenopausal women (Hassager *et al.*, 1989). With regard to the total body, the lean body mass (measured by dual-photon absorptiometry) increased 4 kg on average and the fat mass decreased accordingly. These changes were observed in the limbs and in the trunk, with the relative changes greater in the limbs than in the trunk (Table

Table 13.1 Multivariate analysis of the effects of anabolic steroids and calcitonin on the relative risk (RR) of hip fracture (+95% CI) in women aged 50 years or more from Sienna, Parma and Rome

Treatment combination				
Caltitonin	*Anabolic steroids*	*RR*	*95% CI*	*p =*
No	No	1.00		
No	Yes	0.01	0.00–0.42	0.04
Yes	No	0.71	0.49–1.03	0.07
Yes	Yes	0.09	0.01–0.67	0.02

Kanis, J. (1993) Osteoporosis. Proceedings of the 4th International Symposium on osteoporosis, Hong Kong.

Table 13.2 Changes in body composition (mean ± SD) during the treatment with nandrolone decanoate of 39 osteoporotic but otherwise healthy postmenopausal women

	Nandrolone decanoate group (n = 16)		*Placebo group (n = 16)*		*Significance of difference between changes*
	Initial (kg)	*Change (kg)*	*Initial (kg)*	*Change (kg)*	
LBM					
Head + trunk	24.6 ± 1.7	1.3 ± 1.7*	26.0 ± 2.8	-0.4 ± 1.3	p < 0.01
Arms	3.7 ± 0.5	0.6 ± 0.6†	3.8 ± 0.6	0.1 ± 1.0	p < 0.05
Legs	9.6 ± 1.3	1.9 ± 1.2†	9.9 ± 2.0	0.2 ± 1.4	p < 0.01
Total body	37.9 ± 2.5	3.8 ± 2.5†	39.7 ± 4.8	-0.2 ± 2.2	p < 0.001
FM					
Head + trunk	13.3 ± 4.6	-1.5 ± 1.9*	11.6 ± 6.2	-0.4 ± 2.0	p < 0.12
Arms	3.1 ± 1.0	-0.9 ± 0.5†	3.0 ± 1.7	-0.3 ± 0.4*	p < 0.05
Legs	8.3 ± 2.7	-2.5 ± 1.5†	8.4 ± 3.2	-1.2 ± 1.4*	p < 0.01
Total body	24.7 ± 7.4	-4.9 ± 2.8†	23.0 ± 10.6	-1.9 ± 2.8**	p < 0.01
Body weight	64.5 ± 8.4	-0.1 ± 3.0	65.1 ± 13.8	-1.3 ± 3.4	NS

*Significance of difference between the initial value and the value at 1 year. p < 0.01.
† p < 0.001.
**p < 0.05.

13.2). Since non-osseous lean body mass consists of both muscle and non-muscle lean tissue (viscera, etc.), the observed increase in non-osseous lean body mass could be caused by a change in either of these compartments. The 24-hour urinary creatinine excretion can be used as a rough estimate of the total body muscle mass (Heymsfield *et al.*, 1983). In the above-mentioned study, one year of nandrolone decanoate treatment resulted in an increase in the 24-hour urinary creatinine excretion corresponding to an increase in muscle mass of 3–4 kg (Heymsfield *et al.*, 1983).

Theoretically, part of the increase in urinary creatinine excretion may be caused by metabolic changes rather than changes in the muscle mass *per se*. Testosterone, which nandrolone decanoate resembles in some ways, does in fact stimulate the rate-limiting enzyme (glycine amidino-transferase) in the creatinine production (Walker, 1979). The quantitative importance of this relation is, however, unknown. If the observed increase in urinary creatinine was caused solely by metabolic alteration, one would expect an initial increase followed by a plateau. If the increase was caused solely by a change in muscle mass, a slower and more prolonged increase would be expected. In the above-mentioned study the 24-hour urinary creatinine excretion was only measured before and after the treatment but since the creatinine clearance remained unchanged, the serum concentration of creatinine could be used as an estimate of the urinary creatinine excretion rate. The serum creatinine was already significantly increased at three months of nandrolone decanoate treatment, but it continued to increase throughout the study period. This, and the greater relative increase in non-osseous lean body mass in the limbs than in the trunk, suggests that the increase in non-osseous lean body mass was at least partly due to an increase in muscle mass. Furthermore, the fat content in the forearm (measured by single-photon absorptiometry) continued to decrease gradually during the treatment (Figure 13.4). The total loss in forearm fat at one year of treatment corresponded to a decrease in total body fat of 5 kg (Hassager *et al.*, 1988), i.e. in the same magnitude as that found by the dual-photon absorptiometry measurement.

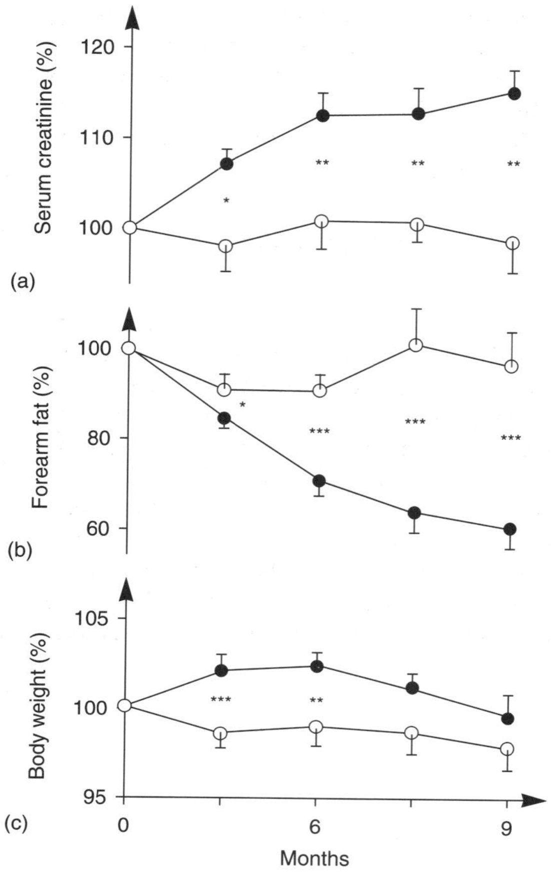

Figure 13.4 (a) Changes in serum creatinine. (b) The thickness of the fat layer in the distal forearm. (c) Body weight during treatment with ND (n = 19, ●) or placebo (n = 17, ○). Values are given in percent of the initial values as mean ± 1 SEM. *$p < 0.05$; **$p < 0.01$; ***$p < 0.001$. Reproduced with permission from Hassager *et al.* (1989).

It is still debated whether treatment with anabolic steroids can increase muscle strength among young and healthy subjects (Haupt and Rovere, 1984). It seems to be most efficient in subjects who have trained to the point where they are in a catabolic state (Haupt and Rovere, 1984), but much higher doses than those used in the present study are needed to change the body composition in young healthy subjects (Forbes, 1985). The hypothesis is perhaps valid that a dose of anabolic steroid, too small to alter the body composition in young healthy subjects, could change the body composition of an elderly osteoporotic woman who is probably in a slight but chronic catabolic state. Attempts to improve nitrogen balance by the use of anabolic steroids in other catabolic states has, however, largely failed to be of practical value (Wilson and Griffin, 1980).

The change in soft tissue composition towards a leaner and more muscular body found in the above-mentioned study agrees with the findings of Aloia *et al.* (1981), who reported a 10% increase in total body potassium in osteoporotic women during treatment with methandrostenolone. In a study of osteoporotic women treated with nandrolone decanoate, Need *et al.* (1987) reported an increase in serum creatinine of the same order.

EFFECTS ON SERUM LIPIDS AND LIPOPROTEINS

Taggart *et al.* (1982) have shown that stanozolol dramatically decreases the serum HDL cholesterol and increases the serum LDL cholesterol, without changing the total serum cholesterol. Other oral anabolic steroids (danazol (Allen and Frazer, 1981) and oxandrolone (Cheung *et al.*, 1980)) have been shown to decrease HDL cholesterol similarly. Anabolic steroids have also been shown to increase insulin resistance (Wym, 1977; Bruce *et al.*, 1992). These alterations in metabolic factors might increase the atherogenic risk (Grodon *et al.*, 1977). The only effect of nandrolone decanoate on serum lipids and lipoproteins was a decrease in HDL cholesterol (Hassager *et al.*, 1989) (Figure 13.5). Thus, from an atherogenic point of view, nandrolone decanoate seems to be safer than oral anabolic steroids, when given IM (avoiding the first-pass effect on the liver), especially for long-term therapy. However its effects on insulin resistance present a concern for long-term use in relatively younger women.

SIDE EFFECTS

Treatment with nandrolone decanoate has shown a marginal increase in serum aspartate aminotransferase (ASAT). The clinical significance of this is unknown, but it must be borne in mind that different hepatic lesions, e.g.

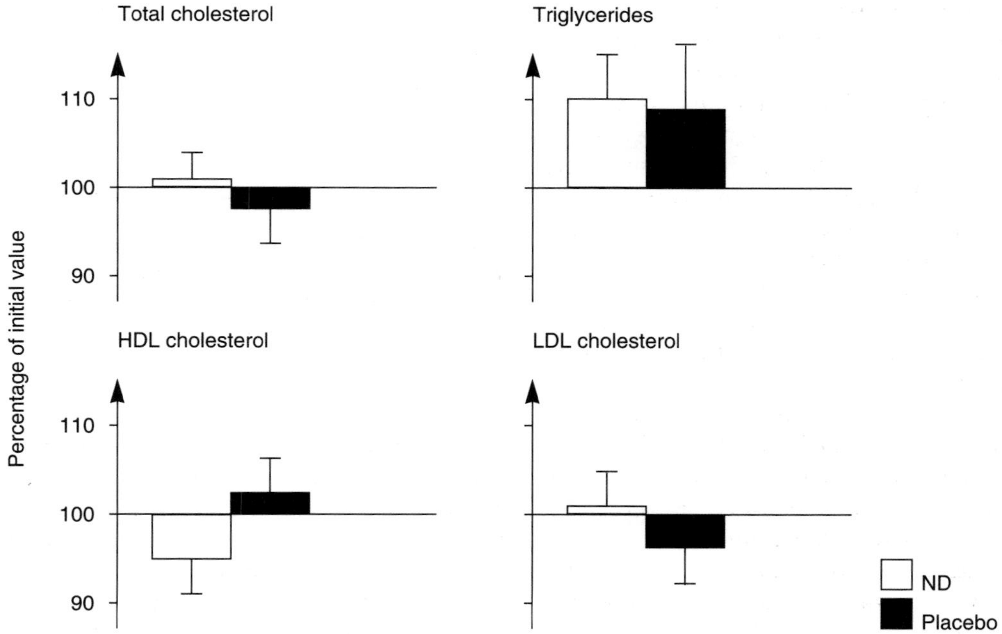

Figure 13.5 Cumulated treatment response (mean of four examinations) on serum lipids and lipoproteins following ND (□, n = 19) and placebo (■, n = 17) treatment. Values are given as mean ± 1 SEM and expressed in percent of initial values. Reproduced with permission from Hassager *et al.* (1989).

hepatomas and peliosis hepatis, have been noted in patients during long-term treatment with oral anabolic steroids in high doses (Haupt and Rovere, 1984). These diseases are serious but rare.

The development of clinical adverse reactions, such as increase in facial hair, acne and hoarseness, during treatment with anabolic steroids has been reported (Chesnut *et al.*, 1983; Haupt and Rovere, 1984). Although it has been claimed that nandrolone decanoate has minimal virilizing side effects when used in the recommended dosage (Dequeker and Guesens, 1985), 80% of the women in the present study complained of hoarseness after one year of therapy. However, the compliance of the patients treated with nandrolone remained high (95%).

EFFECTS ON CORTICOSTEROID-INDUCED BONE LOSS

Long-term corticosteroid administration in humans results almost invariably in osteopenia and increased tendency to fracture (Baylink, 1983). Corticosteroid-induced osteoporosis seems to be due to both a direct inhibition of bone formation and increased bone resorption (Jowsey and Riggs, 1970; Meunier *et al.*, 1984) as a consequence of secondary hyperparathyroidism (Suzuki *et al.*, 1983; Gennari *et al.*, 1984), caused in turn by decreased intestinal absorption of calcium (Klein *et al.*, 1977, Nordin *et al.*, 1981). There are contradictory reports about the beneficial effects on bone mass of calcium supplements and pharmacological doses of vitamin D (Nilsen *et al.*, 1978; Hahn *et al.*, 1979; Dykman *et al.*, 1984).

Bisphosphonates have been reported to counteract bone loss by inhibiting bone resorption in corticosteroid-treated patients (Reid *et al.*, 1988). However, a further rapid inhibition of bone formation induced by these agents might cancel out its long-term efficacy.

Anabolics have been reported to have a positive effect in postmenopausal osteoporosis and it has been suggested that this beneficial effect is due to both inhibition of bone resorption and stimulation of bone formation (Geusens and Dequeker, 1986; Need *et al.*, 1987). These findings seem to indicate that anabolic steroids might represent the ideal treatment for corticosteroid-induced osteoporosis.

Studies have correspondingly indicated that nandrolone decanoate was able to prevent the corticosteroid-induced decrease in bone mass (Adami *et al.*, 1987) (Figure 13.6).

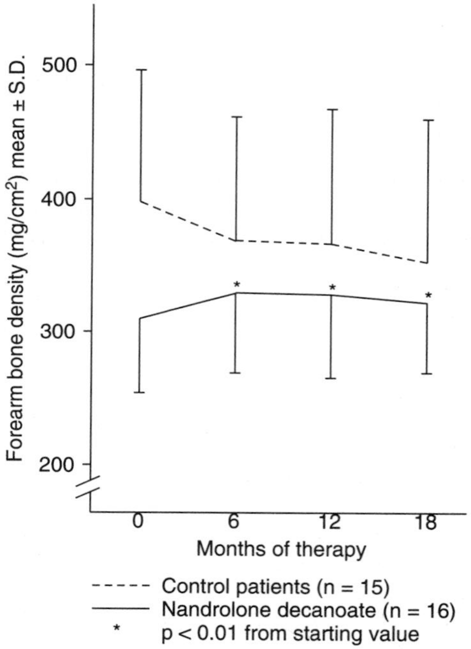

Figure 13.6 The effect of nandrolone decanoate on bone density in patients treated with corticosteroid.

REFERENCES

Adami, S., Fossaluzza, V., Rossini, M. *et al.* (1987) Preventive and therapeutic effects of nandrolone decanoate in the patients with corticosteroid induced osteoporosis. In: *Osteoporosis 1987*, (eds Christiansen, C. *et al.*), Osteopress ApS, Copenhagen, pp. 25–9.

Allen, J.K. and Frazer, I.S. (1981) Cholesterol, high density lipoprotein and danazol. *J Clin Endocrinol Metab* **53**: 149–53.

Aloia, J.F., Kapoor, A., Vawani, A. *et al.* (1981) Changes in body composition following therapy of osteoporosis with methandrostenolone. *Metabolism* **30**: 1076–9.

Baylink, D.J. (1983) Glucocorticoid-induced osteoporosis. *N Engl J Med* **309**: 306–8.

Benéton, M.C., Yates, A.J., Rogers, S., McCloskey, E.V. and Kanis, J.A. (1991) Stanozolol stimulates remodelling of trabecular bone and net formation of bone at the endocortical surface. *Clin Sci* **81**: 543–9.

Bruce, R., Godsland, I., Stevenson, J.C. *et al.* (1992) Danazol induces resistance to both insulin and glucagon in young women. *Clin Sci* **82**: 211–17.

Chesnut III, C.H., Nelp, W.B., Baylink, D.J. *et al.* (1977) Effect of methandrostenolone on postmenopausal bone wasting as assessed by changes in total bone mineral mass. *Metabolism* **26**: 267–77.

Chesnut III, C.H., Ivey, J.L., Gruber, H.D. *et al.* (1983) Stanozolol in postmenopausal osteoporosis: therapeutic efficacy and possible mechanisms of action. *Metabolism* **32**: 571–80.

Cheung, M.C., Albers, J.J., Wahl, P.W. *et al.* (1980) High density lipoproteins during hypolipidemic therapy. A comparative study of four drugs. *Atherosclerosis* **35**: 215–28.

Dequeker, J. and Geusens, P. (1985) Anabolic steroid and osteoporosis. *Acta Endocrinol* **271** (Suppl 110): 45–52.

Dykman, T.R., Haralson, K.M., Gluck, O.S. *et al.* (1984) Effect of oral 1,25 dihyroxyvitamin D and calcium on glucocorticoid-induced osteopenia in patients with rheumatic diseases. *Arth Rheum* **27**: 1336–43.

Forbes, G.B. (1985) The effect of anabolic steroids on lean body mass: the dose response curve. *Metabolism* **34**: 571–3.

Gennari, C., AgnusDei, D., Gonnelli, S. and Nardi, P. (1989) Effects of nandrolone decanoate therapy on bone mass and calcium metabolism in women with established post-menopausal osteo-porosis: a double-blind placebo-controlled study. *Maturitas* **11**: 187–97.

Gennari, C., Imbimbo, B., Montagnani, M. *et al.* (1984) Effects of prednisone and deflazacort on mineral metabolism and parathyroid hormone activity in humans. *Calcif Tissue Int* **36**: 245–52.

Geusens, P. and Dequeker, J. (1986) Long term effect of nandrolone decanoate, 10-hydroxyvitamin D_3, or intermittent calcium infusion therapy on bone mineral content, bone remodeling and fracture rate in symptomatic osteoporosis: a double blind controlled study. *Bone Mineral* **1**: 347–51.

Geusens, P., Dequeker, J., Verstraeten, A., Nijs, J. and van Holsbeeck, M. (1986) Bone mineral context, cortical thickness and fracture rate in osteoporotic women after withdrawal of treatment with nandralone decanoate, 1-alpha hydroxyvitamin D_3, or intermittent calcium infusions. *Maturitas* **8**: 281–9.

Gresik, E.W., and Barka, T. (1983) Epidermal growth factor, renin, and protease in hormonally responsive duct cells of the mouse sublingual gland. *Anat Rec* **205**: 169–75.

Grodon, T., Castelli, W.P., Hjortland, M.C. *et al.* (1977) High density lipoprotein as a protective factor against coronary heart disease. *Am J Med* **62**: 707–15.

Hahn, T.J., Halstead, L.R., Teitelbaum, S.L. and Hahn, B.H. (1979) Altered mineral metabolism in glucocorticoid-induced osteopenia. Effect of 25-hydroxyvitamin D administration. *J Clin Invest* **64**: 655–65.

Hassager, C., Borg, J. and Christiansen, C. (1988) Measurement of the subcutaneous fat in the distal forearm by single photon absorptiometry. *Metabolism* **38**: 159–65.

Hassager, C., Jensen, J.T., Johansen, J.S. *et al.* (1991) Collagen synthesis in postmenopausal women during therapy with anabolic steroid and female sex hormones. *Metabolism* **40**: 205–8.

Hassager, C., Jensen, L.T., Pødenphant, J., Riis, B.J. and Christiansen, C. (1990) The carboxy terminal propeptide of type I procollagen in serum as a marker of bone formation: the effect of nandrolone decanoate and female sex hormones. *Metabolism* **39**: 1167–9.

Hassager, C., Jensen, L.T., Pødenphant, J., Thomsen, K. and Christiansen, C. (1994) The carboxy-terminal pyridinoline cross-linked telopeptide of type 1 collagen in serum as a marker of bone resorption: the effect of nandrolone decanoate and hormone replacement therapy. *Calcif Tissue Int* **54**: 30–3.

Hassager, C., Pødenphant, J., Riis, B.J. *et al.* (1989) Changes in soft tissue body composition and plasma lipid metabolism during nandrolone decanoate therapy in postmenopausal osteoporotic women. *Metabolism* **38**: 238–42.

Haupt, H.A. and Rovere, G.D. (1984) Anabolic steroids: a review of the literature. *Am J Sports Med* **12**: 469–84.

Heymsfield, S.B., Arteaga, C., McManus, C. *et al.* (1983) Measurement of muscle mass in humans: validity of the 24-hour urinary creatinine method. *Am J Clin Nutrition* **37**: 478–94.

Hodgkinson, A., Aaron, J.E., Horsman, A., McLachlin, M.S.F. and Nordin, B.E.C. (1978) Effect of oophorectomy and calcium deprivation on bone mass in the rat. *Clin Sci Mol Med* **54**: 439–46.

Ishii, D.N. and Shooter, E.M. (1975) Regulation of nerve growth factor synthesis in mouse submaxillary glands by testosterone. *J Neurochem* **25**: 843–51.

Johansen, J.S., Hassager, C., Pødenphant, J. *et al.* (1989) Treatment of postmenopausal osteoporosis. Is the anabolic steroid nandrolone decanoate a candidate? *Bone Mineral* **6**: 77–86.

Jowsey, J. and Riggs, B.L. (1970) Bone formation in hypercortisonism. *Acta Endocrinol* **63**: 21–87.

Kalu, D.N., Liu, C.C., Hardin, R.R. and Hollis, B.W. (1989) The aged rat model of ovarian hormone deficiency bone loss. *Endocrinology* **124**: 7–16.

Kanis, J.A., Johnell, O., Gullberg, B. *et al.* (1992) Evidence for efficacy of drugs affecting bone metabolism in preventing hip fracture. *Br Med J* **305**: 1124–8.

Kasperk, C.H., Fitzsimmons, R.J., Strong, D. *et al.* (1990) *J Clin Endocrinol Metab* **56**: 85–92.

Kenyon, A.T., Knowlton, K., Sandiford, I. *et al.* (1940) A comparative study of the metabolic effects of testosterone propionate in normal men and women and in eunuchoidism. *Endocrinology* **26**: 26–45.

Klein, R.G., Arnaud, S.B., Gallagher, J.C., DeLuca, H.F. and Riggs, B.L. (1977) Intestinal calcium absorption in exogenous hypercortisonism. Role of 25-hydroxivitamin D and corticosteroid dose. *J Clin Invest* **60**: 253–9.

Kockakian, C.D. (1976) *Handbook of Experimental Pharmacology*, 43, Springer-Verlag, Berlin.

Kopera, H. (1985) The history of anabolic steroids and a review of clinical experience with anabolic steroids. *Acta Endocrinol* (*Copenh.*) **110** (Suppl 271): 11–18.

Malluche, H.H., Faugere, M.C., Rush, M. and Freidler, R. (1986) Osteoblastic insufficiency is responsible for maintenance of osteopenia after loss of ovarian function in experimental beagle dogs. *Endocrinology* **119**: 2649–54.

Meunier, P.J., Dempster, D.W., Edouard, C. *et al.* (1984) Bone histomorphometry in corticosteroid-induced osteoporosis and Cushing's Syndrome. *Adv Exp Med Biol* **171**: 191–200.

Need, A.G., Horowitz, M., Walker, C.J. *et al.* (1989) Cross-over study of fat-corrected forearm mineral content during nandrolone decanoate therapy for osteoporosis. *Bone* **10**: 3–6.

Need, A.G., Morris, H.A., Hartley, T.F. *et al.* (1987) Effects of nandrolone decanoate on forearm mineral density and calcium metabolism in osteoporotic postmenopausal women. *Calcif Tissue Int* **41**: 7–10.

Nilsen, K.H., Jayson, M.I.V. and Dixon, A.S. (1978) Microcrystalline calcium hydroxyapatite compound in corticosteroid-treated rheumatoid patients: a controlled study. *Br Med J* **2**: 1124–30.

Nordin, B.E.C., Marshall, D.H., Francis, R.M. and Crilly, R.G. (1981) The effects of sex steroid and corticosteroid hormones on bone. *J Steroid Biochem* **15**: 171–4.

Reid, I.R., King, A.R., Alexander, C.J. and Ibbertson, H.K. (1988) Prevention of steroid-induced osteoporosis with (3-amino-1-hydroxypropylidene)-1,1-bisphosphonate (APD). *Lancet* **i**: 143–6.

Saville, P.D. (1969) Changes in skeletal mass and fragility with castration in the rat; a model of osteoporosis. *J Am Geriatr Soc* **17**: 155–67.

Schot, L.D.C., Brunekreet, K., Spanygers, C. and Bouillon, R. (1989) Anabolic and anticatabolic effects of nandrolone decanoate of bone and ovariectomized rats. In: *Osteoporosis 1990*, (eds Christiansen, C. *et al.*), Osteopress APS, Copenhagen, pp. 19–23.

Schot, L.P.C. and Schuurs, A.H.W.M. (1987) Stimulation of bone formation by the anabolic steroid Deca-Durabolin (DD) in osteoporotic female rats. In: *Osteoporosis 1987*, (eds Christiansen, C. *et al.*), Osteopress Aps, Copenhagen, pp. 969–71.

Suzuki, Y., Ichikawa, Y., Saito, E. and Homma, M. (1983) Importance of increased urinary calcium excretion in the development of secondary hyperparathyroidism of patients undergoing glucocorticoid therapy. *Metabolism* **32**: 151–6.

Taggart, H.M., Applebaum-Bowden, D., Haffner, S. *et al.* (1982) Reduction in high density lipoproteins by anabolic steroid (stanozolol) therapy for postmenopausal osteoporosis. *Metabolism* **31**: 1147–52.

Turner, R.T., Francis, R., Wakley, G.K. and Evans, G.L. (1989b) *J Bone Miner Res* **4** (Suppl 1): S337.

Turner, R.T., Hannon, K.S., Demers, L.M., Buchanan, J. and Bell, N.H. (1989a) Differential effects of gonadal function on bone histomorphometry in male and female rats. *J Bone Miner Res* **4**: 557–63.

Turner, R.T., Vandersteenhoven, J.J. and Bell, N.H. (1987) The effect of ovariectomy and 17 beta-oestradiol on cortical bone histomorphometry in growing rats. *J Bone Miner Res* **2**: 115–22.

Walker, J.B. (1979) Creatinine: biosynthesis, regulation, and functions. *Adv Enzymol* **50**: 177–242.

Wilson, J.D. and Griffin, J.E. (1980) The use and misuse of androgens. *Metabolism* **29**: 1278–95.

Wronski, T.H., Lowry, P.L., Walsh, C.C. and Ignasezewski, L.A. (1985) Skeletal alterations in ovariectomized rats. *Calcif Tissue Int* **37**: 317–24.

Wym, V., (1977) Metabolic effects of danazol. *J Int Med Res* **5** (Suppl 3): 25–35.

FLUORIDE THERAPY FOR POSTMENOPAUSAL OSTEOPOROSIS 14

M. Kleerekoper and D.A. Nelson

INTRODUCTION

In 1937, Roholm reported that the bones of people exposed to industrial fluoride had become abnormally dense. This original work demonstrated that the severity of the skeletal changes was correlated with the extent and duration of the exposure. Moderate exposure caused an increase in density with greater exposure (greater amounts, longer duration) resulting in obvious periosteal new bone formation and calcification of tendons and ligaments. Pursuing this observation, Rich and Ensinck (1961) are credited with performing the first clinical experiments with sodium fluoride (NaF) when they reported that 60 mg/day orally for 14 or more weeks resulted in positive calcium balance in patients with Paget's disease of bone, or with postmenopausal or steroid-induced osteoporosis. This was confirmed two years later by Bernstein *et al.* (1963) who used 50–200 mg/day in their studies, and also noted that the therapy was effective in relieving bone pain.

The first report of a favorable radiographic response to therapeutically administered NaF appears to be that of Cohen and Gardner (1964) who used the drug in patients with multiple myeloma. Essentially, as a desperation measure in patients incapacitated by the skeletal complications of their disease, they administered 100 mg/day to 12 patients, only two of whom survived therapy for more than two years. In an addendum to that publication, they reported an additional three patients who received 90 mg/day along with 6 mg/day of calcium lactate. A positive radiographic response was seen as early as three months in one of these patients, substantially faster than the 10 or more years of industrial exposure to fluoride that is required before fluorosis is seen radiographically (Largent, 1961). In the three decades since these pioneering studies with this drug that clearly causes increases in bone density, more than 400 studies have been reported in the peer-reviewed literature and almost certainly an equal number of publications in the non-peer-reviewed literature. Clearly, there has been sufficient time and effort to have learned with certainty whether or not NaF is suitable therapy for osteoporosis. Regrettably, at the time of writing, there remains complete uncertainty and controversy concerning the role, if any, of NaF in the management of osteoporosis. This chapter will review many of these studies, focusing on areas where there is seeming consensus about NaF, areas of conflicting reports and, in particular, areas where clearly insufficient good work has been completed.

Osteoporosis. Edited by John C. Stevenson and Robert Lindsay. Published in 1998 by Chapman & Hall, London. ISBN 0 412 48870 1

ABSORPTION, METABOLISM AND PLASMA LEVELS OF FLUORIDE

Fluoride is normally present in the food chain in humans from a variety of sources, predominantly the water supply and the use of fluoridated water in processing of foods, as well as from toothpastes and mouthwashes. Absorption, mainly in the form of hydrofluoric acid, is fairly rapid from the stomach. Approximately 75–90% of orally administered fluoride is absorbed, but high concentrations of cations (calcium, magnesium, aluminum) can limit this absorption. Absorption also decreases with age and it has been suggested that absorption may be even further impaired in some patients with osteoporosis who do not respond to therapy. Once absorbed, fluoride exists in plasma in an ionic and organically bound form. The ion is removed from the extracellular fluid by uptake in mineralized tissues (bone and teeth) and by renal excretion. Uptake by bones and teeth is greatest during growth and development and during periods of mineralization in the mature adult skeleton. During mineralization, fluoride replaces the hydroxyl ion in the crystal lattice, giving rise to fluorapatite. Fluoride is removed from bone by resorption and the net accumulation of fluoride in the skeleton is the balance between absorption, uptake, resorption and renal excretion. In older adults with decreased absorption and decreased renal excretion, net accumulation appears to increase. From the normal food chain, plasma levels in adults (18–80) range from 0.5 to 2.3 μM (Husdan *et al.*, 1976).

As noted, NaF is readily absorbed from the stomach except in the presence of large quantities of the cations calcium, magnesium and aluminum, with concomitant calcium administration reducing fluoride absorption by 20–35% (Jowsey and Riggs, 1978; Nagant de Deuxchaisnes *et al.*, 1990). As discussed below, it is important to provide adequate calcium when attempting to treat osteoporosis with NaF. Care should be taken to space the ingestion of these two drugs at least one hour apart. Also discussed below is the problem of gastrointestinal distress that often complicates NaF therapy with certain preparations that have been used. Many patients will get prompt relief from these symptoms with antacids, most of which contain aluminum or magnesium. This would also limit the absorption of NaF. Finally, care should be taken to consider lowering the dose of NaF in persons with impaired renal function, since there are case reports of fluoride toxicity when seemingly appropriate doses have been given to patients with mild renal impairment (Gerster *et al.*, 1983).

In 1986, Pak *et al.* reported on the serum fluoride levels obtained with a slow release preparation of NaF, 25 mg twice a day, in women with postmenopausal osteoporosis. Values were between 5 and 10 μM (95–190 ng/ml), and reported to be 'above the subtherapeutic level in serum of 95 ng/ml'. They also reported that 'the lower limit of the toxic level of fluoride has been set at 10 μM (or 190 ng/ml), since fluorosis has been reported above this concentration'. The reference for these alleged established values for the 'therapeutic window' for serum fluoride levels was a review by Taves published in 1970. Much of the data relates to small numbers of animal experiments (sheep, cattle, rats). Even casual reading of that publication reveals that, in 1970, 'There (was) only one patient treated with fluoride in whom we have serum fluoride concentrations and evidence of new bone formation. The available data suggests that a fasting serum fluoride of 5–10 μM will avoid generalized toxic effects and yet induce positive calcium balance and increased bone. However, this estimate is based on much too little data and should be considered only a reasonable starting point for further investigation'. Regrettably, this widely quoted 5–10 μM range has not yet been systematically studied and any statements about the 'therapeutic window' must be regarded with significant skepticism.

The issue of safe, therapeutic and toxic blood levels of fluoride is of more than trivial importance. Water fluoridation programs have been in effect in many communities now for upwards of 30 years. There are a number of disturbing reports of an increased prevalence of hip fractures in communities with high water fluoride content (naturally or as a result of an active fluoridation program). These studies have recently been reviewed in the report of a National Institutes of Health workshop (Gordon and Corbin, 1992). (Interestingly, that report also quotes the 95–190 ng/ml range, without attribution.) Serum levels of fluoride appear to increase with age as a result of more prolonged exposure and also because of age-related declines in renal function. It is entirely possible, but by no means more than speculation for now, that many of our older citizens are accumulating a toxic burden of fluoride. If the therapeutic window for fluoride were indeed more firmly established, one could consider screening exposed communities for potential fluoride toxicity. While somewhat farfetched as this book is being published, the potential increases with each decade of water fluoridation programs. As Taves stated in 1970, the currently accepted values must be regarded as a reasonable starting point for further investigation.

One of the most frequent side effects of fluoride administration is gastrointestinal distress which is felt to be a chemical gastritis resulting from the direct effect of hydrofluoric acid on gastric mucosa. This appears to be dependent on both the dose of fluoride administered and the form in which the drug is ingested. Several groups have attempted to minimize this by utilizing enteric-coated tablets or slow-release preparations. In general, the absorption and bioavailability are greatest with rapidly soluble preparations absorbed from the stomach, worst with enteric-coated preparations, with slow-release products being intermediate (Hasvold and Ekren, 1981; Nagant de Deuxchaisnes *et al.*, 1990; Pak *et al.*, 1986). There is also a greater individual variance in bioavailability with enteric-coated and slow-release preparations (Hasvold and Ekren, 1981). The effect of concomitant administration of food and calcium supplements on fluoride absorption and bioavailability also varies greatly from preparation to preparation (Briancon *et al.*, 1990; Devogelaer *et al.*, 1991). This further underscores the importance of establishing the relationship, if any, between sodium fluoride levels and therapeutic efficacy. Pending these studies being completed, some investigators have evaluated urine excretion of fluoride as a means of monitoring the response to therapy. Not surprisingly, one group has reported that the best response was seen in patients with the highest urine fluoride (Duursma *et al.*, 1990), while the opposite observation was reported by another group (Kraenzlin *et al.*, 1990).

It is not particularly surprising that it has proven so difficult to establish a clear relationship between blood levels or urinary excretion of fluoride and therapeutic efficacy. Orally administered fluoride is deposited in the skeleton at a rate that depends on the absorption and the pre-existing body burden of the ion, the rate of skeletal remodeling and the urinary clearance of fluoride. Furthermore, it would seem reasonable to assume that total skeletal mass, as well as the proportion of cancellous and cortical skeletal mass, would affect blood and urine levels of fluoride. As therapy continues, all of these variables will be changing. It would seem appropriate to obtain a 24-hour urine fluoride and fasting serum fluoride on all patients enrolled in future clinical trials with this drug. Serial measurements of blood and urine fluoride should be obtained whenever serial measurement of bone mass is obtained in these trials. To minimize intraindividual variation in absorption and clearance of orally administered fluoride, blood samples should be drawn in the fasting state before the morning dose of therapy. With this information it will be possible to prospectively determine whether or not monitoring blood or urine fluoride is an important adjunct to fluoride therapy.

MECHANISM OF ACTION

Fluoride appears to have two quite distinct effects on skeletal metabolism, both of which independently and jointly may affect the therapeutic potential of NaF in osteoporosis. While it has not been definitely established that fluoride enhances recruitment of osteoblasts rather than the function of existing cells, the bulk of evidence appears to favor the osteoblast recruitment hypothesis. Fluoride inhibits the activity of osteoblastic acid phosphatase/phosphotyrosyl protein phosphatase and this has been postulated to be the proximate cause of the mitogenic potential of this ion (Lau *et al.*, 1989). Osteoblastic cells from osteoporotic subjects demonstrating a positive histologic response to NaF have greater maximal DNA synthesis than similarly derived osteoblastic cells from untreated subjects or from fluoride nonresponders (Marie *et al.*, 1990). Most importantly, fluoride has little, if any, stimulatory effect on osteoclasts and may even decrease the activity of these cells at levels commonly attained in the plasma of patients treated with NaF (Bellows *et al.*, 1990). In the normal bone remodeling cycle (see Chapters 3 and 4), the stimulus to osteoblast recruitment is prior bone resorption. This property, to promote osteoblast recruitment without prior stimulation of osteoclastic activity, is seen only with fluoride and aluminum (Quarles *et al.*, 1989). Since this is the only mechanism for developing long-term (>3 years) positive skeletal balance (direct stimulation of osteoclasts without osteoblastic stimulation), fluoride has tremendous potential for therapy for osteoporosis.

The second mechanism whereby fluoride affects the skeleton lies in the affinity of the ions for apatite crystal, replacing the hydroxyl group to form fluorapatite. The crystal lattice of fluorapatite is quite different from that of hydroxyapatite (Figure 14.1), and the changes render the crystal more stable (Gron *et al.*, 1966; Eanes and Reddi, 1979). This enhanced stability makes the skeletal structures more resistant to osteoblastic resorption (Grynpas and Cheng, 1988), further altering the normal remodeling cycle. Since remodeling appears to be such an integral part of skeletal health, these two properties of fluoride, increased formation of bone that is more resistant to remodeling, are in apparent conflict. This may, at least in part, explain why it has

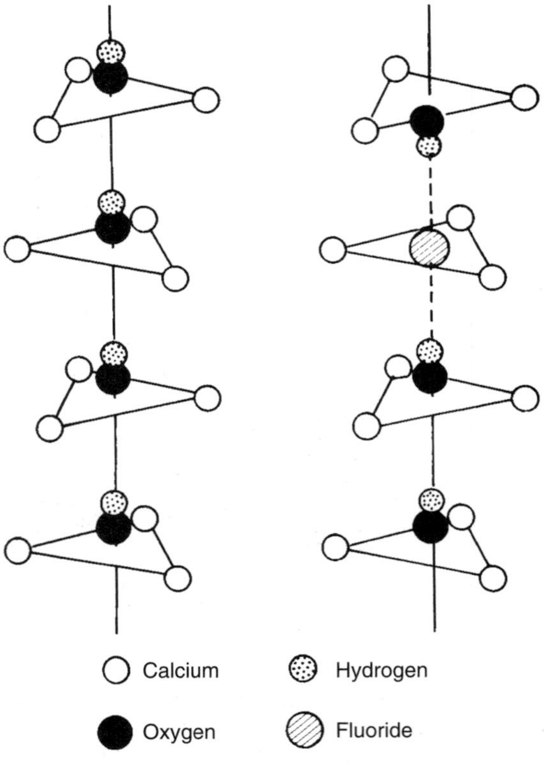

Figure 14.1 Schematic comparison of the crystal lattice structure of hydroxyapatite (left) and fluorapatite (right). Reproduced with permission from Eanes and Reddi (1979).

proven so difficult to demonstrate therapeutic efficacy of this drug in osteoporosis.

The net effect of these conflicting actions is to produce bone that is quite abnormal. Doses of NaF less than 30 mg/day have no consistent effect on skeletal histology, while 80 or more mg/day results in marked abnormalities with the bone matrix being irregularly fibrous and woven rather than lamellar and irregularly distributed osteocytes in enlarged lacunae surrounded by halos of low mineral density (Reutter *et al.*, 1970). The enhanced matrix deposition results in excess osteoid which is poorly mineralized. In some patients this mineralization defect may be of sufficient severity to satisfy criteria for generalized or focal osteomalacia (Figure 14.2) (Parsons *et al.*, 1977; Parfitt, 1990). Frank clinical osteomalacia has been reported when NaF is administered without calcium supplements (Compston *et al.*, 1980), although even 1500 mg/day of supplemental calcium is not sufficient to prevent the development of histologic osteomalacia (Kleerekoper *et al.*, 1990). This osteomalacia is not vitamin D dependent nor does it respond to vitamin D therapy (Compston *et al.*, 1980). In fact, several studies have demonstrated that conconcurrent administration of vitamin D blunts the skeletal response to NaF (Olah *et al.*, 1978; Delmas *et al.*, 1984; Erikson *et al.*, 1985). There is no consensus on the effect of duration of treatment on the histologic changes induced by NaF. We have reported significant changes as early as six months in a group of patients with low turnover osteoporosis (Kleerekoper *et al.*,

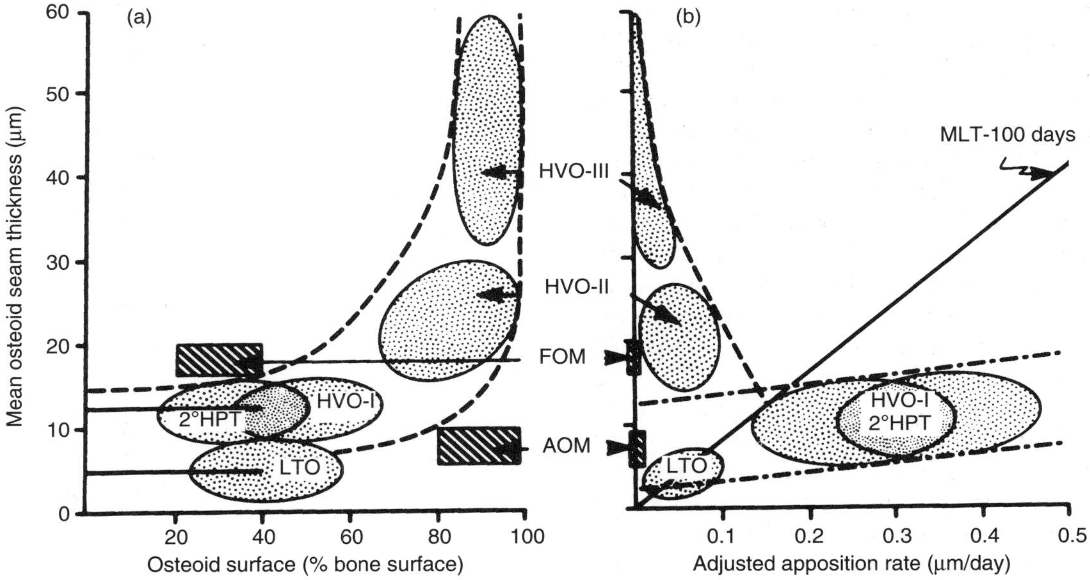

Figure 14.2 Histomorphometric characteristics of different types of osteomalacia. (a) Relationship between increasing osteoid surface and mean osteoid thickness. (b) Relationship between adjusted appositional rate and mean osteoid seam thickness. In focal osteomalacia (FOM) seen in some patients on fluoride therapy, the osteoid seam width is greater than anticipated for both the surface extent of osteoid and the adjusted apposition rate. Other patients on fluoride therapy may exhibit a more usual relationship between these parameters and develop generalized osteomalacia. HVO: hypovitaminosis D; HPT: hyperparathyroidism; LTO: low-turnover osteoporosis; FOM: focal osteomalacia; AOM: atypical osteomalacia; MLT: mineralization lag time. Reproduced with permission from Rao (1993).

1981) and effects as early as two months have been reported in individual patients (Kullencordt *et al.*, 1970). We have demonstrated that bone formation rate and osteoblast vigor are often impaired after three years of continuous therapy (Kleerekoper *et al.*, 1990), while Lundy (1989) has reported that this resolves with several more years of continued therapy.

One of the postulated mechanisms whereby reduction in cancellous bone volume results in osteoporotic fracture is disruption of the internal architecture (Parfitt *et al.*, 1983; Kleerekoper *et al.*, 1985). NaF, despite its ability to increase cancellous bone volume, cannot restore the original, biomechanically competent architecture. Osteoblasts can only deposit newly synthesized bone matrix on existing bone surfaces. Thus, NaF and any other molecule capable of stimulating ostoblastic activity only have potential to thicken existing trabeculae (Aaron *et al.*, 1990) and not restore connectivity. Thus, the relationships between bone mass and mechanical strength that characterize normal bone and bone in untreated osteoporosis, are likely to be non-operative in fluoride-treated bone. This, of course, may not be unique to fluoride therapy and may apply to any therapy for osteoporosis and may explain, at least in part, why it has proven so difficult to develop a suitable therapy for this disease.

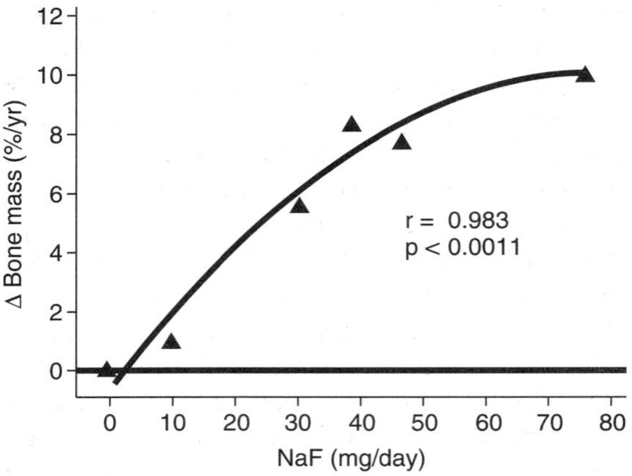

Figure 14.3 The effect of increasing fluoride dose on spinal bone mass. Reproduced with permission from Kleerekoper and Batena (1991).

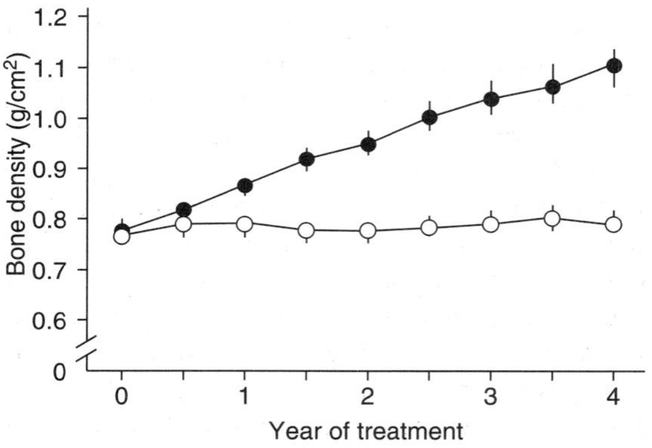

Figure 14.4 The effect of fluoride (solid circles) 75 mg/day plus calcium 1500 mg/day on bone mass is linear over four years of therapy and significantly greater than the effect of calcium 1500 mg/day alone (open circles). Reproduced with permission from Riggs *et al.* (1990).

EFFECT OF NaF ON BONE MASS

It has been firmly established that NaF increases spinal bone mass, in dose-dependent manner, with the lowest effective dose being 30 mg/day (Figure 14.3) (Hansson and Roos, 1987; Kleerekoper *et al.*, 1991). The response appears to be linear with time for at least 4–6 years in one prospective study (Figure 14.4) (Riggs *et al.*, 1990, 1994). In an uncontrolled study with patients treated for upwards of ten years, where spinal bone mass was not measured at baseline (because the study was initiated before we had the ability to obtain this measurement), we were able to demonstrate a linear relationship between bone mass and the duration of therapy prior to the measurement (Kleerekoper *et al.*, 1991). Given the proposed mechanisms of action of NaF described above, it is not surprising that bone mass continues to increase as long as drug therapy is continued and osteoblast recruitment is enhanced. This is in contrast to therapy with antiresorptive drugs such as calcitonin, where there is only limited capacity to increase bone mass (Gennari *et al.*, 1985). In that circumstance, as resorption is inhibited, osteoblastic bone formation continues until pre-existing resorption cavities are filled in with new bone. Once this has occurred, the stimulus to new bone formation has effectively been dampened by inhibition of bone resorption. This property of NaF to apparently continue to enhance recruitment of osteoblasts for 6–10 years without delay in effectiveness may be alerting us to important concepts concerning the pathogenesis of osteoporosis. While there may be reduction in osteoblast vigor with prolonged therapy (Kleerekoper *et al.*, 1990), this does not appear to affect the ability to increase bone mass. Quite possibly, osteoblast recruitment is even further enhanced to compensate for this. Whatever the precise mechanism, it is clear from these studies of fluoride therapy that osteoporotic patients retain the potential to generate new osteoblasts for many years after the disease has become clinically apparent. This suggests that defective signaling between resorption and formation (uncoupling of the bone remodeling cycle) is a crucial factor in the pathogenesis of osteoporosis. Clues to effective therapy clearly lie in further understanding these mechanisms.

While antiresorptive therapy, theoretically and experimentally (Civitelli *et al.*, 1980), is most effective when the rate of remodeling is increased, there is no apparent relationship between pre-treatment bone remodeling rate and response to NaF (Hodsman and Droost, 1989). Nonetheless, not all patients respond to NaF with an increase in bone mass (Lane *et al.*, 1984; Kleerekoper *et al.*, 1991) or volume (Briancon and Meunier, 1981; Hodsman and Droost, 1989). Most series report that 70% of NaF-treated patients respond with an increase in bone formation, volume, and mass. Duursma *et al.* (1987) reported that a rise in serum alkaline phosphatase reliably predicts a positive response to NaF but, as is the case with so many of the observations concerning NaF therapy in osteoporosis, this has not been a consistent finding (Briancon and Meunier, 1981; Erikson *et al.*, 1985; Dambacher *et al.*, 1986; Duursma *et al.*, 1987; Hasling *et al.*, 1987; Pak *et al.*, 1989). Pak *et al.* (1989) have reported a slight but progressive rise in both serum osteocalcin and urinary hydroxyproline excretion on fluoride therapy, but there is still too little information available to ascertain whether these markers of bone turnover might predict the response to therapy. Hodsman and Droost (1989) were forced to conclude that 12–24 months of therapy may be needed before a treated patient could be correctly classified as a responder or non-responder.

There is consensus that NaF increases spinal bone mass in a dose-dependent manner, but there is considerable disagreement about the effect of the drug on appendicular bone mass. Since NaF increases bone mass by deposition of newly formed bone on existing bone surfaces, given the small surface : volume ratio of cortical bone compared to cancellous bone, it is not surprising that any effects on appendicular skeletal mass will be much smaller than on spinal bone mass. In this regard all of the studies are in agreement, differing only in the direction of the small changes noted. In our studies, including the placebo-controlled trial (Kleerekoper *et al.*, 1991), we have been unable to demonstrate any loss of forearm bone mass (greater than would be expected from advancing age and no different from placebo) during up to ten years of therapy. Using a seemingly identical protocol, Riggs *et al.* (1990) reported that bone was lost from the radial midshaft at a rate significantly faster than in the placebo group. Most groups report no effect of NaF on forearm bone mass (Christiansen *et al.*, 1980; Riggs *et al.*, 1982; Devogelaer *et al.*, 1984; Ruegsegger *et al.*, 1985; Farley *et al.*, 1987), but the most surprising result is that of Hodsman and Droost (1989). In those who responded to NaF with an increase in spinal bone mass, there was an annual decrement of almost 8% per year in forearm bone mass. Non-responders had no change in either forearm or spinal bone mass. This has led to the 'rob Peter to pay Paul' concept that NaF increases spinal bone mass only at the expense of peripheral bone mass. With respect to the forearm, this is of little clinical consequence but, as discussed below, assumes greater importance in relation to the potential of NaF to increase the likelihood of hip fracture. With the current availability of non-invasive bone mass measurement at the proximal femur, this should be an easy question to answer. Regrettably, the work has yet to be done. Riggs *et al.* (1990), proponents of a deleterious effect of NaF on appendicular bone mass and an increased propensity to hip fracture, reported no change in femoral bone mass in their controlled trial. It is unlikely on theoretical grounds, and unproven by experiment, that NaF has any major impact on appendicular bone mass.

SODIUM FLUORIDE AND VERTEBRAL FRACTURES

In Chapter 3, the relationship between bone mass and osteoporotic fractures is discussed in detail. In brief, the lower the bone mass, the greater the risk of fracture and the prevalence of fracture increases as bone mass declines. Intuitively, one would therefore expect that fracture rates would decline as bone mass increases. Surprisingly, this has never been demonstrated in any prospective studies and nowhere is this more evident than in studies with NaF, seemingly the most effective drug for increasing bone mass. Table 14.1 lists the clinical trials that have attempted to demonstrate prospectively that, not only does NaF increase bone mass but it also decreases the vertebral fracture rate. Most obvious from this table is the different outcome of placebo-controlled trials compared to trials that are either uncontrolled or have compared NaF to other therapies. It should be noted that in this context, we assume that calcium supplementation is equivalent to placebo.

There has been three peer-reviewed publications of placebo-controlled trials (Dambacher *et al.*, 1986; Riggs *et al.*, 1990; Kleerekoper *et al.*, 1991), each of which has failed to demonstrate that NaF is more effective than placebo in reducing the vertebral fracture rate. The placebo-controlled trial reported by Buckle (1989), in abstract only, did demonstrate a significant reduction in vertebral fractures in those on NaF. The

Table 14.1 Effect of sodium fluoride on vertebral fracture rate

Reference	*NaF dose (mg/day)*	*Control*	*Follow-up (years)*	*VFR[a] control (n)*	*NaF (n)*
Riggs *et al.* (1990)	78	Calcium	2.5	525 (101)	462 (101)
Dambacher *et al.* (1986)	80	Placebo	3	417 (12)	1139 (12)
Kleerekoper *et al.* (1991)	75	Calcium	2.5	529 (38)	733 (46)
Mamelle *et al.* (1988)	50	Various	2	640 (136)	480 (180)
Heaney (1990)	50–60	None	3.5		304 (33)
Pak *et al.* (1989)[b]	50	None	3.1		10 (21)
Pak *et al.* (1989)[b]	50	None	2.7		70 (23)
Tilley *et al.* (1990)	50	None	3.7		46 (26)

[a] Vertebral fracture rate per 1000 patient years of observation
[b] Also received calcitriol 2 μg/day for two weeks before each cycle of NaF

difference between this and the trials for which more details are available is not readily apparent. Mamelle *et al.* (1988) compared NaF to several other therapies for osteoporosis, none of which has documented efficacy. Their study involved 94 physicians in France who selected the 'control' medication after random assignment to NaF or control has been made. The results were reported in several ways in the initial publication and in a follow-up letter to the editor (Mamelle *et al.*, 1990). Most, but not all, of their analyses did show that NaF was significantly more effective than the other therapies in reducing vertebral fracture rate. The many difficulties in conducting a relatively small study in so many centers and the internal inconsistencies in the results have prompted these investigators to conduct a more formal controlled trial of NaF therapy.

It would appear from these controlled trials that NaF is just not effective in reducing vertebral fracture rate in postmenopausal osteroporosis. It must be added that Riggs *et al.* (1994) reanalyzed their data focusing on differences between those who were or were not compliant with therapy and patients on an open-label extension of the study. They found a very complex relationship between the total exposure to fluoride and the antifracture efficacy with too low and too high exposure being deleterious. This observation provides extremely valuable insight into how future clinical trials with sodium fluoride should be conducted but does not really permit conclusions about current effectiveness of the drug.

The results from the uncontrolled studies listed are in sharp contrast, with a beneficial effect of NaF being almost universally reported. So consistent is this observation that it has prompted Heaney (1990) to conclude that controlled clinical trials of antifracture efficacy in postmenopausal osteoporosis are so difficult to conduct that we should gauge effectiveness of therapy from many years of clinical observation without the benefit of formal trials. As the principal investigator and co-investigator of one of the placebo-controlled fluoride trials (Kleerekoper *et al.*, 1991), I would wholeheartedly agree that these trials are difficult to conduct, as we have previously reported (Tilley *et al.*, 1990). However, we cannot conclude that we should simply decide that NaF is effective in reducing vertebral fracture on the basis of the uncontrolled studies and ignore the controlled trials. The only valid conclusion, in our opinion, is that despite the surprise and disappointment, therapeutic efficacy of NaF in reducing vertebral fracture rate in postmenopausal osteoporosis remains unproven.

The more important questions now relate to possible explanations for the apparent failure of the substantial increase in bone mass to be translated into a substantial reduction in fracture rate. There is obviously no simple answer to this. In the simplest sense, perhaps Heaney is correct. The experiment cannot be successfully completed, but the answer is likely to be far more complex. NaF can restore bone mass to within the normal range, but as described elsewhere, the microarchitecture of cancellous bone in the vertebral body and the biomechanical integrity of vertebral cortical and cancellous bone are important co-factors in establishing integrity of vertebrae. There is no evidence that NaF can restore cancellous bone microarchitecture to normal, so that while bone mass and volume may indeed be normalized by NaF, the new bone may be deposited in sites that do not restore biomechanical integrity. Regrettably, there have been limited formal biomechanical studies of fluoride-treated osteoporotic bone. Studies performed on adult human bone exposed to industrial fluoride suggest that there is a 25% increase in compressive strength and a 25% loss of elastic modulus in tensile loading, with a resultant 40% loss of bending strength (Riggins *et al.*, 1976). Carter and Beaupre (1990) have used these limited data to develop a theoretical model explaining the failure of NaF to reduce vertebral fracture rate.

While the precise biologic role of the concept of bone remodeling has not been firmly established, it seems reasonable to conclude that the process has an integral role in maintaining skeletal health. Parfitt (1993) has suggested that a low turnover state may be associated with increased fragility or brittleness of bone by retarding repair of microdamage. If that hypothesis is correct, the increased resistance to resorption that is a feature of the fluorapatite crystal lattice (Grynpas and Cheng, 1988), may result in increased skeletal fragility. Thus, as mentioned above, the two effects of NaF on the skeleton (increased volume, decreased normal remodeling) may have opposing effects on strength of the skeleton.

Whatever the reason(s) for the apparent failure of fluoride to reduce vertebral fractures, the ion alters skeletal metabolism and is incorporated into the skeleton. This makes it imperative that clinical trials of NaF be conducted in the conventional, placebo-controlled manner.

SLOW-RELEASE SODIUM FLUORIDE

The pharmacology of the slow-release preparation investigated by Pak *et al.* has already been discussed. This preparation deserves a separate discussion with respect to controlled clinical trials. The doses used were much smaller than in the studies discussed above, at least with respect to the amount of fluoride absorbed. From the literature it is unclear whether the results obtained are due to the specifics of the preparation or simply to the lower exposure to fluoride with this preparation. Regrettably few, if any, true dose-finding studies have been performed with this drug and no head-to-head comparisons with other fluoride preparations. The results reported in 1995 and 1996 (Pak *et al.*, 1995; 1996) demonstrate a very favorable response with respect to vertebral fracture rate. However, this benefit was only seen in those with minimal disease, specifically bone mass ≥65% of peak adult bone mass. Furthermore, the antifracture efficacy was not demonstrated in previously fractured vertebrae.

Controversy surrounds slow-release sodium fluoride just as it has plagued other sodium fluoride preparations for three decades. The French group that reported the favorable effects with an enteric-coated preparation (Kleerekoper, 1992) have recently completed a controlled trial with a different slow-release preparation to that used by Pak *et al.* That study, to date only reported in abstract form, failed to demonstrate any antifracture efficacy. The Food and Drug Administration (FDA) in the United States reviewed the results of the Pak data towards the end of 1995. An advisory panel recommended approval of the drug but this was prior to the French report. To date, the FDA has not finally acted on a recommendation to approve or disapprove slow-release sodium fluoride for clinical use.

SODIUM FLUORIDE AND HIP FRACTURES

One of the more hotly debated current public health issues is whether or not fluoridation of water supplies is associated with an increased prevalence of hip fractures (Gordon and Corbin, 1992; Pak *et al.*, 1995). A discussion of this important but still unresolved issue is beyond the scope of this chapter which has a focus on the therapeutic use of NaF in osteoporosis.

In 1984, Gutteridge *et al.* reported that NaF was associated with an alarming increased occurrence of spontaneous fractures of the proximal femur. This led to a retrospective review of a large number of NaF-treated patients in four centers in the United States and one in France which concluded that the prevalence of proximal femur fractures was not increased by NaF (Riggs *et al.*, 1987). As with so many aspects of this work, the controversy continues but definitive studies have yet to be undertaken. In the two United States controlled trials (Riggs *et al.*, 1990;

Kleerekoper *et al.*, 1991), NaF was associated with an increased occurrence of the painful lower extremity syndrome, a syndrome that is felt by many to represent fluoride-induced stress fractures (Leroux *et al.*, 1983; Schnitzler and Solomon, 1985; O'Duffy *et al.*, 1986; Schnitzler and Solomon, 1986; van Linthoudt and Ott, 1987; Bayley *et al.*, 1990; Gutteridge *et al.*, 1990; Schnitzler *et al.*, 1990). This syndrome occasionally affects the proximal femur, although more commonly the calcaneus is affected (Leroux *et al.*, 1983; Schulz *et al.*, 1984; Schnitzler and Solomon, 1986). Patients complain of sudden onset of intense, disabling pain over the affected portion of the skeleton and there is associated redness and tenderness. The syndrome remits within 6–8 weeks of discontinuing fluoride therapy and its recurrence when therapy is reinstituted is quite variable and unpredictable. Radiographs of the affected skeleton are negative at presentation, but a radionuclide bone scan reveals intense isotope uptake. Follow-up radiographs taken 2–6 weeks after the onset of symptoms reveal a linear band of sclerosis suggestive of a healing stress fracture. The radiographic and scintigraphic appearances of these lesions suggest that the cortex is not involved in the process and few, if any, of these lesions progress to complete fracture.

The only histologic study of one of these lesions (Schnitzler and Solomon, 1986) was interpreted to demonstrate changes compatible with fracture repair. However, a similar histologic picture might in fact result from an intense osteoblastic response to NaF (i.e. the desired effect) and Schultz *et al.* (1984; 1986; 1990) feel that this is the more plausible explanation for the syndrome. We favor this hypothesis for several reasons. The syndrome never affects the upper limbs and must reflect an interaction between load bearing and NaF, yet the unusual sites of load-bearing stress fractures (not associated with NaF therapy) are infrequently sites of involvement in the painful lower extremity pain syndrome. Furthermore, healing of these stress fractures is almost always associated with radiographic changes that affect the cortex, so that the lesions of the painful lower extremity syndrome differ from usual stress fractures in at least two important aspects.

The classification of these lesions as stress fractures has important implications for the discussion of fluoride (used as therapy for osteoporosis or as a water additive) as a cause of hip fractures. Riggs *et al.* (1990) elected to regard them as stress fractures and report that, in their clinical trial, NaF was associated with a significant increased occurrence of peripheral fractures, including hip fractures. We elected to regard these lesions as not being stress fractures and reported that, in our clinical trial, NaF was not associated with an increased occurrence of hip fractures (Kleerkoper *et al.*, 1991). In addition to not being certain of the etiology and long-term clinical significance of the painful lower extremity syndrome, we pointed out that there was no anatomic overlap in the Riggs study between sites of complete peripheral fractures and sites of involvement of the painful lower extremity syndrome. Regrettably, proponents of water fluoridation as a cause of hip fracture (Sowers *et al.*, 1990; Danielson *et al.*, 1992) point to this study for biologic plausibility for their observations. While the effect of NaF on vertebral fracture rate remains unresolved, this controversy about the effect of NaF on hip fractures needs even more prompt resolution.

OTHER SIDE EFFECTS OF NaF

The most specific side effect of NaF therapy is the painful lower extremity syndrome described above. The most common side effect is gastrointestinal discomfort similar to that seen with non-steroidal anti-inflammatory drugs. This may take the form of pain, bloating, nausea, or change in bowel habit – both diarrhea and constipation. This appears to be a chemical gastritis resulting directly from the effects of hydrofluoric acid on the gastric mucosa. The frequency with which this occurs is apparently dependent on the dose and formulation of the NaF being used. Doses as low as 50 mg/day of enteric-coated tablets or capsules are associated with a 20–30% incidence of gastrointestinal discomfort, increasing to nearly 50% when 75 mg/day of non-enteric coated capsules are used (Duursma *et al.*, 1987; Mamelle *et al.*, 1988; Pak *et al.*, 1989; Riggs *et al.*, 1990; Kleerekoper *et al.*, 1991). Frank hematemesis or melena rarely ocurs, but the completed controlled clinical trials did not document any occurrence of bleeding or any significant change in hemoglobin. Symptoms usually subside spontaneously within 24–48 hours after interrupting therapy and are helped by concomitant use of antacids. Therapy may be restarted in 6–8 weeks, usually at a lower dose, gradually increasing to the required dose. These symptoms can be minimized by ingesting the NaF with food or calcium supplements which may or may not have an effect on absorption and toxic blood levels. Where there is more concrete information on therapeutic and toxic blood levels of fluoride, we will be in a far better position to manage clinically this frequent side effect.

Ideally, all patients should be given NaF in a manner that does not result in gastrointestinal symptoms while attaining a therapeutic blood level. This would certainly improve compliance with therapy and may be the most crucial factor in the difficulties with demonstrating antifracture efficacy of NaF. It clearly cannot be the whole issue because most patients do ingest and absorb sufficient drug to result in substantial gains in bone mass.

CONCLUSION

Sodium fluoride has been studied as a therapy for osteoporosis for more than 30 years, but its precise role in this disease remains controversial. The drug clearly increases bone mass better than any therapeutic options currently available. Equally clearly, it has proven extremely difficult to document clearly antifracture efficacy. Perhaps the role of NaF should be to increase bone mass before the first vertebral fracture has occurred. This study has, in fact, been initiated (Pouilles *et al.*, 1991), but the postulate must be viewed with extreme caution because of the controversy and uncertainty surrounding the issue of NaF therapy and hip fractures. From a public health point of view, it would be calamitous to prevent vertebral fractures only at the expense of hip fractures.

More studies are needed on the meaning of blood levels of fluoride in response to therapy and the development of meaningful therapeutic and toxic ranges as a means of monitoring compliance and comparing different doses and formulations. The issue of responders and non-responders needs resolution. Not only will this prevent non-responders being placed at risk of side effects from NaF without potential for benefit, but it might also help unravel clues to the pathogenesis of different forms of osteoporosis and aid in the design of rational therapies for this disease.

In almost all areas touched on in this chapter, there appear to be more unresolved questions than answers. While this is the case, sodium fluoride must remain experimental therapy for osteoporosis and its use should be restricted to properly designed and conducted controlled clinical trials.

REFERENCES

Aaron, J.E., de Vernejouil, M-C. and Kanis, J.A. (1990) Trabecular microanatomy and fluoride therapy. *Bone* **11**: 376 (abstr).

Bayley, T.A., Harrison, J.E., Murray, T.M. *et al.* (1990) Fluoride-induced fractures: Relation to osteogenic effect. *J Bone Miner Res* **5**: S217–22.

Bellows, C.G., Heersche, J.N.M. and Aubin, J.E. (1990) The effects of fluoride on osteoblast progenitors *in vitro*. *J Bone Miner Res* **5**: S101–5.

Bernstein, D.S., Guri, C.D., Cohen, P., Collins, J.J. and Tamvakapoulos, S. (1963) The use of sodium fluoride in metabolic bone disease. *J Clin Invest* **42**: 916.

Briancon, D., D'Aranda, P., Quillet, P. *et al.* (1990) Comparative study of fluoride bioavailability following the administration of sodium fluoride alone and in combination with different calcium salts. *J Bone Miner Res* **5**(1): S71–73.

Briancon, D. and Meunier, P.J. (1981) Treatment of osteoporosis with fluoride, calcium and vitamin D. *Orthop Clin North Am* **12**: 629–48.

Buckle, R.M. (1989) 3 year study of sodium fluoride on vertebral fracture incidence in osteoporosis. *J Bone Miner Res* **4**: S186 (abstr).

Carter, D.R. and Beaupre, G.S. (1990) Effects of fluoride treatment on bone strength. *J Bone Miner Res* **5**: S177–84.

Civitelli, R.T., Gonneli, S., Zacche, F. *et al.* (1980) Bone turnover in post-menopausal osteoporosis: Effect of calcitonin treatment. *J Clin Invest* **82**: 1268–74.

Christiansen, C., Christensen, M.S., McNair, P. *et al.* (1980) Prevention of early postmenopausal bone loss: Controlled 2 year study in 315 normal females. *Eur J Clin Invest* **10**: 273–9.

Cohen, P. and Gardner, F.H. (1964) Induction of subacute skeletal fluorosis in a case of multiple myeloma. *N Engl J Med* **271**: 1129–33.

Compston, J.E., Chadha, S. and Merrett, A.L. (1980) Osteomalacia developing during treatment of osteoporosis with sodium fluoride and vitamin D. *Br Med J* **281**: 910–11.

Dambacher, M.A., Ittner, J. and Ruegsegger, P. (1986) Long-term fluoride therapy of postmenopausal osteoporosis. *Bone* **7**: 199–205.

Danielson, C., Lyon, J.L., Egger, M. *et al.* (1992) Hip fractures in fluoridation in Utah's elderly population. *JAMA* **268**: 781–2.

Delmas, P.D., Casez, J.P., Voivin, G.Y. *et al.* (1984) Cyclic fluoride therapy for postmenopausal osteoporosis. In: *Osteoporosis, Proceedings of the Copenhagen International Symposium*, (eds C. Christiansen, D. Arnaud and B.E.C. Nordin), Stiftsborgtrykkery Aalborg, pp. 689–91.

Devogelaer, J.P., Nagant de Deuxchaisnes, C., Stein, F. (1991) Bioavailability of enteric-coated sodium fluoride tablets as affected by the administration of calcium supplements at different time intervals. *J Bone Miner Res* **5**(1): S75–79.

Devogelaer, J.P., Resimont, P., Huaux, J.P. *et al.* (1984) Effect of sodium fluoride on bone mineral content of the radius in postmenopausal osteoporosis. In: *Osteoporosis, Proceedings of the Copenhagen International Symposium*, (eds C. Christiansen, D. Arnoud and B.E.C. Nordin), pp. 689–91.

Duursma, S.A., Glerum, J.H, Van Dijk, A. *et al.* (1987) Responders and non-responders after fluoride therapy in osteoporosis. *Bone* **8**: 131–6.

Duursma, S.A., Raymakjers, J.A., De Raadt, M.E. *et al.* (1990) Urinary fluoride excretion in responders and non-responders after fluoride therapy in osteoporosis. *J Bone Miner Res* **5**(1): S43–7.

Eanes, E.D. and Reddi, A.H. (1979) The effect of fluoride on bone mineral apatite. *Metab Bone Dis Rel Res* **2**:3–10.

Erikson, E.F., Mosekilde, L. and Melsen, F. (1985) Effects of sodium fluoride, calcium, phosphate and vitamin D_2 for 5 years on bone balance and remodeling in osteoporotics. *Bone* **6**: 381–9.

Farley, S.M.G., Wergedal, J.E., Smith, L.C. *et al.* (1987) Fluoride therapy for osteoporosis: Characterization of the skeletal response by the serial measurements of serum alkaline phosphatase activity. *Metabolism* **36**: 211–18.

Gennari, R., Chierichetti, S.M., Bigazzi, S. *et al.* (1985) Comparative effects on bone mineral content of calcium and calcium plus salmon calcitonin given in two different regimens in post-menopausal osteoporosis. *Curr Ther Res* **38**: 455–64.

Gerster, J., Charhon, S.A., Jaeger, P. *et al.* (1983) Bilateral fractures of femoral neck in patients with moderate renal failure receiving fluoride for spinal osteoporosis. *Br Med J* **287**: 723–5.

Gordon, S.L. and Corbin, S.B. (1992) Summary of workshop on drinking water fluoride influence on hip fracture on bone health. *Osteopor Int* **2**: 109–17.

Gron, P., McCann, H.G. and Bernstein, D. (1966) Effect of fluoride on human osteoporotic bone mineral: A chemical and crystallographic study. *J Bone Joint Surg* **48A**: 892–8.

Grynpas, M.D. and Cheng, P.T. (1988) Fluoride reduces the rate of dissolution of bone. *Bone and Mineral* **5**(1): 1–9.

Gutteridge, D.H., Price, R.I., Kent, G.N. *et al.* (1990) Spontaneous hip fractures in fluoride-treated patients: Potential causative factors. *J Bone Miner Res* **5**(1): S205–15.

Gutteridge, D.H., Price, R.I., Nicholson, G.C. *et al.* (1984) Fluoride in osteoporotic vertebral fractures-trabecular increase, vertebral protection, femoral fractures. In: *Osteoporosis, Proceedings of the Copenhagen International Symposium*, (eds C. Christiannsen, D. Arnaud and B.E.C. Nordin), Stiftsborgtrykkery Aalborg, pp 705–7.

Hansson, T. and Roos, B. (1987) The effect of fluoride and calcium on spinal bone mineral content: a controlled, prospective (3 years) study. *Calcif Tissue Int* **40**: 315–17.

Hasling, C., Nielsen, H.E., Melsen, F. and Mosekilde, L. (1987) Safety of osteoporosis treatment with sodium fluoride, calcium phosphate and vitamin D. *Mineral Electrolyte Metab* **13**: 96–103.

Hasvold, O. and Ekren, T. (1981) New approach to the treatment of bone disease with fluoride. *Fed Proc* **29**: 1185–7.

Heaney, R.P. (1990) How can we tell if a treatment works: Further thoughts on the randomized controlled trial. *Osteopor Int* **1**: 215–7.

Hodsman, A.B., Droost, D.J. (1989) The response of vertebral bone mineral density during the treatment of osteoporosis with sodium fluoride. *J Clin Endocr Metab* **69**: 932–8.

Husdan, H., Vogl, R., Oreopoulos, D., Gryfe, C. and Rapoport, A. (1976) Serum ionic fluoride: Normal range and relationship to age and sex. *Clin Chem* **22**: 1884–8.

Jowsey, J. and Riggs, B.L. (1978) Effect of concurrent calcium ingestion on intestinal absorption of fluoride. *Metabolism* **27**: 971–4.

Kleerekoper, M. (1992) Please pass the roach poison again. *JAMA*, **268**: 781–2.

Kleerekoper, M. and Balena, R. (1991) Fluoride and osteoporosis. *Ann Rev Nutr* **11**: 309–24.

Kleerekoper, M., Balena, R., Foldes, J. *et al.* (1990) Histomorphometric changes in iliac bone induced by sodium fluoride therapy depend on cumulative dose. *J Bone Miner Res* **5**: S140 (abstr).

Kleerekoper, M., Frame, B., Villaneuva, A.R. *et al.* (1981) Treatment of osteoporosis with sodium fluoride alternating with calcium and vitamin D. In: *Osteoporosis: Recent Advances in Pathogenesis and Treatment*, (eds H.F. DeLuca, H.M. Frost and W.S.S. Jee), pp 441–8.

Kleerekoper, M., Peterson, E., Nelson, D.A. *et al.* (1991) A randomized trial of sodium fluoride as a treatment for postmenopausal osteoporosis. *Osteopor Int* **1**: 155–62.

Kleerekoper, M., Villanueva, A.R., Stancium, J. *et al.* (1985) The role of three dimensional trabecular microstructure in the pathogenesis of vertebral compression fractures. *Calcif Tissue Int* **37**: 594–7.

Kraenzlin, M.E., Kraenzlin, C., Farley, S.M.G., Fitzsimmons, R.J., Baylink, D.J. (1990) Fluoride pharmacokinetics in good and poor responders to fluoride therapy. *J Bone Miner Res* **5**(1): S49–52.

Kuhlencordt, F., Kruse, H.P., Eckermeier, L. *et al.* (1970) The histological evaluation of bone in fluoride treated osteoporosis. In: *Fluoride in Medicine*, (ed. T.L. Vischer), Hans Huber, Bern, pp. 169–74.

Lane, J.M., Healey, J.H., Schwartz, E. *et al.* (1984) Treatment of osteoporosis with sodium fluoride and calcium: Effects on vertebral fracture incidence and bone histomorphometry. *Orthop Clin North Am* **15**: 729–45.

Largent, E.J. (1961) *Fluorosis: The Health Aspects of Fluorine Compounds*. Ohio State University Press, Columbus.

Lau, K.H.W., Farley, J.R., Freemen, T.K. *et al.* (1989) A proposed mechanism of the mitogenic action of fluoride on bone cells: Inhibition of the activity of an osteoblastic acid phosphatase. *Metabolism* **38**: 858–68.

Leroux, J.L., Blotman, F., Claustre, J. *et al.* (1983) Fractures du calcaneum au cours du traitement de l'osteoporose par le fluor. *Sem Hosp Paris* **59**: 3140–2.

Lundy, M.W., Wergedal, J.E., Teubner, E. *et al.* (1989) The effect of prolonged fluoride therapy for osteoporosis: Bone composition and histology. *Bone* **10**: 321–7.

Mamelle, N., Dusan, R., Martin, J.L. *et al.* (1988) Risk-benefit of sodium fluoride treatment in primary vertebral osteoporosis. *Lancet* **ii**: 361–5.

Mamelle, N., Muenier, P.J. and Netter, P. (1990) Fluoride and vertebral fractures. *Lancet* **336**: 243 (Letter).

Marie, P.J., de Vernejoul, M.C. and Lomri, A. (1990) Fluoride induced stimulation of bone formation is associated with increased DNA synthesis by osteoblastic cells *in vitro*. *J Bone Miner Res* **5**(2): S140.

Nagant de Deuxchaisnes, C., Devogelaer, J.P. and Stein, F. (1990) Comparison of the bioavailability of the NaF capsules used in the NIH-sponsored trials as compared to that of NaF enteric-coated tablets commercially available in Europe. *J Bone Miner Res* **5**(1): S251.

O'Duffy, J.D., Wahner, H.W. O'Fallon, W.M. *et al.* (1986) Mechanism of acute lower extremity pain syndrome in fluoride-treated osteoporotic patients. *Am J Med* **80**: 561–6.

Olah, A.J., Reutter, F.Q. and Dambacher, M.A. (1978) Effects of combined therapy with sodium fluoride and high doses of vitamin D in osteoporosis. A histomorphometric study of the iliac crest. In: *Fluoride and Bone*, (eds B. Courvasier, A. Donath and C.A. Band), Hans Huber, Bern, pp. 242–8.

Pak, C.Y., Adams-Huet, B. Sakhaee, K. *et al.* (1996) Comparison of nonrandomized trials with slow-release sodium fluoride with a randomized placebo-controlled trial in postmenopausal osteoporosis. *J Bone Miner Res*, **11**: 160–8.

Pak, C.Y., Sakhaee, K., Adams-Huet, B. *et al.* (1995) Treatment of postmenopausal osteoporosis with slow-release sodium fluoride. Final report of a randomized controlled trial. *Ann Intern Med* **123**: 401–8.

Pak, C.Y.C., Sakhaee, K., Gallagher, C. *et al.* (1986) Attainment of therapeutic fluoride levels in serum without major side effects using slow-release preparation of sodium fluoride in postmenopausal osteoporosis. *J Bone Miner Res* **1**: 563–71.

Pak, C.Y.C., Sakhaee, K., Zerwekh, J., *et al.* (1989) Safe and effective treatment of osteoporosis with intermittent slow release sodium fluoride: Augmentation of vertebral bone mass and inhbition of fractures. *J Clin Endocrinol Metab* **68**: 150–9.

Parfitt, A.M. (1990) Osteomalacia and related disorders. In: *Metabolic Bone Disease and Clinically Related Disorders*, 2nd edn, (eds. L.V. Avioli and S.M. Krane), Philadelphia, W.B. Saunders, Philadelphia, pp. 329–96.

Parfitt, A.M. (1993) Bone age, mineral density, and fatigue damage. *Calcif Tissue Int* **53** (Suppl1): S82–S85.

Parfitt, A.M., Mathews, C.H.E., Villaneuva, A.R. *et al.* (1983) Relationships between surface, volume and thickness of iliac trabecular bone in aging and in osteoporosis: Implications for the microanatomic and cellular mechanisms of bone loss. *J Clin Invest* **72**: 1369–409.

Parsons, V., Mitchell, C.J., Reeve, J. *et al.* (1977) The use of sodium fluoride, vitamin D and calcium supplements in the treatment of patients with axial osteoporosis. *Calcif Tissue Res* **22**: S236–40.

Pouilles, J.M., Tremellieres, Causse, E. *et al.* (1991) Fluoride therapy in post-menopausal osteopenic women: Effect on vertebral and femoral bone density and prediction of bone response. *Osteopor Int* **1**: 103–9.

Quarles, L.D., Gittlemena, H.J. and Drezner, M.K. (1989) Aluminum induced de novo bone formation in the beagle. A parathyroid hormone dependent event. *J Clin Invest* **83**: 1644–50.

Rao, D.S. (1993) Metabolic bone disease in gastrointestinal and biliary disorders. In: *Primer on the Metabolic Bone Diseases and Disorders of Mineral Metabolism*, 2nd edn, (ed M.J. Favus), Raven Press, New York, pp. 268–73.

Reutter, F.W., Siebenmann, R. and Pajorola, M. (1970) In: Fluoride in Medicine, (ed. T.L. Fischer), Hans Huber, Bern, pp. 143–52.

Rich, C. and Ensinck, J. (1961) Effect of sodium fluoride on calcium metabolism of human beings. *Nature* **191**: 184–5.

Riggins, R.S., Rucker, R.C., Chan, M.M. *et al.* (1976) The effect of fluoride supplementation on the strength of osteopenic bone. *Clin Orthop Rel Res* **114**: 352–7.

Riggs, B.L., Baylink, D.J., Kleerekoper, M. *et al.* (1987) Incidence of hip fractures in osteoporotic women treated with sodium fluoride. *J Bone Miner Res* **2**: 123–6.

Riggs, B.L., Hodgson, S.F., O'Fallon, W.M. *et al.* (1990) Effect of fluoride treatment on the fracture rate in post-menopausal women with osteoporosis. *N Engl J Med* **322**: 802–9.

Riggs, B.L., O'Fallon, W.M., Lane, A. and Hodgson, S.F. (1994) Clinical trial of fluoride therapy in postmenopausal women: extended observations and additional analysis. *J Bone Miner Res* **9**: 265–75.

Riggs, B.L., Seaman, E., Hodjson, S.F. *et al.* (1982) Effect of the fluoride calcium regimen on vertebral fracture occurrence in postmenopausal osteoporosis: Comparison with conventional therapy. *N Engl J Med* **306**: 446–50.

Roholm, K. (1937) Fluorine Intoxication. A Clinical-Hygienic Study, with a Review of the Literature and some Experimental Observations. H.K. Lewis, London.

Ruegsegger, P., Ruegsegger, E., Itner, J. *et al.* (1985) Natural course of osteoporosis and fluoride therapy – a longitudinal study using quantitative computed tomography. *J Comput Assist Tomogr* **9**: 626–7.

Schnitzler, C.M. and Solomon, L. (1985) Trabecular stress fractures during fluoride therapy for osteoporosis. *Skel Radiol* **14**: 276–9.

Schnitzler, C.M. and Solomon, L. (1986) Histomorphometric analysis of a calcaneal stress fracture: A possible complication of fluoride therapy for osteoporosis. *Bone* **7**: 193–8.

Schnitzler, C.M., Wing, J.R., Mesquita, J.M. *et al.* (1990) Risk factors for the development of stress fractures during fluoride therapy for osteoporosis. *J Bone Miner Res* **5**(1): S195–200.

Schulz, E.E., Engstrom, H., Sauser, D.D. *et al.* (1986) Osteoporosis: Radiographic detection of fluoride-induced extra-axial bone formation. *Radiology* **159**: 457–62.

Schulz, E.E., Flowers, C., Sauser, D.D. *et al.* (1990) The causes of bone scintigram hot spots in fluoride-treated osteoporotic patients. *J Bone Miner Res* **5**(1): S195–200.

Schulz, E.E., Libanati, C.R., Farley, S.M. *et al.* (1984) Skeletal scintigraphic chnges in osteoporosis treated with sodium fluoride: Concise communication. *J Nucl Med* **25**: 651–5.

Sowers, M.R., Clark, M.K., Jannausch, M.L. *et al.* (1990) A prospective study of bone mineral content and fracture in communities with differential fluoride exposure. *Am J Epidemiol* **133**: 548–9.

Taves, D.R. (1970) New approach to the treatment of bone disease with fluoride. *Fed Proc* **29**: 1185–7.

Tilley, B.C., Kleerekoper, M., Peterson, E.L. *et al.* (1990) Designing clinical trials of treatment for osteoporosis: recruitment and follow-up. *Calcif Tissue Int* **47**: 327–31.

van Linthoudt, D. and Ott, H. (1987) Supra-acetabular and femoral head stress fracture during fluoride treatment. *Gerontology* **33**: 302–6.

PARATHYROID HORMONE AS AN ANABOLIC TREATMENT

15

F. Cosman and R. Lindsay

INTRODUCTION

Most physicians view parathyroid hormone (PTH) as an agent catabolic to the skeleton, capable of liberating skeletal calcium in order to maintain serum calcium levels within a tight homeostatic range. During times of relative calcium stress or deficiency, whether due to nutritional vitamin D deprivation, decreased calcium absorption efficiency or renal calcium wasting, where serum calcium levels are decreased, adaptive increases in PTH and consequent increases in skeletal resorption occur (Silver, 1993). Dynamic studies in humans, such as those using EDTA to lower serum calcium, show consistent increases in PTH secretion (Cheema *et al.*, 1989; Cosman *et al.*, 1994). In addition to stimulating bone resorption, other mechanisms by which PTH accomplishes its homeostatic function include increasing distal renal tubular calcium reabsorption and promoting $1,25(OH)_2D$ formation, thereby increasing gastrointestinal calcium absorption (Silver, 1993).

This chapter reviews the *in vitro*, animal and human data suggesting that PTH can also exert an anabolic action on the skeleton.

PARALLELS WITH PRIMARY HYPERPARATHYROIDISM

In cases of endogenous primary hyperparathyroidism, where mean PTH levels are chronically elevated, hypercalcemia usually occurs. In mild cases, it is conceivable that hypercalcemia could be maintained by effects on renal and gastrointestinal calcium handling alone without a significant catabolic effect on the skeleton. Although PTH in primary hyperparathyroidism does activate skeletal turnover (Riggs *et al.*, 1965; Baron and Magee, 1983), whether there is actually an overall increase in net bone resorption in this disorder is unclear. The effects of primary hyperparathyroidism on bone mass are also dependent on skeketal site. Bone mass in appendicular skeletal sites composed primarily of cortical bone is reduced (Kleerekoper *et al.*, 1983; Martin *et al.*, 1986; Richardson *et al.*, 1986; Rao *et al.*, 1988; Silverberg *et al.*, 1989), while bone mass in sites containing more cancellous bone is variable with our group showing preservation (Silverberg *et al.*, 1989) and other groups showing reductions at both lumbar spine (Seeman *et al.*, 1982; Richardson *et al.*, 1986) and distal forearm (Martin *et al.*, 1986). Likewise, data concerning fracture prevalence in this disorder, as it is currently seen clinically, are conflicting, with some studies indicating increased fracture rates (Dauphine *et al.*, 1975; Peacock *et al.*, 1984; Martin *et al.*, 1986; Kochersberger *et al.*, 1987) and others not (Rao *et al.*, 1988; Wilson *et al.*, 1988; Lafferty and Hubay, 1989).

Histomorphometric studies on the iliac

Osteoporosis. Edited by John C. Stevenson and Robert Lindsay. Published in 1998 by Chapman & Hall, London.
ISBN 0 412 48870 1

crest have consistently shown a reduction in cortical thickness (Kleerekoper *et al.*, 1983; Parfitt, 1986, 1989; Parisien *et al.*, 1990) but no reduction in cancellous bone volume (Mosekilde and Melsen, 1978; Melsen and Mosekilde, 1981; Kleerekoper *et al.*, 1983; Eriksen, 1986; Delmas *et al.*, 1986; Delling, 1987; de Vernejoul *et al.*, 1988; Parfitt, 1989; Parisien *et al.*, 1990). Hypotheses to explain this conservation of cancellous bone mass include coupled increases in bone turnover with increased osteoblastic activity and a prolonged formation period (Baron and Magee, 1983; Delling, 1987) or decreased depth of erosion cavities, with complete refilling by osteoblastic production (Mosekilde and Melsen, 1978; Eriksen, 1986).

POSSIBLE MECHANISMS OF ACTION

Although work done over 30 years ago on fixed bone sections suggested that osteoclasts expressed PTH receptors (Rao *et al.*, 1983), an elegant series of studies by Chambers *et al.* and others (Chambers *et al.*, 1985; McSheehy and Chambers, 1986; Perry *et al.*, 1987; Morris *et al.*, 1990) indicated that osteoblasts were the only bone cells which responded directly to physiologic doses of PTH. Briefly, these experiments demonstrated that when osteoclasts were separated from other bone cells, they were unable to resorb bone in response to PTH stimulation, but when osteoblasts were added back into the assay, bone resorption was seen. More recent work, however, has again raised the possibility that PTH receptors might also exist on osteoclasts and may actually inhibit bone resorption directly (Duong *et al.*, 1990; Agarwala and Gay, 1992). These observations suggest that PTH activity on bone is quite complex, perhaps being mediated through opposing effects on osteoclasts and osteoblasts. The presence of at least two different intracellular signal transduction pathways, cyclic AMP-dependent protein kinase A and calcium-dependent protein kinase C, in osteoblasts (Rosenblatt, 1986; Yamaguchi *et al.*, 1987; Cosman *et al.*, 1989; Fujimori *et al.*, 1992) and in osteoclasts (Klein *et al.*, 1988; Murrills *et al.*, 1992; Su *et al.*, 1992; Teti *et al.*, 1992) increases the possibility of a dual regulatory system and adds great diversity to the potential effects of parathyroid hormone.

Even on the osteoblast alone, PTH effects are somewhat conflicting. Bovine 1-34PTH increases osteoblast number and osteoid formation in embryonic mouse radii (Herrmann-Erlee *et al.*, 1976). Furthermore, PTH increases tritiated thymidine incorporation into DNA in bone organ culture systems, cultured osteoblasts and osteoblast-like cells, again indicating that PTH stimulates osteoblast replication (Majeska and Rodan, 1981; DeBartolo *et al.*, 1982; Partridge and Martin, 1984; MacDonald *et al.*, 1986; Canalis *et al.*, 1989). In contrast, in some osteoblast cell preparations, PTH inhibits collagen synthesis (Hefley *et al.*, 1986; Partridge *et al.*, 1989; Vargas and Raisz, 1990) and decreases alkaline phosphatase activity in some (Wong *et al.*, 1977; Majeska and Rodan, 1981) but not all studies (McPartlin *et al.*, 1984; Puzas and Brand, 1985) and decreases osteocalcin synthesis (Beresford *et al.*, 1984) in some systems. The duration of cell exposure to PTH has an important influence on its effect. Inhibitory effects on collagen synthesis occur upon continuous prolonged PTH exposure (Dietrich *et al.*, 1976; Partridge *et al.*, 1989) whereas stimulatory effects on collagen synthesis can occur with shorter exposure (Canalis *et al.*, 1989).

PTH stimulation of bone formation may be mediated by local growth factors. Potential mediators include insulin-like growth factors (IgF) and transforming growth factor B (TGFβ). PTH stimulates IgF release from fetal and mouse calvarial cells (Canalis *et al.*, 1989; Linkhart and Mohan, 1989). IgFs can then increase collagen production by both increasing synthesis of type I procollagen mRNA (Canalis *et al.*, 1989) and stimulating osteoblast proliferation (McCarthy *et al.*,

1989). Inactive TGFβ is contained in large quantities in the bone matrix and upon PTH stimulation of bone resorption, is activated by the acidic milieu of the subosteoclast resorption zone. TGFβ is a known potent stimulator of bone formation both *in vitro* (Centrella *et al.*, 1986; Dijke *et al.*, 1990) and *in vivo* (Noda and Camilliere, 1989; Mackie and Trechsel, 1990). Several studies indicate, however, that resorption is not required to allow the anabolic action of PTH to occur. In rats, intermittent PTH administration causes an increase in bone apposition rate without a change in resorption surface (Tam *et al.*, 1982) and the anabolic action of PTH is not diminished by antiresorptive agents such as calcitonin and bisphosphonate (Hock *et al.*, 1989).

In summary, anabolic actions of PTH may be accomplished through stimulatory effects on osteoblasts (cell proliferation and cell production) and inhibitory effects on osteoclasts, may use two different intracellular transduction pathways and may involve local bone growth factors. The dominance of an anabolic rather than a catabolic effect *in vitro* and *in vivo* can, at least in part, be attributed to the mode and duration of administration of PTH.

ANIMAL STUDIES

Evidence that PTH, in the form of parathyroid extract, could increase bone formation in the rat date back to as early as 1929 (Bauer *et al.*, 1929). Histologic data (Selye, 1932; Pugsley and Selye, 1933; Burrows, 1938; Heller *et al.*, 1950), dry femur weight measurements (Shelling *et al.*, 1933), radiologic imaging (Kalu *et al.*, 1970; Walker, 1971) and calcium balance studies (Cramer *et al.*, 1961; Schulz *et al.*, 1971) subsequently confirmed that PTH could have an anabolic action in bone.

Over the last decade, the availability of purified PTH fragments has led to a renewed interest in the anabolic actions of PTH. Although a few studies have shown positive effects on bone formation and calcium absorption in the dog (Podesek *et al.*, 1980, 1983), the majority of the experiments have been performed in rats, in both intact animals as well as in the ovariectomized rat which serves as a model of postmenopausal osteoporosis. These studies are well summarized (Table 15.1) in a recent review (Dempster *et al.*, 1993).

In the intact animal, most investigators have found dose-dependent increments in cancellous bone with less pronounced or nonexistent changes in cortical bone (Gunness-Hey and Hock, 1984; Hori *et al.*, 1988; Hock *et al.*, 1988, 1989; Gunness-Hey *et al.*, 1988; Hock and Fonseca, 1990). Most of the analyses were performed on parts of the tibia or femur, but similar data have also been found for vertebrae (Liu and Kalu, 1990; Tuukkanen *et al.*, 1990; Liu *et al.*, 1991). Treatment periods as short as 12 days with daily PTH injections can result in increased cancellous bone mass (Wronski *et al.*, 1988). Both male and female rats respond to PTH (Hock *et al.*, 1988; Liu *et al.*, 1991). Bone formed under the influence of PTH appears to be of normal quality with increments in quantity of bone accompanied by increases in biomechanical strength of vertebrae (Hori *et al.*, 1988; Su *et al.*, 1992; Shen *et al.*, 1993).

Studies investigating the anabolic effect of PTH in the ovariectomized rat model of osteoporosis have been equally promising. In contrast to conventional antiresorptive agents which prevent further bone loss, intermittent administration of PTH increases bone mass (Kalu, 1991; Frost and Jee, 1992) and restores bone mass after ovariectomy (Hori *et al.*, 1988; Hock *et al.*, 1988; Tada *et al.*, 1990; Mellish *et al.*, 1990; Kalu *et al.*, 1990; Liu *et al.*, 1991; Shen *et al.*, 1992) as well as after orchidectomy in the male rat (Hock *et al.*, 1988).

The opposing effects of PTH on the skeleton in animal experiments, anabolic versus catabolic, can be explained in part by the mode and duration of administration. In dogs infused continuously with low-dose

Table 15.1 Quantitation of the anabolic action of PTH on rat bones

Animals	PTH	Dose μg/kg/d	Length of trmt	Oper	Bone	Percentage change in TBV	Percentage change in Ash wt or calcium	Percentage change in BMD	Reference
6 mo ♀ Wis	bPTH 1–34	75[1]	3 wk	int	Whole body	–	20	–	Hefti *et al.* (1982)
300 g ♂ SD	bPTH 1–84	0.4–102[1]	12 d	int	Femur	0–60	–	–	Tam *et al.* (1982)
4–6 wk ♂ SD	hPTH 1–34	20–100	12 d	int	Femur	–	6–60	–	Gunness–Hey and Hock (1984); Gera *et al.* (1987) Gunness-Hey *et al.* (1988)
10 wk ♀ SD	hPTH 1–34	6.0	26 wk	int	Femur	–	4	–	Hori *et al.* (1988)
				ovx		–	15		
5 wk ♂ SD	hPTH 1–34	80	12 d	int	Femur	–	34 (Trab) 12 (Cort)	–	Hock *et al.* (1988)
				ochx	Femur	–	37 (Trab) 19 (Cort)	–	
5 wk ♀ SD	hPTH 1–34	80	12 d	int	Femur	–	18 (Trab) 5 (Cort)	–	Hock *et al.* (1988)
				ovx	Femur	–	14 (Trab) 10 (Cort)	–	
4 wk ♂ SD	hPTH 1–34	80	12 d	int	Femur	100	31 (Trab) 20 (Cort)	–	Gunness-Hey and Hock (1989); Hock and Fonseca (1990); Hock *et al.* (1989)
8 mo ♀ Wis	hPTH 1–34	60	35 d[2]	PTX	Vert	70 (Trab)	–	–	Tada *et al.* (1990)
				+ovx			30 (Cort)	–	
				+cx	Tibia	300 (Trab) 12 (Cort)	– –	–	

3 mo ♀ SD	hPTH 1–34	80, 160	35 d	ovx	Femur	–	34	13	Kalu *et al.* (1990)
					Vert	70	49	12	
					Tibia	550	–	–	
4 mo ♀ SD	hPTH 1–34	1.5	28 d[3]	ovx	Tibia	46	–	4	Mellish *et al.* (1990)
3 mo ♀ SD	hPTH 1–34	80	20 d[4]	ovx	Femur	–	50	4	Liu and Kalu (1990)
					Tibia	271 (Trab) 4 (Cort)	–	–	Liu *et al.* (1991)
					Vert	–	12	5	
70 d ♂ Wis	hPTH 1–34	4–120	30 d	int	Vert	13–59	0–32	–	Mosekilde *et al.* (1991)
	hPTH 1–84	10–300	30 d	int	Vert	11–45	5–24	–	
3 mo ♂	bPTH 1–34	80	21 d	int	Vert	–	–	9	Wronski *et al.* (1988)
23 mo ♂			21 d	int	Vert	–	–	14	Wronski *et al.* (1988)
24 mo ♀	hPTH 1–34	80	21 d	int	Vert	–	–	16	Wronski *et al.* (1988)
24 mo ♀	hPTH 1–34	160	14 d	ovx	Femur	178	–	44	Ibbotson *et al.* (1982)
5 mo ♀	rPTH 1–34	40	28 d	ovx	Tibia	175	–	0	Shen *et al.* (1992)
					Femur	198	–	2	
						165	–	9	

1. Unit of PTH/rat/day.
2. Treatment begins 11 wks after the operation.
3. Treatment begins 4 wks after the operation.
4. Treatment begins 40 days after the operation

Abbreviations: TBV = trabecular bone volume; BMD = bone mineral density; vert = lumbar vertebrae; Trab = trabecular bone; Cort = cortical bone; int = intact; ovx = ovariectomy; ochx = orchidectomy; cx = hemicordectomy; Oper = operation; SD = Sprague Dawley; Wis = Wistar.

1-34hPTH, increments in bone resorption and osteoid surface were seen without an increase in bone volume (Malluche *et al.*, 1982). In another series of studies in the greyhound dog, continuous 1-34PTH infusion increased only the osteoclast surface without increasing bone volume. In contrast, daily PTH injections increased both formation and resorption surfaces, with consequent increases in calcium accretion and cancellous bone volume (Podesek *et al.*, 1980, 1983). A similar set of investigations performed in the rat (Tam *et al.*, 1982) showed that when 1-34PTH was given by infusion, both formation and resorption surfaces increased but in this case, net bone loss was seen at the higher PTH doses. When PTH was given by daily injection in this species, bone formation but not resorption surfaces increased and there was an increment in cancellous bone volume (Tam *et al.*, 1982). Other studies in the rat have confirmed these observations (Hock and Gera, 1992). These data indicate that the anabolic effect of PTH may not require a prior increase in bone resorption. In fact, coadministration of PTH with an antiresorptive agent does not block the anabolic effect of PTH (Hock *et al.*, 1989; Shen *et al.*, 1992) and may even increase the magnitude of the effect (Shen *et al.*, 1992).

HUMAN STUDIES

Preliminary data on administration of human PTH(1-34) in the mid-1970s showed dose-dependent effects. High doses (750 U per day) resulted in net bone resorption, while lower doses (450 U) improved calcium balance and calcium accretion (Reeve *et al.*, 1976a; Slovik *et al.*, 1981). A small number of largely uncontrolled and non-randomized investigations with heterogeneous patient populations have susbsequently appeared in the literature (Table 15.2; Dempster *et al.* 1993).

In the first trial, 21 osteoporotic patients (women and men) were treated with hPTH(1-34) in an average daily dose of 400–500 U (subcutaneously administered) for 6–24 months at seven separate British centers. Patients served as their own controls. Increases in skeletal turnover were reflected by increases in serum alkaline phosphatase and urinary excretion of hydroxyproline, calcium and phosphate. Radiocalcium kinetic studies showed dramatic increments in new bone accretion (mean 144%) with smaller increases in bone resorption (Reeve *et al.*, 1981). In the iliac crest, mean cancellous bone volume increased 92% and mean osteoid-covered surface increased 50%. Despite these positive findings, intestinal calcium absorption and overall calcium balance did not increase consistently. To explain this discrepancy, it was argued that PTH administration might redistribute bone mineral from the cortical to the cancellous skeleton, rather than causing a net increase in bone mass. This theory had minimal scientific support, based on femoral bone density determinations in only seven individuals (Hesp *et al.*, 1981), but remains a possible explanation, particularly if subjects were somewhat calcium deficient. In addition, it was postulated that calcium absorption did not increase, perhaps due to an insufficient $1,25(OH)_2D$ response to PTH, also a hypothesis with little supportive evidence. These theories led to subsequent investigations of PTH in combination with either $1,25(OH)_2D$ or antiresorptive agents.

Slovik *et al.* (1986) treated eight osteoporotic men with daily s.c. hPTH(1-34) 400–500 U in addition to oral $1,25(OH)_2D$ 0.25 μg/day for one year. Vertebral trabecular density, measured by single-energy CT, increased on average 98% in the four patients in whom it was performed. Radius density by single-photon absorptiometry did not change. Calcium balance and calcium absorption increased in the four patients tested.

The same group investigated 15 osteoporotic women given the same regimen of hPTH(1-34) and $1,25(OH)_2D$ (Neer *et al.*, 1993) compared with a similar control group (n = 15) treated with calcium alone over a 12–24-month period. Spinal trabecular density (CT)

Table 15.2 Clinical studies employing PTH in the treatment of osteoporosis

Patients Sex/ age range	Duration of treatment	PTH fragment dose/regimen	Coadministered agents	Results	Reference
16 ♀ 49–78 5 ♂ 52–61	6–24 mo	Variable but mostly 400–500 U hPTH (1–34)	None	No change in calcium balance 70% increase of cancellous bone volume in iliac crest, bone loss in the distal femur	Reeve *et al.* (1980b) Reeve *et al.* (1976b) Reeve *et al.* (1976a) Reeve *et al.* (1981) Reeve *et al.* (1980a) Hesp *et al.* (1981)
8 ♂ 37–62	1 yr	hPTH (1–34) 400–500 U/day	0.25 μg/day 1,25$(OH)_2D_3$ 600–1200 mg/day calcium	98% increase in vertebral trabecular BMD (QCT), no change in radius mid shaft BMD (SPA) Calcium retention improved by 120 mg/day	Slovik *et al.* (1986)
15 ♀	1–2 yrs	Control	1000–2000 mg/day calcium	1.7% ↓ in cortical bone No changes in vertebral BMD	Neer *et al.* (1993)
15 ♀	1–2 yrs	hPTH (1–34) 400–500 U/day	0.25 μg/day 1,25$(OH)_2D_3$ 1000–2000 mg/day calcium	32% ↑ in vertebral trabecular BMD (QCT) 12% ↑ in spinal BMD (DPA) 5.7% ↓ in cortical bone	
11 ♀/1 ♂ 64/67	1 yr	hPTH (1–34) 500 U/day	9F given estrogen 8/12 months 2F/1M given nandrolone 25 mg/3 wk	Calcium retention improved by 64 mg/day Trabecular vertebral bone density ↑ (QCT) by 50% Cancellous bone volume in iliac crest ↑ by 42%	Bradbeer *et al.* (1992) Reeve *et al.* (1980a) Reeve *et al.* (1991) Reeve *et al.* (1993)
6 ♂/2 ♀ 33–67	14 mo	hPTH (1–38) 720–750 U/day 8 wks/14 wk cycle Total of 4 cycles	6/14 wk cycle nasal calcitonin 200 U/day	Vertebral BMD (QCT) ↑ by 12–89% (mean approx. 15%)	Hesch *et al.* (1989)

increased 32% and total spinal bone density (by dual-photon absorptiometry) increased 12% in the PTH+1,25$(OH)_2$D-treated group. There were no changes in spinal bone density in the calcium-treated group. In contrast, cortical bone density (site unspecified) decreased 5.7% in the treatment group but only 1.7% in the control group.

Hesch *et al.* (1980) treated eight osteoporotic patients (six men, two women) with the 1-38 fragment of hPTH subcutaneously administered for a total of 32 out of 56 weeks. In addition, calcitonin was given intranasally (200 U/day) for 24 of the 56-week study period. In this protocol, PTH was being used both as an anabolic agent and as a skeletal activator although the duration of administration suggests that the anabolic effect would dominate. Vertebral trabecular density (QCT) increased in all patients (mean 15%) while no change was seen in forearm BMD (SPA). Since there was no control group receiving calcitonin or PTH alone, it was unclear whether or not this regimen was more effective than either of these agents separately.

Another study combining PTH with antiresorptive therapy was performed by Reeve *et al.* (1980a) who used s.c. hPTH(1-34) 500 U/day in 12 osteoporotic subjects (11 women, one man). Nine of the 12 were also treated with hormonal replacement therapy for eight of the 12 months and the other three patients were treated with nandrolone in addition to hPTH. The hPTH-treated patients were compared with 12 patients treated with sodium fluoride (dose not specified). Spinal trabecular bone density (by QCT) increased approximately 50% on average in the PTH+HRT-treated group, with a smaller increment in fluoride-treated patients. Total spinal bone density (by DPA) increased in both groups, with a larger increment in the fluoride-treated patients (mean 13%). The majority of the integral vertebral density increase in the PTH-treated group could be attributed to an increase in the trabecular component. Radial bone density (by CT) did not change in either group at either the proximal or distal site. Radioisotopic analysis in the PTH-treated patients revealed increments in bone formation and calcium balance improved in most patients (Reeve *et al.*, 1991, 1993). Cancellous bone volume of the iliac crest increased by 42% and there was no consistent change in cortical width. Both trabecular width and width of new cancellous bone packets increased significantly (Bradbeer *et al.*, 1992; Reeve *et al.*, 1993).

PTH has also been used in at least three ADFR (Frost, 1979, 1984) protocols (A: Activate remodeling, D: Depress resorption, F: allow Formation to occur freely, R: Repeat cycle). In this application, the PTH is generally used for a short period to activate a cohort of bone-remodeling units to allow inhibition of a larger number of active remodeling units during the resorption phase. The theory is that the formation phase will then proceed with 'overfilling' of these remodeling units and net bone formation will occur. This use of PTH should be distinguished from the purely anabolic uses described above. ADFR remains a theoretical approach to osteoporosis treatment but has never been shown to be effective in any protocol devised thus far.

Reeve *et al.* (1984, 1987) gave hPTH(1-34) 1500 U/day for 1 week followed by 3 weeks of oral 1,25$(OH)_2$D 0.25 μg. The cycle was repeated 15 times. No mean change in bone density was found and paired iliac biopsies revealed no increases in cancellous bone volume. Hesch *et al.* (1989) treated eight osteoporotic patients with hPTH(1-38) 400 U/day for two weeks followed by EHDP during the second and third weeks of the cycle. Over the next 12 weeks, no medications were given. This entire regimen was repeated six times. There was no histological evidence of an increase in bone mass. In the third ADFR study, Hodsman and Fraher (1990) treated 20 osteoporotic patients with 400 U PTH(1-38) for two weeks, followed by eight weeks of s.c. salmon calcitonin in 10 patients and no further medication in the other 10 patients. Both groups were off medication for four more weeks and the entire cycle was repeated once. In the groups treated cyclically with PTH+calcitonin, no change in bone mass occurred. In the group treated with intermittent cyclical PTH alone, bone mass in the spine (by DPA) increased by a mean of 13%, while bone mass in the forearm (SPA) decreased by a mean of 11%.

NOTE IN PROOF

Since this chapter was originally written, three important human studies were published involving use of PTH as an anabolic agent (Finkelstein *et al.*, 1994; Hodsman *et al.*, 1997; Lindsay *et al.*, 1997).

Finkelstein *et al.* (1994) performed a placebo controlled, randomized study in premenopausal women with endometriosis (n = 40) rendered acutely estrogen deficient by GnRH agonist therapy (Nafarelin) as treatment for endometriosis. At the same time that Nafarelin was started, hPTH(1–34) 500 U/day, was administered daily by subcutaneous injection for 6 months in 20 patients and no other treatment was given to the other 20 patients enrolled in the study. PTH prevented vertebral bone loss compared with a reduction of 2.8% in anteroposterior bone density of the spine in the Nafarelin alone group (by DXA). However, there were similar bone losses in both groups in the femoral neck and no change in either group in the radius. The same group reported preliminary results of an extension of this protocol to 1 year (Finkelstein *et al.*, 1995). Anteroposterior and lateral spine densities increased 3% and 9% respectively over baseline in the PTH plus Nafarelin group, compared with losses of 5% and 6% in the Nafarelin alone group. Furthermore, there was **no** bone loss from the femoral neck in the PTH treated group compared with a loss of 5% in the Nafarelin alone group. As seen in the 6 month study, there were no changes in the radius of either group.

Hodsman *et al.* (1997) presented results of a study of cyclical PTH alone versus cyclical PTH plus pulse calcitonin in 30 women with postmenopausal osteoporosis. Human PTH(1–34) was given at a high dose (800 IU) cyclically, one month out of every 3, with or without cyclical calcitonin given for 6 weeks of each 3-month cycle. Bone mass increased approximately 8–10% over two years in the spine (by DXA) with no significant difference in the PTH alone versus PTH plus calcitonin group. Although there was a suggestion of an increase in the femoral neck of the hip in the PTH alone group, there were no significant changes at this site in either group of patients.

Our group has studied 50 women who had been on hormone replacement therapy (HRT) for an average of 9 years for treatment of postmenopausal primary osteoporosis. After assuring that bone mass was stable on HRT over a period of at least 1 year, patients were randomized to remain on HRT alone or stay on HRT in addition to receiving PTH(1–34), 400 IU daily by subcutaneous injection. Over a three year period in 35 patients who have so far completed the study, bone mass increased 13% in the lumbar spine, 2.6% in the total hip and 7.8% in the total body (Lindsay *et al.*, 1997). Forearm bone mass did not change in either group. Moreover, incident vertebral deformity measured by either a 15% or a 20% reduction in anterior, middle or posterior height on lateral spine radiograph was lower in the PTH+HRT group compared with the HRT alone group ($p < 0.04$ for 15% deformity and $p = 0.12$ for 20% deformity). This is the first demonstration in humans that the increment in bone mass induced by PTH is associated with an increment in bone strength. These results confirm animal data also produced by our group showing that PTH induced increments in bone mass of rats is associated with increased compressive strength (Shen *et al.*, 1995).

CONCLUSION

If the increment in bone mass due to PTH administration persists after discontinuation of PTH and the quality of the bone formed is normal, one might expect a reduction in fracture risk (at least in the spine) of more than 50%. PTH may therefore have a role at least in the treatment of spinal osteoporosis. The risk and side effects associated with PTH appear minimal, in contrast to sodium fluoride, the only other agent known to be anabolic to the skeleton. A preparation which could be administered in a way other than injection, such as a nasal spray, could increase the potential utility of this therapeutic agent.

REFERENCES

Agarwala, N. and Gay, C.V. (1992) Specific binding of parathyroid hormone to living osteoclasts. *J Bone Miner Res* **7**: 531.

Baron, R. and Magee, S.S. (1983) Estimation of trabecular bone resorption by histomorphometry: evidence for prolonged reversal phase with normal resorption in post menopausal osteoporosis and coupled increased resorption in primary hyperparathyroidism. In: *Clinical Disorders of Bone and Mineral Metabolism*, (eds Frame, B. and Potts, J.T.), Excerpta Medica, Amsterdam, pp. 191–5.

Bauer, W., Aub, J.C. and Albright, F. (1929) Studies of calcium phosphorus metabolisms: study of bone trabeculae as ready available reserve supply of calcium. *J Exp Med* **49**: 145–62.

Beresford, J.N., Gallagher, J.A., Poser, J.W. and Russell, R.G.G. (1984) Synthesis of osteocalcin by human bone cells *in vitro*. Effects of $1,25(OH)_2D_3$, PTH and glucocorticoids. *Metabol Bone Dis Rel Res* **5**: 229.

Bradbeer, J.M., Arlot, M.E., Meunier, P.J. and Reeve, J. (1992) Treatment of osteoporosis with parathyroid peptide (hPTH 1-34) and oestrogen: increase in volumetric density of iliac cancellous bone may depend on reduced trabecular spacing as well as increased thickness of packets of newly formed bone. *Clin Endocr* **37**: 282–9.

Burrows, R.B. (1938) Variations produced in bones of growing rats by parathyroid extracts. *Am J Anat* **62**: 237–90.

Canalis, E., Centrella, M., Burch, W. and McCarthy, T.L. (1989) Insulin-like growth factor I mediates selective anabolic effects of parathyroid hormone in bone cultures. *J Clin Invest* **83**: 60–5.

Centrella, M., Massague, J. and Canalis, E. (1986) Human platelet-derived transforming growth factor-b stimulates parameters of bone growth in fetal rat calvariae. *Endocrinology* **119**: 2306–12.

Chambers, T.J., McSheehy, P.M.J., Thomson, B.M. and Fuller, K. (1985) The effect of calcium-regulating hormones and prostaglandins on bone resorption by osteoclasts disaggregated from neonatal rabbit bone. *Endocrinology* **116**: 234–9.

Cheema, C., Grant, B.F. and Marcus, R. (1989) Effects of estrogen on circulating free and total 1,25 dihydroxyvitamin D and on the parathyroid vitamin D axis in postmenopausal women. *J Clin Invest* **83**: 537–42.

Cosman, F., Morrow, B., Kopal, M. and Bilezikian, J.P. (1989) Stimulation of inositol phosphate formation in ROS 17/2.8 cell membranes by guanine nucleotide, calcium and parathyroid hormone. *J Bone Miner Res* **4**: 413.

Cosman, F., Nieves, J., Horton, J., Shen, V. and Lindsay, R. (1994) Effects of estrogen on response to EDTA infusion in postmenopausal osteoporotic women. *J Clin Endocrinol Metab* **78**: 939–43.

Cramer, C.F., Suiker, A.P., Copp, D.H., Greep, R.O. and Talmage, R.V. (eds) (1961) *The Parathyroids*, Charles C. Thomas, Springfield pp. 158–66.

Dauphine, R.T., Riggs, B.L. and Scholtz, D.A. (1975) Back pain and vertebral crush fractures: an unemphasized mode of presentation for primary hyperparathyroidism. *Ann Intern Med* **83**: 365–7.

DeBartolo, T.F., Pegg, L.E., Shasserre, C. and Hahn, T.J. (1982) Comparison of parathyroid hormone and calcium ionophore A23187: effects on bone resorption and nucleic acid synthesis in cultured fetal rat bone. *Calcif Tissue Int* **34**: 495.

Delling, G. (1987) Bone morphology in primary hyperparathyroidism. A qualitative and quantitative study of 391 cases. *Appl Pathol* **55**: 147–59.

Delmas, P.D., Meunier, P.J., Faysse, E. and Saubier, E.C. (1986) Bone histomorphometry and serum bone gla-protein in the diagnosis of primary hyperparathyroidism. *World J Surg* **10**: 572–8.

Dempster, D.W., Cosman, F., Parisien, M., Shen, V. and Lindsay, R. (1993) Anabolic actions of parathyroid hormone on bone. *Endocr Rev* **14**: 690–709.

De Vernejoul, M.C., Benamount, M.P. and Cancela, L. (1988) Hyperparathyroidie primitive vue en rhumatologie: Signes cliniques et relations entre les signes histologiques osseux et les parametres biologiques. *Rev Rhum* **55**: 489–94.

Dietrich, J.W., Canalis, E.M., Maina, D.M. and Raisz, L.G. (1976) Hormonal control of bone collagen synthesis *in vitro*. Effects of parathyroid hormone and calcitonin. *Endocrinology* **98**: 943–9.

Dijke, P., Iwata, K., Goddard, C. *et al.* (1990) Recombinant transforming growth factor type beta 3: biological activities and receptor-binding properties in isolated bone cells. *Mol Cell Biol* **10**: 4473–9.

Duong, L.T., Grasser, W., DeHaven, P.A. and Sato, M. (1990) Parathyroid hormone receptors identified on avian and rat osteoclasts. *J Bone Miner Res* **5**: s203.

Eriksen, E.F. (1986) Normal and pathological remodeling of human trabecular bone: three dimensional reconstruction of the remodeling sequence in normals and in metabolic bone disease. *Endocr Rev* **7**: 379–408.

Finkelstein, J.S., Klibanski, A., Schaefer, E.H. *et al.* (1994) Parathyroid hormone for the prevention of bone loss induced by estrogen deficiency. *N Engl J Med* **331**: 1618–23.

Finkelstein, J., Klibanski, A. and Neer, R. (1995) Prevention of bone loss from the hip and spine with parathyroid hormone in estrogen-deficient women. [Abstract]. *J Bone Miner Res* **11**: S460.

Frost, H.M. (1979) Treatment of osteoporosis by manipulation of coherent cell populations. *Clin Orthop Rel Res* **143**: 227–44.

Frost, H.M. (1984) The ADFR concept revisited. *Calcif Tissue Int* **36**: 349–53.

Frost, H.M. and Jee, W.S.S. (1992) On the rat model of human osteopenias and osteoporosis. *Bone Mineral* **18**: 227–36.

Fujimori, A., Cheng, S., Avioli, L.V. and Civitelli, R. (1992) Structure–function relationship of parathyroid hormone: activation of phospholipase-C, protein kinase-A and -C in osteosarcoma cells. *Endocrinology* **130**: 29–36.

Gera, I., Hock, J.M., Gunness-Hey, M., Fonseca, J. and Raisz, L.G. (1987) Indomethacin does not inhibit the anabolic effect of PTH on the long bones of rats. *Calcif Tissue Int* **40**: 206–11.

Gunness-Hey, M., Gera, I. Fonseca, J., Raisz, L.G. and Hock, J.M. (1988) 1,25 dihydroxyvitamin D_3 alone or in combination with PTH does not increase bone mass in young rats. *Calcif Tisue Int* **43**: 284–8.

Gunness-Hey, M. and Hock, J.M. (1984) Increased trabecular bone mass in rats treated with synthetic human PTH. *Metab Bone Dis Rel Res* **5**: 177–81.

Gunness-Hey, M. and Hock, J.M. (1989) Loss of the anabolic effect of PTH on bone after discontinuation of hormone in rats. *Bone* **10**: 447–52.

Hefley, T.J., Krieger, N.S. and Stern, P.H. (1986) Simultaneous measurement of bone resorption and collagen. *Anal Biochem* **153**: 166–71.

Hefti, E., Trechsel, U., Bonjour, J.P., Fleisch, H. and Schenk, R. (1982) Increase of whole body calcium and skeletal mass in normal and osteoporotic adult rats treated with PTH. *Clin Sci* **62**: 389–96.

Heller, M., Mclean, F.C. and Bloom, W. (1950) Cellular transformations in mammalian bones induced by parathyroid extract. *Am J Anat* **87**: 315–39.

Herrmann-Erlee, M.P., Heersche, J.N., Hekkelman, J.W. *et al.* (1976) Effects of bone *in vitro* of bovine parathyroid hormone and synthetic fragments representing residues 1-34, 2-34 and 3-34. *Endocrinol Res Commun* **3**: 21–35.

Hesch, R.D., Busch, U., Prokop, M. *et al.* (1989) Increase of vertebral density by combination therapy with pulsatile 1-38hPTH and sequential addition of calcitonin nasal spray in osteoporotic patients. *Calcif Tissue Int* **44**: 176–80.

Hesp, R., Hulme, P., Williams, D. and Reeve, J. (1981) The relationship between changes in femoral bone density and calcium balance in patients with involutional osteoporosis treated with human parathyroid hormone fragment (hPTH 1-34). *Metab Bone Dis Rel Res* **2**: 331–4.

Hock, J.M. and Fonseca, J. (1990) Anabolic effect of human synthetic PTH depends on growth hormone. *Endocrinology* **127**: 1804–10.

Hock, J.M. and Gera, I. (1992) Effects of continuous and intermittent administration and inhibition of resorption on the anabolic response of bone to PTH. *J Bone Miner Res* **7**: 65.

Hock, J.M., Gera, I., Fonseca, J. and Raisz, L.G. (1988) Human PTH (1-34) increases bone in ovariectomized and orchidectomized rat rats. *Endocrinology* **122**: 2899–903.

Hock, J.M., Hummert, J.R., Boyce, R., Fonseca, J. and Raisz, L.G. (1989) Resorption is not essential for the stimulation of bone growth by hPTH-(1-34) in rats in vivo. *J Bone Miner Res* **4**: 449–58.

Hodsman A.B. and Fraher, L.J. (1990) Biochemical responses to sequential human parathyroid hormone (1-38) and calcitonin in osteoporotic subjects. *Bone Mineral* **9**: 137–52.

Hodsman, A.B., Fraher, L.J., Watson, P.H. *et al.* (1997) A randomized controlled trial to compare the efficacy of cyclical parathyroid hormone versus cyclical parathyroid hormone and sequential calcitonin to improve bone mass in postmenopausal women with osteoporosis. *J Clin Endocrinol Metab* **82**: 620–8.

Hori, M., Uzawa, T., Morita, K. *et al.* (1988) Effect of human parathyroid hormone (PTH(1-34)) on experimental osteopenia of rats induced by ovariectomy. *Bone Mineral* **3**: 193–9.

Ibbotson, K.J., Orcutt, C.M., D'Souza, S.M. *et al.* (1992) Contrasting effects of PTH and IGF-1 in an aged OVX rat model of postmenopausal osteoporosis. *J Bone Miner Res* **7**: 425–31.

Kalu, D.N. (1991) The ovariectomized rat model of postmenopausal bone loss. *Bone Mineral* **15**: 175–92.

Kalu, D.N., Echon, R. and Hollis, B.W. (1990) Modulation of ovariectomy-related bone loss by parathyroid hormone in rats. *Mech Ageing Dev* **56**: 49–62.

Kalu, D.N., Pennock, J., Doyle, F.H. and Foster, G.V. (1970) Parathyroid hormone and experimental osteosclerosis. *Lancet* **i**: 1363–6.

Kleerekoper, M., Villaneuva, A.R. and Mathews, C.H.E. (1983) PTH mediated bone loss in primary and secondary hyperparathyroidism. In: *Clinical Disorders of Bone and Mineral Metabolism*, (eds Frame, B. and Potts, J.T.), Excerpta Medica, Amsterdam, pp. 200–3.

Klein, R.F., Nissenson, R.A. and Strewler, G.J. (1988) Forskolin mimics the effects of calcitonin but not parathyroid hormone on bone resorption *in vitro*. *Bone Mineral* **4**: 247–56.

Kochersberger, G., Buckley, N.J. and Leight, G.S. (1987) What is the clinical significance of bone loss in primary hyperparathyroidism? *Arch Intern Med* **147**: 1951–53.

Lafferty, F.W. and Hubay, C.A. (1989) Primary hyperparathyroidism: a review of the long term surgical and non-surgical morbidities as a basis for a ration approach to treatment. *Arch Intern Med* **149**: 789–96.

Lindsay, R., Nieves, J., Formica, C. *et al.* (1997) Parathyroid hormone increases vertebral bone mass and may reduce vertebral fracture incidence in estrogen treated postmenopausal women with osteoporosis. *Lancet* **350**: 550–5.

Linkhart, T.A. and Mohan, S. (1989) Parathyroid hormone stimulates release of insulin-like growth factor-I (IGF-I) and IGF-II from neonatal mouse calvaria in organ culture. *Endocrinology* **125**: 1484.

Liu, C.C. and Kalu, D.N. (1990) Human parathyroid hormone (1-34) prevents bone loss and augments bone formation in sexually mature ovariectomized rats. *J Bone Miner Res* **5**: 973–81.

Liu, C.C., Kalu, D.N., Salerno E. *et al.* (1991) Preexisting bone loss associated with ovariectomy in rats is reversed by PTH. *J Bone Miner Res* **6**: 1071–80.

McCarthy, T.L., Centrella, M. and Canalis, E. (1989) Regulatory effects of insulin-like growth factor I and II on bone collagen synthesis in rat calvarial cultures. *Endocrinology* **124**: 301.

MacDonald, B.R., Gallagher, J.A. and Russell, R.G.G. (1986) Parathyroid hormone stimulates the proliferation of cells derived from human bone. *Endocrinology* **118**: 2445–9.

Mackie, E.J. and Trechsel, U. (1990) Stimulation of bone formation in vivo by transforming growth factor-b: remodeling of woven bone and lack of inhibition by indomethacin. *Bone* **11**: 295–300.

McPartlin, J., Skrabanek, D. and Powell, D. (1984) Bone alkaline phosphatase: quantitative cytochemical characterization and response to parathyrin *in vitro*. *Biochem Soc Trans* **123**: 894–8.

McSheehy, P.H.J. and Chambers, T.J. (1986) Osteoblastic cells mediate osteoclastic responsiveness to parathyroid hormone. *Endocrinology* **118**: 824–8.

Majeska, R.J. and Rodan, G.A. (1981) Low concentrations of parathyroid hormone enhance growth of cloned osteoblast-like cells *in vitro*. *Calcif Tissue Int* **33**: 323.

Malluche, H.H., Sherman, D., Meyer, W. *et al.* (1982) Effects of long term infusion of physiologica doses of 1-34 PTH on bone. *Am J Physiol* **242**: F197–F202.

Martin, P., Bergmann, P. and Gillett, C. (1986) Partially reversible osteopenia after surgery for primary hyperparathyroidism. *Arch Intern Med* **146**: 689–91.

Mellish, R.W.E., Shen, V., Birchman, R. *et al.* (1990) Quantitative analysis of trabecular bone in ovariectomized rats after intermittent administration of low dose human parathyroid hormone fragment (1-34) and 17β-estradiol. In *Osteoporosis 1990*, (eds Christiansen, C. and Overgand, K.), Handestrykkeriet Aalborg APS, Aalborg, pp. 1335–7.

Melsen, F. and Mosekilde, L. (1981) The role of bone biopsy in the diagnosis of metabolic bone disease. *Orthop Clin North Am* **12**: 571–601.

Morris, C.A., Mitnick, M.E., Weir, E.C., Horowitz, M. and Kreider, B.L. (1990) The parathyroid hormone-related protein stimulates human osteoblast-like cells to secrete a 9000-dalton bone-resorbing protein. *Endocrinology* **126**: 1783–85.

Mosekilde, L. and Melsen, F. (1978) A tetracycline-base histomorphometric evaluation of bone resorption and bone turnover in hyperthyroidism and hyperparathyroidism. *Acta Med Scand* **204**: 97–102.

Mosekilde, L., Soggard, C.H., Danielson, C.C., Torring, O. and Nilsson, M.H.L. (1991) The anabolic effects of human PTH on rat vertebral body mass are also reflected in the quality of bone, assessed by biomechanical testing: a comparison study between hPTH (1-34) and hPTH (1-84). *Endocrinology* **129**: 421.

Murrills, R.J., Stein, L.S., Horbert, W.R. and Dempster, D.W. (1992) Effects of phorbol myristate acetate on rat and chick osteoclasts. *J Bone Miner Res* **7**: 415.

Neer, M., Slovik, D.M. Daly, N., Potts, Jr, J.T. and Nussbaum, S.R. (1993) Treatment of post-menopausal osteoporosis with daily parathyroid hormone plus calcitriol. *Osteoporosis Int* **1** (Suppl): S204–S205.

Noda, M. and Camilliere, J. (1989) In vivo stimulation of bone formation by transforming growth factor-b. *Endocrinology* **124**: 2991–4.

Parfitt, A.M. (1986) Accelerated cortical bone loss: primary and secondary hyperparathyroidism. In: *Current Concepts of Bone Fragility*, (eds Uhtoff, H. and Stahl, E.), Springer Verlag, Berlin, pp. 279–85.

Parfitt, A.M. (1989) Surface specific bone remodeling in health and disease. In: *Clinical Disorders of Bone and Mineral Metabolism*, (ed. Kleerekoper, M.), Mary Ann Liebert, New York, pp. 7–14.

Parisien, M., Silverberg, S.J., Shane, E. *et al.* (1990) The histomorphometry of bone in primary hyperparathyroidism: preservation of cancellous bone structure. *J Clin Endocrinol Metab* **70**: 930–8.

Partridge, N.C., Dickson, C.A., Kopp, K. *et al.* (1989) Parathyroid hormone inhibits collagen synthesis at both ribonucleic acid and protein levels in rat osteogenic sarcoma cells. *Mol Endocrinol* **3**: 232–9.

Partridge, N.C. and Martin, T.J. (1984) Studies on the effects of parathyroid hormone on growth of UMR 106 osteogenic sarcoma cells. *Calcif Tissue Int* **3**: 468.

Peacock, M., Horsman, A., Aaron, J.E. *et al.* (1984) The role of parathyroid hormone in bone loss. Proceedings of the Copenhagen International Symposium on Osteoporosis, (eds Christiansen, C. *et al.*), Aalborg Stiftsbotrykkeri, Copenhagen, pp. 463–7.

Perry, H.M., Skogen, W., Chappel, J.C. *et al.* (1987) Conditioned medium from osteoblast-like cells mediates parathyroid hormone induced bone resorption. *Tissue Int* **40:** 298–300.

Podesek, R., Edouard, C., Meunier, P.J. *et al.* (1983) Effects of two treatment regimes with synthetic human parathyroid hormone fragment on bone formation and the tissue balance of trabecular bone in greyhounds. *Endocrinology* **112**: 1000–6.

Podesek, R., Stevenson, R., Zanelli, G.D. *et al.* (1980) Treatment with human parathyroid hormone fragment (hPTH 1-34) stimulates bone formation and intestinal calcium absorption in the greyhound: comparison with data from the osteoporosis trial. In: *Hormonal Control of Calcium Metabolism*, Excerpta Medica, Amsterdam, pp. 118–23.

Pugsley, L.I. and Selye, H. (1933) The histological changes in the bone responsible for the action of parathyroid hormone on the calcium metabolism of the rat. *J Physiol* **79**: 113–17.

Puzas, J.E. and Brand, J.S. (1985) Bone cell phosphotyrosine phosphatase: characterization and regulation by calcitropic hormones. *Endocrinology* **116**: 2463–8.

Rao, L.G., Murray, T.M. and Heersche, J.N.M. (1983) Immunohistochemical demonstration of parathyroid hormone binding to specific cell types in fixed rat bone tissue. *Endocrinology* **113**: 805–10.

Rao, D.S., Wilson, R.J., Kleerekoper, M. and Parfitt, A.M. (1988) Lack of biochemical progression or continuation of accelerated bone loss in mild asymptomatic primary hyperparathyroidism: evidence for biphasic disease course. *J Clin Endocrinol Metab* **67**: 1294–8.

Reeve, J., Arlot, M., Bernat, M. *et al.* (1980a) Treatment of osteoporosis with human parathyroid hormone fragment 1-34: a positive final tissue balance in trabecular bone. *Metab Bone Dis Rel Res* **2** (Suppl): 355–60.

Reeve, J., Arlot, M., Bernat, M. *et al.* (1981) Calcium-47 kinetic measurements of bone turnover compared to bone histomorphometry in osteoporosis: the influence of human parathyroid fragment (hPTH 1-34) therapy. *Metab Bone Dis Rel Res* **3**: 23–30.

Reeve, J., Arlot, M.E., Bradbeer, J.N. *et al.* (1993) Human parathyroid peptide treatment of vertebral osteoporosis. *Osteoporosis Int* **3** (Suppl): 199–203.

Reeve, J., Bradbeer, J.N., Arlot, M. *et al.* (1991) hPTH 1-34 Treatment of osteoporosis with added hormone replacement therapy: biochemical, kinetic and histological responses. *Osteoporosis Int* **1**: 162–70.

Reeve, J., Arlot, M., Price, T.R. *et al.* (1987) Periodic courses of human 1-34 parathyroid peptide alternating with calcitriol paradoxically reduce bone remodeling in spinal osteoporosis. *Eur J Clin Invest* **17**: 421–8.

Reeve, J., Hesp, R., Williams, D. *et al.* (1976b) Anabolic effect of low doses of a fragment of human parathyroid hormone on the skeleton in postmenopausal osteoporosis. *Lancet* **i**: 1035–8.

Reeve, J., Meunier, P., Parsons, J.A. *et al.* (1980b) Anabolic effect of human parathyroid hormone fragment on trabecular bone in involutional osteoporosis: a multicentre trial. *Br Med J*: 1340–4.

Reeve, J., Podesek, R.D., Price, T.R. *et al.* (1984) Studies of a "short-cycle" ADFR regime using parathyroid peptide hPTH 1-34 in idiopathic osteoporosis and in a dog model. In: *Osteoporosis 1984*, (eds Christiansen, C., Arnaud, C.D., Nordin, B.E.C. *et al.*), Aalborg Stiftsbogtrykkeri, Copenhagen, pp. 567–73.

Reeve, J., Tregear, GW. and Parsons, J.A. (1976a) Preliminary trial of low doses of human parathyroid hormone 1-34 peptide in treatment of osteoporosis. *Calcif Tissue Int*. **21**: 469–77.

Richardson, M.L., Pozzi-Mucelli, R.S., Kanter, A.S. *et al.* (1986) Bone mineral changes in primary hyperparathyroidism. *Skeletal Radiol* **15**: 85–95.

Riggs, B.L., Kelly, P.J., Jowsey, J. and Keating, F.R. (1965) Skeletal alterations in hyperparathyroidism: determination of bone formation, resorption and morphologic changes by microradiography. *J Clin Endocrinol Metab* **25**: 777–83.

Rosenblatt, M. (1986) Peptide hormone antagonists that are effective *in vivo*. *N Engl J Med* **315**: 1004.

Schulz, A., Remagen, W. and Grosse, P. (1971) Effects of parathyroid extract on calcium metabolism and on bone morphology in the intact rat. Z Ges Exp Med **155**: 87–97.

Seeman, E., Wahner, H.W., Offord, K.P. *et al.* (1982) Differential effects of endocrine dysfunction on the axial and the appendicular skeleton. *J Clin Invest* **69**: 1302–9.

Selye, H. (1932) On the stimulation of new bone-formation with parathyroid extract and irradiated ergosterol. *Endocrinology* **16**: 547–58.

Shelling, D.H., Asher, D.E. and Jackson, D.A. (1933) Calcium and phosphorus studies: effects of variations and dosage of parathormone and of calcium and phosphorus and diet on concentrations of calcium and inorganic phosphorus in serum and on histology and chemical composition of bones of rats. *Bull Johns Hopkins Hosp* **53**: 348–9.

Shen, V., Dempster, D.W., Birchman, R., Xu, R. and Lindsay, R. (1992) Loss of cancellous bone mass and connectivity in ovariectomized rats can be restored by combined treatment with parathyroid hormone and estradiol. *J Clin Invest* **91**: 2479–87.

Shen, V., Birchman, R., Xu, R. *et al.* (1995) Effects of reciprocal treatment with estrogen and estrogen plus parathyroid hormone on bone structure and strength in ovariectomized rats. *J Clin Invest* **96**: 2331–8.

Silver, J. (1993) Regulation of parathyroid hormone synthesis and secretion. In: *Disorders of Bone and Mineral Metabolism*, (eds Coe, F.L. and Favus, M.J.) Raven Press, New York, pp. 83–106.

Silverberg, S.J., Shane, E. and de la Cruz, L. (1989) Skeletal disease in primary hyperparathyroidism. *J Bone Miner Res* **4**: 283–91.

Slovik, D.M., Neer, R.M. and Potts, J.T.J. (1981) Short-term effects of synthetic human parathyroid hormone (1-34) administration on bone mineral metabolism in osteoporotic patients. *J Clin Invest* **68**: 1261–71.

Slovik, D.M., Rosenthal, D.I., Doppelt, J.H. *et al.* (1986) Restoration of spinal bone in osteoporotic men by treatment with human parathyroid hormone (1-34) and 1,25-dihydroxyvitamin D. *J Bone Miner Res* **1**: 377–81.

Su, Y., Chakraborty, M., Nathanson, M.H. and Baron, R. (1992) Differential effects of the 3′,5′-cyclic adenosine monophosphate and protein kinase C pathways on the response of isolated rat osteoclasts to calcitonin. *Endocrinology* **131**: 1497–502.

Tada, K., Yamamuro, T., Okumura, H., Kasai, R. and Takahashi, H. (1990) Restoration of axial and appendicular bone volumes by h-PTH (1-34) in parathyroidectomized and osteopenic rats. *Bone* **11**: 163–9.

Tam, C.S., Heersche, J.N.M., Murray, T.M. and Parsons, J.A. (1982) Parathyroid hormone stimulates the bone apposition rate independently of its resorptive action: differential effects of intermittent and continuous administration. *Endocrinology* **110**: 506.

Teti, A., Colucci, S., Grano, M., Argentino, L. and Zallone, A.Z. (1992) Protein kinase C affects microfilaments, bone resorption and [Ca3+]o sensing in cultured osteoclasts. *Am J Physiol* **263**: C130–C139.

Tuukkanen, J., Jalovaara, P. and Vaananen, K. (1990) Calcitonin treatment of immobilization osteoporosis in rats. *Acta Physiol Scand* **141**: 119–24.

Vargas, S.J. and Raisz, L.G. (1990) Simultaneous assessment of bone resorption and formation in cultures of 22-day fetal rat parietal bones: effects of parathyroid hormone and prostaglandin E2. *Bone* **11**: 61–5.

Walker, D.G. (1971) The induction of osteoporotic changes in hypophysectomized, thyroparathyroidectomized and intact rats of various ages. *Endocrinology* **89**: 1389–406.

Wilson, R.J., Rao, D.S., Ellis, B., Kleerekoper, M. and Parfitt, A.M. (1988) Mild asymptomatic primary hyperparathyroidism is not a risk factor for vertebral fractures. *Ann Intern Med* **109**: 959–62.

Wong, G.L., Luben, R.A. and Cohn, D.V. (1977) 1,25-Dihydroxycholecalciferol and parathormone: effects on isolated osteoclast-like and osteoblast-like cells. *Science* **197**: 663.

Wronski, T.J., Cintron, M. and Dann, L.M. (1988) Temporal relationship between bone loss and increased bone turnover in ovariectomized rats. *Calcif Tissue Int* **43**: 179–83.

Yamaguchi, D.T., Hahn, T.J., Iida-Klein, A., Kleeman, C.R. and Muallem, S. (1987) Parathyroid hormone-activated calcium channels in an osteoblast-like clona osteosarcoma cell line. cAMP-dependent and cAMP-independent calcium channels. *J Biol Chem* **262**: 7711–18.

Physical Activity

& osteoporosis

Never ?

Generated

Caused.

PHYSICAL ACTIVITY AND OSTEOPOROSIS 16

R. Marcus and B.J. Kiratli

INTRODUCTION

The relationship of physical activity to bone mass and prevention of osteoporosis continues to provoke great interest. On the basis of current knowledge, optimism is justified that regular physical activity will help to maintain a higher bone mass throughout life and decrease the long-term risk for fracture due to bone fragility. By mechanisms that are not yet defined, bone mineral increases in response to application of mechanical stress and decreases when stress is removed. The profound importance of physical activity to skeletal health can be seen in the effects of decreased activity and immobilization as well as those of increased activity. In this chapter we review the influence of physical activity on bone mass and the role of exercise in preventing and treating osteoporosis.

We give primary attention to newer information regarding both immobilization and exercise and emphasize recent exercise intervention studies over older cross-sectional comparative literature. Although some animal work is cited, we concentrate primarily on human studies. For a comprehensive review of this topic the reader is referred to Snow-Harter and Marcus (1991).

THE RELATIONSHIP OF MECHANICAL LOADING TO BONE MASS

The skeleton is constantly subjected to forces generated by muscle contraction and by direct impact on the ground. These forces lead to alterations in bone shape and, to a large degree, determine bone strength. Exactly 100 years ago the German scientist Julius Wolff stated the theory, now called Wolff's Law, that bone accommodates the forces applied to it by altering its amount and distribution of mass. This concept has been expanded to a general theory of bone regulation, in which mechanical loading is the primary stimulus (Rubin and Lanyon, 1984; Carter and Fyhrie, 1987; Frost, 1987), subject to modulating influences of hormonal, dietary and other factors. Carter and Fyhrie (1987) and Whalen and Carter (1988) have proposed that the steady-state apparent density of a unit of bone directly reflects its customary loading history, which itself represents the sum of all daily loading events to which it is subjected. The principle explains the differences in mass in different areas of a given bone, differences in mass from one bone to the next and differences in the same bone among individuals.

BONE STRAIN

As a deformable object, bone has mechanical properties similar to any structural material (Cornwall, 1984). All forces imposed on bone produce strain and the amount of strain that a material can withstand determines its strength. Strain is defined as the change in dimension divided by the original dimension.

Osteoporosis. Edited by John C. Stevenson and Robert Lindsay. Published in 1998 by Chapman & Hall, London.
ISBN 0 412 48870 1

In engineering terms, one 'strain' unit is equivalent to a 1% change and one microstrain represents 10^{-6} 'strain'. Physiologic loading generally produces strains up to 2000–3000 μstrain, whereas excessive strain may precipitate fracture. Ordinary strains within bone stimulate the cellular activities that regulate bone configuration and density. If the strain experience for a given bone remains constant over time, the bone will maintain an equilibrium state. If strain increases or decreases, bone is gained or lost until a new equilibrium is reached. The work of Rubin and Lanyon (1984) and Whalen *et al.* (1987) suggests that the strain magnitude and rate (Δstrain ÷ Δtime) outweigh the number of cycles as determinants of skeletal response to loading.

FATIGUE DAMAGE

Bone accumulates areas of fatigue damage as a consequence of repetitive daily loading. Carter *et al.* (1981) concluded that repetitive loading at impacts equivalent to running would produce fatigue damage after 100 000 cycles or about 100 miles and Burr *et al.* (1985) found that repetitive physiological loading of the dog ulna produced visible microdamage. It is considered likely that the process of bone remodeling serves a protective surveillance and scavenger role to remove areas of fatigue damage as they develop.

The continuous process of breakdown and renewal called bone remodeling is described in other chapters of this volume and will not be detailed here. Suffice it to state that remodeling is thought to be the final pathway by which adult humans gain or lose bone. Although remodeling is a coupled process in which bone formation is preceded by and dependent on an episode of bone resorption, it is inherently inefficient. That is to say, the amount of bone replaced by osteoblasts does not quite equal the amount that was removed. Under ordinary circumstances, therefore, anything that increases the overall rate of bone remodeling will increase the rate of bone loss (Marcus, 1987).

Since mechanical loading increases remodeling activity, an inefficient process that should promote bone loss, the positive association of physical activity with bone mass appears to be paradoxical. It is likely that remodeling induced by mechanical loads differs from that induced by dietary inadequacy, hormonal changes or other means. Several explanations have been offered, including the possibilities that loading directly stimulates osteoblastic activity without prior resorption or that systemic hormonal responses to physical activity may constrain the degree to which bone is removed during resorption, thereby shifting remodeling dynamics to favor net bone accretion with each cycle. At present, the solution to this problem is not known.

THE ROLE OF BONE GEOMETRY

Virtually the entire body of literature dealing with physical activity and bone health has focused on bone mass. Since bone strength is determined also by its quality and architecture, bone mineral measurements provide only partial information regarding bone fragility. To some degree, this explains the substantial overlap in bone mineral content that is found between fractured and non-fractured individuals (Hui *et al.*, 1988). The geometrical contributions to bone strength differ somewhat for cortical and trabecular bone. In cortical bone, the distribution of bone around the longitudinal bending axis constitutes an important geometrical determinant of bone strength. This parameter is called the cross-sectional moment of inertia (CSMI). Of two bones with the same mineral content, that with the higher CSMI has greater bending strength. In trabecular bone, orientation of vertical and horizontal trabeculae is critical to strength. In young adults, the load-bearing trabecular bone is characterized by thick vertical plates and columns which are crossed by thinner horizontal trabeculae. Maximum strength is gained by the connnection of all trabecular elements (Parfitt, 1984). With age, trabecular connectivity is progressively disrupted (Parfitt *et al.*, 1983), reflecting disappearance of entire trabecular elements. Such loss of connectivity contributes substantially to structural failure and the risk for fracture. Unfortunately, we currently have no satisfactory non-invasive technique to assess this aspect of bone health.

RELATIONSHIP OF DISUSE TO BONE MASS

The earliest evidence of bone loss following immobilization came from observations of increased urinary calcium and hydroxyproline output in spinal cord-injured (SCI) patients and patients with poliomyelitis in the 1940s and 1950s. When these observations were initially made, no direct methods for quantifying bone mass were available. More recently, increased excretion of calcium and hydroxyproline has been substantiated with measurements of bone mineral density in both retrospective and prospective studies of various conditions of reduced physical activity in humans, including individuals immobilized from illness or injury, astronauts exposed to microgravity and volunteers subjected to prolonged bedrest.

Although hypogravic and hypoactive conditions are found in all of these situations, important differences exist among the situations of weightlessness (space flight), recumbency (prolonged bedrest) in otherwise healthy young men and paralysis or paresis (resulting from spinal cord injury, poliomyelitis or stroke). Space flight removes gravitational forces and is accompanied by reduced activity; prolonged bedrest, imposed on healthy subjects, includes both reduced weight bearing and decreased muscular activity. Neither astronauts nor volunteers at bedrest lose normal muscular tone although activity is certainly decreased. Paralyzed patients, in contrast, experience normal gravity but absence of upright posture and associated weight bearing. In addition, voluntary muscle activity and normal muscle tone is eliminated in these patients although a form of muscle tension may be preserved in those with spastic, involuntary contractions. Thus, comparisons of the skeletal responses to 'disuse' between these conditions might be expected to yield discrepancies.

In fact, many of the same physiologic changes observed in SCI patients, and attributed to loss of muscle tension and weight bearing, are observed in astronauts and bedrest subjects. This consistency of results between the healthy human subjects and paralyzed patients indicates that observed bone responses result primarily from reduced mechanical loading, rather than from trauma or other non-mechanical causes.

In a variety of study designs using both human and animal models, it has been demonstrated that bone loss occurs in areas of the skeleton from which mechanical loads are reduced or eliminated. Most evidence indicates that this response is localized to the unloaded region(s). Prospective data on astronauts and bedrest subjects indicate that this loss is detectable soon after onset of immobilization and that bone is lost at approximately 1% per month. Retrospective studies of subjects with chronic paralysis exhibit no relationship between bone mass and duration of paralysis. Thus, it appears that bone loss with disuse is not continuous but occurs only as an initial response to unloading. After this, the bone seems to adjust to a new 'normal' stress environment and homeostasis is re-established at this reduced bone mass.

WEIGHTLESSNESS AND INACTIVITY IN SPACE FLIGHT

Demineralization with space flight has been examined in Gemini missions (4–14 days) and Skylab missions (SL2: 28 days; SL3: 59 days; SL4: 84 days). Data obtained by X-ray aluminum equivalency of the calcaneus from the Gemini flights are summarized by Vose (1974). Losses of approximately 3% were observed in astronauts on all flights (one exception was a 9% loss in one individual after eight days in space). Although these changes are consistent with metabolic data, they are also within the error of the measurement technique. Data from the longer Skylab flights are reviewed by Anderson and Cohn (1984) and Whedon (1984). Densitometric measurements (by photon absorptiometry) of the calcaneus indicated variable results over the three flights: no change over 28 days, 7.4% loss over 59 days, and 4.5% and 7.9% decline over 84 days. Similar losses (5–8% decrease over 175 days) were reported from Soviet studies. No significant changes were observed in radius and ulna bone mass during any of the flights.

With return to normal gravity, bone deposition occurred in the calcaneus. Calcaneal bone mass returned to normal after 87 days following 59 days in space. However, normal bone mass was not regained in 95 days after a longer period in space (84 days, Skylab flight). Furthermore, a five-year follow-up study indicated that astronauts, after flights of 28 to 84 days in space, had bone mass significantly below preflight values (Tilton *et al.*, 1980). The five-year differences were also compared between the astronauts and controls; although losses were observed over time in both groups, greater losses were observed in the astronauts and only these were significant.

EXPERIMENTAL BEDREST IN HEALTHY YOUNG MEN

In bedrest subjects, loss of bone mass from the calcaneus occurred at a rate 10 times greater than the rate of loss of total body calcium, calculated from balance studies; 25–45% loss was found in this bone after 36 weeks of bedrest (Donaldson *et al.*, 1970). In earlier work, Dietrick and coworkers (1948) had estimated 1–2% loss per month in total skeletal mineral. No loss was observed in radius bone mineral with prolonged bedrest, and similar losses of 26–39% over 24–30 weeks were observed in the heel by Hulley *et al.* (1971). This was taken as evidence that weight-bearing bones were more susceptible to bone resorption than the rest of the skeleton and contributed disproportionately to calcium excretion. With reambulation, bone mineral in the calcaneus was regained at a rate similar to the rate of loss (Donaldson *et al.*, 1970; Hulley *et al.*, 1971).

IMMOBILIZATION ASSOCIATED WITH ILLNESS OR INJURY

Bone atrophy following spinal cord injury (SCI) and paralysis has been documented in a number of different studies. Radiographic and densitometric (photon absorptiometry) techniques have been used to determine the specific sites of bone loss, to estimate the amount of change and to ascertain the time course of the response.

Using both radiographs of the lower arm and densitometric measurements of the wrist and forearm shaft, Griffiths *et al.* (1976) compared paraplegic and quadriplegic patients to non-injured individuals. No evidence of cortical loss was found, but significant trabecular loss was observed. This was more marked in the quadriplegics but was also observed in some of the paraplegics; the authors expressed surprise at this result as increased stress during lifting maneuvers might be expected to preserve skeletal mass in these patients. Nikolic *et al.* (1977) found metacarpal cortical indices (total thickness of cortical bone divided by the diameter) to be normal in paraplegics but decreased in quadriplegics, whereas femoral cortical indices were generally reduced in both.

When radiographic comparisons were made between the affected and unaffected upper extremities of hemiplegic stroke patients (Panin *et al.*, 1971), the cortical thicknesses of humeri, radii and third metacarpal bones were found to be significantly smaller on the affected side. It was also determined that the extent of cortical thinning was related to the degree of residual motor function in patients who recovered some motor ability, but no effects were detectable due to spasticity. These data indicate the importance of local muscular stresses and strains alone in maintenance of normal bone mass or the upper limbs.

Densitometric measurements comparing the normal and affected arms of hemiplegic stroke patients were used to differentiate the effects of immobilization and residual activity on trabecular and cortical bone (Prince *et al.*, 1988). The decline in cortical bone depended primarily on the duration of immobilization while decline in trabecular bone with duration of paralysis was influenced by muscle stresses imposed by spasticity and functional motor ability. The predominance of trabecular bone response over cortical was demonstrated by Iverson *et al.* (1989) in a study comparing arms and legs of hemiparetic/hemiplegic patients by whole-body bone densitometry. The decrease (difference in bone mass between affected and unaffected limbs, divided by the unaffected limb) in the mostly trabecular distal arm bone (13%) significantly exceeded that in the mostly cortical proximal site (8%). Further, there was a greater loss in the arms (10%) than in the legs (4%). To explain the latter result, the authors proposed that a hospitalization-dependent decrease in overall activity led to a decline in bone mass of the unaffected leg as well; this would effectively reduce the 'loss', determined by the affected bone mass as a proportion of unaffected bone mass.

Bone density in the lower extremities of paraplegic and quadriplegic patients with durations of injury between two and 25 years was found to be significantly below normal values, measured in the tibia and femur (Hancock *et al.*, 1980; Biering-Sorensen and Bohr, 1988; Kiratli, 1989; Biering-Sorenson *et al.*, 1990). Loss of bone mass of the tibia was twice as great as loss in the femur; tibia values were 50% of predicted normal values while femur values were 25% below normal. No influence on bone mass was detected due to spasticity or use of standing braces. Further, lumbar spine bone mass was not found to be different from expected control values in either retrospective or prospective studies (Kiratli, 1989; Biering-Sorensen *et al.*, 1990). It is suggested that the loading experienced by the lumbar spine with upright sitting posture and possibly during transfers is sufficient to protect against bone loss. In a study of total body bone response (Garland, 1991) significant losses were observed in the upper extremity, pelvis and throughout the lower extremity during the first 16 months postinjury, compared with controls. There was no evidence of further loss observed at any sites in individuals with chronic paralysis (>5 years postinjury), compared with 16-month postinjury values. Finally, no differences were observed in bone mass of the trunk or head among control, newly injured and chronically injured SCI individuals.

Most of the bone decline with paralysis occurs during the first year after injury and no continued change was observed in patients with 'relatively long-standing' paralysis. Based on data from cross-sectional studies, bone loss was not related to duration of injury in patients injured between two and 40 years earlier (Griffiths *et al.*, 1976; Hancock *et al.*, 1980). In contrast, Prince *et al.* (1988) suggest that bone loss continues up to 15 years after immobilization by stroke.

Localized skeletal responses are demonstrated in studies of various other patient populations. Vertebral bone loss was described in a longitudinal study by Krølner and Toft (1983) of patients immobilized due to low backache and disc protrusion. In these patients, bone mineral content declined at a rate of approximately 1% per week over the study period (11–61 days); reambulation led to gain in vertebral bone and restoration of normal values after four months. In an examination of patients with frozen shoulder syndrome, Lundberg and Nilsson (1968) determined that the immobilized humerus had significantly reduced bone mineral content when compared to the unaffected side; this result was not dependent on duration of rigidity, was more pronounced in males and was not restored with remobilization of one year. Decreases in femoral bone mass parameters were also observed in amputees (Jenkins and Cochran, 1969; O'Malley *et al.*, 1980) when the intact leg was compared with the stump of the amputated leg. Increased medullary diameters and decreased cortical widths indicated cortical thinning, with greater differences observed distally. These changes indicated the importance of loss of muscle attachments near the measurement sites.

Increased fracture risk is another well-established complication of long-term spinal cord injury (Guttmann, 1976). Long bone fractures occur in individuals with chronic SCI often in the absence of any discernible trauma, such as during a transfer or range of motion exercises. The majority of fractures occur in the lower extremity, with the highest prevalence in the femur. Although fracture prevalence in SCI patients has been estimated to be as high as 15% (Comarr and Hutchinson, 1962), most estimates report approximately 5% (Freehafer and Mast, 1965; Nottage, 1981; Ragnarsson and Sell, 1981; Ingram *et al.*, 1989). This might not seem a significant prevalence, but several concurrent factors augment the severity of the injury. A slow healing process, non-union and other complications are more common in SCI than in non-SCI patients following fracture and surgical intervention (such as open reduction and internal fixation) is often not attempted, mostly because of the expectation of pre-existing osteopenia and heightened risk for further complications. The presence of a non-healed or healed but malaligned fracture may interfere in performance of activities of daily living, even without the potential sequelae of infection, heterotopic bone formation or subsequent fracture. Furthermore, in the absence of sensation, SCI individuals are often unaware that a fracture has occurred and thus do not seek medical attention until more extensive and serious symptoms are present.

INTERVENTIONS TO ACHIEVE INCREASED LOADING AND MINIMIZE BONE LOSS

Although early weight bearing is often recommended (Yashon, 1978; Ragnarsson and Sell, 1981) as useful to prevent the development of osteoporosis and joint stiffness after SCI, few data have been collected which demonstrate the efficacy of this therapy and little research has been directed toward the therapeutic use of mechanical loading to prevent bone loss in paralyzed patients. No alterations in calcium loss were observed in studies of patients paralyzed with poliomyelitis who were rocked in bed, exercised underwater or ambulated on crutches (Whedon and Shorr, 1957; Plum and Dunning, 1958).

The influences of muscular activity and weight bearing on bone metabolism were evaluated by Claus-Walker and coworkers (1975) in 32 quadriplegic patients. Patients were divided into two groups: those 'actively engaged in daily living' and those confined to bed. No description was given of the amount and types of activities which comprised 'daily living', but these were considered as muscular activity in the discussion of the results. Mean levels of urinary hydroxyproline were significantly lower in the active patients, although there were no significant differences in urinary calcium excretion between the groups. In addition, patients left in bed for extended periods had longer duration of hypercalciuria and hyper-hydroxyprolinuria than those who were involved in rehabilitation exercises. The authors concluded that recumbency favored bone resorption while muscular activity favored bone formation and that metabolism of collagen and bone after onset of paralysis was 'greatly influenced by the patient's physical activity'. However, Maynard and Imai (1977) report that passive weighting through sitting and tilt-table treatments had no effect in reducing hypercalcemia in SCI patients.

Following assisted ambulation in paralyzed patients, urinary calcium excretion was decreased and calcium balance became positive (Kaplan *et al.*, 1978). The length of time since injury was a factor in the magnitude of the response. Patients with injuries less than three months earlier showed greater changes in calcium metabolism than those with injuries more than six months earlier.

Spastic (involuntary) muscular contraction, frequently found with upper motor neuron SCI, has not been found to influence bone loss while voluntary muscle contraction, in partial paralysis, has seemed to reduce the loss (Panin *et al.*, 1971; Ragnarsson and Sell, 1981).

A number of physical treatments have been tested for prevention of bone resorption in experiments on immobilized volunteers. These have been designed to replicate or replace the influences of weight bearing and/or muscular activity. The results of the various studies have been inconsistent and contradictory.

In 1949, Whedon *et al.* reported the effects of an oscillating bed (from horizontal to a 20° foot-down position) on elevated urinary calcium in healthy subjects immobilized in body casts. Hypercalciuria was decreased in subjects undergoing this treatment for 8–21 hours a day. It was assumed that this resulted from increased compression on the lower extremity imposed by the downward tilt.

Issekutz *et al.* (1966) conducted a series of experiments on 14 subjects during bedrest for up to 42 days. Supine isotonic exercises on a bicycle ergometer of four hours/day had no effect on urinary calcium excretion. Sitting for eight hours/day (and bedrest for the remaining 16 hours) also had no effect on calcium output. However, three hours per day of quiet standing resulted in reduction of hypercalciuria. The pattern of change in calcium excretion was different from that of recovery and reambulation. With standing, a slow, fluctuating decline was observed, which did not drop below the pre-bedrest level. During recovery of 14–16 ours 'up- and about', the reduction in calcium excretion was steady and in several cases continued below the initial baseline. The interpretation of these results was that since standing was effective in modulating calcium loss and 'vigorous' exercise was ineffective, the hypercalciuria with bedrest resulted from the prolonged supine position and elimination of weight bearing rather than from physical inactivity.

No significant effects were detected on calcium metabolism or calcaneal mineral loss in bedrest subjects treated with various physical countermeasures (Hantmann *et al.*, 1973; Schneider and McDonald, 1984). These included 'exercise' (passive) with a pulley, static and intermittent longitudinal compression, lower body negative pressure and impact loading with longitudinal compression. In both the static and intermittent longitudinal compression conditions, 80% body weight was applied. There were two conditions of impact loading with compression. One involved adding a 20 lb (9 kg) impact 40 times per minute for eight hours per day. The second condition added a 36 lb (16 kg) impact for six hours per day. Explanations for the negative results were that the applied forces did not adequately simulate normal ambulation and/or that other factors are important in bone tissue activity.

However, in another study (V.S. Schneider, described in Anderson and Cohn (1984)), there was evidence that impact loading and compression at 80% of body weight increased or maintained calcaneal bone mineral in bedrest subjects although there were no effects on negative calcium balance. In addition, the impact delivered by the 'drop technique' from standing on tiptoe to heels was found to be associated with improved calcium balance.

In general, the attempts to find countermeasures to bone loss with prolonged bedrest have focused on replacement of weight bearing. This seems a reasonable approach because, in this model of immobilization, weight bearing is the primary influence which has been removed. Although movement of the body and limbs is restricted and recruitment of the postural muscles of the back and legs reduced, muscular contractions are certainly not eliminated. Therefore, bone loss with recumbency appears to result primarily from decreased compressive loading.

In order to verify that the bone loss observed in disuse models results from mechanical unloading, data are presented on the skeletal responses in these models to mechanical loading. There is evidence that bone loss may be reversed or prevented with normal external loads (reambulation or remobilization), but the data are less conclusive on the bone response to artificial loading regimes. Further, the ability of the skeletal system to remodel and increase mass after loss will depend heavily on the type of tissue affected and the extent of skeletal reduction. Specifically, if the decrement is due to resorption of trabeculae, no restitution of bone mass will be possible in these areas. Conversely, changes in cortical bone may be reversible with remodeling.

RELATIONSHIP OF EXERCISE TO BONE MASS

The inability to measure accurately or precisely a person's habitual physical activity remains a major impediment to proper understanding of the relationship between activity and bone health. Most validated instruments for assessing activity patterns were designed to estimate aerobic or metabolic activity, such as daily energy expenditure, rather than skeletal loading. A few attempts at estimating daily loads have given primary emphasis to recreational exercise and have neglected occupational or other activities that may also be important. For example, an individual who frequently opens a heavy door during the workday may derive more skeletal loading from that single activity than from any of his recreational pursuits. At present, therefore, it is necessary to discuss this general topic only in terms of recreational exercise. In this regard, it is somewhat reassuring that a recent study by Snow-Harter *et al.* (1992b) found that bone density in men was more closely related to recreational activities than to non-recreational miles walked per day.

CROSS-SECTIONAL STUDIES

Examination of active and sedentary populations at single points in time confirms a positive relationship between habitual activity and bone density. Literature in support of this conclusion is voluminous and, except for a few studies that illustrate particular aspects of this issue, will not be exhaustively cited. In composite, however, these studies show that 'active' or athletic subjects have significantly increased bone mineral density compared to that of sedentary controls, a difference that ranges from about 8% to 30%, almost without regard for the type of exercise (Snow-Harter and Marcus, 1991). It should be pointed out that the great majority of this literature is based on extraordinary levels of physical activity. It has been far more difficult to establish a skeletal effect of activity in sedentary to moderately active populations.

The skeletal benefit of exercise appears to be at least partly site specific. For example, in tennis players, bone density is significantly greater at the dominant radius (Huddleston *et al.*, 1980; Pirnay *et al.*, 1987). However, some evidence favors a systemic effect of activity, for example the finding that distance runners may have relatively high mineral content in the arms as well as at load-bearing sites (Dalen and Olsson, 1974; Brewer *et al.*, 1983).

Traditional views hold that exercise must be weight bearing to produce skeletal benefit. Weight-bearing activities by definition expend energy to withstand the effects of gravity. Representative examples include walking, running, dancing and jumping. Recent studies suggest that loads other than those generated by gravity, such as muscular pull, actively stimulate bone deposition. Young women who supplemented aerobic exercise with weight training for one hour per week had higher spine densities than women who participated in aerobic exercise only (Davee *et al.*, 1990). Orwoll and colleagues (1989) found higher radial and vertebral bone mineral density (BMD) among men who swam regularly as their only exercise than in sedentary men and Jacobson *et al.* (1984) found that bone density of female intercollegiate swimmers was higher than that of sedentary college students. Although swimming is certainly not a weight-bearing activity, its contributions to BMD could occur through loads created from high intensity muscular activity.

Other literature suggests that muscle strength, physical fitness and body weight all predict spine and hip BMD in premenopausal women (Pocock *et al.*, 1980). Considering the fact that the loss of bone parallels age-related declines in muscle mass and strength and in aerobic fitness, it is not unreasonable to postulate that physical activity may ameliorate age-related bone loss. Jacobson *et al.* (1984) reported bone density values in older athletic women that were equivalent to those of younger athletic women. Further, a 0.7% decrease per year in spine density was observed in a population of sedentary women older than 50 years which was not seen in a group of more active subjects. 'Athletic' was the term used to describe adult women who exercised at least three times per week, eight or more months of the year, for a minimum of three years, but the type of exercise was not defined. Talmage *et al.* (1986) found a negative correlation betwen bone density and age in a group of non-athletic women, with apparent acceleration of loss between ages 45 and 55. By contrast, an athletic group demonstrated weaker correlations of bone density with age and no accelerated loss from 45 to 55 years.

Although one is tempted to conclude from these studies that activity itself increases bone mass, their cross-sectional nature leaves open the possibility of ascertainment bias. In most reports, 'athletic' subjects must satisfy defined exercise inclusion criteria. A typical criterion might be to run 20 miles each week for more than five years. Since most adults who initiate an exercise program stop training before reaching such ambitious target levels, it is not unreasonable to consider that individuals who persist for sufficient time to qualify as a 'runner' or 'weight lifter' may succeed by virtue of some baseline physical characteristic, for example, a higher bone mass prior to the onset of training. Many of these studies may also be confounded by failing to allow for anthropometric and ethnic factors. For example, the conventional bone mineral density measurement, BMD (g/cm^2), is based on the projected area of the bone and does not take into account differences in bone thickness. Since all bones show some degree of geometric proportionality, longer and wider bones will also be thicker and tall individuals will have an artifactually higher areal BMD than short people, even if true volumetric mineral density is the same (Carter *et al.*, 1992). Similarly, body weight is related to bone mass (Bevier *et al.*, 1989; Snow-Harter *et al.*, 1990) and few, if any, of the cross-sectional exercise studies have corrected bone density measurements for differences in weight or body mass index.

EXERCISE INTERVENTION TRIALS

The most effective defense against these biases is the randomized intervention trial. Some exercise trials have been conducted, with results that generally, but not uniformly, support the conclusion that exercise promotes bone mass. However, the changes in bone density achieved in these studies are less impressive than what might be predicted from the cross-sectional literature. There are several reasons for this. Little attention has been given in the design of such studies to understanding the type, intensity, frequency or duration of exercise most likely to improve bone mass. Some trials were designed with primary emphasis on aerobic training and flexibility, rather than on effective skeletal loading. Measurements have been made in skeletal regions, such as the forearm, that were not loaded by the training protocol, e.g. running. Training duration may have been insufficient. Most exercise trials have not been randomized. There has frequently been poor subject compliance and a lack of adequate controls. Finally, there has been almost no documentation of changes in other forms of habitual activity that may have occurred when exercise training was introduced. For example, a woman who ran three miles each day might have decreased her running mileage, walked less or otherwise modified her daily loading after starting a vigorous weight-training program. Such a modification might have a profound influence on the apparent response to the exercise stimulus.

EXERCISE STUDIES IN YOUNG ADULTS

Several trials have explored the impact of exercise on bone mass at the time that peak bone mass is reached. In one of very few studies in young men, Leichter and colleagues (1989) reported positive changes in tibial BMD following short-duration (14 weeks), very high intensity (eight hours per day) physical training. Studies in young women have not given consistent results. Gleeson *et al.* (1990) found that one year of weight training marginally increased lumbar spine density. Although a significant difference in spine mineral was found between weight trainers and controls, the observed increase of 0.8% in bone mass over baseline values did not achieve significance. Rockwell *et al.* (1990) reported that women completing one year of weight training *lost* approximately 4% of lumbar spine mineral and they questioned the safety of weight training. Most recently, Snow-Harter *et al.* (1992a) conducted an eight-month exercise trial for healthy college women who were randomly assigned to a control group or to progressive training in either jogging or weight lifting. Weight training produced a significant increase in muscle strength for all muscle groups, whereas no change in strength was observed in the control or running groups. In contrast, aerobic performance improved only in the running group. Lumbar BMD increased significantly in both the runners and weight trainers by 1.3% and 1.2%, respectively. These results did not differ from each other, but were both significantly greater than results in control subjects, in whom bone mineral did not change. No measure of bone mineral at the proximal femur changed significantly in any group. Of particular interest in this study was the documentation of a wide variety of non-training physical activities during the course of the protocol. Such activities included hours per day of standing, walking, sitting and nonprotocol recreational exercise. No significant change in other habitual activities was observed in any group. Thus, the observed changes in bone mineral appear to reflect increased mechanical loading specifically due to the exercise program.

In view of important differences that distinguish these three studies from each other, it may be useful to compare them in detail. The majority of Gleeson's participants were said to be sedentary, but 10 exercisers and nine controls regularly participated in strenuous exercise prior to initiating the protocol. Whether this recreational activity continued throughout the study period is not stated. Rockwell's participants were also relatively sedentary, although several took part in regular exercise prior to the start of the protocol. It was stated that habitual activities continued throughout the study, but quantitative activity estimates were not recorded. Snow-Harter's subjects were active college women. Although they did not participate in competitive athletics, self-reported hours of walking and recreational activity were probably greater than those of the other two studies. These did not change significantly over the duration of the study.

The training schedule of Gleeson included upper and lower extremity exercises that did not specifically load the spine and emphasized relatively low loads and high repetitions. This schedule could result in a greater effect on muscle endurance than on dynamic strength. It is difficult to compare the reported strength gains with those observed in the other two studies, since maximal strength scores were not given and the improvement was reported as upper and lower limb composites. Thus, despite its longer duration and greater number of subjects, a lower intensity of training and measurement precision may have adversely affected the outcome. In Rockwell, the training stimulus was based on 70% of maximal strength and included exercises that specifically loaded the spine. However, workouts were scheduled only twice each week, compared to 3–4 times per week in Gleeson and Snow-Harter. Although individual strength gains were not reported, it appears that strength improved substantially in all muscle groups. Snow-Harter employed a program of progessively increasing intensity, both in the running and in the weight-training groups. The weight-training stimulus was particularly intense, beginning at about 70% of maximum strength and increasing to >80% of updated maximal strength during the last two months of the intervention. The results of Snow-Harter *et al.* (1992a) argue that a supervisd program or progressive resistance training does not decrease bone mass and can actually increase lumbar spine mineral in young women.

Among these three studies there was uniform failure to observe any effect of exercise on bone mineral at the proximal femur. This is a surprising result, since several of the strength-training exercises specifically load the hip. It is possible that the greater abundance of cortical bone at this site may require more prolonged training for a detectable response. It may also be that habitual loading of the hip during such daily activities as standing and walking is so great that the increments in daily loading history produced by the exercise intervention were not important.

EXERCISE STUDIES IN MIDLIFE

As exemplified by the women athlete with amenorrhea, loss of normal reproductive hormone secretion leads to bone loss and increased fracture risk even when exercise levels are high (Drinkwater *et al.*, 1984; Marcus *et al.*, 1985). It is of obvious interest, therefore, to know whether an exercise program for recently menopausal women can offer skeletal protection. Pruitt *et al.* (1992) assigned women within seven years of menopause to a nine-month program of weight training or a control group. No subject had taken estrogen replacement therapy. Training involved muscle groups in the upper and lower extremities and in the trunk and was sufficiently intense to increase strength in all muscle groups. Whereas the control subjects lost 3.6% of bone density at the lumbar spine, no loss was observed in the training group. No significant changes were seen in either group at the femoral neck or distal radius.

Heikkinen *et al.* (1991) randomly incorporated an exercise program into the management of women taking different combinations of estrogen and progestin and found no effect of 12 months of exercise at the lumbar spine in any group. The exercise regimen in this program was stated to be of 'moderate' intensity but actually amounted to only a single session each week under supervision. That an interaction between estrogen status and exercise level may actually exist may be inferred from the studies of Notelovitz *et al.* (1991). These authors assigned a group of women who had undergone a surgical menopause to estrogen replacement alone or estrogen replacement plus a weight-training program for one year. Whereas BMD at the lumbar spine was maintained in the estrogen-alone group, the weight-training group experienced an increase of 8.3%. At the radial shaft, exercisers increased BMD by 4.1% in comparison to no significant change in the hormone-only group It is of particular interest to note that in an earlier unpublished study, these same investigators found no effect of the resistance training program on a group of menopausal women who were not taking estrogen replacement (Notelovitz, M., personal communication).

Thus, exercise as a single modality may help to conserve bone in recently menopausal women, but for significant meaningful increases in bone mass to occur, it may be necessary to carry out exercise in a state of estrogen repletion.

EXERCISE STUDIES IN OLDER SUBJECTS

Several exercise trials have trained postmenopausal women with calisthenics and light aerobic activity for eight to 48 months (Smith *et al.*, 1981, 1984, 1989; Krølner *et al.*, 1983). In one report, significant changes in total body calcium and lumbar spine density were found in under 12 months (Krølner *et al.*, 1983). Smith *et al.* (1981, 1984, 1989) have conducted two prospective studies. In one (1981), women with an average age of 81 years were placed into control, physical activity, calcium supplement and combined activity/supplement groups. After 36 months, the activity and calcium groups increased radial bone mineral by 2.3% and 1.6%, whereas the combined exercise/calcium and control groups decreased radial bone mineral by 0.32% and 3.29%, respectively. In considering the reasons that the combination group failed to increase bone mass, the authors found that subjects randomized to that group were 2.6 years older than those in other groups and may have had a higher overall rate of decline in physical and mental function. In another study, Smith and colleagues (1989) enrolled 200 women, aged 35–65 years, in a similar 48-month exercise program. Exercise during the first year consisted of weight-bearing activity, whereas emphasis was placed on upper body strength during successive years. Results demonstrated lower rates of loss of radial and ulnar bone mineral in the exercisers compared to controls. From these results, the independent contributions of weight-bearing activity and strength training to bone mineral density cannot be determined.

In other prospective studies which have examined the effects of weight bearing on bone density, White *et al.* (1984) observed no changes in the forearm bone density of postmenopausal women after six months of dancing. However, in a nine-month study of runners, Williams and colleagues (1984) found a significant increase in bone density of the calcaneus. These data and those previously mentioned indicate that the site selected for measurement is critical to the results obtained.

Nielsen *et al.* (1992) reported the results of a comparison of gymnastics, swimming and dancing in a group of elderly women (62–80 years). Despite a rise in circulating osteocalcin concentrations in the gymnastic group, no significant changes were observed in bone mineral density at the forearm or lumbar spine in any group. Interpretation of this study is severely hampered by the fact that it was only five months in duration, that the subjects were permitted to select their activity assignment and that their actual load experience is not described.

Whether gains in bone density are maintained when an exercise program has been terminated has been addressed by Dalsky and colleagues (1988). After nine months of weight-bearing and non-weight-bearing exercise with resistance, postmenopausal women showed an increase of 5.2% in spinal bone mineral content. This value increased to 6.1% after an additional 13 months of exercise, whereas a non-randomized group of sedentary controls exhibited no change in bone mineral content. Following a 13-month detraining period, bone mass was only 1.1% above baseline. This return toward baseline exemplifies the dynamic nature of the skeletal system and reinforces the view that long-term maintenance of activity is essential to achieving sustained benefit.

Cavanaugh and Cann (1988) examined the effect of weight-bearing exercise on spinal trabecular mineral in postmenopausal women assigned either to no activity or to a one-year program of regular brisk walking. The walkers actually lost trabecular bone (5.6%) while the control group lost 4% over the same interval. These results directly contradict those of Dalsky *et al.* (1988) and may be related to differences in experimental protocol. In addition to walking, Dalsky's exercise group jogged and performed exercises that specifically loaded the vertebrae. Thus, it appears that the additional loading provided by jogging and resistance exercise may give a more potent osteogenic stimulus than brisk walking. In this regard, the forces produced at the lumbar vertebrae during walking equal one body weight (BW) (Cappozzo, 1984; Cromwell *et al.*, 1989), whereas loads on the lumbar vertebrae during weight-lifting activity have been reported to be as much as 5–6 times body weight (Granhad *et al.*, 1987).

EXERCISE FOR THE PATIENT WITH ESTABLISHED OSTEOPOROSIS

Among the several goals of an exercise program for osteoporotic patients, increased bone mineral density, while desirable, should be considered a secondary outcome. Most importantly, exercise should not be harmful; it should increase a patient's functional capacities and it should minimize the risk for subsequent fracture. Health professionals who work with osteoporotic patients recognize that back-strengthening exercise constitutes a powerful intervention for reducing pain and increasing functional capacity. Chow *et al.* (1989) described an exercise rehabilitation program for patients with osteoporosis that was aimed at improving functional capacity and providing social interactions in addition to improving strength and flexibility. Compliance in this program was high and led to significant improvements in aerobic capacity and bone mass. No patient developed a fracture as a result of the program, which is particularly important because many physicians express reluctance to prescribe exercise for osteoporotic patients out of concern for injury and additional fracture. This view may be counterproductive in the long run, since avoidance of activity will certainly aggravate bone loss and place the skeleton at even greater jeopardy.

Little information is available concerning the effect of exercise on bone mass of osteoporotic patients. Krølner *et al.* (1983) evaluated the effect of exercise on bone mineral density of women who had previously experienced a Colles fracture. The results showed a 3.5% increase in lumbar spine BMD in the exercise group compared to a 2.7% loss for the controls. In another controlled trial, Simkin *et al.* (1987) administered a five-month program of thrice-weekly dynamic loading exercise to the distal forearm to older osteoporotic women. Bone mineral content of the distal radius increased by 3.8% in the training group, whereas bone density declined by 1.9% in the controls.

In one of the few exercise studies in patients with vertebral compression, Sinaki and Mikkelsen (1984) found that resistance exercise to strengthen the back extensor muscles reduced new vertebral fractures compared to a control group, whereas a substantial increase in vertebral deformities was observed in subjects assigned to a program that included flexion activity. For patients with vertebral osteoporosis, therefore, it appears that activities that place an anterior load on vertebral bodies, as with back flexion, are particularly harmful and patient education must emphasize their danger. Even modest weights may be deleterious to the spine because their effect is amplified by leverage. For example, if one lifts a 5 kg weight from a shopping cart using arms that are 50 cm in length, the load is balanced by paraspinous muscles that may be no more than 1 cm long. Thus the load on the vertebral body may be magnified 50-fold to a value of 250 kg (Wt × length = Wt′ × length′, or 5 × 50 = 250 × 1).

For a severely osteopenic patient, one may appropriately ask what the real benefits could be from the limited improvement documented by these studies. Although the skeletal changes were modest, one should not overlook the possibility that exercise may have produced benefits that were not directly reflected in BMD. Hayes *et al.* (1991) presented evidence that most older individuals have insufficient bone strength at the proximal femur to withstand the impact of a fall. Since the great majority of hip fractures result directly from a fall, strategies aimed at reducing falls may be more effective at reducing the incidence of hip fracture than those aimed specifically at increasing bone mineral (Hayes *et al.*, 1991). Muscle weakness is an important predictor of falls risk (Nevitt *et al.*, 1989; Schultz, 1992) and decreased muscle mass and strength are consequences of normal human aging. It has now been established that progressive resistance exercise can increase muscle strength and promote muscle fiber hypertrophy in older men and women, even in the 10th decade (Frontera *et al.*, 1988; Charette *et al.*, 1991).

Preliminary evidence suggests that increased lower extremity strength may reduce falls risk by improving postural stability. Gross and Marcus (unpublished data) evaluated the act of rising from a chair by healthy elderly and young women. Kinematic and reaction force data were obtained using a video-based motion analysis system and force plates fixed into the chair seat and floor. The elderly women then participated in a 12-week strength-training program that emphasized hip and knee musculature, after which the chair tests were repeated. Initial muscle strength was very low in these women, ranging from 37% to 70% of values observed in young women. Instability during the rise from a chair was maximum at the moment of loss of chair contact. The center of body mass was located at its most posterior point at this time, sometimes lying beind the feet. With strength training, muscle strength increased significantly. Stability improved and the center of mass was located more anteriorly. Results of this pilot study indicate that strength training alters movement strategy in a way that favors increased static and dynamic stability. Many falls in the elderly occur at times of 'transfer', that is, changing from one position to another. Thus, a widely disseminated program of leg-strengthening exercise could lower the risk of falling and reduce hip fracture incidence even if no changes in bone mineral were achieved (Hayes *et al.*, 1991). The importance of proper attention to safety cannot be overemphasized in this discussion. Although experimental data indicate the danger of loading the spine in flexion, there is very little scientific support for other recommendations. Nonetheless, a few reasonable principles can be offered (Table 16.1).

PRACTICAL CONSIDERATIONS

Although we still do not fully understand the optimal components for an exercise prescription, it is possible from the foregoing discussion to reach a few general conclusions. The changes in skeletal integrity associated with immobilization greatly exceed those brought about by increasing the activity of an already

Table 16.1 Principles of strength training for patients with osteoporosis

1.	Avoid back flexion and trunk torque
2.	Strengthen back extensors
3.	Use small weights
4.	Increase very slowly to reasonable maximal loads (4–6 kg)
5.	Exercise all body regions
6.	Emphasize proper technique for routine daily activities

mobile person. In adults, exercise-related gains in bone mass appear to be modest. For increases in bone mass to be sustained, exercise needs to be continued. The skeleton adapts to the loads which are imposed on it and a reduction in loading, even after many years of activity, will predictably lead to a decrease in bone mass. The material reviewed in this chapter has dealt exclusively with the skeleton. Exercise directed at other aspects of health, such as flexibility or aerobic fitness, may require different types or intensities of exercise to achieve optimal results. However, exercise is not a way of life for most adults. Men and women commonly state that regular exercise is not necessary at their age; they frequently have unrealistic expectations regarding the health benefits of their usual daily activities and they seriously exaggerate the risks of vigorous exercise. It is very unlikely, therefore, that many people will carry out multiple exercise programs to achieve diverse physiological ends. If there is any chance for widespread acceptance of exercise by the population, it will be necessary to define a few sensible and relatively simple exercise strategies that can be carried out by people of average capacity and motivation without major requirements for time or financial investment. Finally, although considerable scientific efforts continue to be directed at the relationship between physical activity and health, for new insights to yield practical benefits it will be necessary to invest a similar effort into motivating a sedentary population to incorporate exercise into daily life.

NOTE IN PROOF

Material reviewed for this chapter includes papers published through 1993.

REFERENCES

Anderson, S. and Cohn, S. (1984) Final Report Phase III: Research Opportunities in Bone Demineralization, National Aeronautics and Space Administration (NASA) Houston.

Bevier, W., Wiswell, R., Pyka, G. *et al.* (1989) Relationship of body composition, muscle strength, and aerobic capacity to bone mineral density in older men and women. *J Bone Miner Res* **4**: 421–32.

Biering-Sørensen, F., Bohr, H. and Schaadt, O. (1990) Longitudinal study of bone mineral content in the lumbar spine, the forearm and the lower extremities after spinal cord injury. *Eur J Clin Invest* **20**: 330–5.

Biering-Sorensen, R. and Bohr, H. (1988) Bone mineral content of the lumbar spine and lower extremities years after spinal cord lesion. *Paraplegia* **26**: 293–301.

Brewer, V., Meyer, B., Keele, M. *et al.* (1983) Role of exercise in prevention of involutional bone loss. *Med Sci Sports Exerc* **15**: 445–9.

Burr, D., Martin, R., Schaffler, M. *et al.* (1985) Bone remodeling in response to in vivo fatigue damage. *J Biomech* **18**: 189–200.

Cappozzo, A. (1984) Compressive loads in the lumbar vertebral column during normal level walking. *J Orthop Res* **1**: 292–301.

Carter, D., Bouxsein, M. and Marcus, R. (1992) New approaches for interpreting projected bone densitometry data. *J Bone Miner Res* **7**: 137–45.

Carter, D., Caler, W. and Spengler, D. (1981) Fatigue behavior of adult cortical bone: the influence of mean strain and strain range. *Acta Orthop Scand* **52**: 481–90.

Carter, D. and Fyhrie, D., (1987) Trabecular bone density and loading history: regulation of connective tissue biology by mechanical energy. *J Biomech* **20**: 785–94.

Cavanaugh, D. and Cann, C. (1988) Brisk walking does not stop bone loss in postmenopausal women. *Bone* **9**: 201–4.

Charette, S., McEvoy, L., Pyka, G. *et al.* (1991) Muscle hypertrophy response to resistance training in older women. *J Appl Physiol* **70**: 1912–16.

Chow, R., Harrison, J. and Dornan, J. (1989) Prevention and rehabilitation of osteoporosis program: exercise and osteoporosis. *Int J Rehab Res* **12**: 49–56.

Claus-Walker, J., Spencer, W.A., Carter, R.E. *et al.* (1975) Bone metabolism in quadriplegia: dissociation between calciuria and hydroxyprolinuria. *Arch Phys Med Rehabil* **56**: 327–32.

Comarr, A.E. and Hutchinson, R.H. (1962) Extremity fractures of patients and spinal cord injuries. *Am J Surg* **103**: 732–9.

Cornwall, M.W. (1984) Biomechanics of noncontractile tissue. *Phys Ther* **64**: 1869–73.

Cromwell, R., Schultz, A., Beck, R. *et al.* (1989) Loads on the lumbar trunk during level walking. *J Orthop Res* **7**: 371–7.

Dalen, N. and Olsson, K. (1974) Bone mineral content and physical activity. *Acta Orthop Scand* **45**: 170–4.

Dalsky, G., Stocke, K. and Ehsani, A. (1988) Weight-bearing exercise training and lumbar bone mineral content in postmenopausal women. *Ann Int Med* **108**: 824–8.

Davee, A., Rosen, C. and Adler, R. (1990) Exercise patterns and trabecular bone density in college women. *J Bone Miner Res* **5**: 245–50.

Deitrick, J.E., Whedon, G.D. and Shorr, E. (1948) Effects of immobilization upon various metabolic and physiologic functions of normal men. *Am J Med* **4**: 3–35.

Donaldson, C.L., Hulley, S.B., Vogel, J.M. *et al.* (1970) Effect of prolonged bed rest on bone mineral. *Metabolism* **19**: 1071–84.

Drinkwater, B.K., Milson, K. Chesnut, C.I. *et al.* (1984) Bone mineral content of amenorrheic and eumenorrheic athletes. *N Engl J Med* **311**: 277–81.

Freehafer, A. and Mast, W. (1965) Lower extremity fractures in patients with spinal cord injury. *J Bone Joint Surg* **47A**: 683–94.

Frontera, W., Meredith, C., O'Reilly, K. *et al.* (1988) Strength conditioning in older men: skeletal muscle hypertropy and improved function. *J Appl Physiol* **64**: 1038–44.

Frost, H. (1987) The mechanostat: a proposed pathogenic mechanism of osteoporosis and the bone mass effects of mechanical and nonmechanical agents. *Bone Mineral* **2**: 73–86.

Garland, D. (1991) A clinical perspective on common forms of acquired heterotopic ossification. *Clin Orthop* **263**: 13–26.

Gleeson, P., Protas E., LeBlanc A. *et al.* (1990) Effects of weight lifting on bone mineral density in premenopausal women. *J Bone Miner Res* **5**: 153–8.

Granhad, H., Jonson, R. and Hansson, T. (1987) The loads on the lumbar spine during extreme weight lifting. *Spine* **12**: 146–9.

Griffiths, H.J., Bushueff, B. and Zimmerman, R.E. (1976) Investigation of the loss of bone mineral in patients with spinal cord injury. *Paraplegia* **14**: 207–12.

Guttmann, L. (1976) *Spinal Cord Injuries: Comprehensive Management and Research*, Blackwell Scientific Publications, Oxford.

Hancock, D.A., Reed, G.W., Atkinson, P.J. *et al.* (1980) Bone and soft tissue changes in paraplegic patients. *Paraplegia* **17**: 267–71.

Hantmann, D.A., Vogel, J.M., Donaldson, C.L. *et al.* (1973) Attempts to prevent disuse osteoporosis by treatment with calcitonin, longitudinal compression and supplementary calcium and phosphate. *J Clin Endocrinol Metab* **36**: 845–58.

Hayes, W., Piazza, S. and Zysset, P. (1991) Biomechanics of fracture risk prediction of the hip and spine by quantitative computed tomography. *Radiol Clin North Am* **29**: 1–18.

Heikkinen, J., Kurtila-Matero, E., Kyllonen, E. *et al.* (1991) Moderate exercise does not enhance the positive effect of estrogen on bone mineral density in postmenopausal women. *Calcif Tissue Int* **49** (Suppl): S83–S84.

Huddleston, A., Rockwell, D., Kulund, D. *et al.* (1980) Bone mass in lifetime tennis athletes. *J Am Med Assoc* **244**: 1107–9.

Hui, S.L., Slemenda, C. and Johnston Jr C.C. (1988) Age and bone mass as predictors of fracture in a prospective study. *J Clin Invest* **81**: 1804–9.

Hulley, S.B., Vogel, J.M. and Donaldson, C.L. (1971) Effect of supplemental calcium and phosphorus on bone mineral changes in bed rest. *J Clin Invest* **50**: 2506–18.

Ingram, R., Suman, R. and Freeman, P. (1989) Lower limb fractures in the chronic spinal cord injured patient. *Paraplegia* **27**: 133–9.

Issekutz, B., Blizzard, J., Birkhead, N. *et al.* (1966) Effect of prolonged bed rest on urinary calcium output. *J Appl Physiol* **21**: 1013–20.

Iversen, E., Hassager, C. and Christiansen, C. (1989) The effect of hemiplegia on bone mass and soft tissue body composition. *Acta Neurol Scand* **79**: 155–9.

Jacobson, P., Beaver, W., Grubb, S. *et al.* (1984) Bone density in women: college athletes and older athletic women. *J Orthop Res* **2**: 328–32.

Jenkins, D.P. and Cochran, T.H. (1969) Osteoporosis: the dramatic effect of disuse of an extremity. *Clin Orthop* **64**: 128–34.

Kaplan, P.E., Gandhavadi, B., Richards, L. *et al.* (1978) Calcium balance in paraplegic patients: influence of injury and ambulation. *Arch Phys Med Rehabil* **59**: 447–50.

Kiratli, B.J. (1989) Skeletal adaptation to disuse: longitudinal and cross-sectional study of the response of the femur and spine to immobilization (paralysis). PhD dissertation, University of Wisconsin-Madison.

Krølner, B. and Toft, B. (1983) Vertebral bone loss: an unheeded side effect of therapeutic bed rest. *Clin Sci* **64**: 537–40.

Krølner, B., Toft, B., Nielsen, S. *et al.* (1983) Physical exercise as prophylaxis against involutional vertebral bone loss: a controlled trial. *Clin Sci* **64**: 541–6.

Leichter, I., Simkin, A., Margulies, J. *et al.* (1989) Gain in mass density of bone following strenuous physical activity. *J Orthop Res* **7**: 86–90.

Lundberg, B. and Nilsson, B. (1968) Osteopenia in the frozen shoulder. *Clin Orthop* **60**: 187–91.

Marcus, R. (1987) Normal and abnormal bone remodeling in man. *Ann Intern Med* **38**: 129–41.

Marcus, R., Cann, C., Madvig, P. *et al.* (1985) Menstrual function and bone mass in elite women distance runners: endocrine metabolic features. *Ann Intern Med* **102**: 158–63.

Maynard, F.M. and Imai, K. (1977) Immobilization hypercalcemia in spinal cord injury. *Arch Phys Med Rehabil* **58**: 16–24.

Nevitt, M., Cummings, S., Kidd, S. *et al.* (1989) Risk factors for recurrent nonsyncopal falls. A prospective study. *J Am Med Assoc* **261**: 2663–8.

Nielsen, H., Brixen, K., Kristensen, L. *et al.* (1992) Effects of different kinds of exercise on bone mass and bone metabolism in elderly women. *Eur J Exp Musculoskel Res* **1**: 41–6.

Nikolic, V., Vladovia, P., Sajko, D. *et al.* (1977) Bone mass and the safety factor of bone strength in lower extremities of patients with paraplegia. *Calcif Tissue Res* **22** (Suppl): 303–6.

Notelovitz, M., Martin, D., Tesar, R. *et al.* (1991) Estrogen therapy and variable-resistance weight training increase bone mineral in surgically menopausal women. *J Bone Miner Res* **6**: 583–90.

Nottage, W. (1981) A review of long-bone fractures in patients with spinal cord injuries. *Clin Orthop Rel Res* **155**: 65–70.

O'Malley, S., Huang, H., Kenrick, M. *et al.* (1980) A CT of bone changes in lower extremities of human amputees. Fourth International Conference on Bone Measurement, (ed. Mazess, R.B.), National Institutes of Health, Washington DC.

Orwoll, E., Ferar, J., Oviatt, S. *et al.* (1989) The relationship of swimming exercise to bone mass in men and women. *Arch Intern Med* **149**: 2197–200.

Panin, N., Gorday, W.J. and Paul, B.J. (1971) Osteoporosis in hemiplegia. *Stroke* **2**: 41–7.

Parfitt, A.M. (1984) Age-related structural changes in trabecular and cortical bone: cellular mechanisms and biomechanical consequences. *Calcif Tissue Int* **36**: 123–8.

Parfitt, A.M., Mathews, H., Villanueva, A. *et al.* (1983). Relationships between surface, volume and thickness of iliac trabecular bone in aging and in osteoporosis. *J Clin Invest* **72**: 1396–409.

Pirnay, F., Bodeux, M., Crielaard, J. *et al.* (1987) Bone mineral content and physical activity. *Int J Sport Med* 8: 331–5.

Plum, F. and Dunning, M.F. (1958) The effect of therapeutic mobilization on hypercalciuria following acute poliomyelitis. *Arch Intern Med* **101**: 528–36.

Pocock, N., Eisman, J., Gwinn, T. *et al.* (1980) Muscle strength, physical fitness and weight but not age predict femoral neck bone mass. *J Bone Miner Res* **4**: 441–7.

Prince, R.L., Price, R.I. and Ho, S. (1988) Forearm bone loss in hemiplegia: a model for the study of immobilization osteoprosis. *J Bone Miner Res* **3**: 305.

Pruitt, L., Jackson, R., Bartels, R. *et al.* (1992) Weight-training effects on bone mineral density in early postmenopausal women. *J Bone Miner Res* **7**: 179–85.

Ragnarsson, K. and Sell, G. (1981) Lower extremity fractures after spinal cord injury: a retrospective study. *Arch Phys Med Rehabil* **62**: 418–23.

Rockwell, J., Sorensen, A., Baker, S. *et al.*

(1990) Weight training decreases vertebral bone density in premenopausal women: a prospective study. *J Clin Endocrinol Metab* **71**: 988–93.

Rubin, C. and Lanyon, L. (1984) Regulation of bone formation by applied dynamic loads. *J Bone Joint Surg* **66A**: 397–402.

Schneider, V. and McDonald, J. (1984) Skeletal calcium homeostasis and countermeasures to prevent disuse osteoporosis. *Calcif Tissue Int* **36** (Suppl): S151–S154.

Schultz, A. (1992) Mobility impairment in the elderly: challenges for biomechanics research. *J Biomech* **25**: 519–28.

Simkin, A., Ayalon, J. and Leichter, I. (1987) Increased trabecular bone density due to bone-loading exercises in postmenopausal osteoporotic women. *Calcif Tissue Int* **40**: 59–63.

Sinaki, M. and Mikkelsen, B. (1984) Postmenopausal spinal osteoporosis: flexion versus extension exercises. *Arch Phys Med Rehabil* **65**: 593–6.

Smith, E., Gilligan, C., McAdam, M. *et al.* (1989) Deterring bone loss by exercise intervention in premenopausal and postmenopausal women. *Calcif Tissue Int* **44**: 312–21.

Smith, E., Reddan, W. and Smith, P. (1981) Physical activity and calcium modalities for bone mineral increase in aged women. *Med Sci Sport Exerc* **13**: 60–4.

Smith, E., Smith, P., Ensign, C. *et al.* (1984) Bone involution decrease in exercising middle-aged women. *Calcif Tissue Int* **36**: S129–S138.

Snow-Harter, C., Bouxsein, M., Lewis, B. *et al.* (1992a) Effects of resistance and endurance exercise on bone mineral status of young women: a randomized exercise intervention trial. *J Bone Miner Res* **7**: 761–9.

Snow-Harter, C., Bouxsein, M., Lewis, B. *et al.* (1990) Muscle strength as a predictor of bone mineral density in young women. *J Bone Miner Res* **5**: 589–95.

Snow-Harter, C. and Marcus, R. (1991) Exercise, bone mineral density, and osteoporosis. *Exerc Sport Sci Rev* **19**: 351–88.

Snow-Harter, C., Whalen, R., Myburgh, K. *et al.* (1992b) Bone mineral density, muscle strength, and recreational exercise in men. *J Bone Miner Res* **7**: 1291–96.

Talmage, R., Stinnett, S., Landwehr, J. *et al.* (1986) Age-related loss of bone mineral density in non-athletic and athletic women. *Bone Mineral* **1**: 115–25.

Tilton, F., Degioanni, J. and Schneider, V. (1980) Long-term follow-up of Skylab bone demineralization. *Aviat Space Environ Med* 1209–13.

Vose, G. (1974) Review of roentgenographic bone demineralization studies of the Gemini space flights. *Am J Roentgenol* **121**: 1–4.

Whalen, R. and Carter, D. (1988) Influence of physical activity on the regulation of bone density. *J Biomech* **21**: 825–37.

Whalen, R., Carter, D. and Steele, C. (1987) The relationship between physical activity and bone density. *Trans Orthop Res Soc* **12**: 464.

Whedon, G. (1984) Disuse osteoporosis: physiological aspects. *Calcif Tissue Int* **36** (Suppl): S146–S150.

Whedon, G., Deitrick, J. and Shorr, E. (1949) Modification of the effects of immobilization upon metabolic and physiologic functions of normal men by the use of an oscillating bed. *Am J Med* **6**: 684–711.

Whedon, G.D. and Shorr, E. (1957) Metabolic studies in paralytic acute anterior poliomyelitis. II: Alterations in calcium and phosphorus metabolism. *J Clin Invest* **36**: 966–81.

White, M., Martin, R., Yeater, R. *et al.* (1984) The effects of exercise on the bones of postmenopausal women. *Int Orthop* **7**: 209–14.

Williams, J., Wagner, J., Wasnich, R. *et al.* (1984) The effect of long-distance running upon appendicular bone mineral content. *Med Sci Sport Exerc* **16**: 223–7.

Yashon, D. (1978) *Spinal Injury*, Appleton-Century-Crofts, New York.

PHYSICAL MEDICINE AND REHABILITATION

17

F.J. Bonner

INTRODUCTION

Physical medicine and rehabilitation strategies are essential in the treatment of osteoporosis as a means of relieving symptoms and restoring function. These strategies are based on the clinical knowledge of the patient's degree of impairment and functional limitations and they are directed towards specific goals of pain relief, physical restoration and prevention of further impairment. Physical rehabilitation involves the development of a person to their fullest potential consistent with their pathological or anatomical impairment and environmental limitations. Realistic goals for rehabilitation are determined by the patient and those concerned with the patient's care. Rehabilitation is provided by a team of professionals to obtain optimal function despite the residual disability the patient may have. Rehabilitation is provided to patients even though their impairment may be caused by a pathological process that cannot be reversed even with the best of modern medical treatment (Christiansen, 1991).

The diagnosis of osteoporosis implies reduction in bone mass beyond that which is considered normal for patient's age and sex and the consequent impairment of the skeleton's ability to withstand stress. The most severe consequence of this condition results in fracture and disability (Frost, 1985). Until recently, routine use of bone mass measurements has not been standard medical practice. Therefore, it is most common for patients to present for care only when their bone loss results in fracture functional limitation and disability. When the disease results in acute and chronic pain with impairments in ambulation, posture, flexibility and respiration, disability becomes apparent. At this stage, osteoporosis is not a silent disease, but rather a major life crisis-threatening disability and handicap with loss of independence, chronic pain and nursing home placement (Lyles *et al.*, 1993).

Osteoporosis frequently occurs as a comorbidity with other disabling conditions. Clinical experience indicates that over 60% of the patients admitted for acute inpatient rehabilitation from an acute hospital setting have severe osteoporosis (Fitzsimmons *et al.*, 1995). The reasons for rehabilitation admission include diagnoses such as stroke, amputation, chronic obstructive pulmonary disease, arthritis, joint replacement and fractures. It is extremely uncommon, however, for osteoporosis to be listed in the hospital chart as comorbidity. This failure points to the need for increased awareness of this disease by the entire medical community.

Osteoporosis. Edited by John C. Stevenson and Robert Lindsay. Published in 1998 by Chapman & Hall, London.
ISBN 0 412 48870 1

OUTCOME OF FRACTURE

In the United States, there are almost 250 000 osteoporosis-related hip fractures per year. These patients suffer long-term morbidity from associated illnesses related to their convalescence such as deep vein thrombosis, pulmonary embolism and pneumonia. About 15% of these patients will die in the first year and 20–25% will be institutionalized. Up to another 35% will be dependent on another person or assistive device to aid in their daily activities. Most studies in which researchers examined the sequelae of osteoporosis fractures have focused on hip fractures (Ettinger *et al.*, 1988). However, repeated vertebral compression fractures are also associated with significant impairments in physical, functional and psychosocial ability in older women. Patients can experience loss of height, thoracic kyphosis with possible restrictive lung disease, limitation of motion of the spine, generalized weakness, disturbed balance, protruding abdomen, reduced ambulation, chronic pain and lowered self-image (Chow *et al.*, 1989).

Fractures of the wrist increase in women at menopause and plateau around 65 years of age. These fractures cause short-term morbidity and functional impairment, but are usually not a source of great disability such as that associated with hip fractures and vertebral fractures. Other fractures associated with osteoporosis are proximal humerus, pelvis, tibial plateau and ribs (Melton and Riggs, 1985). These may result in temporary or permanent impairment with chronic pain associated with progressive deformity and marked reduction in quality of life. Following fractures, patients frequency adopt a more sedentary and lonely lifestyle. These patients will limit their activity and tend to remain at home not only due to pain, but also for fear of future fractures. This fear, in the presence of progressive deformities, pain, inactivity, disturbed balance and boredom, contributes to depression and progressive functional decline (Harrison *et al.* 1993).

REHABILITATION INTERVENTIONS

Because of these multiple impairments, care can ideally be provided by a modern rehabilitation team. The need to co-ordinate the activity of different rehabilitation professionals in addressing comprehensive needs of individuals with disability distinguishes the rehabilitation model from the medical model (Strasser *et al.*, 1994). This interdisciplinary team activity is the cornerstone of modern rehabilitation philosophy and practice. The team approach is central to the notion of rehabilitation and requires the involvement of a variety of professionals in a goal-directed, complex medical intervention. The patient with disability may best be served by intervention of an interdisciplinary team co-ordinated by a physician knowledgeable in osteoporosis and rehabilitation strategies.

Although the data are sparse, there is evidence to suggest significant benefit from rehabilitation interventions. The concept of providing multidisciplinary rehabilitative care to patients with osteoporosis was put forth by Vaughan over 20 years ago (Vaughan, 1976). Steiger (1977) reported alleviation of pain in patients with vertebral compression fractures as a result of proper instruction in body mechanics and use of a lumbar corset.

More recently, Chow reviewed the outcome of rehabilitation programs for patients with osteoporosis. These programs provided exercise sessions combined with educational seminars and social activities for osteoporotic women with either a traumatic fracture or below normal bone mass. The exercise sessions were performed in both a supervised (two times per week) and unsupervised setting. There was strong compliance with the program manifested by the fact that 78 out of the 139 who enrolled over two years remained in the program for at least four years. This suggests that the patients found the program beneficial. Additionally, patients who improved in fitness suffered less back pain. Parameters of function in activities in daily living (ADL) were not reported and the role and composition of the interdisciplinary team is unclear (Harrison *et al.*, 1993). The need for a comprehensive approach to patients with osteoporosis was promulgated by Vaughan, who stated goals of optimizing physiological, social and psychological patient outcomes. She recognized the need for specific, multidisciplinary treatment plans that address the patient's emotional responses to osteoporosis, pain, limitation of activity, frequent non-traumatic fractures and depression (Vaughan, 1976).

Dequeker recommends goal-oriented exercise programs to reduce further bone loss, improve general health and decrease susceptibility to falls (Dequeker and Geusens, 1990). He further states that rehabilitation programs are indicated for all osteoporosis sufferers with programs being appropriately tailored for the patient's clinical state and living conditions. He suggests no contraindications other than cautioning: 'provided appropriate exercise programs are used'. Goals for osteoporosis should be substantially different from an exercise program whose primary goal is prevention of low bone mass.

At this time, there is no literature available which addresses the functional outcome of osteoporotic patients who have undergone a comprehensive multidisciplinary rehabilitation program.

PROGRAM EVALUATION

The practice of medical rehabilitation has utilized various measurement scales to evaluate the effectiveness of treatment (Katz *et al.*, 1963; Mahoney and Barthel, 1965; Schoening and Iversen, 1968; Keith *et al.* 1984; McGinnis *et al.*, 1984). Although no specific functional measurement scale has been reported for disability associated with osteoporosis, many scales have been developed, most of these for specific diagnostic and age groups. The use of these scales is encouraged as in practice therapists tend to modify existing measures to suit a given clinical situation.

Emphasis for the future is to adapt existing scales using a universal disability framework which shifts the measure to those self-care activities required for daily function rather than to specific (ADL) skills affected by certain diseases.

Several studies are under way internationally to evaluate and compare existing scales. Currently, the Functional Independence Measure (FIM) is favored by many (National Health Policy Forum, 1991).

These scales rely heavily on ADL assessment to establish goals and monitor a patient's progress through a rehabilitation program. Through the ADL assessment the patient's functional status can be quantified and risk factors for falls can be assessed. The activities considered most important to functional independence include dressing, toileting, washing and mobility. These activities are assessed in the following manner.

DRESSING

The person is observed dressing and undressing. Advice is given when difficulties arise. This can involve modifications to clothes, i.e. using Velcro fasteners or advice on simple devices to make the task easier and safer. Women who are particularly interested in fashion and embarrassed with deformity caused by their osteoporosis are advised by their occupational therapist on designer fashions that are now available for handicapped persons. Footwear assessment must always be included.

WASHING

This includes bathing, washing, showering, brushing teeth, applying make-up and hair care. With safety and avoidance of falls constantly in mind, the therapist goes through the various activities giving appropriate energy-saving advice. Items such as non-skid mats on floors, bath and shower with strategically placed seats and grab rails are discussed. Transfer equipment may also be necessary for the bath and shower.

TOILETING

Poor hygiene leads to social isolation, but may be solved. Direct questioning on bladder control and bowel habit frequently identifies problems. The patient often feels more comfortable discussing this with the therapist. In the elderly, problems can range from mild stress incontinence to an unstable irritable bladder and occasionally a neurogenic bladder. These problems must be referred for accurate diagnosis and medical management, enabling the patient to become socially continent. In some, this may involve intermittent self-catheterization or an indwellng catheter, though the latter is avoided as much as possible because of associated complications. Constipation is common and is aggravated by immobility, calcium intake and irregular bowel habit. Many will have associated arthritis with limitation of motion of the hips and will require an elevated toilet seat or commode.

MOBILITY

This will range from the ability to walk independently to the use of a wheelchair because of severe pain, balance disturbance from kyphosis and weakness of the upper and lower extremities. The patient's mobility is usually assessed by the physical therapist. Tests such as arising from a chair, turning and spinal range of motion are administered to the patient. During this assessment, the therapist will evaluate transfer ability, standing and sitting balance and ambulation. The occupational therapist will evaluate the patient's mobility by assessing ability to do standing kitchen activities, laundry and housekeeping.

SITE FOR PROVISION OF REHABILITATION SERVICES

Modern rehabilitation centers make great efforts to simulate the real world by using custom-designed environments in assessing ADL. These units (Figures 17.1, 17.2) are designed to help patients relearn skills and regain their confidence and mobility before they face real-life situations. This is particularly important for a patient after a hip fracture when confidence and self-image are low and there is great fear of institutional care. Most patients wish to live in their own house, but need to be proficient and safe in self-care and other various activities. These include the

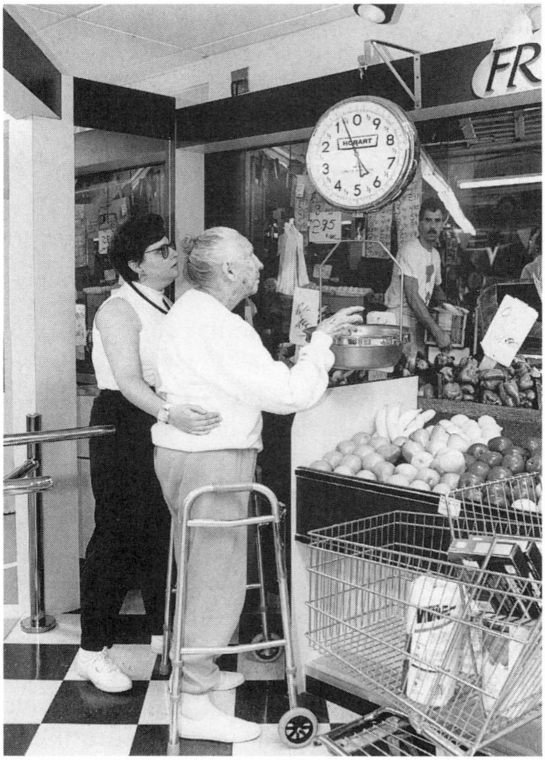

Figure 17.1 Therapist working with patient on functional activities in a specially designed setting: 'Easy Street', Mt Sinai Hospital, Philadelphia.

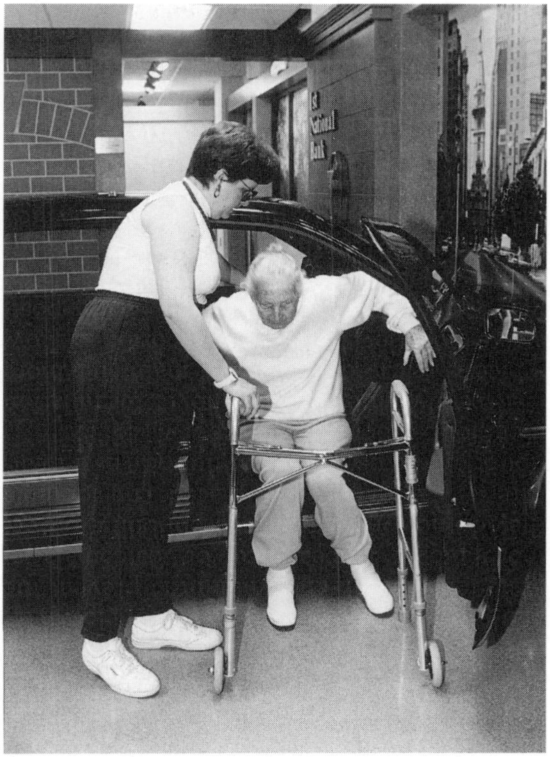

Figure 17.2 Specially designed setting allowing for practice of car transfers: 'Easy Street', Mt Sinai Hospital, Philadelphia.

need to do cooking, laundry, cleaning, shopping and driving. The ADL assessment allows for reliable evaluation of these tasks, enabling reasonable recommendations concerning living site.

Rehabilitation services for the patient with osteoporosis may be provided in a variety of settings. Outpatient care may be given in an outpatient rehabilitation facility or a day hospital. Both of these settings should provide comprehensive, intensive and structured therapy utilizing a team approach. Inpatient treatment is provided in a comprehensive medical rehabilitation (CMR) hospital or a CMR unit in an acute-care hospital. Whereas programs of rehabilitation are being provided in subacute settings, in the presence of comorbidity, the complexity of the osteoporosis treatment program demands a CMR hospital or hospital-based CMR unit. The less intense, subacute programs provided in nursing homes may serve as a pre- or post-CMR setting where less patient participation is required and less intense programs are offered.

The emphasis on functional status by the rehabilitation team is critical to assessment regarding the patient's ability to live independently. This assessment in turn may govern where the patient lives following discharge. Elderly patients who live alone and are responsible for their own self-care must be judged to be safe in their home environment. Even though a patient following hip or vertebral fractures achieves a level of mobility requiring only close supervision or contact guarding, it would not be reasonable to have this patient return home without supervision (Aitken, 1982).

ROLE OF TEAM MEMBERS

The rehabilitation team is usually under the direction of a physiatrist (a physician who specializes in physical medicine and rehabilitation). The multidisciplinary rehabilitation team may consist of up to eight types of professionals including physical therapist (PT), occupational therapist (OT), rehabilitation nurse, medical social worker, dietitian and psychologist. The team should remain flexible and capable of accommodating other professionals such as vocational counselor, speech pathologist, recreation therapist, etc. where applicable. Whatever the team composition, it is essential that they work in harmony and that each member accepts that there is an overlap in roles with other team members. The team attempts to implement its goals for physical restoration of the patient through specific strategies. With the multidisciplinary approach, interventions are employed that will enhance the functional capacity of the affected system as well as improve systems unaffected by the pathological condition. These include building muscle strength, improving balance and initiation of specific physical activity programs (Delisa *et al.*, 1993). Through the use of appropriate exercise and bracing, deformity and disability can be minimized. Maintenance of function may require the use of adaptive equipment as well as modification of the home and work environment. All disciplines involved in the multidisciplinary team can contribute their expertise to assist the patient in reaching goals for functional improvement and/or pain relief.

The physical therapist is responsible for the implementation of the therapeutic exercise prescription. Therapeutic exercise may be defined as organized activities of bodily movement prescribed to improve a disability or to maintain the state of well-being. They may vary from highly selected activities restricted to specific muscles or parts of the body to general and vigorous activities used to restore a convalescing patient to the peak of physical condition. In osteoporosis, the therapeutic exercise prescribed will depend on the strength, balance and flexibility of the patient, as well as on the patient's bone mass. This bone mass may be ascertained through measurement or may be inferred as the result of fracture history. The therapeutic exercise goals for healthy postmenopausal female with minimal reduction in bone mass will be substantially different from the program prescribed for an elderly, frail, kyphotic female with significant comorbidity (Frost, 1972).

Additionally, the physical therapist assumes responsibility for application of modalities for relief of pain and providing the patient with appropriate assistive equipment such as a broad-based cane, walker or wheelchair. The physical therapist works with the patient to insure that spinal orthoses fit properly and are comfortable. Instruction in body mechanics is given by both the physical therapist and occupational therapist.

Usually, the occupational therapist provides upper-extremity devices such as splints for use following wrist fracture, gives training in ADL and promotes safety awareness. The occupational therapist may also make safety recommendations for modification of the home and review methods of energy conservation with the patient. Adaptive equipment that can promote independent living skills is demonstrated to the patient. These items are particularly helpful for those who have suffered hip and vertebrae fractures. They include an adjustable-height tub bench, a raised toilet seat, grab bars, non-skid stickers on tub and shower, long-handled shoehorn, long-handled bath sponge, stocking air (for putting on stockings), elastic shoe laces, reachers, walker bag, etc.

During the course of the patients' rehabilitation program, home safety and accessibility should be evaluated. This may be accomplished by the therapist or nurse visiting the home with the patient or by reviewing floor plans of the home with the patient and family. At this time, recommendations can be made for installation of grab bars, sturdy handrails on both sides of stairs, easy-to-reach light switches, coverage of porch steps with gritty, weatherproof paint, generous placement of telephones and a professional alert system in case of a fall.

The patient is encouraged to have well-fitting shoes with good heel and arch supports and soft rubber soles. Caution is given regarding loose-fitting slippers and shoes with sloping soles or heels.

Wearing long nightgowns and robes should be discouraged because they too many cause tripping and falling. The advantage of dressing while sitting is pointed out, as is the necessity of maintaining an uncluttered path from the bed to the bathroom.

The dietitian will provide education for the patient on foods that are rich in bioavailable calcium or calcium supplementation. Working with both the dietitian and occupational therapist, the patient can perform supervised meal preparation incorporating these foods into the meal.

Psychologists work with osteoporosis patients who have difficulty coping with pain and who have frequent fractures and limitation of activity. These patients may become withdrawn and show signs of depression and other negative emotional responses, requiring psychological management.

The rehabilitation nurse specializes in direct care of patients with disability arising from physical impairment. The nurse may assist with dietary and medication management and act as a resource to both the patient and the rehabilitation team.

The social worker interacts with the patient, family and rehabilitation team. Information regarding a patient's total living situation, finances, employment and community resources are provided by the social worker (Delisa *et al.*, 1993).

The goal of the team is the optimal functional and physical restoration of the patient to a level most compatible with their pathological disorder. This rehabilitation team is most-effective when they work with physician leadership in a harmonious atmosphere. It is important for members of the team to be prepared to modify their goals based on the reports of other team members.

HISTORY AND PHYSICAL EXAMINATION

The history is an important part of the evaluation. There should be special focus on calcium intake, exercise, menopause and history of back pain, fractures and a family history of osteoporosis. Bowel and bladder difficulties should be reviewed. Past medical history may reveal previous thyroid disorder, rheumatoid arthritis, diabetes mellitus, seizures or liver disease. A review of current medications, especially antihypertensives, psychotropics, sedatives, analgesics, antihistamines, diuretics and steroids should be included (Ray and Marie, 1987).

The importance of the social history cannot be overemphasized, especially in the elderly female who may require assistance in her living environment or nursing home placement. The amount of alcohol intake and smoking are both positively correlated with bone loss and should be noted (Williams *et al.*, 1982).

A general physical examination should incorporate attention to height and weight, station, posture, gait and balance. Changes in height may be assessed by measuring arm span which is usually within 1.5′ of height. This measurement can provide a useful indication of progressive disease. Screening for vision and hearing are an important part of this examination (Tinetti, 1986; Felson *et al.*, 1989). Proprioception and general mobility of spine and joints of upper and lower extremities should be assessed. Manual muscle testing should be performed on upper and lower extremities and an assessment of abdominal and spinal muscular strength should be made (Felson *et al.*, 1989). The amount of kyphosis, chest expansion and relationship of the lower ribs to the iliac crest should be recorded.

Guarding of the paravertebral muscles and pain on palpation of the spinous processes may indicate a vertebral fracture. As a result of the findings of the history and physical examination, a program may be designed which will maintain or increase function, prevent deformity, manage pain and provide adequate mechanical support for the spine.

REHABILITATION FOLLOWING ACUTE FRACTURES

Osteoporosis is a disease that progresses from minimal impairment of the skeleton's ability to bear stress to a disease characterized by frailty, deformity, chronic pain and handicap. Postmenopausal women may therefore present to the physician with risk factors for osteoporosis but without low bone mass. This group of patients requires education on osteoporosis prevention with emphasis on reduction of risk factors and maintenance of bone mass. Others will present with significant risk factors, low bone mass and fracture with acute or chronic disability. This group of women will suffer varying degrees of disability and handicap and will require full assessment by a rehabilitation team. Most commonly, patients with osteoporosis initially present with pain resulting from fractures.

Patients with osteoporosis suffer fractures which cause acute pain. This pain is usually self-limited. These fractures occur in one of three common sites: distal radius, proximal femur and/or spinal fractures. The patient with the hip fracture will initially be under the primary care of an orthopedic surgeon. After stabilization of the fracture, these patients require pain management and gait training with appropriate assistive devices. Special precautions to prevent deep venous thrombosis should be taken. Benefit from rehabilitation service is maximized by early intervention with physical and occupational therapy programs.

Fractures of the wrist are the most common fractures in women before the age of 75. These fractures increase in number after menopause and although they usually occur in relatively healthy active women, they may be the first sign of an underlying problem such as low bone mass (Cummings *et al.*, 1985). The primary goal of treatment is return of pain-free, normal function of the hand and wrist. Initial casting usually extends above the elbow and restricts movement of both elbow and wrist. During the period of immobilization, usually 6–8 weeks, strength and flexibility should be maintained in the upper extremities. Active and passive range of motion exercises should be provided for the fingers and shoulder on the affected side.

These exercises to hand, wrist, forearm, elbow and shoulder should be continued following cast removal. At this time, a local wrist splint may be used to support and protect the wrist. As a result of the wrist fracture, particularly on the dominant side, the patient may require assistance with activities of daily living such as getting dressed, combing hair and brushing teeth.

Acute vertebral fracture may occur with little discomfort, poor localization of pain and complaints of generalized lumbosacral discomfort. Usually the pain is severe, most intense at the fracture level. It often follows a minor injury or physical activity that ordinarily would not be expected to cause a fracture (Lukert, 1994). The osteoporotic patient complaining of acute pain resulting from vertebral fracture should be managed with rest, immobilization of fracture site and analgesic agents. Because these vertebral fractures generally heal well, management is directed at pain control and providing adequate rest and immobilization of the fracture site (Figure 17.3). The unwanted side effects associated with analgesic agents may complicate treatment. Pharmacological interventions used for acute fractures include codeine, morphine, Percodan and other narcotic-like analgesics. Within 1–2 weeks, other analgesic agents such as salicylates and acetaminophen should be used in conjunction with other pain therapies (Ferrell and Ferrell, 1991). These compounds are to be used sparingly and with extreme caution. Pain management utilizing rest, orthoses and physical agents should be undertaken first, with pharmacologic agents serving as adjunctive therapy. Activities that

- Supine – bedrest 7–10 days
- Short-term narcotics ±
- Muscle relaxants
- Prevent constipation and urinary retention
- Maintain respiratory function (painmeds)
- Breathing exercise
- Encourage p.o. fluids – monitor for ileus
- Pain-relieving modalities: hot packs, ice, TENS
- Mobilize 7–10 days

Figure 17.3 Treatment of acute vertebral fracture.

aggravate the pain should be avoided. The use of a sheepskin, egg crate or gel flotation pad on the mattress frequently enhances patient comfort. During the initial treatment involving bedrest, a stool softener and laxative will help prevent straining during defecation. Use of a bedside commode may prove easier than a bedpan and requires less energy expenditure. With the initiation of bedrest, a program of progressive activity is indicated. Graduated bed activities progressing to sitting in bed, bedside sitting and progressive ambulation should be provided by the therapist.

Heated therapeutic pools are becoming more widespread and allow for gravity-free ambulation and exercise programs. With increasing activities, pain control may be aided by an orthosis and assistive devices such as a cane or walker. Patients with recurrent fractures and severe kyphosis frequently utilize a wheelchair and ambulate only for transfer (Sinaki, 1988).

The program should incorporate both short- and long-term goals which are reviewed with the patient. Patient education concerning proper posture, body mechanics, increasing strength and aerobic capacity is an essential component of short-term intervention. The patient needs to understand that osteoporosis is a progressive disease and if unchecked, it can cause severe disability. Prevention of falls and fractures through an ongoing program that maintains proper nutrition, strength and aerobic capacity is coupled with adequate support for the spine and pain management as objectives for long-term goals.

REHABILITATION OF OSTEOPOROSIS-RELATED DISABILITY

Intervention must be based upon the degree of frailty and fitness, functional limitations, skeletal involvement and comorbidity. The non-pharmacological intervention program can best be determined through knowledge of risk factors, bone mass, patient history and physical examination. Based on these factors, a program appropriate to the patient's degree of involvement may be initiated. A program of physical activity in the form of therapeutic exercise is almost always incorporated into the treatment plan (Kottke *et al.*, 1984).

The therapeutic exercise should be tailored to the patient's level of fitness and anticipated propensity to fractures. Objective measures such as bone density and manual muscle testing can help assignment of a given patient to an entry level on a clinical pathway (Figure 17.4). Patients may be grouped according to degree of impairment with or without disability. The beneficial effects of exercise are sought to attenuate bone loss and to increase strength and balance to prevent falls and avoid fracture (Figure 17.5).

The following five general principles should be considered when recommending therapeutic exercise (NOF Scientific Advisory Board, 1991):

1. *Principle of specificity*. Exercise should stress the specific physiological system being trained. Activities selected should stress sites most at risk for fracture in patients without low bone mass. Patients with very low bone mass and multiple fractures need skeletal protection while building strength and increasing balance and flexibility. Activities involving spinal flexion should be avoided in this group of patients.
2. *Principle of progression*. There must be a progressive increase in the intensity of the exercise for continued improvement. Applied loads must consider the capacity of the bone to sustain mechanical stress. Progression in resistance is important for goals of bone health and improved functional capacity.
3. *Principle of reversibility*. The positive effect of exercise will slowly be lost if the program is discontinued.
4. *Principle of initial values*. Those who initially have low capacity will have the greatest

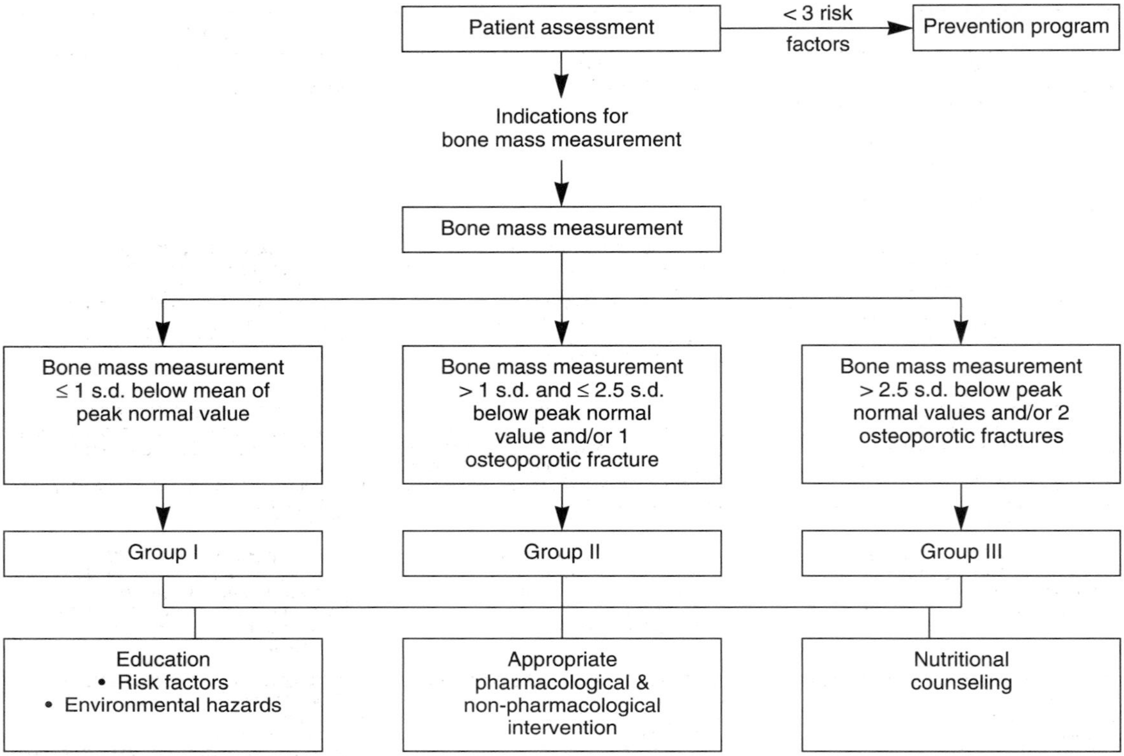

Figure 17.4 Rehabilitation of the female patient with osteoporosis.

functional improvement from a given program.

5. *Principle of diminishing returns.* There is a biological ceiling to exercise-induced improvements in function. As this ceiling is approached, greater effort is needed to achieve minimal gain.

CHRONIC PAIN MANAGEMENT

The management of the patient with osteoporosis will often include the management of acute and chronic pain (Frost, 1972; Ferrell and Ferrell, 1991). Whereas a patient with osteoporosis may complain of pain, their symptoms may be associated with other diagnoses such as arthritis, cancer, herpes zoster, polymyalgia rheumatica, pancreatic tumor and abdominal aortic aneurysm. It is important to treat the pain complaint promptly. If the patient experiences pain over prolonged periods, they may suffer consequences such as depression, sleep disturbance and functional decline (Figure 17.6).

Although chronic back pain is a common complaint of the elderly, the extent to which osteoporosis contributes to this pain is questionable. In a study involving 242 women of 55 years of age, 30% had complaints of back pain but there was no relationship between this pain and spinal curvature. In a group of older women (age 60–79), back pain affected a similar 30% but was twice as likely to occur in women with kyphosis or a loss in height exceeding 4 cm (Ettinger *et al.*, 1994). There is not an absolute relationship, however, between osteoporosis and kyphosis.

It is recognized that kyphosis may be

GROUP I	GROUP II	GROUP III
STRETCHING	**STRETCHING**	**STRETCHING**
• Pectoral • Shoulders abducted to 90 degrees and hands behind head, hold for 30 sec., repeat 15x; increase time up to 1 minute. Overhead extension incorporated – deep breathing. • Manual stretching for soft tissue restriction	• Same as Group I.	• Same as Group I.
BACK EXTENSION STRENGTHENING	**BACK EXTENSION STRENGTHENING**	**BACK EXTENSION STRENGTHENING**
• Initially – done prone or sitting in a chair. • May continue on resistive equip. Initially demonstrated by a trained professional. • Instructed in daily home program or 3–5x/wk program on resistive equip.	• Initially – sitting in a chair; may progress to prone position. • May continue on resistive equip. – supervised by a trained professional with a slow progression. • Daily Home Program or 3–5x/wk on resistive equip.	• Demonstration by professional. • Initially, sitting in chair. • May progress to supervised light resistance with slow progression. • Progress to daily home program.
ISOMETRIC ABDOMINAL STRENGTHENING	**ISOMETRIC ABDOMINAL STRENGTHENING**	**ISOMETRIC ABDOMINAL STRENGTHENING**
• Lie supine with both knees bent, lift both legs to 90 degrees of hip flexion and knee flexion, then lower, keeping back flat throughout. With hips and knees at 90 degrees, lower and straighten legs keeping back flat.	• Lie supine with one knee bent and the opposite leg straight. Lift the straight leg 4 inches, hold 10 seconds, do 15 times. • May sit or stand and contract abdominal and pelvic muscles.	• Sit or stand and contract abdominal and pelvic muscles, hold 30 sec., repeat 15x. • May lie supine as above if medically appropriate. • Pelvic Tilts
UPPER EXTREMITY STRENGTHENING	**UPPER EXTREMIIY STRENGTHENING**	**UPPER EXTREMITY STRENGTHENING**
• Theraband – 2–4 lbs. moderate resistance (red, green). • Shoulder – overhead extension. • Push-ups	• Medium resistive exercise with 1–2 lbs. or yellow theraband. • Wall push offs (minimal impact). • Putty hand exercises.	• Assistive range of motion exercises, progress to yellow theraband. • Monitored resistance wand exercise. • Putty hand exercise for postural hypotension.
WEIGHT BEARING AND LOWER EXTREMITY STRENGTHENING	**WEIGHT BEARING AND LOWER EXTREMIIY STRENGTHENING**	**WEIGHT BEARING AND LOWER EXTREMITY STRENGTHENING**
• Walking • Jogging/Running • Nordic Track • Low-Impact Aerobics Step Aerobics • 30 min., 3–5x/week • Leg Presses	• Acute – Pool therapy • Walking • Nordic Track • Low-Impact Aerobics • Step Aerobics • 30 min., 3–5x/wk • Isometric quad. exercise and ankle pumps for postural hypotension.	• Pool therapy • Walking • 30 min., 3–5x/wk • Isometric quad. exercise and ankle pumps for postural hypotension.
BALANCE TRAINING AND TRANSFER TECHNIQUES	**BALANCE TRAINING AND TRANSFER TECHNIQUES**	**BALANCE TRAINING AND TRANSFER TECHNIQUES**
• Demonstrate unsupported standing balance. • Unsupported single limb stand more than 30 seconds. • Frenkel's Exercise • Fall Prevention Program	• Same as Group I. • Instruct on proper transfer activity. • Consider hip protectors. • Gait training with appropriate assistive device if needed.	• Same as Group I, but goal for single limb stand to 15 seconds. • Gait training with appropriate assistive device if needed. • Monitor transfer activity – bed, chair, toilet, tub, car. • Consider hip protectors.
PROPER LIFTING TECHNIQUES	**PROPER LIFTING TECHNIQUES**	**PROPER LIFTING TECHNIQUES**
• All weights held close into body. • Use legs to lift, not back. • Avoid spinal flexion. • Ergonomics – Work; Home	• Same as Group I. • Precaution with loads over 10 lbs.	• Same as Group I. • Avoid loads over 10 lbs.
POSTURE CORRECTION	**POSTURE CORRECTION**	**POSTURE CORRECTION**
• Self-correction – flat back exercises. • Wall stretch Chin tucks Shoulder rolls • Manual stretching for soft tissue restriction.	• Same as Group I but may benefit from corset or P.T.S. (Postural Training System). • May require instruction and reinforcement for efficient breathing	• Same as for Group II, but may require TLSO or molded body jacket.
PAIN CONTROL	**PAIN CONTROL**	**PAIN CONTROL**
	• Rest • Hot packs, cold packs, TENS • May benefit from P.T.S. • Abdominal corset or TLSO • Pharmacologic • Psychological support	• Same as Group II, may require facet and/or inter-costal nerve blocks.

Figure 17.5 Physical medicine program for patients with osteoporosis, commenced after stabilization of fracture.

- Acute fractures (spine, hip, wrist)
- Microfractures
- Mechanical effects of deformity – changes in soft tissues
- Facet joint
- Iliocostal syndrome
- Radicular
- Other – arthritis, metastasis, etc.

Figure 17.6 Mechanisms of pain.

secondary to chronic poor posture and age-related changes in muscle, ligaments and intervertebral discs. Seventy percent of women over 60 years may demonstrate kyphosis without evidence of vertebral deformity. With aging, there is a progression of kyphosis (Gandy and Payne, 1986) but however, back pain does not appear to be associated with the kyphosis unless vertebral deformity is such that there is a reduction in the height of the vertebral body greater than four SD from normal (Ettinger *et al.*, 1992).

Investigations of causes of back pain using bone scintigraphy revealed a high incidence of facet joint disease in osteoporotic women with previous vertebral fracture. Abnormalities were noted in association with collapsed vertebral bodies in a majority of these women, but very few showed evidence of degenerative disc disease. The most prominent abnormalities were noted in the facet joint at the level of the vertebral collapse. Smaller lesions were commonly found in the facets above and below the level of collapse (Ettinger *et al.*, 1994).

Complaints of back pain in the patient with previous osteoporotic vertebral fractures may be associated with or due to other causes unrelated to osteoporosis. Back pain with neurological symptoms in the lower extremities may occur when vertebral fractures result in retropulsed fragments (Ryan *et al.*, 1992).

COSTAL-ILIAC IMPINGEMENT SYNDROME

Loss of height resulting from vertebral collapse may cause the lower ribs to impinge on the iliac crest (Wynne *et al.*, 1985). This leads to pain from mechanical irritation which may be located in the lower back and loin and may radiate into the leg. Known as the costal-iliac impingement syndrome, diagnosis may be made by palpating the lower ribs and the iliac crest (Figure 17.7). Lateral bending and rotation elicit pain and confirm the diagnosis. Injection of lidocaine into the margin of the iliac crest and lower ribs allows for performance of these maneuvers with markedly decreased pain and readily confirms the diagnosis. Further injections into these areas with sclerosing material may give more prolonged relief (Kallings, 1993). In severe cases, resection of the lower ribs has been beneficial (Hirschberg *et al.*, 1992). The use of a wide cloth belt to compress the lower ribs, thereby allowing them to avoid contact with the iliac crest by sinking into the pelvic cavity, is reported to be a benefit.

Pain management of chronic back pain

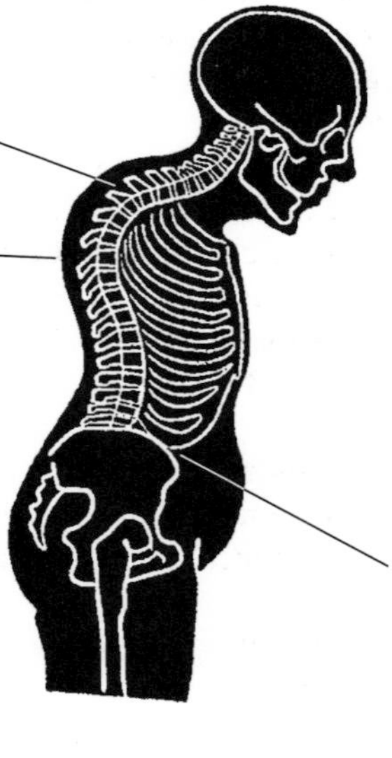

Figure 17.7 Impingement syndrome.

associated with osteoporotic vertebral fracture should include a program of strengthening paravertebral, abdominal and gluteal muscles, improving balance, flexibility and providing postural correction. Relief of stress on the spine through use of proper body mechanics is encouraged. In severe cases, an orthosis can be of benefit. An assessment of activities of daily living may lead to the use of other techniques and devices that can help the patient to avoid situations which aggravate pain.

Physical agents such as heat, ice, transcutaneous electrical nerve stimulation and acupuncture can be helpful. Non-narcotic agents such as ibuprofen, acetaminophen and asprin should be used sparingly and with knowledge of potential side effects. Calcitonin has been reported to be of benefit in the treatment of bone pain resulting from osteoporotic fractures (Gennari *et al.*, 1991; Rifat *et al.*, 1992). Hypnosis, behavioral modification, biofeedback and counseling have been beneficial in treatment of chronic pain. Injection of sclerosing material is used to relieve back pain. When vertebral fractures are associated with significant deformity, injection of sclerosing agents into the facet joint at the fracture site, as well as into the joints above and below, may be of additional benefit.

An extended range of management options is available to treat patients with chronic pain from severe spinal deformity. It is essential that this management be physician directed (Wolff *et al.*, 1991). A multidisciplinary team approach is beneficial to insuring maintenance of function in this population. Non-pharmacologic interventions utilized to manage chronic back pain include:

- *hypnosis*: this has been effectively utilized to improve functional ability and increase self-esteem in chronic pain sufferers (Appel, 1992);
- *acupuncture*: the practice of inserting extremely thin needles into various areas of the body offers an additional therapeutic tool in the management of pain (Lundeberg, 1993);
- *biofeedback*: behavioral modification programs, designed to change responses to pain involving various relaxation techniques, are used for patients with chronic pain to enable patients to relax and control muscle tension, particularly in the paraspinal musculature (Freeman *et al.*, 1980);
- *transcutaneous electrical nerve stimulation (TENS)*: brief electrical impulses are thought to stimulate nerve endings beneath the skin, interfering with the passage of pain signals in the nervous systems (Nolan, 1988; Simmonds and Kumar, 1994).

DEVELOPMENT OF SPINAL ARTHRITIS

Vertebral collapse is followed by an increase in lumbar lordosis which is accentuated by additional fractures. This lordosis places mechanical stress on ligaments, muscles and apophyseal joints. Continued progression of fracture leads to severe kyphosis and loss of height may cause pain from pressure of the ribs on the iliac crest. The combination of these changes leads to further stress on articular facets and hastens the development of degenerative arthritis.

CONSERVATIVE PAIN MANAGEMENT

Chronic back pain in the osteoporotic patient is managed by adequate recumbent bedrest for periods of 20–30 minutes twice daily. This program is supplemented by encouraging adjustments in lifestyle, medications, physical agents, orthoses and other therapies considered useful for chronic pain. These interventions are employed after ruling out other causes of back pain in the elderly and after assessment of the effect depression is having on the symptoms.

SPINAL SUPPORTS

Supports for the spinal column have been used for hundreds of years. These supports are usually in the form of corsets, braces and molded jackets. Generally, they are referred to as orthoses, '. . . an appliance or apparatus used to support, align, or hold parts of the body in correction position' (Dorlands Medical Dictionary, 1994). The distinction between braces and corsets is that braces have a transverse rigid (metal, plastic) part, whereas corsets do not. Frequently, corsets will have pockets for vertical insertion of plastic or metal stays which do not add to the function of the corset but maintain the corset in proper positions. Jackets may be custom fabricated with either hard or soft plastic material or are available in ready-made sizes. The terminology for these orthoses is based upon the spinal segments they control. For example, the Taylor thoracolumbosacral orthosis is an example of a brace used for spinal immobilization of the thoracic and lumbar spine (Licht and Kamanetz, 1966).

The degree and types of skeletal pain and disability among patients with osteoporosis present a complicated challenge to provide adequate mechanical support (Frost, 1972). When many solutions are available to answer a given problem, it usually means that there is no single good solution. Such is the case with mechanical supports for the osteoporotic spine.

These orthoses may be used for pain relief and stabilization for both the acute fracture and the long-term care of the osteoporotic spine. The use of an orthosis in the treatment of acute spine fracture may reduce pain and immobilize the spine, thereby promoting healing. Use in the long-term treatment of the osteoporotic spine may assist weakened spinal musculature, alleviate chronic pain and prevent further fracture. Additionally, orthoses may be prescribed for special situations where it is anticipated that vertebral loads may be increased.

These orthoses are prescribed for the osteoporotic patient based on predetermined goals. Spinal orthoses are used to alter the biomechanics of the spine by applying external forces. Compression forces on vertebral bodies may be transferred to the posterior spinal elements (Cailliet, 1988), while at the same time restricting movement and stabilizing the spine.

Recently, an orthosis (Posture Training System) (Figure 17.8) has been introduced which assists spinal extension and whereas it does not provide immobilization, it does provide stabilization and some transfer of vertebral compression (Kaplan and Sinaki, 1993).

An understanding of the biomechanics and kinesiology of the spine is essential to the rational prescription of these orthotic appliances (Levin, 1984). Chronic low back pain in patients with vertebral compression fractures is sometimes attributed to increased lumbar lordosis (Parfitt, 1978). The thoracic kyphosis resulting from progressive vertebral fracture causes a shift in gravitational forces necessary for a balanced vertebral column. By rotation of the pelvis upward on the femoral heads, the lumbosacral angle is increased, causing an increased lumbar lordosis but bringing the spine into balance. Decreasing this angle will decrease lumbar lordosis and facilitate a compensatory reduction in thoracic kyphosis (Cailliet, 1988). The angle can be modified by controlling the position of the pelvis on the femoral heads. When alteration of this angle has occurred, changing the relationships of vertebral elements, there is a concomitant lengthening and shortening of soft tissues surrounding the spine. The surrounding spinal musculature, particularly the gluteal groups, is essential to control. The use of an orthosis may serve to stabilize the angle.

Flexion and extension motions are possible in the lumbar spine to a far greater extent than in the thoracic spine. This difference is due to the orientation of the facet joints (Cailliet, 1988). In the lumbar spine, these joints are aligned vertically, whereas in the thoracic spine the alignment is horizontal. This alignment, together with the restriction of the rib cage and overlapping spinous process, impedes flexion and extension but does allow for rotation and lateral flexion.

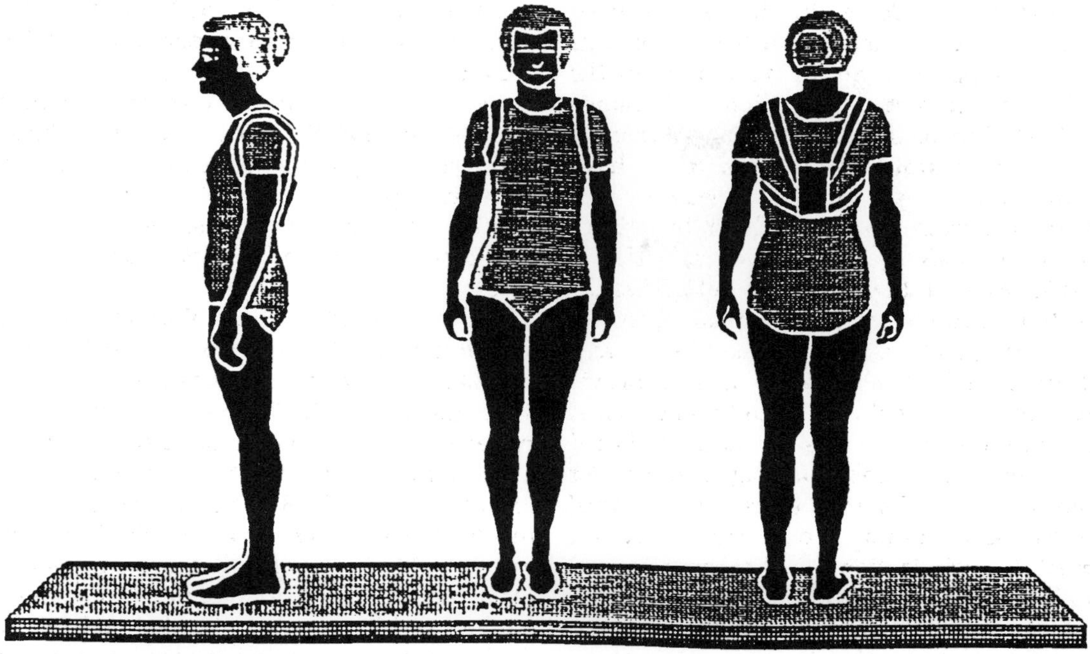

Figure 17.8 Posture Training System.

Spinal orthoses are therefore limited to restricting rotation and lateral bending in the thoracic spine and flexion and extension in the lumbar spine (Licht and Kamenetz, 1966). Spinal orthoses may fix the spine in various positions. All thoracolumbosacral orthoses provide some degree of fixation, forcing spinal extension. By fixing the thoracolumbar spine in positions such as extension, the orthosis can transfer some portion of compression loading on vertebral bodies.

In summary, spinal orthoses are used in the osteoporotic patient to decrease the lumbosacral angle, decrease anterior wedging, add support to a fragile vertebral column and provide pain relief and decrease compression fractures. There are several types of spinal orthosis used in the treatment of osteoporosis (Licht and Kamanetz, 1966). The most commonly prescribed devices are:

1. *Corsets (Figure 17.9).* Function primarily by providing abdominal compression which acts as a supplement for the support of abdominal musculature. This compression converts the abdominal cavity to a nearly rigid walled cylinder of soft tissue and viscera through which stresses can be distributed to shoulder and ribs (Bartelink, 1957). They may also maintain the degree of lumbar lordosis, reducing stress transmitted to intervertebral discs. Lumbosacral corsets are used to stabilize the spine and reduce back pain. They act as a reminder to the patient to maintain adequate posture. Some corsets provide a posterior pocket into which a heat-moldable plastic plate can be placed. It is claimed that this plate provides additional stabilization for the low back. Often lumbosacral corsets are fabricated from a contoured flexible cloth or elastic garment that encompasses the

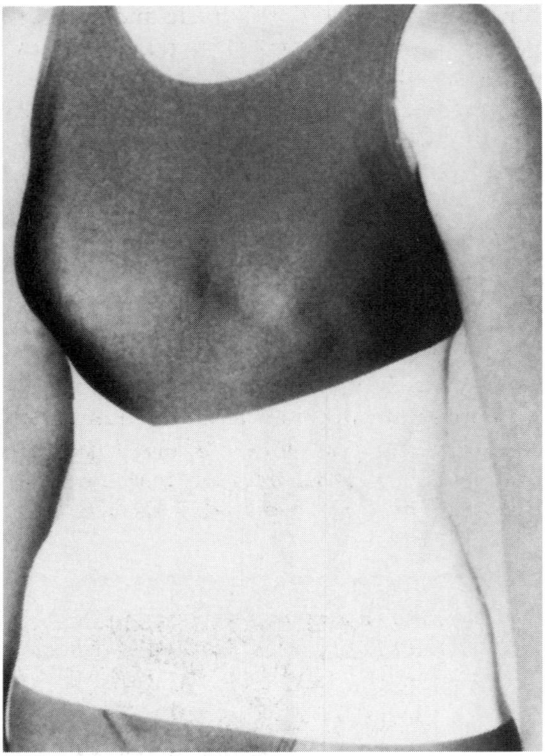

Figure 17.9 Lumbosacral corset.

torso and pelvis and is adjustable circumferentially. This type of corset is also available as a thoracolumbosacral orthosis with shoulder straps. The addition of the straps provides for hyperextension of the thoracic spine. This type of corset is popular in the treatment of acute vertebral fracture.

2. *Thoracolumbosacral (TLSO) orthosis (Figure 17.10)*. Repositions the anterior longitudinal ligaments and pulls the flattened vertebral body back to a more anatomical position (Hipps, 1967).
   - *The Taylor brace (Figure 17.11)*. This is fabricated from metal and leather and consists of a pelvic band, interscapular bands, two extended posterior uprights with a corset front and overlapping straps. This brace restricts motion in flexion and extension and provides hyperextension of the thoracic spine (Licht and Kamanetz, 1966).
   - *The Knight-Taylor brace (TLSO) (Figure 17.12)*. This is the same as the Taylor brace except for the provision of lateral metal uprights that restrict motion in the lateral plan.
   - *The Jewett orthosis (Figure 17.13)*. Hyperextension TLSO consisting of an adjustable metal frame with three point pressure rods applied at sternal, suprapubic and lumbar areas. The function of this brace is to hyperextend the thoracic spine.
   - *The CASH orthosis (Figure 17.14)*. (Cruciform Anterior Sternal Hyperextension) This functions similarly to the Jewett, but it is more easily adjustable and is configured with a circumferential

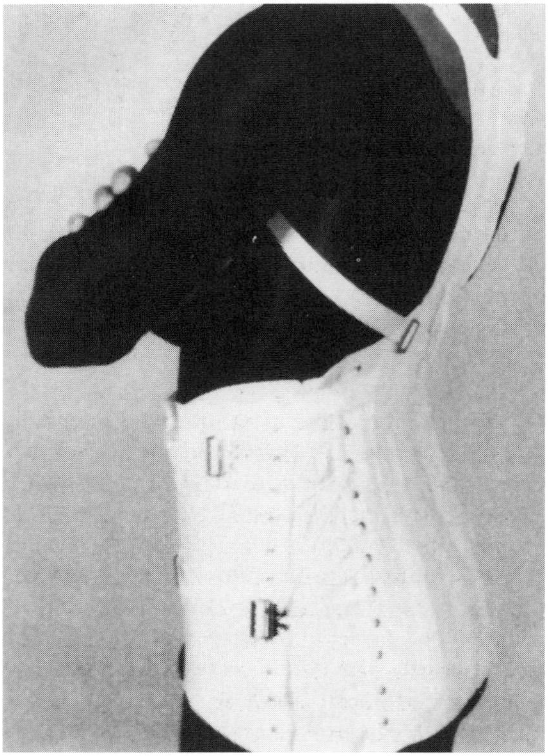

Figure 17.10 Thoracolumbar corset, side view.

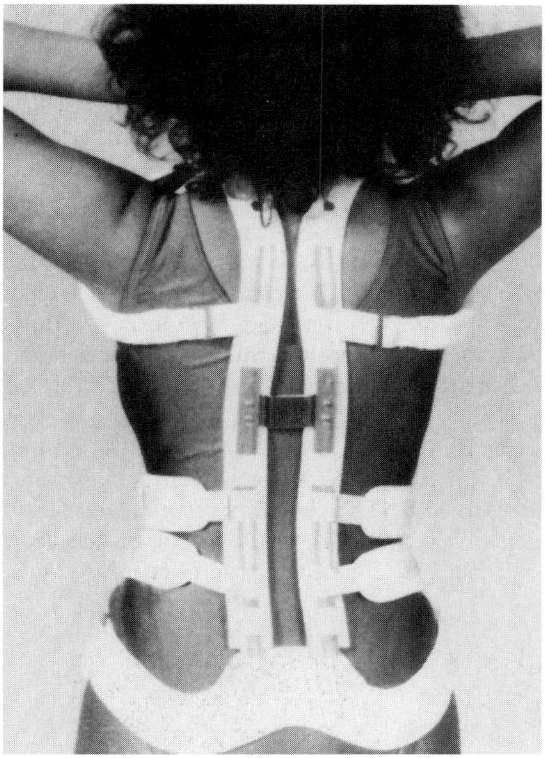

Figure 17.11 Taylor orthosis.

waist belt to which a pad is attached posteriorly at mid-back level (Licht and Kamenetz, 1966).

- *Molded plastic orthoses (Figure 17.15).* This is an anterior molded hyperextension orthosis consisting of a plastic shell extending from sternal notch to pubic bone. It can be trimmed for a breast cutout. A lumbar pad is provided posteriorly and it is joined to the anterior portion by hook and loop fasteners. This orthosis hyperextends the thoracolumbar spine and provides a wide distribution of pressure. Its use is particularly beneficial in a thin elderly female.

3. *Molded plastic body jacket (Figure 17.16).* This is fabricated from heat-molded rigid plastic which is custom fitted, trimmed and bivalved. This jacket provides maximum immobilization of the thoracic and lumbar spine and may be fitted for patients with scoliosis who could not tolerate other forms of bracing. It can be effective in pain control for both acute and chronic symptoms and does provide some stabilization to the spine. It is expensive, hot to wear, very restrictive of chest exercise and can be uncomfortable.
4. *The Posture Training System (PTS).* Recently described by Kaplan and Sinaki (1993), this uses the mechanical advantage of gravity and the biomechanics of the spine to promote unloading of vertebral bodies and consequently pain relief. It has a pocket into which weights up to a maximum of two pounds may be placed. This pocket is

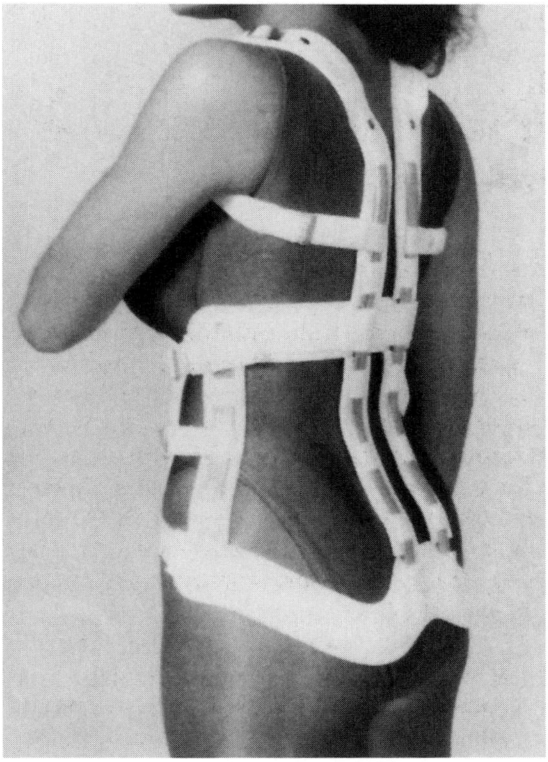

Figure 17.12 Knight-Taylor orthosis; note lateral upright.

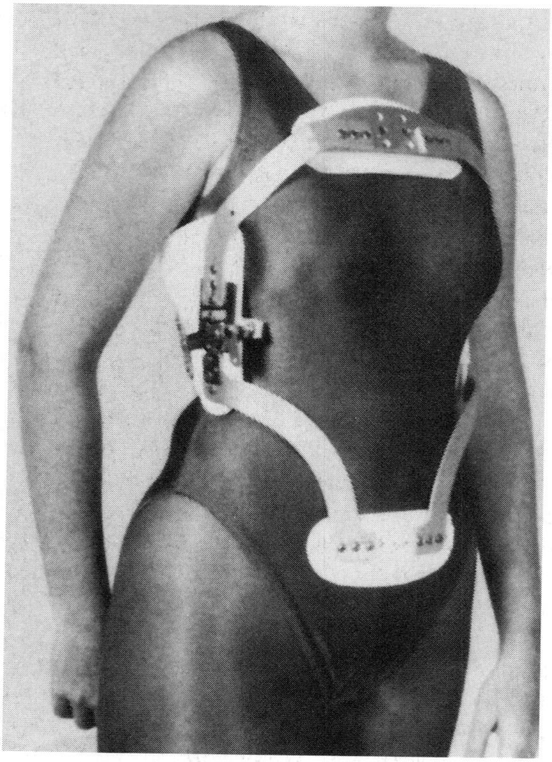

Figure 17.13 Jewett orthosis.

> placed posteriorly below the inferior angle of the scapula so that it promotes and aids spinal extension. Flexion caused by kyphosis in the upper trunk is partially counteracted, thereby assisting the patient in achieving an upright posture. Compression forces in the lower thoracic spine are reduced. This device is not meant to provide spinal immobilization inherent in the use of braces. With the concomitant use of an abdominal bind, goals of spinal support, stabilization and transfer of loads and reduction of compression forces can be achieved. This device (with corset) is soft and comfortable, promoting patient compliance.

The Jewett brace does not reduce lumbar and thoracic flexion in patients with vertebral compression fractures (Sinaki, 1988). Extension bracing with a TLSO combined with early mobilization has been effective in the treatment of selected patients with fractures of the thoracolumbar spine (Levin, 1984). Nonetheless, the decision on which orthosis to use remains subject to debate.

The amount of restriction of spinal motion and the amount of comfort afforded by an orthosis are the major considerations in the orthotic prescription. Studies have demonstrated that not only is the lumbosacral spine not immobilized by bracing (Sinaki, 1982), but spinal motion may be increased at the segments adjacent to the upper and lower ends of the brace. If full immobilization of the spine is to be achieved, fixation to the pelvis is required and this would require extending

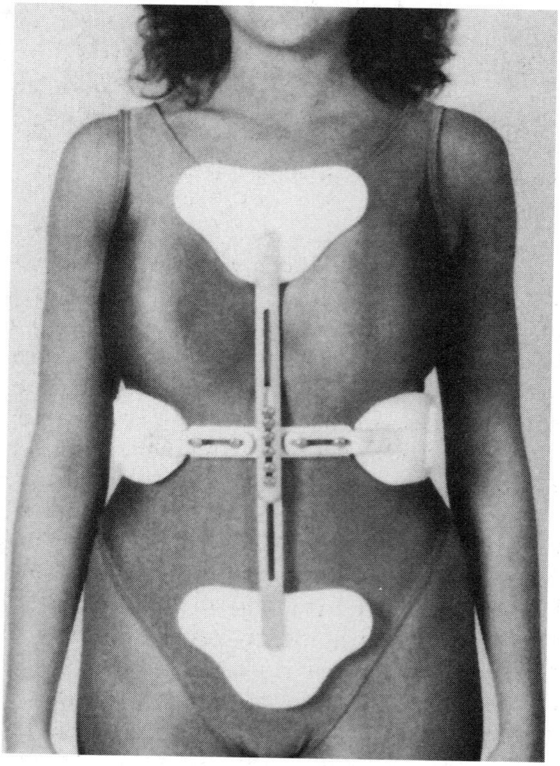

Figure 17.14 Cruciform anterior sternal hyperextension (CASH) orthosis.

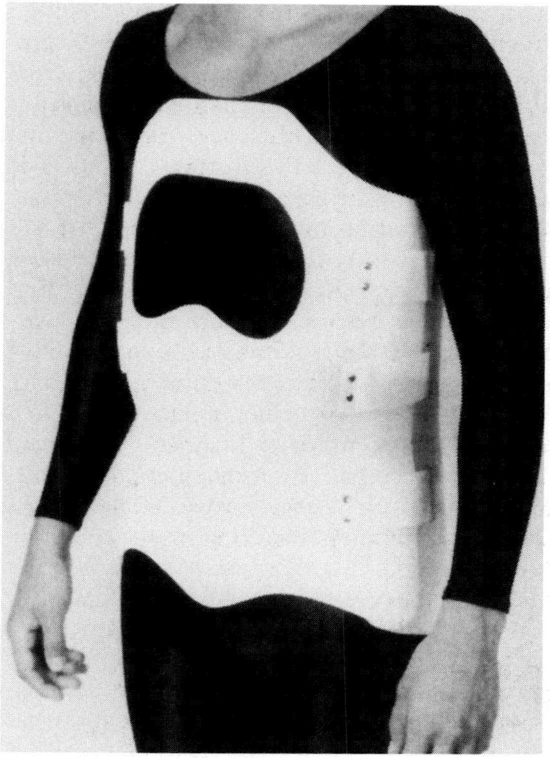

Figure 17.15 Molded plastic orthosis.

the orthosis below the pelvis to the thigh. Commonly prescribed orthoses achieved restriction of up to 20% in flexion and up to 48% in extension, lateral bending and twisting (Lantz and Schultz, 1986). A comparison study analyzed the restriction of motion in three planes and assessed perceived comfort among four common braces. The sample consisted of 33 subjects and the braces include the Raney jacket, the camp lace-up corset, a molded-polypropylene thoracolumbosacral orthosis (TLSO) and a common elastic corset. The Raney jacekt provided maximal restriction but was the most uncomfortable brace tested. The most comfortable brace was the elastic corset, which also was the least restrictive of all braces tested. In deciding which orthosis is more appropriate, the degree of patient compliance must be balanced with the amount of immobilization desired to control pain and prevent fractures (Buchalter *et al.*, 1989).

A prospective study of bracing thoracic and lumbar spine fractures supported the advantages of a bracing regimen as an alternative to prolonged immobilization in bed or early operative fusion. Rigid bracing has resulted in a higher correlation with pain relief (Willner, 1985).

Patient compliance with use of these braces and corsets is generally poor. These devices are considered to be cumbersome, uncomfortable, difficult to put on and take off and often a cause of skin irritation. Particularly in the elderly population, orthotic use may have a negative impact on gait, with increased

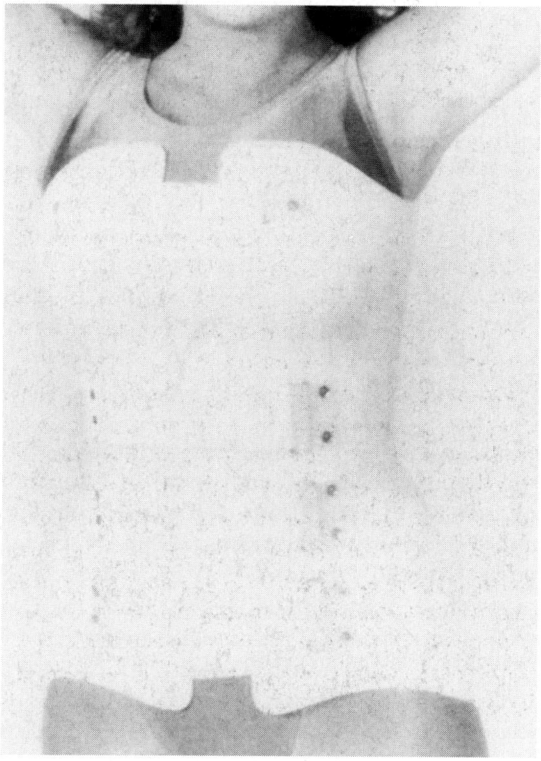

Figure 17.16 Molded plastic body jacket.

oxygen consumption and difficulties with balance. Whereas corsets are generally more comfortable than braces, because they function through increasing intra-abdominal pressure, they may be contraindicated in patients with orthopnea from chronic obstructive pulmonary disease (COPD), hiatal and inguinal hernias and obesity. The use of an orthosis must be accompanied by a program of therapeutic exercise so that muscle weakness may be avoided (Sinaki and Mikkelsen, 1984). The abdominal musculature and the erector spinae are most vulnerable to weakness resulting from spinal orthotic use.

The Posture Training System and the canvas thoracolumbar corset with shoulder straps are usually comfortable and have a sound rationale for use in patients with acute vertebral fractures. In patients with severe osteoporosis and multiple compression fractures, the use of a body jacket made from a plastic mold may be required for stability and relief.

Improved function and decreased disability may be achieved through the use of spinal supports and early mobilization following acute vertebral fracture. The use of these orthoses, the Posture Training System and appropriate therapeutic exercise is fundamental to rehabilitation of patients with osteoporosis (Hipps, 1967; Kaplan and Sinaki, 1993).

FALL AND FRACTURE PREVENTION

The members of the rehabilitation team may play a major role in prevention of fractures through providing both individual patient and community programs. The National Safety Council estimates that injuries are the sixth most common cause of death in the elderly, surpassing both diabetes mellitus and pneumonia. The most widespread cause of injury in this age group is falls which not only account for half of the deaths due to injury in the elderly, but are also one of the major causes of osteoporotic fractures. In women greater than 70 years of age, falling is predictive of future osteoporotic fractures (Lotz and Hayes, 1990). Like the incidence of hip fracture, the risk of falling and fall-related injuries increases with age in both sexes. Potential causes of falls can be categorized as intrinsic factors (e.g. arthritis, neuromuscular decline and visual impairment) or extrinsic (environmental) factors. It is these falls coupled with low bone mass that lead to disability and morbidity for both men and women.

Efforts to decrease the general incidence of fractures from a fall prevention perspective must address intrinsic host-related factors, as well as environmental factors. Functional assessment of patients can identify those at highest risk of falling. Recurrent fallers are more likely to demonstrate poor back flexibility, decreased lower extremity strength, poor distant vision, symptoms when turning or extending their neck, difficulty arising from a chair, difficulty sitting down, instability on first standing, staggering or turning, short or discontinued steps (Tinetti *et al.*, 1988). It has been demonstrated that lower extremity strengthening as well as flexibility could be improved with an exercise program (Lichtenstein *et al.*, 1989). Specific exercise programs tailored to an individual should be able to decrease their tendency to fall, especially when that individual is given appropriate assistive devices.

Generally, the presumption that targeted exercise programs can decrease falling has not been borne out in clinical studies; nonetheless, it does appear prudent to provide a program of increasing strength and balance to the elderly population.

The practice of Tai Chi has been positively correlated with a decreased incidence of falling among the elderly (Kirsteins *et al.*, 1991). Tai Chi is a martial art which stresses balance and static stretching as a form of exercise. With Tai Chi, the practitioner performs a pattern of stances which emphasize fluidity of motion. These stance changes are integrated with body posture alteration and weight shifting. The Chinese believe that these movements enhance the flow of one's life force (Chi) through the different meridians of one's body. These movements would also tend to strengthen spinal extensor musculature as well as improve lower extremity flexibility.

Risk factors for increased trauma resulting from a fall include the height of the fall, the hardness of the landing surface, increased frequency of falls and impaired energy absorption (Melton and Riggs, 1985). Whereas the percentage of falls resulting in injury varies widely, most people do not sustain serious injury from a fall (Perry, 1982). In the light of the high potential energy generated by a fall, it seems as though there should be a far greater number of fractures. A 50-year-old female who falls from a standing position generates 65 times the energy required to shatter a normally mineralized femur (Gardsell *et al.*, 1989). The fracture may be caused in part because local shock absorbers such as fat and muscle are lacking or because normal protective responses are impaired. This is particularly pertinent to the elderly with decreased strength, balance and co-ordination, as well as changes in body composition. With comorbidity, the risk of serious injury from a fall increases from 8% to 40% (Rubenstein *et al.*, 1988).

Studies have shown that hip protectors for preventing fractures offer much promise. Lauritzen (1992) provided external hip protectors, fixed in special underwear, to 167 women in a nursing home setting. Over a period of time, there was a significant decrease in hip fractures among the women wearing the hip protectors.

Extrinsic causes of fall include alcohol use, poorly lit areas, stairs, throw rugs and slippery surfaces (Rubenstein *et al.*, 1988). In-home occupational therapy evaluation for environmental intervention is an integral part of fall prevention. Grab bars for the toilet, shower and bath and removal of throw rugs and improved lighting may all be helpful.

CONCLUSION

The heterogeneous etiology of osteoporotic fracture requires a multidimensional approach. While interventions directed at increasing bone mineral density, strength and balance are the cornerstone of this problem, addressing host and environmental factors related to fallng are an important part of prevention. As the unadjusted relative risk of fracture doubles every 5–10 years, an intervention which forestalls fracture by five years could effectively half the incidence of fracture (Cummings *et al.*, 1965).

Efforts to decrease the general incidence of fragility fractures from a fall prevention perspective must address intrinsic host-related factors as well as environmental factors. Functional assessment of patients can identify those at highest risk of falling. The profile of the patient likely to fall is that of an individual with lower exremity weakness, failing vision, difficulty arising from a chair as well as sitting in a chair, staggering when turning and exhibiting short or discontinued steps. Tinetti *et al.* (1988) demonstrated that lower extremity strengthening as well as flexibility could be improved with an exercise program. Specific exercise programs tailored to an individual should be able to decrease their tendency to fall, especially when that individual is given the appropriate assistive devices and has the benefit of other rehabilitation interventions.

REFERENCES

Aitken, M.F. (1982) Self-concept and functional independence in the hospitalized elderly. *Am J Occup Ther* **35**: 243–50.

Appel, P.R. (1992) The use of hypnosis in physical medicine and rehabilitation. *Psychiatr Med* **10**: 133–48.

Bartelink, D.L. (1957) The role of abdominal pressure in relieving the pressure on the lumbar intervertebral discs. *J Bone Joint Surg* **39B** (4): 718–25.

Buchalter, D., Kahanovitz, N., Viola, K. *et al.* (1989) Three-dimensional spinal motion measurements. Part 2: A noninvasive assessment of lumbar brace immobilization of the spine. *J Spinal Disorders* **1**(4): 284–6.

Cailliet, R. (1988) *Low Back Pain Syndrome*, F.A. Davis, Philadelphia.

Chow, R., Harrison, J. and Dornan Jr (1989) Prevention and rehabilitation of osteoporosis program: exercise and osteoporosis. *Int J Rehabil Res* **12**(1): 49–56.

Christiansen, C. (1991) Introduction: Consensus Development Conference on Osteoporosis. *Am J Med* **91**: 5B–1S.

Cummings, S.R., Kelsey, J.L., Nevitt, M.C. *et al.* (1985) Epidemiology of osteoporosis and osteoporotic fractures. *Epidemiol Rev* **7**: 178–208.

Delisa, J.A., Gans, B.M. and Currie, D.M. (1993) *Rehabilitation Medicine: Principles and Practice*, 2nd edn, J.B. Lippincott, Philadelphia.

Dequeker, J. and Guesens, P. (1990) Treatment of established osteoporosis and rehabilitation: current practice and possibilities. Elsevier Scientific Publishers, Ireland, pp. 121–36.

Ettinger, B., Black, J.E., Smith, R. *et al.* (1988) An examination of the association between vertebral deformities, physical disabilities, and psychosocial problems. *Maturitas* **10**: 283–92.

Ettinger, B., Black, D.M., Nevitt, M.C. *et al.* (1992) Contribution of vertebral deformities to chronic back pain and disability. The Study of Osteoporotic Fractures Research Group. *J Bone Miner Res* **7**(4): 449–56.

Ettinger, B., Black, D.M., Palermo, L. *et al.* (1994) Kyphosis in older women and its relation to back pain, disability and osteopenia: the study of osteoporosis fractures. *Osteoporosis Int* **4**: 55–60.

Felson, D.T., Anderson, J.J., Hannan, M.T. *et al.* (1989) Impaired vision and hip fracture. *J Am Geriatr Soc* **37**(6): 495–500.

Ferrell, B.A. and Ferrell, B.R. (1991) Principles of pain management in older people. *Comprehensive Ther* **17**: 53–8.

Fitzsimmons, A., Bonner, F. and Lindsay, R. (1995) Failure to diagnose osteoporosis. *Am J Phys Rehabil* **74**(3): 240–2.

Freeman, C.W., Calsyn, D.A., Paige, A.B. *et al.* (1980) Biofeedback with low back pain patients. *Am J Clin Biofeedback* **3**: 118.

Frost, H.M. (1972) Managing the skeletal pain and disability of osteoporosis. *Orthop Clin North Am* **3**(3): 561–70.

Frost, H.M. (1985) The pathomechanics of osteoporosis. *Clin Orthop Rel Res* **200**: 198–226.

Gandy, S. and Payne, R. (1986) Back pain in the elderly: updated diagnosis and management. *Geriatrics* **41**: 59–72.

Gardsell, P., Johnell, O. and Nilsson, B.E. (1989) The predictive value of fracture, disease, and falling for fragility fractures in women. *Calcif Tissue Int* **45**(6): 327–30.

Gennari, C., Agnusdci, D. and Camporeale, C. (1991) Use of calcitonin in the treatment of bone pain associated with osteoporosis. *Calcif Tissue Int* **49**(21): S9–S13.

Harrison, J., Chow, R., Dornan Jr, Goodwin, S., Strauss and The Bone and Mineral Group of the University of Toronto (1993) Evaluation of a program for rehabilitation of osteoporotic patients (PRO): 4-year follow-up; *Osteoporosis Int* **3**: 13–17.

Hipps, H.E., (1967) Back braces: types, functions, and how to order and use them. *Med Clin North Am* **51**(5): 1315–43.

Hirschberg, G.G., Williams, K.A. and Byrd, J.G. (1992) Medical management of iliocostal pain. *Geriatrics* **47**(9): 62–6.

Kallings, P. (1993) Nonsteroidal anti-inflammatory drugs. *Vet Clin North Am Equine Practice* **9**: 523–41.

Kaplan, R.S. and Sinaki, M. (1993) Posture training support: preliminary report on a series of patients with diminished symptomatic complications of osteoporosis. *Mayo Clin Proc* **68**: 1171–6.

Katz, S., Ford, A.B. and Moskowitz, R.W. (1963) Studies of illness in the aged. *J Am Med Assoc* **185**: 914–19.

Keith, R.A., Granger, C.V., Hamilton, B.B. and Sherwin, F.S. (1984) The functional independent measure: a new tool in rehabilitation medicine. In: *Advances in Clinical Rehabilitation*, (eds Eisenberg, M.B. and Grezesiak, R.C.), Springer-Verlag, New York, pp. 6–18.

Kirsteins, A.E., Dietz, F. and Swang, S.M. (1991) Evaluating the safety and potential use of a weight-bearing exercise, Tai-Chi Chuan, for rheumatoid arthritis patients. *Am J Phys Rehabil* **70**(3): 136–41.

Kottke, T.E., Caspersen, C.J. and Hill, C.S. (1984) Exercise in the management and rehabilitation of selected chronic diseases. *Preventive Med* **13**: 47–65.

Lantz, S. and Schultz, A. (1986) Lumbar spine orthosis wearing I. Restriction of gross body motions. *Spine* **11**(8): 834–7.

Lauritzen, J.S. (1992) Protection against hip fractures by energy absorption. *Danish Med Bull* **39**: 91–3.

Levin, A.M. (1984) Spinal orthoses. *Am Family Phys* (US) **29**(3): 277–80.

Licht, S. and Kamanetz, H. (1966) *Orthotics Etcetera*, Elizabeth Licht, Connecticut.

Lichtenstein, M.J., Shields, S.L., Shiavi, R.G., *et al.* (1989) Exercise and balance in aged women: a pilot controlled clinical trial. *Arch Phys Med Rehabil* **70**: 138–43.

Lotz, J.C. and Hayes, W.C. (1990) The use of quantitative computer tomography to estimate risk of fracture of hip from falls. *J Bone Joint Surg* **72**: 689–700.

Lukert, B.P. (1994) Vertebral compression fractures: how to manage pain, avoid disability. *Geriatrics* **49**(2): 22–6.

Lundeberg, T. (1993) Peripheral effects of sensory nerve stimulation (acupuncture) in inflammation and ischemia. *Scand J Rehabil Med* **29**: 61–86.

Lyles, K.W., Gold, D.T., Shipp, K.M. *et al.* (1993) Association of osteoporotic vertebral compression fractures with impaired functional status. *Am J Med* **94**: 595–601.

Mahoney, F.L. and Barthel, D.W. (1965) Functional evaluation. The Barthel index. Maryland State *Med J* **14**: 61–5.

McGinnis, G.E., Seward, M., DeJong, G. and Osberg, J.S. (1984) Program evaluation of PM&R departments using self reported Barthel. *Arch Phys Med Rehabil* **67**: 123–5.

Melton III, L.J. and Riggs, B. (1985) Risk factors for injury after a fall. *Clin Geriatr Med* **1**(3): 525–39.

National Health Policy Forum (1991) An Update on Functional Assessment: Perspectives From Consumers, Practitioners, Policymakers, and Payers, NHPF, Washington, D.C.

National Osteoporosis Foundation Scientific Advisory Board (1991) Position Paper on Exercise and Osteoporosis.

Nolan, M.F. (1988) Selected problems in the use of transcutaneous electrical nerve stimulation for pain control and appraisal with proposed solutions. *Phys Ther* **68**: 1694–8.

Parfitt, A.M. (1978) *What Are the Causes of Pain in Osteoporosis*, (ed. Heaney, R.), Biomedical Information Corporation, New York, p. 12.

Perry, B.C. (1982) Falls among the elderly: a review of the methods and conclusions of the epidemiologic studies. *J Am Geriatr Soc* **30**: 367.

Ray, W. and Marie, R. (1987) Psychotropic drug use and the risk of hip fracture. *N Engl J Med* **3167**: 363–8.

Rifat, S.F., Kiningham, R.B. and Peggs, J.F. (1992) Calcitonin in the treatment of osteoporotic bone pain. *J Family Practice* **35**(1): 9393–6.

Rubenstein, L.Z., Robbins, A.S. and Shulman, B.L. (1988) Falls and instability in the elderly. *J Am Geriatr Soc* **36**: 266.

Ryan, P.J., Evans, P., Gibson, T. and Fogelman, I. (1992) Osteoporosis and chronic back pain: a study with single-photon emission computed tomography bone scintigraphy. *J Bone Miner Res* **7**(12): 455–60.

Schoening, H.A. and Iversen, I.A. (1968) Numerical scoring of self-care status: a study of the Kenny self-care evaluation. *Arch Phys Med Rehabil* **49**: 221–9.

Simmonds, M.J. and Kumar, S. (1994) Pain and the placebo in rehabilitation using TENS and laser. *Disabil Rehabil* **16**: 13–20.

Sinaki, M. (1982) Post-menopausal spinal osteoporosis. Physical therapy and rehabilitation principles. *Mayo Clin Proc* **57**: 699–703.

Sinaki, M. (1988) Exercise and physical therapy. *Osteoporosis, Etiology, Diagnosis and Management*, pp. 457–79.

Sinaki, M. and Mikkelsen, B.A. (1984) Postmenopausal spinal osteoporosis: flexion versus extension exercises. *Arch Phys Med Rehabil* **65**: 593–6.

Steiger, U. (1977) Rehabilitation von Patienten mit Osteoporose. *Ther Umsch/Rev Ther* **34**: 648–54.

Strasser, D., Falconer, J., Martino-Saltzmann, D. and the Rehabilitation Team (1994) Staff perceptions of the hospital environment, the interdisciplinary team environment, and interprofessional relations. *Arch Phys Med Rehabil* **75**: 177–82.

Tinetti, M. (1986) Performance oriented assessment of mobility problems in elderly patients. *J Am Geriatr Soc* **34**: 119–26.

Tinetti, M.E., Speechley, M. and Guiter, S.F. (1988) Risk factors for falls among elderly persons living in the community. *N Engl J Med* **319**(16): 1701–7.

Vaughan, C. (1976) Rehabilitation in postmenopausal osteoporosis. *Rehabilitation* **12**(7): 652–7.

Williams, A.R., Weiss, N.S., Ure, C.L. *et al.* (1982) Effect of weight, smoking, and estrogen use on

the risk of hip and forearm fractures in postmenopausal women. *Obstet Gynecol* **60**(6): 695–9.
Willner, S. (1985) Effect of a rigid brace on back pain. *Acta Orthop Scand* **56**: 40–2.
Wolff, M., Michel, T.H., Krebs, D.E. *et al.* (1991) Chronic pain – assessment of orthopedic physical therapists' knowledge and attitudes. *Phys Ther* **71**: 207–14.
Wynne, A.T., Nelson, M.A. and Nordin, B.E.C. (1985) Costoiliac impingement syndrome. *Br Soc Bone Joint Surg* **67B**(1): 124–5.

ORTHOPAEDIC MANAGEMENT 18

P.R. Allen

INTRODUCTION

The orthopaedic management of osteoporosis is almost entirely concerned with its most obvious manifestation, namely a fracture. In order for a fracture to occur, a bone must be subjected to a force greater than that which it can resist. This resistance, the inherent stength of a bone, may be normal and the applied force therefore must be high. When the inherent strength of bone is less than normal, lower forces will produce a fracture. This broad generalization is an oversimplification of both the mechanism of a fracture and the nature of bone strength.

MECHANISM OF FRACTURE

Bone is a composite material made up of a series of close-packed irregularly shaped cylinders (osteons) and irregularly shaped fragments of bone which fill the spaces between the osteons. The interfaces between the structures are devoid of collagen fibres and are called cement lines. Also present are numerous interconnected pores which connect the osteocytic lacunae. The collagen fibres are either randomly arranged (woven bone) or layered (lamellar bone). Thus bone behaves mechanically as an anisotropic material with differing properties in different directions. Studies on compact bone specimens have shown that tensile loading results in relatively flat fracture surfaces, perpendicular to the loading direction (Wright and Hayes, 1976). The loading may be compressive, tensile or torsional but the stress required to cause the fracture depends on many variables including the rate at which load is applied (Currey, 1975; Wright and Hayes, 1976), orientation of the specimen (Pope and Outwater, 1974; Reilly and Burstein, 1975) and the bone microstructure (Reilly and Burstein, 1975; Wright and Hayes, 1976). One of the parameters used to describe the toughness of a material containing a flaw is the critical stress intensity factor. A positive correlation between bone density and critical stress intensity factor has been shown similar to that found between bone density and ultimate tensile strength (Wall *et al.*, 1972; Wright and Hayes, 1976). Therefore, an increase in bone density leads to increased strength and thus has implications when bone density declines, with increased susceptibility to fracture. An additional cause of loss of strength in such individuals is an increased susceptibility to crack initiation from initial cavities or flaws in the bone microstructure.

NATURE OF BONE STRENGTH

Cortical and cancellous bone both contribute to mechanical strength of bone. The compact nature of cortical bone confers important mechanical properties. Even in vertebrae where trabecular bone predominates, cortical bone is a major determinant of compressive

Osteoporosis. Edited by John C. Stevenson and Robert Lindsay. Published in 1998 by Chapman & Hall, London.
ISBN 0 412 48870 1

strength (Vesterby *et al.*, 1991). In cancellous bone the trabecular arrangement influences its strength. Vertebrae have a cubic lattice of thick vertical columns and thin interconnecting horizontal struts while other sites have a more random structure. In osteoporosis the trabeculae may thin but maintain their overall structure. On the other hand, there may be penetration or erosion of trabeculae, leading to reduction in strength and susceptibility to fracture. However, as trabecular thinning occurs, the likelihood of penetration increases and the two processes are to some extent interdependent (Compston *et al.*, 1989).

OSTEOPOROTIC FRACTURES

Osteoporotic fractures occur as a result of reduced bone strength as described above. The three fractures commonly associated with osteoporosis are fractures of the distal forearm (Colles fractures, etc.), vertebral fractures and hip fractures. However, fractures attributed to osteoporosis occur commonly at other skeletal sites (Seeley *et al.*, 1991). Fractures of the proximal humerus, distal femur, proximal tibia, tibial plateau fractures, pelvis and ankle fractures all have an increased incidence in the postmenopausal female and all such fractures occupy a large proportion of the trauma workload of all orthopaedic units in the United Kingdom. In one study of atraumatic fractures in men and women over 60 years old, the dominant sites of fracture were hip (18.9%), distal radius (18.5%), ribs and humerus (11.9% in each case), ankle and foot (9.1% and 6.6% respectively) and spine (3.8%). The low incidence of vertebral fractures in this study may reflect the strict criteria applied to diagnose a new symptomatic vertebral fracture (Nguyen *et al.*, 1993).

FRACTURES OF THE DISTAL RADIUS

The most common type of wrist fracture was first described by Dr Abraham Colles in 1814. This fracture occurs at the distal radius with or without involvement of the ulna and in displaced fractures this usually involves the distal radioulnar joint. It produces a classic 'dinner fork' deformity as a result of dorsal and lateral angulation with rotational deformity in supination (Figure 18.1). Other fractures occur in the wrist, e.g. Smith's fracture, Barton's fracture, with the opposite displacement but the Colles fracture remains the most frequently occurring, with an increasing incidence in women after the menopause. The frequency increases sixfold between the ages of 35–39 and 60–64 and then levels off (Owen *et al.*, 1982). The incidence is lower in men and there is a smaller rise in the elderly. Many accident and emergency departments in the United Kingdom experience sudden dramatic increases during periods of ice and snow. The estimated cost of treatment based on an average of three outpatient attendances and two GP consultations is approximately £170 (Vessey, M., 1993, personal communication).

Treatment

In the United Kingdom, fractures of the distal radius are usually treated by accident and emergency doctors who may be trainees, general practitioners or accident and emergency specialist consultants. The patient is then reviewed and the treatment continued under the supervision of the orthopaedic specialist.

Initially, the displaced fracture is reduced under general anaesthesia or various types of regional anaesthesia, of which a local haematoma block is the most convenient (Case, 1985). The reduced position is then maintained by a padded plaster slab which may be converted to a full surrounding plaster support after approximately 7–10 days when the initial swelling has settled. This is usually removed after about 5–6 weeks and rehabilitation is then commenced. Unstable comminuted Colles fractures have been

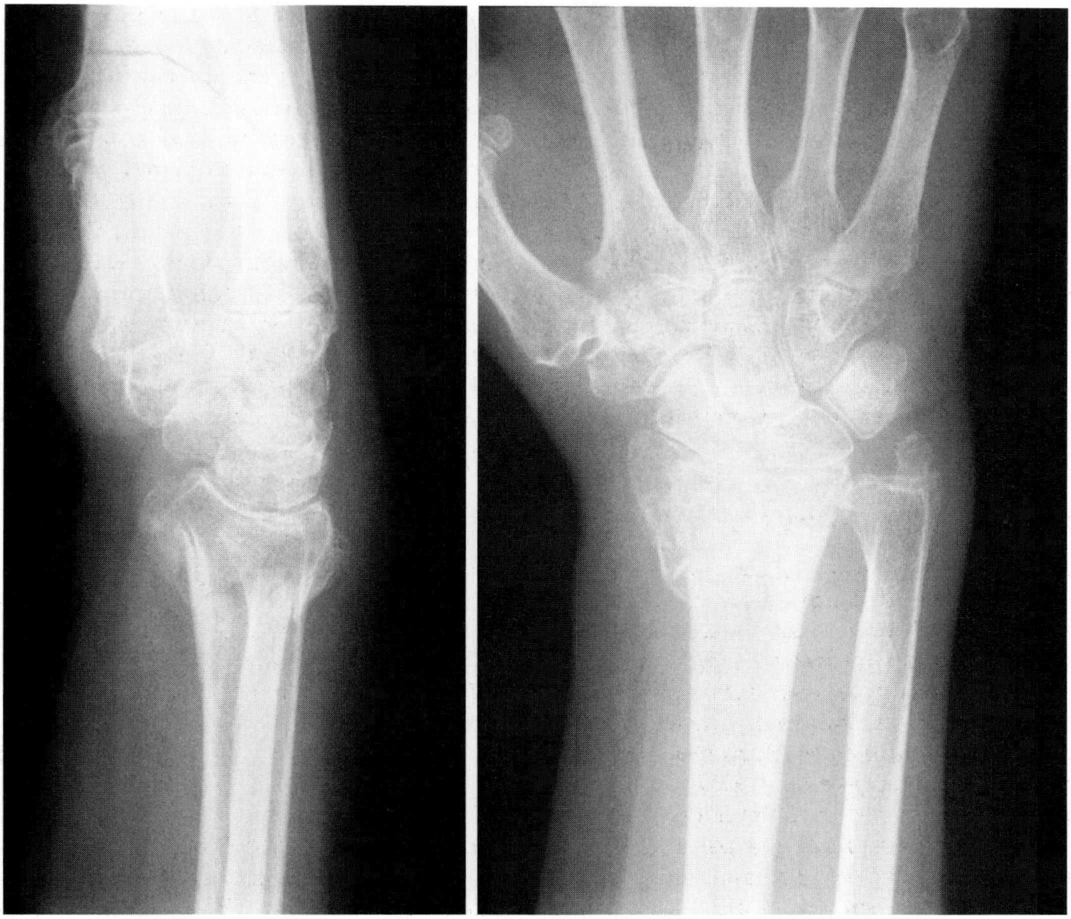

Figure 18.1 A healed Colles fracture with mild residual deformity.

treated with alternative methods of immobilization, including external fixation, buttress plates and screws or simply percutaneous pinned fixation (Coney *et al.*, 1979; Müller *et al.*, 1979; Clancey, 1984). There is conflicting evidence on whether the final position of reduction significantly affects the end result. Smale (1965) observed that good function may be present in spite of marked residual bony deformity and some authors report encouraging recovery as early as six months after the fracture (Pool, 1973; Sarmiento *et al.*, 1975; Stuart *et al.*, 1984). Other authors noted that over 17% of patients had poor function one year after injury (Gartland and Werley, 1951; Bacorn and Kurtkze, 1953; Golden, 1963). This poor function has been attributed to bony deformity and hence the importance of obtaining an anatomical reduction has been repeatedly emphasized (Gartland and Werley, 1951; Van der Linden and Ericksen, 1981; Stuart *et al.*, 1984). However, Dias *et al.* (1987) concluded that the major determinant of functional outcome was the severity of the soft tissue injury. Certainly, it has been shown in patients over 60 years old that if the initial reduction is lost, remanipulation does not achieve a lasting improvement (McQueen *et al.*, 1986).

Although the general opinion is that Colles fractures do not produce the same morbidity as hip fractures, there is a definite functional impairment in Colles fractures, particularly those with significant displacement and soft tissue injury. Dias *et al.* (1987) found that the result was the same whether patients were mobilized early or late and in their study a poor functional result occurred in 10% of patients in both groups. Limitation of movement and weakness of the hand on the affected side are two important features of functional deficit in such patients. Other complications such as median nerve palsy and late rupture of extensor policus longus also occur in a small proportion of patients and recently there has been shown to be a significant morbidity in the form of algodystrophy. Atkins *et al.* (1990) showed that 37% of patients following Colles fractures had evidence of an algodystrophy, although this study assessed patients between two and six weeks after plaster removal and a significant proportion of these had some degree of recovery.

Thus, there is a significant morbidity in patients following Colles fractures in the short term. However, Colles fractures are still considered to have less long-term morbidity when compared with the two other major fractures of osteoporosis, namely vertebral and hip fractures. There are a proportion of patients who would appear to have a long-term functional impairment of their wrist and hand, but longer term studies are required to assess the size of the problem.

VERTEBRAL FRACTURES

The incidence of vertebral fractures increases after the menopause but unlike distal radial fractures, it continues to rise steadily beyond the age of 65.

As in the distal forearm, vertebral bodies contain large amounts of trabecular bone and the rate and timing of cortical and trabecular bone loss explain the pattern of fractures at these two sites and in the hip, with its later increased incidence (Nordin *et al.*, 1984).

Vertebral fractures are of the crush type occurring in the vertebral body. Up to half of vertebral fractures are asymptomatic and therefore are often detected late from radiographs. Lateral spinal radiographs remain the commonest method of determining the presence or absence of deformity of the vertebral bodies (Figure 18.2) although vertebral morphometry, such as with dual-energy X-

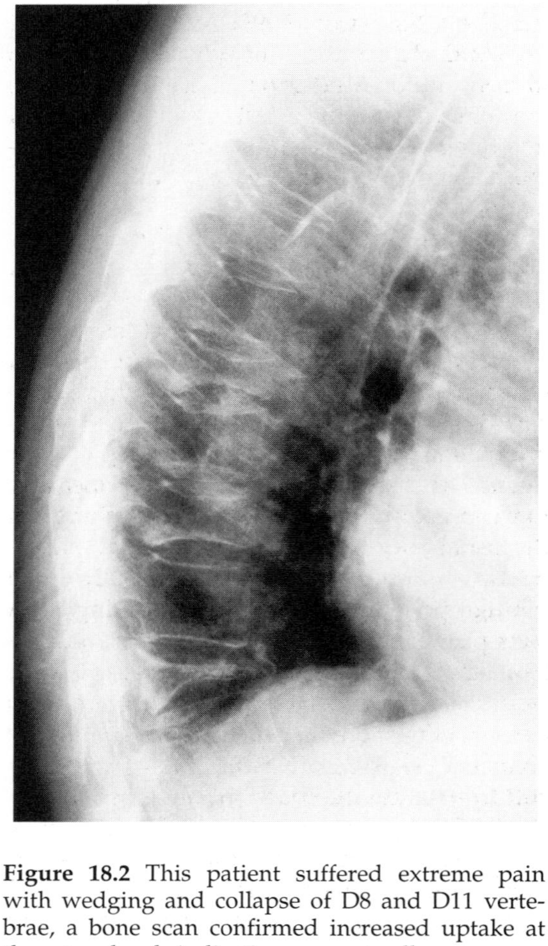

Figure 18.2 This patient suffered extreme pain with wedging and collapse of D8 and D11 vertebrae, a bone scan confirmed increased uptake at these two levels indicating a recent collapse.

ray absorptiometry, may become more widespread. Vertebral deformities are typically classified into one of three types: compression (collapse of the entire vertebral body), anterior wedge (collapse of the anterior border) and bioconcavity (collapse of the central portion of the body). However, there are some difficulties in classification because of the variation in normal vertebral body shape in different individuals and within individual spinal columns. Recent guidelines, however, suggest that prevalent deformities be defined on the basis of a reduction of three standard deviations or more from reference values of height ratios (National Osteoporosis Foundation Working Group on Vertebral Fractures, 1993). Other causes of vertebral deformities include Scheuerman's disease and osteoarthritis. These may confuse the clinical picture, but a triage system involving both subjective, radiological assessment and morphometry may improve the diagnosis.

The orthopaedic surgeon will meet vertebral osteoporosis with the acute vertebral fracture following minor trauma. In this situation, the clinical findings of local tenderness in conjunction with radiographs showing an obvious vertebral crush fracture at the corresponding level of tenderness leave little doubt about the diagnosis, although other causes of pathological fractures, especially metastatic disease, will need to be excluded in the usual way with a general clinical examination, routine serology and possibly bone scintigraphy. In the patient presenting with back pain in the absence of trauma, it may be less obvious that osteoporosis is present. Acute back pain has a large number of causes and in the absence of obvious vertebral abnormalities on plain radiographs, it is difficult to estimate the contribution of osteoporosis in this group of patients. Chronic back pain may be even more difficult to assess and it has been estimated that only 1–2% of all cases of chronic persistent back pain are caused by medical conditions, including metabolic diseases (Asherson, 1984). However, this probably does not truly reflect the contribution of vertebral fractures and osteoporosis to chronic back pain and recent studies have pointed out that subsequent deformities resulting from vertebral collapse may lead to chronic pain (Ettinger *et al.*, 1992). These authors showed that in vertebral osteoporosis 50.2% of individuals with evidence of severe vertebral deformity had lost 4 cm in height compared with 23% of those without deformity.

TREATMENT

The initial management of osteoporotic vertebral fractures is mainly concerned with pain control and rest. Spinal orthotic supports may have some part to play in the short-term or even long-term management but surgery is not usually regarded as a treatment option. The orthopaedic surgeon therefore has very little to contribute after the initial diagnosis compared with all those involved in rehabilitation.

Although vertebral fractures are common after the menopause, the morbidity in terms of chronic pain, spinal deformities with associated respiratory deficiency and abdominal compression is difficult to quantify. Unlike distal forearm and hip fractures, there is no surgery involved, with its attendant risks and economic costs. However, there is no doubt significant morbidity does occur following vertebral fractures and the initial management itself has been estimated as involving an average of two general practitioner consultations and two outpatient visits, resulting in a cost of between £170 and £420 per patient which does not, of course, consider any long-term treatment involving the physiotherapist and both pharmaceutical and community care costs (Vessey, M. personal communication). Also, it has been shown that women who have vertebral fractures have twice the expected risk of developing hip fractures in the future and there is a higher association with intertrochanteric fractures than femoral neck fractures (Katowitz *et al.*, 1994).

HIP FRACTURES

Hip fractures, including both intracapsular (subcapital and transcervical) and exracapsular (basicervical, intertrochanteric and subtrochanteric), represent the largest group of fractures associated with osteoporosis. They are the subject of a profusion of publications annually which reflects their major effect on orthopaedic practice and on patient morbidity and mortality.

The latest figures show that overall, in the United Kingdom alone, approximately 60 000 hip fractures occur each year (RCP, 1989). It has been estimated that the global load of hip fracture will treble to over 6 million cases a year by 2050 (Cooper *et al.*, 1992). In the United Kingdom, patients admitted to hospital with fractured femoral necks occupy 20% of all trauma and orthopaedic beds and 4% of beds in all specialties used by patients aged 65 and over (Robbins and Donaldson, 1984). Current trends show an increase in incidence of fractures of the femoral neck which is greater than that which might be expected as a result of the increasing number of elderly people in the population (Lewis, 1981; Boyce and Vessey, 1985).

Considerable resources are deployed in the management of patients with fractures of the proximal femur. The average length of hospital stay for hip fractures is 30 days. The cost of hip fractures varies from a minimum of £2230 to a maximum of £6210. Direct hospital costs of femoral neck fractures have been estimated at £160 million per year (Wallace, 1987). These economic considerations reflect the more important effects of proximal femoral fractures, namely a considerble morbidity and mortality. This morbidity and mortality may be affected by surgical management but comparative studies are few and far between.

TREATMENT

Astley Cooper first made a distinction between fractures of the femoral neck and other fractures about the hip, drawing attention to the loss of blood supply to the proximal fragment (Cooper, 1823) as the blood supply to the femoral head arises mainly from the circumflex vessels which enter at the head–neck junction through a vascular ring. Fractures at this level will interrupt the blood supply and affect the healing of such fractures (Trueta, 1957). The classification of hip fractures is therefore divided into two broad categories: intracapsular and extracapsular fractures. The potential complications of intracapsular fractures, namely non-union, avascular necrosis and instability, and of extracapsular fractures, namely malunion and instability, have influenced the treatment of each type of hip fracture.

In both groups of hip fractures, it has been recognized that delay in mobilization and rehabilitation increases the morbidity and mortality (Todd *et al.*, 1995). The surgical principle is to stabilize the fracture, thus enabling the patient to mobilize as soon as possible. As the two categories of hip fracture behave differently, this surgical management can be considered separately.

Intracapsular fractures

There have been several classifications of femoral neck fractures (Faltin, 1924; Pauwells, 1935) but Garden's classification (Garden, 1961), based on the degree of displacement, has been used most widely. Garden Stage 1 (incomplete), an impacted valgus fracture, is the only fracture where non-operative treatment has been advocated but the possibility of disimpaction (Crawford, 1960) and lower union rate in this non-operated group compared with operated cases (Bentley, 1968) suggest that even these fractures are best treated surgically.

The surgical methods of treating intracapsular fractures are influenced by the likelihood of disruption of the blood supply and, if this occurs, the potential for revascularization. These two possible complications of a fractured femoral neck may lead to avascular necrosis or non-union, but are less likely to occur when the fracture itself is undisplaced or minimally displaced. The incidence of avascular necrosis in impacted (Garden 1) fractures was 14% and 18% in conservative and operative cases respectively in Bentley's series. This contrasts with displaced fractures where the incidence of avascular necrosis may be as high as 35% (Massey, 1973). The small volume of osteoporotic bone in the femoral head makes internal fixation of this fracture difficult. The risk of losing the reduction with a relatively large triflanged nail, as advocated by Smith-Petersen *et al.* (1931), has been considerably reduced by the use of small screws or pins (Moore, 1934; Knowles, 1936; Deyerle, 1959), telescoping nails and screws to allow the fracture to stabilize (Pugh, 1955; Massey, 1958; Badgley, 1960; Clawson; 1964) and more recently compression screws or cannulated lag screws. Various fixation devices are inserted by visualizing the fracture and the position of the implant in the head of a femur with the use of an image intensifier. This reduces the surgical trauma which would be necessary if the fracture and the hip joint itself were to be exposed.

Patients are carefully positioned on a special fracture table which enables traction to be applied to the affected leg and reduction of the fracture to be achieved. The patient's sacrum rests on a narrow support and the patient's buttocks are effectively suspended between the sacral support and the foot support, thus allowing access for the image intensifier to view the hip fracture in both the AP and lateral planes (Figure 18.3). The C arm of the image intensifier is thus repeatedly swung through 90° to allow correct positioning of the implant within the femoral head. Modern biplanar image intensifiers have two X-ray tubes set at 90° to each other and it is possible to achieve instantaneous positioning of the implant in two planes which reduces operating time. Thus reduction with impaction and rigid fixation can be achieved (Figure 18.4).

Despite the numerous modifications of implants and the use of fluoroscopy techniques, loss of reduction, non-union and avascular necrosis continue to occur such that the reoperation rate remains a problem with this type of treatment, particularly with displaced fractures.

The alternative surgical management of the displaced femoral neck fracture is to abandon any attempt at fixation and to replace the head with a femoral prosthesis. This allows early mobilization and has been advocated for all elderly patients with such fractures (D'Arcy and Devas, 1976). Although this method of treatment avoids the complications of internal fixation, it has its own complications, including dislocation of the prosthesis, deep wound infection and in the longer term prosthetic loosening and acetabular erosion.

The early femoral prostheses used for replacement of the femoral head were introduced by Moore and Bohlam (1943), Moore (1957) and Thompson (1965). These early cementless designs were introduced following the development of a chrome cobalt alloy, vitalium. The introduction of cement has reduced the loosening rate (Mears and Creuss, 1973) and dislocation has also been reduced with the anterolateral approach (Devas and Hinves, 1983). Another reported complication with femoral head replacement hemiarthroplasty is acetabular erosion (D'Arcy and Devas, 1976). However, this complication has been reduced using a bipolar prosthesis with a dynamic self-aligning outer head (Devas and Hinves, 1983).

There is still no firm agreement on whether internal fixation or the use of a hemiarthroplasty is less hazardous or has a greater success rate in terms of rehabilitation and early mobilization. Sikorski and

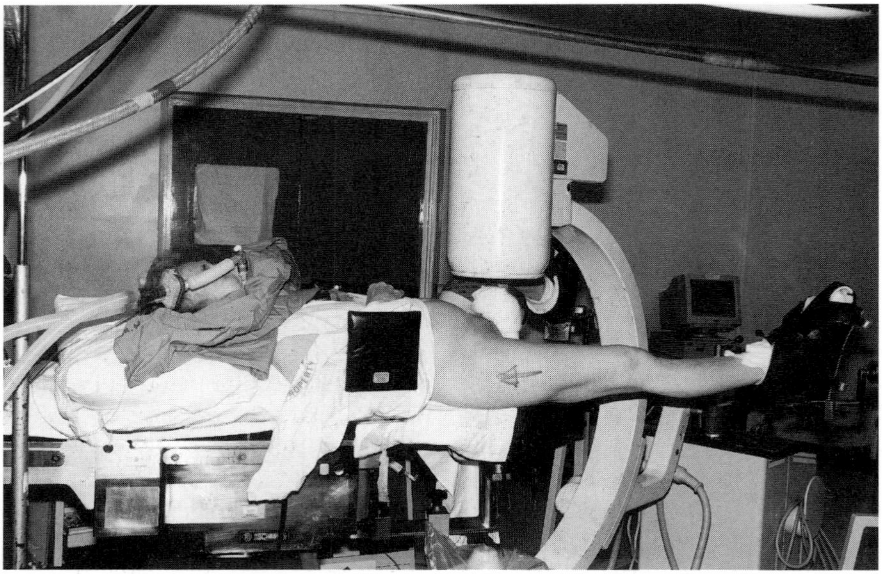

(a)

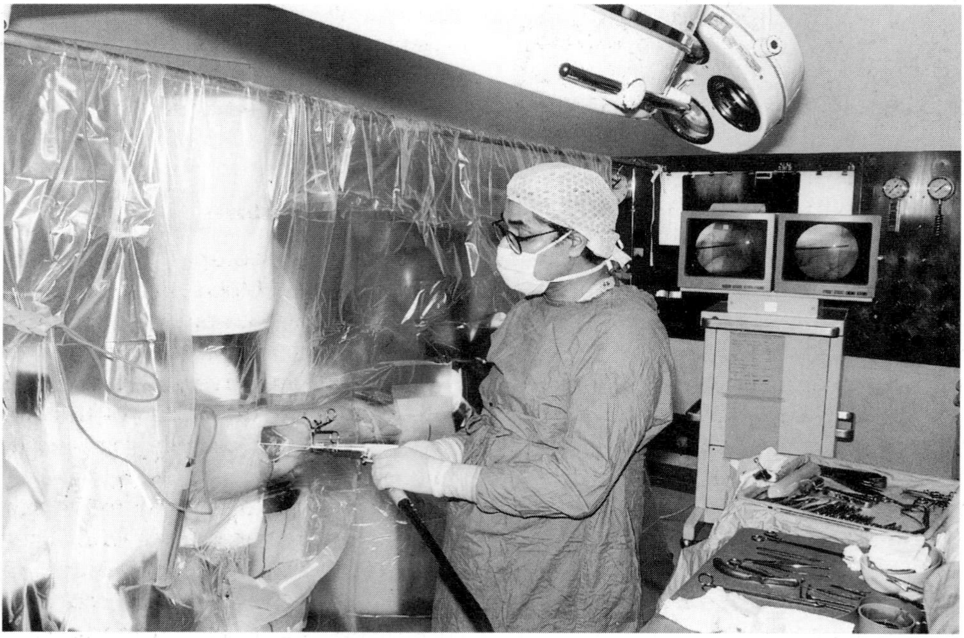

(b)

Figure 18.3 (a) Patient on a fracture table with the image intensifier in position to view the hip in an AP plane. (b) Surgeon inserting a guidewire into the neck of the femur. He can check the position by using the monitor behind him.

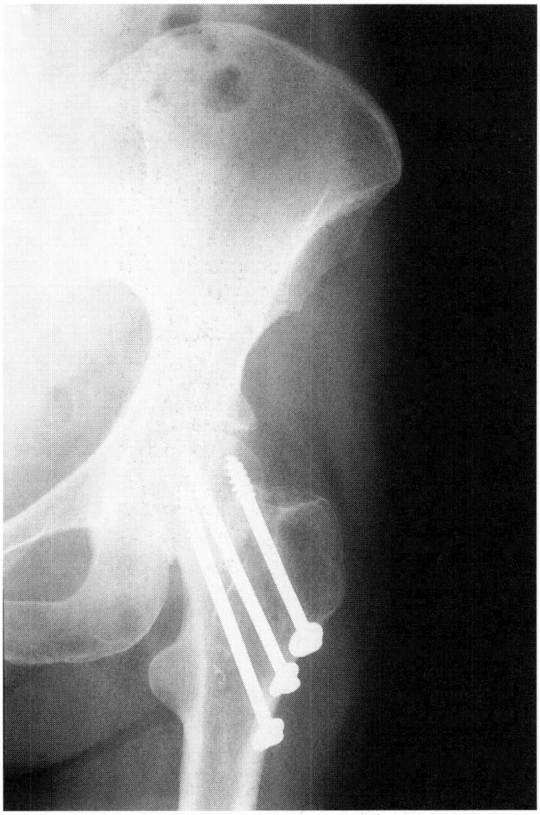

Figure 18.4 An X-ray of a subcapital fracture internally fixed with screws. This fracture in a 63-year-old was not anatomically reduced but still united with no complications.

Barrington (1981), in one of the few prospective randomized studies of internal fixation versus hemiarthroplasty, showed a significant difference in the mortality of the internal fixation and posterior arthroplasty groups, compared with the anterolateral arthroplasty group. These two authors studied patients over 70 with Garden Stage 3 and Stage 4 subcapital femoral neck fractures and randomly selected patients for reduction and internal fixation or hemiarthroplasty using the posterior approach and hemiarthroplasty using the anterolateral approach. The latter group was shown to have a lower mortality such that the authors concluded that a Thompson hemiarthroplasty using an anterolateral approach was the safest operation in this group. Other authors have suggested that hemiarthroplasty is a less safe alternative to internal fixation (Hunter, 1969, 1974) but in these studies the analyses were retrospective.

Another alternative treatment for more active younger patients with Stage 3 and 4 fractures is to perform a primary total hip arthroplasty (Coates and Armour, 1980). This avoids the complication of acetabular erosion but compared with total hip arthroplasty in a standard group of patients with degenerative joint disease as a reason for their operation, the results were disappointing with over half failing at an average follow-up of just under five years (Greenhough and Jones, 1988).

It is probably a good general principle that in a well-aligned and stabilized subcapital fracture internal fixation is preferred to replacement of the femoral head with an implant, but in the older age group (over 70) with displaced subcapital fracture, hemiarthroplasty appears to be the safest operation.

Extracapsular fractures

These fractures occur in cancellous bone which has a good blood supply and avascular necrosis and non-union are therefore not a problem. An extracapsular fracture will unite if treated conservatively but the displaced fractures, even with the use of traction techniques, will tend to unite in varus with shortening.

The same principles apply to the treatment of extracapsular fractures as with intracapsular fractures and early mobilization and rehabilitation are the main objectives which reduce both morbidity and mortality. This is achieved by internal fixation. The main complication of this treatment is loss of reduction, with failure of the implant by penetration of the femoral head by the implant or the implant cutting through the osteoporotic cancellous bone of the head and neck. As with subcapital fractures, the stable intertrochanteric fracture can be treated with a number of different devices all yielding satisfactory results (Cleveland *et al.*, 1959; Dimon and Hughston, 1967; Holt, 1963; Sarmiento and Williams, 1970). However, in the unstable fracture, failure of the implant may occur and even with sliding screw devices (Figure 18.5) failure rates of 5–10% have been reported (Jensen *et al.*, 1978; Kyle *et al.*, 1979; Wolfgang *et al.*, 1982; Bannister *et al.*, 1983). Surgical stabilization other than with anatomical reduction has been advocated to reduce the incidence of failure of a fixation device used. These include medial displacement (Dimon and Hughston, 1967), valgus osteotomy (Sarmiento and Williams, 1970) or the precise placement of the implant which has been recommended as being ideally located centrally in the femoral head (Mulholland and Gunn, 1972; Davis *et al.*, 1990) or posteriorly placed (Laskin *et al.*, 1979). Other devices have been designed such as the Kuntschner Y-nail (Cuthbert and Howat, 1976) and similar implants which avoid a side plate and potential failure at the junction of the plate and sliding screw. However, there still remain a number of comminuted fractures in very osteoporotic bone that will not allow early weight bearing and rehabilitation may be prolonged.

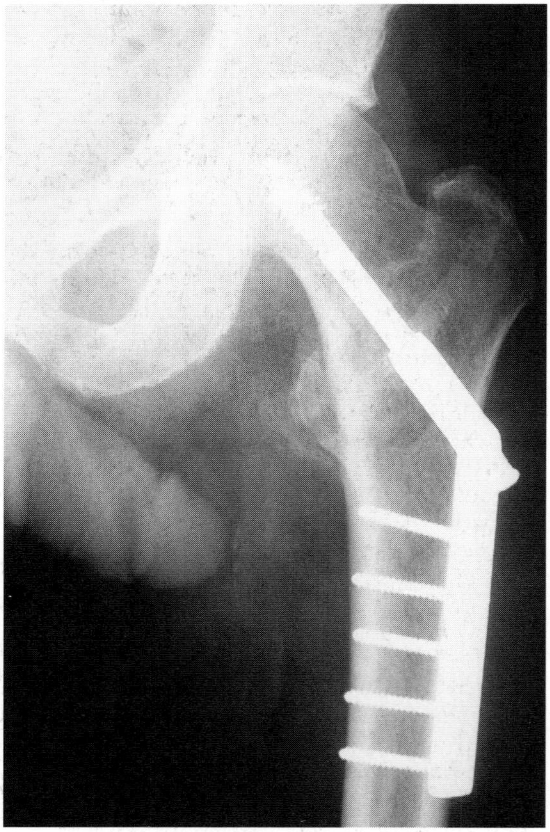

Figure 18.5 An inter-trochanteric fracture internally fixed with a dynamic hip screw and a plate.

Despite the improvements in surgical management and design of implants in the treatment of both types of hip fracture, there remains a high morbidity and mortality. Many elderly patients already have medical conditions which influence the clinical management and prognosis. Coexisting cardiovascular and respiratory disorders may cause delay in surgery while these are corrected and disorders of the locomotor and central nervous system will influence rehabilitation. Holmberg and Thorngren (1987) found that 50% of patients admitted to hospital with fractures of the proximal femur had at least one comorbidity. In a recent multicentre study in the United Kingdom 74% of patients had recorded pre-existing clinical problems (Todd *et al.*, 1995). In another study an impaired mental state correlated closely with survival (Barnes *et al.*, 1976; Gouke, 1985), and its effect on outcome has been shown to be more important than age. Other factors influencing the outcome of hip fractures are existing functional ability and physical mobility. In a study of 1503 cases of fractured necks of femur Barnes *et al.* (1976) found that, at one month postoperation, 1.9% of women who were fully active before operation had died compared with 21.4% of bedridden women. For men the prognosis was even worse, with 7.8% mortality of those fully active before operation and 50% for those bedridden.

The type of fracture also seems to influence the prognosis, with extracapsular fractures carrying a worse prognosis than intracapsular fractures (Lawton *et al.*, 1983). This may be explained by the evidence which suggests that the ratio of extracapsular to intracapsular fracture increased with age and those who have extracapsular fractures have a poorer physical status and are less mobile prefracture than those who have an intracapsular fracture (Lawton *et al.*, 1983; Aitken, 1984). Another factor affecting the outcome of fractured neck of femur is the length of time between sustaining the fracture, admission to hospital and subsequent surgical treatment. Immediately following the injury patients are immobile and may lie for long periods of time in their own homes, either in bed or on the floor, and not only develop pressure sores but also become confused and dehydrated as well as developing hypostatic-pneumonic changes. A long delay in seeking attention may also lead to an exacerbation of existing medical conditions, a worse clinical state on admission and hence a poor prognosis. Villar *et al.* (1986) showed a significant difference in rehabilitation in three months for those having a short compared with a long operative delay and Todd *et al.* (1995), in a study investigating differences between hospitals in clinical management of patients admitted with a fractured hip, showed a significant difference in mortality in 90 days among the different hospitals. Although no single factor accounted for this, a low mortality was thought to be associated with the accumulative effect of several aspects of the organization of treatment and management of the fracture of the hip, including antibiotic prophylaxis and early mobilization. Thromboembolic pharmaceutical prophylaxis was also thought to influence the morbidity and mortality although it was difficult to differentiate between this factor and early mobilization. The current opinion on the management of hip fractures is that the earlier the fracture is detected and internally fixed with the appropriate surgical techniques, the earlier the mobilization and rehabilitation. This will reduce the morbidity and mortality which still remain a considerable problem.

Whilst orthopaedic surgeons continue to struggle to cope with what is becoming an avalanche of all osteoporotic fractures, hip fractures in particular continue to cause concern despite the improvement of surgical management and the more aggressive approach to mobilization and rehabilitation. Only a reduction in the incidence of osteoporosis can possibly stem this tide of patients. Therefore, it is imperative that research into reduction or even cure of this condition be continued.

REFERENCES

Aitken, J.M. (1984) Relevance of osteoporosis in women with fracture of the femoral neck. *Br Med J* **288**: 597–601.

Atkins, R.M., Duckworth, T. and Kanis, J.A (1990) Algodystrophy following Colles fracture. *J Bone Joint Surg* **723**: 105–10.

Bacorn, R.W. and Kurtkze, J.F. (1953) Colles fracture: a study of two thousand cases from the New York State Workman's Compensation Board. *J Bone Joint Surg (Am)* **35a**: 643–58.

Badgley, C.E. (1960) Fractures of the hip joint, some causes for failure, and suggestions for success. A.A.O.S. *Instructional Course Lectures* **17**: 106.

Bannister, G.C., Gibson, A.G.F. and Jewett (1983) Nail plate or A.O. dynamic hip screw for trochanteric fractures? A randomised prospective controlled trial. *J Bone Joint Surg (Br)* **65b**: 218

Barnes, R., Brown, J.T., Garden, R.S. and Nicoll, E.A. (1976) Sub-capital fracture of the femur: a prospective review. *J Bone Joint Surg* **58b**: 2–24.

Bentley, G. (1968) Impacted fractures of the neck of femur. *J Bone Joint Surg* **50b**: 551–61.

Boyce, W.J. and Vessey, M.P. (1985) Rising incidence of fractures of the proximal femur. *Lancet* **i**: 150–1.

Case, R.D. (1985) Haematoma – a safe method of reducing Colles fractures. *Injury J* **16**: 469–70.

Clancey, G.J. (1984) Percutaneous Kirchner-wire fixation of Colles fractures. *J Bone Joint Surg (Am)* **66**: 1008–14.

Clawson, D.K. (1964) Intra-capsular fractures of the femur treated by the sliding screw plate fixation method. *J Trauma* **4**: 753–6.

Cleveland, M., Bosworth, D.M., Thompson, F.G., Wilson, H.J. and Ishizukat (1959) A ten year analysis of intra-trochanteric fractures of the femur. *J Bone Joint Surg* **41a**: 1399–409.

Coates, R.L. and Armour, P. (1980) Treatment of sub-capital femoral fractures by primary total hip replacement. *Injury* **11**: 132–5.

Compston, J.E., Mellish, R.W., Garrahan, N.J. *et al.* (1989) Structural mechanisms of trabecular bone loss in man. *Bone Mineral* **6**: 331–8.

Coney, W.P., Linscheid, R.L. and Dobyns, J.H. (1979) External pin fixation for unstable Colles fractures. *J Bone Joint Surg (Am)* **61**: 840–5.

Cooper, A.P. (1823) *A Treatise on Dislocations and Fractures of the Joints*, 2nd edn, Longman Hunt, London.

Cooper, C., Camplin, G. and Melton, L.J. (1992) Hip fractures in the elderly: a worldwide projection. *Osteoporosis Int* **2**: 285–9.

Crawford, H.B. (1960) Conservative treatment of impacted fractures of the femoral neck. *J Bone Joint Surg* **42a**: 471–9.

Currey, J.D. (1975) The effects of strain rate, reconstruction, and mineral content on some mechanical properties of bovine bone. *J Biomech* **8**: 81.

Cuthbert, H. and Howat, T.W. (1976) The use of the Kuntschner Y-nail in the treatment of intertrochanteric and subtrochanteric fractures of the femur. *Injury* **8**: 135–42.

D'Arcy, J. and Devas, M. (1976) Treatment of fractures of the femoral neck by replacement with the Thompson prosthesis. *J Bone Joint Surg (Br)* **58b**: 279–86.

Davis, T.R.C., Sher, L., Horsman, A. *et al.* (1990) Intertrochanteric fractures: mechanical failure after internal fixation. *J Bone Joint Surg (Br)* **72b**: 26–31.

Devas, M. and Hinves, B. (1983) Prevention of acetabular erosion after hemi-arthroplasty for fractured neck of femur. *J Bone Joint Surg* **65b**: 548–51.

Deyerle, W.M. (1959) Absolute fixation with contact compression in hip fractures. *Clin Orthop* **13**: 279–97.

Dias, J.J., Wray, C.C. and Jones, J.M. (1987) Osteoporosis and Colles fractures in the elderly. *J Hand Surg* (Br) **12**: 57–9.

Dimon, A.H. and Hughston, J.C. (1967) Unstable intra-trochanteric fractures of the hip. *J Bone Joint Surg* **49a**: 400–50.

Ettinger, B., Black, D.M. and Nevitt, M.C. (1992) Contribution of vertebral deformities to chronic back pain and disability. *J Bone Miner Res* **7**: 449–56.

Faltin, R. (1924) The classification of the factors of the upper portion of the femur. *Acta Orthop Scand* **57**: 1–9.

Garden, R.S. (1961) Low angle fixation in fractures of the femoral neck. *J Bone Joint Surg (Br)* **43b**: 647–63.

Gartland Jr, J.J. and Werley, C.W. (1951) Evaluation of healed Colles fractures. *J Bone Joint Surg (Am)* **33a**: 895–907.

Golden, G.N. (1963) Treatment and prognosis of Colles fracture. *Lancet* **i**: 511–15.

Gouke, C.R. (1985) Mortality following surgery for fractures of the neck of femur. *Anaesthesia* **40**: 578–83.

Greenhough, C.G. and Jones, J.R. (1988) Primary and total hip replacement for displaced sub-capital fracture of the femur. *J Bone Joint Surg* **70b**: 639–43.

Holmberg, S. and Thorngren, K.G. (1987) Statistical analysis of femoral neck fractures based on 3053 cases. *Clin Orthop Rel Res* **218**: 32–46.

Holt, E.P. (1963) Hip fractures in the trochanteric region: treatment with a strong nail and early weight bearing. *J Bone Joint Surg* **45a**: 681–705.

Hunter, G.A. (1969) A comparison of the use of internal fixation and prosthetic replacement for fresh fractures of the neck of the femur. *Br J Surg* **56**: 229–32.

Hunter, G.A. (1974) A comparison of the use of internal fixation and prosthetic replacement for fresh fracture of the neck of the femur. *Br J Surg* **61**: 382–4.

Jensen, J.S., Tøndevolde, E. and Mossing, N. (1978) Unstable trochanteric fractures treated with the sliding plate system: a biomechanical study of unstable trochanteric fractures. *Acta Orthop Scand* **49**: 392–7.

Katowitz, M.A., Melton III, L.J., Cooper, C. *et al.* (1994) Risk of hip fracture in women with vertebral fractures. *J Bone Miner Res* **9**: 599–605.

Knowles, F.L. (1936) Fractures of the neck of femur. *Wisconsin Med* **35**: 106–9.

Kyle, R.F., Gustilo, R.B. and Premar, R.F. (1979)

Analysis of 622 trochanteric fractures: a retrospective and prospective study. *J Bone Joint Surg (Am)* **61a**: 216–21.

Laskin, R.S., Grüberm, A. and Zimmerman, A.J. (1979) Intertrochanteric fractures in the hip in the elderly: a retrospective analysis of 236 cases. *Clin Orthop* **141**: 188–95.

Lawton, J.O., Baker, M.R. and Dixon, R.A. (1983) Femoral neck fractures – two populations. *Lancet* **ii**: 70–2.

Lewis, A.F. (1981) Fracture of neck of femur: changing incidence. *Br Med J* **283**: 1217–20.

McQueen, M.M., MacLaren, A. and Charmers, J. (1986) The value of re-manipulating Colles fractures. *J Bone Joint Surg (Br)* **68**: 232–3.

Massey, W.K. (1958) Functional fixation of femoral neck fractures; telescoping nail technique. *Clin Orthop* **12**: 230–55.

Massey, W.K. (1973) Treatment of femoral neck fractures emphasising longterm follow-up observations on aseptic necrosis. *Clin Orthop* **92**: 16–62.

Mears, T.S. and Creuss, R.L. (1973) Evaluation of the use of acrylic cement in anchoring medullary stem femoral head prosthesis in the hip. Proceedings of the First Open Scientific Meeting of the Hip Society, St Louis, C.V. Mosby, p. 137.

Moore, A.T. (1934) Fractures of the hip joint (intracapsular): a new method of skeletal fixation. *J S Carolina Med Ass* **30**: 119–205.

Moore, A.T. (1957) The self-locking metal hip prosthesis. *J Bone and Joint Surg* **39a**: 811–27.

Moore, A.T. and Bohlam, H.R. (1943) Metal hip joint – a case report. *J Bone Joint Surg* **25**: 688–93.

Mulholland, R.C. and Gunn, D.R. (1972) Sliding screw fixation of intertrochanteric femoral fractures. J *Trauma* **12**: 581–91.

Müller, M.E., Allgöwer, M., Schneider, R. and Villenerer, H. (eds) (1979) The A.O. buttress plate for fracture of the distal radius, In: *Manual of Internal Fixation*, Springer-Verlag, Berlin, pp. 196–7.

National Osteoporosis Foundation Working Group on Vertebral Fractures (1993) Assessing Vertebral Fractures, Osteoporosis Foundation, Washington, D.C.

Nguyen, T., Sambrook, P., Kelly, P. *et al.* (1993) Prediction of osteoporotic fractures by postural instability and bone density. *Br Med J* **307**: 1111–14.

Nordin, B.E.C., Crilly, R.G. and Smith, D.A. (1984) Osteoporosis. In *Metabolic Bone and Disease*, (ed. Nordin, B.E.C.) Churchill Livingstone, Edinburgh, pp. 1–7..

Owen, R.A., Melton, L.J., Johnson, K.A., Ilstrup, D.M. and Riggs, B.L. (1982) Incidence of Colles fractures in a North American community. *Am J Public Health* **72**: 605–7.

Pauwells, F. (1935) Der Schenkel Halsbruck ein Mechanischs Problem Grendlagen Des Heilungsvorganges Prognose und Kausale Therapie. Ferdinand Enke Verlag, Stuttgart.

Pool, C. (1973) Colles fracture: a prospective study of treatment *J Bone Joint Surg (Br)* **55b**: 540–4.

Pope, M.H. and Outwater, J.O. (1974) Mechanical properties of bone as a function of position and orientation. *J Biomech* **7**: 61.

Pugh, W.L. (1955) A self-adjusting nail plate for fractures about the hip joint. *J Bone Joint Surg* **37a**: 1085–93.

Reilly, D.T. and Burstein, A.H. (1975) The elastic and ultimate properties of compact bone tissue. *J Biomech* **8**: 393.

Robbins, J.A. and Donaldson, L.J. (1984) Analysing stages of care in hospital stay for fractured neck of femur. *Lancet* **ii**: 1028–9.

Royal College of Phsyicians (1989) Fractured neck of femur, prevention and management. Summary and recommendations of a report from the Royal College of Physicians. *J R Coll Phys Lond* **23**: 8–12.

Sarmiento, A., Pratt, G.W., Bury, N.C. and Sinclair, W.F. (1975) Colles fractures: functional bracing in supination. *J Bone Joint Surg (Am)* **57a**: 311–17.

Sarmiento, A. and Williams, E.M. (1970) The unstable intertrochanteric fracture: treatment with a valgus osteotomy and I-beam nail-plate. *J Bone Joint Surg* **52**: 1309–18.

Seeley, D.G., Browner, W.S., Nevitt, N.C. *et al.* and the Study of Osteoporosis Research Group (1991) Which fractures are associated with low appendicular bone mass in elderly women? *Ann Intern Med* **115**: 837–43.

Sikorski, J.M. and Barrington, R. (1981) Internal fixation versus hemi-arthroplasty for the displaced sub-capital fracture of the femur. *J Bone Joint Surg* **63b**: 357–61.

Smale, G.B. (1965) Longterm follow-up of Colles fractures. *J Bone Joint Surg (Br)* **47b**: 85.

Smith-Peterson, M.N., Cave, E.F. and van Gorder, W. (1931) Intra-capsular fracture of the neck of the femur. *Arch Surg* **23**: 715–59.

Stuart, H.D., Innes, A.R. and Burke, F.D. (1984) Functional cast-bracing for Colles fractures: a comparison between case-bracing and conventional plaster casts. *J Bone Joint Surg (Br)* **66b**: 749–53.

Thompson, F.R. (1965) Indications and contra-indications for the early use of an intra-medullary hip prosthesis. *Clin Orthop* **6**: 9–16.

Todd, C.J., Frieman, C.J., Camilleri-Ferrante, C. *et al.* (1995) Difference in mortality after fractures of the hip: The East-Anglian Audit. *Br Med J* **310**: 904–8.

Trueta, J. (1957) Appraisal of the vascular factor in the healing of fractures of the femoral neck. *J Bone Joint Surg* **39b**: 3–5.

Van der Linden, W. and Ericksen, R. (1981) Colles fracture: how should its displacement be measured and how should it be mobilised? *J Bone Joint Surg (Am)* **63a**: 1285–8.

Vesterby, A., Mosekilde, L., Gunderson, H.J. *et al.* (1991) Biologically meaningful determinants of the *in vitro* strength of lumbar vertebrae. *Bone* **12**: 219–24.

Villar, R.N., Allen, S.M. and Barnes, S.J. (1986) Hip fractures in healthy patients: operative delay versus prognosis. *Br Med J* **293**: 1203–4.

Wall, J.C., Chatterji, S. and Jeffrey, J.W. (1972) Human femoral cortical bone: a preliminary report on the relationship between strength and density. *Med Biol Eng* **10**: 673.

Wallace, W.A. (1987) The scale and financial implications of osteoporosis. *Int Med* **12** (Suppl): 3–4.

Wright, T.M. and Hayes, W.C. (1976) Tensile testing of a bone over a wide range of strain rates: effects of strain rate, microstructure and density. *Med Biol Eng* **14**: 671.

Wolfgang, G.L., Bryant, M.H. and O'Neill, J.P. (1982) Treatment of intertrochanteric fractures of the femur using sliding screw plate fixation. *Clin Orthop* **163**: 148–58.

FUTURE STRATEGIES FOR OSTEOPOROSIS

19

G.R. Mundy

INTRODUCTION

There is no totally satisfactory and universally acceptable treatment for established osteoporosis. This is the reason why pharmaceutical companies have been spending millions of dollars in the search for better modalities of treatment than those available. The task is not easy. There are special problems associated with osteoporosis research which have made the search for new treatments very difficult. A number of special questions which have haunted investigators and to which there are no clear satisfactory answers currently include: Is bone loss in patients with osteoporosis irreversible? Can aging bone cells respond to drug therapy? Is bone architecture irreversibly destroyed in patients with osteoporosis? Are there suitable *in vivo* animal models for evaluating new drugs? Although there are no totally convincing and definitive answers to any of these questions, there is nevertheless reason for optimism. Bone growth can be stimulated in the elderly, as treatment with fluoride and the observation that fracture healing does occur in the elderly, which requires the normal osteoblast function, demonstrate.

Possibly the major problem which bedevils researchers involved in the search for better treatments is the complexities of the biology involved. In order to understand the pathophysiology of osteoporosis, we need to understand the control mechanisms that regulate the normal bone-remodeling process. Bone remodeling takes place in discrete packets throughout the skeleton, known as bone structural units or bone-remodeling units (Hattner *et al.*, 1965; Parfitt, 1979; Mundy, 1990, 1995a). These packets of bone remodeling occur on cancellous bone surfaces in intimate contact with the cellular constituents of the bone marrow cavity and within the Haversian canals which tunnel through cortical bone and which are probably influenced more by systemic factors than the cells on cancellous bone surfaces. The cellular sequence of events is the same whether it occurs on cancellous bone surfaces or in Haversian systems. It begins with osteoclastic bone resorption and concludes with the formation of new bone by bone-forming osteoblasts to replace the packet of bone which has been removed by the activity of osteoclasts. Bone resorption and bone formation rates are balanced in healthy young adults.

Osteoporosis, whether in the younger postmenopausal woman or in the elderly, is due to an imbalance between the processes of bone formation and bone resorption, so that there is a relative increase in resorption over

Osteoporosis. Edited by John C. Stevenson and Robert Lindsay. Published in 1998 by Chapman & Hall, London.
ISBN 0 412 48870 1

formation and the result is progressive bone loss. At different stages in the disease, the primary abnormality may be different. For example, in the immediate postmenopausal period, there is an absolute increase in osteoclastic bone resorption due to estrogen deficiency, whereas in the elderly there is an impairment in osteoblast vigor associated with a decrease in mean wall thickness and bone formation. The important consideration is that these pathogenetic factors (estrogen withdrawal and aging) are superimposed on the normal bone-remodeling sequence to cause the imbalance between resorption and formation.

An excellent experimental example of the normal remodeling sequence is seen when interleukin-1 is studied *in vivo* in rodents (Boyce *et al.*, 1989). Interleukin-1 (IL-1) is a powerful stimulator of osteoclastic bone resorption. (Similar effects would be expected from estrogen withdrawal; in fact, one of the hypotheses for the bone-resorbing effects of estrogen withdrawal is through stimulation of IL-1 production by monocytes.) As a result of three days of IL-1 injections, there is a profound increase in osteoclastic bone resorption which lasts through a period of approximately one week. This is followed by a phase of new bone formation. Osteoclast activity ceases and the packets of bone which have been resorbed by the activity of osteoclasts are replaced by new hyperactive bone-forming osteoblasts. At the end of four weeks, all of the bone which has been removed by the osteoclasts is replaced by osteoblasts.

In addition to the complexities of the bone biology, there are other facets of osteoporosis which make the search for new agents particularly difficult. The heterogenous pathophysiologic nature of the disorder is a major problem. Osteoporosis can be exacerbated by multiple factors which have varying effects on resorption and formation. Osteoporosis is due to a combination of an inadequate peak bone mass associated with accelerated loss of bone mass after midlife. The accelerated loss after midlife may be accentuated by the menopause and by aging, but also by sporadic factors such as alcohol, smoking, certain drugs such as corticosteroids, inadequate calcium nutrition and immobilization. All of these factors have varying effects on rates of resorption and formation, but all favor a relative imbalance between resorption and formation. Another pathophysiologic problem is the marked disturbance in bone architecture which occurs in patients with osteoporosis (Kleerekoper *et al.*, 1985). Osteoporosis is a disorder not just of decreased bone mass but also of a disturbance in bone architecture. Bone is lost from cancellous bone surfaces by increased osteoclastic bone resorption and in time, fragmentation of the horizontal struts occurs with subsequent loss of these struts. This not only markedly impairs the structural integrity of the bone, but also removes the foundations or building blocks on which new bone formation can occur. It has long been debated whether these changes are irreversible and whether bone-stimulatory agents could produce any beneficial effects once this stage has been reached.

These problems notwithstanding, there are four general approaches which have been applied to the therapy of osteoporosis. These are:

1. inhibition of osteoclastic bone resorption;
2. stimulation of bone formation;
3. combination therapy, using agents which inhibit resorption and stimulate formation;
4. coherence therapy or the ADFR approach.

These different approaches will now be considered individually.

RESORPTION INHIBITORS

There are three major therapies which cause inhibition of osteoclastic bone resorption which are used in osteoporosis. These are estrogen, calcitonin and bisphosphonates. At this point in time, only estrogen and calcitonin have been approved by the FDA for use in osteoporosis. All of these drugs inhibit bone resorption and all are fairly effective in this regard. However, for a number of reasons, it is clear that we should aim for better drugs than those currently available. These drugs are not universally acceptable. Estrogens have a large share of the therapeutic market in postmenopausal women in the United States, but are culturally unacceptable in Japan. In contrast, calcitonin has an enormous worldwide market, but a relatively small share of the US market. Even those patients in whom estrogens are not contraindicated for other reasons frequently will not comply with estrogen therapy. There are other problems associated with the use of these agents. With the exception of calcitonin, we do not understand how they work. There are many theories for estrogen's inhibitory effect on osteoclastic bone resorption including both direct and indirect effects on osteoclasts. It has only recently been shown that osteoclasts contain estrogen receptors (Oursler *et al.*, 1991). Whether these will turn out to be responsible for the major effects of estrogen to inhibit osteoclastic bone resorption remains unclear. Estrogen may exert its beneficial effects on osteoclastic bone resorption indirectly by influencing the production of growth factors or osteotropic cytokines by bone cells or mononuclear cells (Pacifici *et al.*, 1987, 1989; Girasole *et al.*, 1992). There is a body of evidence which suggests that estrogens can influence the release of IL-1 by monoctyes (Pacifici *et al.*, 1987, 1989) and *in vitro* evidence which suggests that estrogen can enhance the production of transforming growth factor β and insulin-like growth factor 1 (Keeting *et al.*, 1989; Ernst *et al.*, 1989; Ernst and Rodan, 1991).

More recently, estrogens have been shown to have inhibitory effects on the production of IL-6 by cells with the osteoblast phenotype. Jilka *et al.* (1992) have shown that neutralizing antibodies to IL-6 can prevent the loss of bone which is associated with estrogen withdrawal in mice. Manolagas and Jilka (1995) have suggested that IL-6 and the GP-130 signal transduction mechanism play a critical role in both bone resorption and bone formation during normal bone remodeling. Any one or several of these mechanisms of action may be important when estrogens are administered to women after the menopause.

Bisphosphonates are very effective inhibitors of osteoclastic bone resorption and their usefulness in the management of osteoporosis has now been convincingly demonstrated (Liberman *et al.*, 1995). We do not understand how the bisphosphonates exert their inhibitory effects on bone resorption but current theories suggest that their major effects may be extracellular (Sato *et al.*, 1991). They may bind to bone surfaces and be present at resorbing sites where they are released to inactivate the osteoclasts locally (Blair *et al.*, 1989). Recently, it has been claimed that they may exert inhibitory effects on osteoclasts by inhibiting the action of a protein-tyrosine phosphatase involved in osteoclast function (Schmidt *et al.*, 1996). Hughes *et al.* (1995) have shown that bisphosphonates enhance osteoclast apoptosis both *in vitro* and *in vivo*. It is well established that they are retained in bone and may be released from bone slowly over prolonged periods. Because of their powerful inhibitory effects on bone remodeling, they could 'freeze' the skeleton. Rogers *et al.* (1997) have suggested that at least some of the bisphosphonates inhibit key enzymes such as farnesyl transferase and squalene synthase in the cholesterol biosynthesis pathway, and this may be responsible for bisphosphonate action.

There is another problem with the use of resorption inhibitors for osteoporosis. If their effects are simply to inhibit resorption and not stimulate formation, then they may be expected to stabilize bone mass but not to increase it (Mundy, 1995a). In fact, most studies suggest that the effects of inhibitors of bone resorption on bone mass are to maintain it constant rather than to increase it substantially. There is some evidence that in rodents estrogens may stimulate bone formation so this issue is not entirely resolved. Nevertheless, with the information currently available, if these resorption inhibitors do in fact have a stimulatory effect on bone formation it appears to be fairly minor and it is unlikely that these drugs will increase bone mass substantially unless they are used in conjunction with other agents.

For all of these reasons, it is reasonable to continue to search for better and more effective resorption inhibitors. To date, most resorption inhibitors that have been identified have been found by serendipity to inhibit osteoclastic bone resorption. However, as we understand more of the molecular mechanisms involved in osteoclastic bone resorption, then it may be possible to design rational therapeutic agents. For example, many of the molecular mechanisms involved in the process of osteoclastic bone resorption have recently been clarified. It is known that the attachment of osteoclasts to mineralized matrix is an essential component of the resorption process. This occurs presumably through integrin receptors on the osteoclasts (Horton and Davies, 1989). Antagonists to RGD sequences can inhibit osteoclast attachment and bone resorption (Helfrich *et al.*, 1992a, b). The monoclonal antibodies to the vitronectin receptor are used as markers to identify osteoclasts and to distinguish osteoblasts from multinucleated giant cells.

There are other important molecular mechanisms involved in the bone-resorbing process which could be utilized in the development of new agents. For example, a vacuolar ATPase has been identified which is responsible for pumping protons across the ruffled border of the osteoclast and demineralizing bone (Blair *et al.*, 1989). The proton-producing capacity of the osteoclast is essential for bone resorption. When proton production is inhibited by carbonic anhydrase inhibitors such as acetazolamide or when carbonic anhydrase type II is ineffective, as occurs in one variant of human osteopetrosis (Sly *et al.*, 1983), then impaired osteoclast function ensues. There are other possible inhibitors of osteoclastic bone resorption. It is possible that if we understood more of the molecular mechanisms involved in osteoclastic bone resorption by proteolytic enzymes, then inhibitors to these agents could be developed.

Osteopetrosis has been a very informative disease for osteoclast biology and for indicating specific molecular mechanisms involved in bone resorption. This disease reflects incompetent osteoclasts. It is a heterogeneous condition which occurs in a number of variants in rodents and in man. The molecular mechanisms responsible for osteopetrosis in some of these variants have now been identified. For example, in the defect which occurs in humans associated with renal tubular abnormalities and calcification in the brain, it has been shown that there is a defect in expression of carbonic anhydrase type II, leading to impaired production of protons and subsequent inadequate osteoclastic bone resorption (Sly *et al.*, 1983). In several murine variants, the molecular mechanism responsible has recently been clarified. In the op/op variant of murine osteopetrosis, there is an impairment of osteoclast formation associated with decreased production of colony-stimulating factor-1 (CSF-1) by stromal cells in the osteoclast microenvironment. Impaired production of CSF-1 leads to impaired osteoclast formation (Wiktor-Jedrejzcak *et al.*, 1982; Kodama *et al.*, 1991; Takahashi *et al.*, 1991). This disease can be corrected by treatment with CSF-1 (Felix *et al.*, 1990; Kodama *et al.*, 1991). The fact that it is a microenvironmental defect has been shown by transplantation experiments. When osteoclast precursors are transplanted into lethally irradiated mice with this disease, the osteopetrosis is not reversed. Similarly, mixing and matching experiments in which accessory cells or bone-resorbing osteoclasts from osteopetrotic mice are mixed with normal stromal cells or osteoclast precursors from normal littermates show that the defect is in the stromal cells or accessory cells and not in the osteoclast lineage (Takahashi *et al.*, 1991). These results show that normal production of CSF-1 is required for normal osteoclast formation.

In another variant of osteopetrosis recently described, it has been shown that deficient expression of src tyrosine kinase is responsible (Soriano *et al.*, 1991). In this variant of osteopetrosis, observed in mice made deficient in src tyrosine kinase expression by targeted disruption of the src proto-oncogene by introduction of a null mutation followed by homologous recombination in embryonic stem cells, the src-deficient mice developed classic osteopetrosis. However, unlike the osteopetrosis which occurs in the op/op variant, in this case osteopetrosis is due not to impaired osteoclast formation but rather to impaired osteoclast action. In src-deficient osteopetrosis, there is impaired formation of the ruffled border of the osteoclasts and no resorption lacunae are excavated (Boyce *et al.*, 1992). In this disorder, the defect is in the osteoclast lineage rather than in accessory cells (Lowe *et al.*, 1993). Since the src proto-oncogene encodes an intracullular tyrosine kinase related to the cytoskeleton, these results show that expression of several tyrosine kinases are important for normal osteoclast function, including an intracellular tyrosine kinase encoded by src as well as a receptor kinase encoded by the receptor for CSF-1, also known as the c-fms proto-oncogene. Since these tyrosine kinases can be inhibited by small molecular weight compounds, this information provides the possibility of development of new classes of inhibitors of osteoclastic bone resorption. For example, agents might be developed which could inhibit both receptor tyrosine kinases and intracellular tyrosine kinases required for both osteoclast formation and osteoclast action. The non-specific tyrosine kinase inhibitor herbimycin A has been shown to effectively inhibit bone resorption both *in vitro* and *in vivo* (Yoneda *et al.*, 1993). Such drug combinations should effectively prevent or inhibit bone resorption.

Another variant of osteopetrosis has recently been described which is clearly distinct phenotypically from both src deficiency and M-CSF deficiency. This is observed in mice in which the null mutation for the gene c-fos has been introduced so the mice are c-fos deficient. In these mice there is an abnormality in the osteoclast lineage and a failure of osteoclast formation (Grigoriadis *et al.*, 1994).

BONE GROWTH STIMULATORS

Bone formation at remodeling sites may be stimulated by treatment with agents which directly stimulate osteoblastic function or by evoking the coupling response which links bone formation to prior bone resorption. Two approaches to the latter are the use of resorption inhibitors which in the short term cause an unbalanced increase in bone formation (see above) and the theoretical concept of coherence therapy, which utilizes the coupling phenomenon to lead to a relative increase in bone formation. To date, these approaches have not provided encouraging results. Resorption inhibitors such as estrogen, calcitonin and bisphosphonates lead to very modest increases in bone formation over relatively short periods (up to two years), but not prolonged stimulatory effects on bone formation which are comparable to those seen with direct-acting osteoblast-stimulating agents. As suggested earlier, estrogen, calcitonin and bisphosphonates have all produced positive effects on bone formation in periods of up to two years of approximately 4% as measured by bone mineral density. There even remains the possibility that these agents may have growth-stimulatory effects in addition to their inhibitory effects on bone resorption. In the case of estrogen, there is evidence in rodents that bone formation may be stimulated (Chow *et al.*, 1992). Calcitonin has been thought by some to stimulate bone formation but here the evidence *in vivo* is less convincing.

ADFR OR COHERENCE THERAPY

Frost described the bone-remodeling sequence (Frost, 1979, 1981, 1983). He also introduced the concept that it could be successfully modulated to favor bone formation. He reasoned that if bone-remodeling units at multiple sites could be simultaneously activated by bone resorption stimuli so that osteoclastic bone resorption was synchronized and then an osteoclast inhibitor was used to inhibit osteoclast activity, the coupling phenomenon would occur and there would be an overall stimulus to bone formation not balanced by continued bone resorption. These agents would have to be given sequentially. He called this approach ADFR (for Activate, Depress, Free and Repeat). It received a lot of attention through the 1980s and attempts were made to utilize the concept in the design of clinical trials.

However, there are several problems. Firstly, it has never been shown to work experimentally, so it has not been tested. Secondly, there is no accurate method to determine the timing of administration of the resorption activators or inhibitors. Finally, it is not clear that the stimulus to coupling is not directly proportional to the stimulus to resorption. If the stimulus to bone formation is related quantitatively to the stimulus to resorption, then when resorption is inhibited so too will be the bone formation stimulus. The concept is novel, but our knowledge of the cellular events in bone remodeling and how they are controlled is still not adequate to effectively evaluate it.

Of the direct osteoblast stimulants, three approaches have been tried. These include fluoride, low-dose intermittent parathyroid hormone and bone-derived bone growth regulatory factors.

FLUORIDE

It has been known for 30 years that fluoride stimulates osteoblastic bone formation. People living in areas of endemic fluoride ingestion develop fluorosis, characterized by diffuse osteosclerosis. Fluoride has been used in the treatment of diseases of bone loss such as myeloma and osteoporosis, with striking results, particularly with osteoporosis. Increases in new bone are dramatic both morphologically and by bone mineral density measurements (Riggs *et al.*, 1982; Pak *et al.*, 1989). Bone mineral density indicates there is approximately a 10% increase in bone mass per year and the increase may continue in successive years of treatment. However, with fluoride treatment there is also unfortunate toxicity. The new bone which forms is not of normal quality and fractures easily (Riggs *et al.*, 1990). The reason is not entirely clear but it may occur because fluoride is incorporated into the mineral phase of the new bone and as such increases its brittleness. The result is pain, microfractures, partial fractures and incomplete fractures. The morphologic appearance may show impaired normal mineralization (osteomalacia) unless calcium and vitamin D are coadministered. However, although calcium and vitamin D prevent the morphologic appearance of osteomalacia, they do not prevent the susceptibility to fracture. A large trial has placed considerable doubt on the usefulness of fluoride as a treatment for osteoporosis (Riggs *et al.*, 1990).

Recently, fluoride, in a novel formulation which is released slowly and maintains more stable blood levels, has been reported to show very good results in patients with postmenopausal osteoporosis (Pak *et al.*, 1995; Mundy, 1995b). In these doses, it is suggested that fluoride avoids the blood levels which are associated with side effects such as gastric irritation and at the same time has a very marked beneficial effect on the skeleton. If this work can be confirmed by other groups, it raises the likelihood that fluoride may achieve an important place in the therapeutic armamentarium for osteoporosis.

Although the use of fluoride is controversial at this time, it is still widely used and highly favored by some investigators. The side effects notwithstanding, fluoride undoubtedly has a powerful effect on osteoblast function. The molecular mechanism is not clearly understood. One possibility suggested by Baylink and coworkers (Lau *et al.*, 1989a) is that fluoride exerts its effects by influencing the phosphorylation state of tyrosine residues on intracellular proteins. Many of the bone growth factors exert their mitogenic effects on bone cells through tyrosine phosphorylation – for example, insulin-like growth factor I and transforming growth factor α. Since fluoride is a non-specific inhibitor of tyrosine phosphorylation which dephosphorylates these proteins, then fluoride may be expected to enhance these tyrosine kinase-mediated effects (Lau *et al.*, 1989b). These workers have identified an osteoblast acid phosphatase which they believe may be the target for fluoride. However, fluoride is a non-specific phosphatase inhibitor and it remains to be explained why its stimulatory effects on bone cells are the major effects seen following fluoride treatment if this is indeed the mode of action. More recently, Caverzasio *et al.* (1996) have suggested that fluoride may exert its beneficial effects by targeting a tyrosine kinase in bone cells, possibly in conjunction with aluminum. This would presumably cause an inhibitory effect on a phosphatase, namely to enhance the stimulatory effects of growth regulatory factors which work through tyrosine kinase-mediated mechanisms. Much work needs to be done in identifying the molecular mechanism of the action of fluoride on bone growth stimulation.

LOW-DOSE PARATHYROID HORMONE

It has been realized now for a number of years that when parathyroid hormone is delivered in low dose and intermittently, there is a stimulatory effect on new bone formation. This favors predominantly cancellous bone and has been observed in dogs, rats and man. Although the mechanism is not entirely clear, it may be related to generation of local growth factors within bone such as insulin-like growth factor I and transforming growth factor B (Pfeilschifter and Mundy, 1987; Canalis *et al.*, 1989). These effects are in contrast to what is seen when parathyroid hormone is delivered continuously. Under these circumstances, there is a prominent effect to increase bone resorption. The anabolic response to parathyroid hormone may be of benefit in the treatment of osteoporosis, particularly if it is used in conjunction with 1,25-dihydroxyvitamin D (Reeve *et al.*, 1980, 1989; Slovik *et al.*, 1986). This is still undergoing evaluation.

Some believe that parathyroid hormone-related peptide or analogs also has similar powerful anabolic effects on bone (Stewart, 1996; Vickery *et al.*, 1996).

BONE-DERIVED GROWTH FACTORS

The formation of bone by osteoblasts may be influenced by a multitude of growth regulatory factors for bone cells which are incorporated into the bone matrix (Hauschka *et al.*, 1986). For some of these factors, bone is the largest storehouse in the body. They are released when bone is resorbed and presumably thereby influence subsequent events involved in bone remodeling. These factors include transforming growth factor β (TGFβ), platelet-derived growth factor (PDGF), the heparin-binding growth factors acidic and basic FGF, insulin-like growth factors I and II (IGF-I and IGF-II). They are all potential drugs which could be used as therapeutic agents to stimulate the formation of bone. However, there are problems associated with their potential usefulness as therapeutic agents which make their development problematic.

1. These factors are peptides which must be given by repeated injections.
2. They all have extremely short half-lives when administered systemically.
3. They have ubiquitous effects on many

tissues and are therefore likely to cause significant systemic toxicity.
4. It is unclear if they all stimulate appositional bone growth or bone formation associated with bone remodeling.

The most thoroughly studied for its effects on bone formation is TGFβ. TGFβ is also the most abundant of these growth factors in bone (Seyedin *et al.*, 1986, 1987; Hauschka *et al.*, 1986). It is present in bone in a latent form, bound to binding proteins. It is presumably released when bone is resorbed in an active form to stimulate new bone formation and inhibit osteoclastic bone resorption (Pfeilschifter and Mundy, 1987). TGFβ represents a family of highly homologous proteins, TGFβ1–5. TGFβ1 and TGFβ2 have been found in bone. They appear to have identical effects on bone cell targets. TGFβ is about 10 times as abundant as TGFβ2 in bone. TGFβ3, 4 and 5 are not known to be present in bone. TGFβ has dramatic effects on bone *in vivo*. We tested the effects of TGFB1 injected subcutaneously over the calvarium of normal mice for 2–5 days (Marcelli *et al.*, 1990). Similar experiments have been performed by Noda and Camilliere (1989) in rats and by Mackie and Trechsel (1990). We found that TGFβ1 caused a fivefold increase in periosteal thickness, with marked increases in cellularity, new mineralized woven bone formation and an increase in the numbers of active osteoblasts. These effects were present locally at the site of injection. There was no increase in osteoclastic bone resorption in the periosteum, in contrast to what is seen using similar injections of parathyroid hormone, parathyroid hormone-related protein or interluekin-1, but there was an expansion of the marrow cavity with increased osteoclastic bone resorption and the appearance of large active osteoclasts. These changes were modified by indomethacin treatment. We also tested the effects of TGFβ1 on cortical bone by infusions of TGFβ into the medullary cavity of the femur and observed similar effects. We have found no differences between TGFβ1 and TGFβ2 in their effects in any of our bone assay systems.

Another family of growth regulatory factors related to TGFβ have recently been identified in the bone matrix (Wang *et al.*, 1988; Wozney *et al.*, 1988). These are the bone morphogenetic proteins (BMPs). These peptides have amino acid sequence homology to TGFβ and probably arose from a common ancestral gene. They have been linked to the phenomenon of ectopic bone formation which occurs following injection of demineralized bone matrix in the subcutaneous tissue of the flank of the rat (Urist, 1965). This process occurs over 21 days and begins with the recruitment of mesenchymal cells from tissues surrounding the injection site. These cells firstly differentiate into chondroblasts, then lay down a cartilage matrix which calcifies and is removed by chondroclasts. Local mesenchymal cells then differentiate into osteoblasts which lay down new bone matrix and by three weeks after implantation a small ossicle of bone complete with hematopoietic bone marrow occupies the original implant site. The active component in the bone extract was termed bone morphogenetic protein (BMP) by Urist (1965).

In the last few years, an active principle in the bone matrix has been identified which can mimic these responses. This active principle belongs to a family of six peptides in the extended TGFβ family. Their amino acid sequences and cDNAs have been described (Wozney *et al.*, 1988; Wang *et al.*, 1988; Celeste *et al.*, 1990). These BMPs have a pre, pro and mature region which is dimerized through cysteine disulfides. The pro region is required for proper folding and dimerization. The mature region has the characteristic 7-cys pattern, rather than the 9-cys pattern as is seen with TGFβ1-3. BMPs may be necessary for normal growth and development as well as for the remodeling and repair of bone. Patterns of expression of the TGFβ superfamily of genes, including BMP2, BMP4 and BMP6 (also called Vgr-1), have been described in mesenchymal cells and the developing skeleton of embryonic mice (Lyons *et al.*, 1989; Jones *et al.*, 1991).

Differential expression of these and other genes may be critical elements in the differentiation of chondroblasts and osteoblasts from mesenchymal cells. *In situ* hybridization studies using a specific BMP4 cRNA probe have demonstrated specific expression patterns of BMP4 mRNA during morphogenesis in mouse embryos at various stages of development (Jones *et al.*, 1991). The observation of endogenous expression of BMPs during early embryonic skeletal development, together with the observation that exogenous BMP2, 3, 4 and 5 stimulate ectopic bone formation, support the hypothesis that BMPs are important morphogenetic factors for bone differentiation and development. To date, there is limited information on the potential physiologic effects of the BMPs on bone. It is not known whether they have similar bone-forming effects to those of TGFβ or if they are involved in normal appositional bone growth or in bone remodeling. These data will have to await their availability in sufficient amounts for testing in appropriate systems.

The other growth regulatory factors in bone have also been studied for their bone growth stimulatory effects. The heparin-binding fibroblast growth factors (FGFs) have been found to have mitogenic effects on osteoblasts *in vitro* (Rodan *et al.*, 1987; Globus *et al.*, 1988). More recently, acidic and basic FGF has been shown to have anabolic effects on bone *in vivo* (Mayahara *et al.*, 1993; Dunstan *et al.*, 1995). IGF-I has bone growth stimulatory effects but has not been tested in the same way as TGFβ, so comparisons of *in vivo* effects are difficult. IGF-I may play an important role in the anabolic response to PTH, since in embryonic rat calvariae PTH has been shown to induce IGF-I production when administered intermittently (Canalis *et al.*, 1989). IGF-I has also recently been shown to work in conjunction with PDGF to repair bone defects in alveolar bone associated with periodontal disease (Lynch *et al.*, 1989). IGF-II has not been studied for its effects on bone formation *in vivo* to my knowledge.

CONCLUSION

At the present time the search for new treatments for bone disease is focused on resorption inhibitors and formation stimulators. We have at present effective resorption inhibitors, but none that are totally satisfactory or universally acceptable. Moreover, resorption inhibitors alone may not be enough to combat established osteoporosis. In contrast, we have no acceptable formation stimulators available and this is the current focus of most research efforts. In the future, it appears that combinations of resorption inhibitors and formation stimulators will be the approach most likely to bring maximal benefits.

ACKNOWLEDGEMENTS

I am grateful to Nancy Garrett for her excellent secretarial assistance. Part of the work described here was performed with the aid of NIH grants AR39529, CA40035, DE08569, AR28149, RR01346 and AR07464 from the National Institutes of Health.

REFERENCES

Blair, H.C., Teitelbaum, S.L., Ghiselli, R. *et al.* (1989) Osteoclastic bone resorption by a polarized vacuolar proton pump. *Science* **245**: 855–7.

Boyce, B.F., Aufdemorte, T.B., Garett, I.R. *et al.* (1989) Effects of interleukin-1 on bone turnover in normal mice. *Endocrinology* **123**: 1142–50.

Boyce, B.F., Yoneda, T., Lowe, C., Soriano, P. and Mundy, G.R. (1992). Requirement of pp60c-src expression of osteoclasts to form ruffled borders and resorb bone. *J Clin Invest* **90**: 1622–7.

Canalis, E., Centrella, M., Burch, W. *et al.* (1989) Insulin-like growth factor I mediates selective anabolic effects of parathyroid hormone in bone cultures. *J Clin Invest* **83**: 60–5.

Caverzasio, J., Imai, T., Ammann, P., Burgener, D. and Bonjour, J.P. (1996) Aluminum potentiates the effect of fluoride on tyrosine phosphorylation and osteoblast replication in vitro and bone mass in vivo. *J Bone Miner Res* **11**, 46–55.

Celeste, A.J., Iannazzi, J.A., Taylor, R.C. *et al.* (1990) Identification of transforming growth factor β family members present in bone-inductive protein purified from bovine bone. *Proc Natl Acad Sci USA* **87**: 9843–7.

Chow, J., Tobias, J.H., Colston, K.W. *et al.* (1992) Estrogen maintains trabecular bone volume in rats not only by suppression of bone resorption but also by stimulation of bone formation. *J Clin Invest* **89**: 74–8.

Dunstan, C.R., Garrett, I.R., Adams, R. *et al.* (1995) Systemic fibroblast growth factor (FGF-1) prevents bone loss, increases new bone formation, and restores trabecular microarchitecture in ovariectomized rats. *J Bone Miner Res* **10** (Suppl 1): P279.

Ernst, M. and Rodan, G.A. (1991) Estradiol regulation of insulin-like growth factor-I expression in osteoblastic cells – evidence for transcriptional control. *Mol Endocrinol* **5**: 1081–9.

Ernst, M., Health, J.K. and Rodan, G.A. (1989) Estradiol effects on proliferation, messenger ribonucleic acid for collagen and insulin-like growth factor-I, and parathyroid hormone-stimulated adenylate cyclase activity in osteoblastic cells from calvariae and long bones. *Endocrinology* **125**: 825–33.

Felix, R., Cecchini, M.G. and Fleisch, H. (1990) Macrophage colony stimulating factor restores in vivo bone resorption in the OP/OP osteopetrotic mouse. *Endocrinology* **127**: 2592–4.

Frost, H.M. (1979) Treatment of osteoporoses by manipulation of coherent bone cell populations. *Clin Orthop* **143**: 227–44.

Frost, H.M. (1981) Coherence treatment of osteoporoses. *Orthop Clin North Am* **12**: 649–69.

Frost, H.M. (1983) The ADFR concept revisited. *Calcif Tissue Int* **36**: 349–53.

Girasole, G., Jikla, R.L., Passeri, G. *et al.* (1992) 17β estradiol inhibits interleukin-6 production by bone marrow-derived stromal cells in osteoblasts *in vitro*: a potential mechanism for the anti-osteotropic effect of estrogens. *J Clin Invest* **89**: 883–91.

Globus, R.K., Patterson-Buckendahl, P. and Gospodarowicz, D. (1988) Regulation of bovine bone cell proliferation by fibroblast growth factor and transforming growth factor beta. *Endocrinology* **123**: 98–105.

Grigoriadis, A.E., Wang, Z.Q., Cecchini, M.G. *et al.* (1994). C-Fos: a key regulator of osteoclast-macrophage lineage determination and bone remodeling. *Science* **266**: 443–8.

Hattner, R., Etker, B.N. and Frost, H.M. (1965) Suggested sequential mode of control of changes in cell behavior in adult bone remodelling. *Nature* **206**: 489–90.

Hauschka, P.V., Mavrakos, A.E., Iafrati, M.D. *et al.* (1986) Growth factors in bone matrix. *J Biol Chem* **261**: 12665–74.

Helfrich, M.H., Nesbitt, S.A., Dorey, E.L. *et al.* (1992a) Rat osteoclasts adhere to a wide range of RGD (Arg-Gly-Asp) peptide-containing proteins, including the bone sialoproteins and fibronectin, via a β_3 integrin. *J Bone Miner Res* **7**: 335–43.

Helfrich, M.H., Nesbitt, S.A. and Horton, M.A. (1992b) Integrins on rat osteoclasts: characterization of two monoclonal antibodies (F4 and F11) to rat B3. *J Bone Miner Res* **7**: 345–51.

Horton, M.A. and Davies, J. (1989) Perspectives – adhesion receptors in bone. *J Bone Miner Res* **4**: 803–8.

Hughes, D.E., Wright, K.R., Uy, H.L. *et al.* (1995) Bisphosphonates promote apoptosis in murine osteoclasts in vitro and in vivo. *J Bone Miner Res* **10**: 1478–87.

Jilka, R.L., Hangoc, G., Girasole, G. *et al.* (1992) Increased osteoclast development after estrogen loss – mediation by interleukin-6. *Science* **257**: 88–91.

Jones, C.M., Lyons, K.M. and Hogan, B.L.M. (1991) Involvement of bone morphogenetic protein-4 (BMP-4) and Vgr-1 in morphogenesis and neurogenesis in the mouse. *Development* **111**: 531–42.

Keeting, P.E., Bonewald, L.F., Colvard, D.S. *et al.* (1989) Estrogen-mediated release of transforming growth factor-beta by normal human osteoblast-like cells. *J Bone Miner Res* **4** (Suppl 1): 655.

Kleerekoper, M., Villanueva, A.R., Stanciu, J. *et al.* (1985) The role of three-dimensional trabecular microstructure in the pathogenesis of vertebral compression fractures. *Calcif Tissue Int* **37**: 594–7.

Kodama, H., Yamasaki, A., Nose, M. *et al.* (1991) Congenital osteoclast deficiency in osteopetrotic (op/op) mice is cured by injections of macrophage colony-stimulating factor. *J Exp Med* **173**: 269–72.

Lau, K.H., Farley, J.R. and Baylink, D.J. (1989a) Phosphotyrosyl protein phosphatases. *Biochem J* 257: 23–36.

Lau, K.H., Farley, J.R., Freeman, T.K. *et al.* (1989b) A proposed mechanism of the mitrogenic action of fluoride of bone cells – inhibition. *Metabolism* **38**: 851–68.

Liberman, U.A., Weiss, S.R., Broll, J. *et al.* (1995) Effect of oral alendronate on bone mineral density and the incidence of fractures in postmenopausal osteoporosis. *N Engl J Med* **333**: 1437–43.

Lowe, C., Yoneda, T., Boyce, B.F. *et al.* (1993) Osteopetrosis in src deficient mice is due to an autonomous defect of osteoclasts. *Proc Natl Acad Sci USA* **90**: 4485–9.

Lynch, S.E., Williams, R.C., Polson, A.M. *et al.* (1989) A combination of platelet-derived and insulin-like growth factors enhances periodontal regeneration. *J Clin Periodontol* **16**: 545–8.

Lyons, K., Graycar, J.L., Lee, A. *et al.* (1989) Vgr-1, a mammalian gene related to Xenopus Vg-1, is a member of the transforming growth factor-beta gene superfamily. *Proc Natl Acad Sci USA* **86**: 4554–8.

Mackie, E.J. and Trechsel, U. (1990) Stimulation of bone formation in vivo by transforming growth factor beta – remodeling of woven bone and lack of inhibition by indomethacin. *Bone* **11**: 295–300.

Manolagas, S.C. and Jilka, R.L. (1995) Mechanisms of disease: bone marrow, cytokines, and bone remodeling – emerging insights into the pathophysiology of osteoporosis. *N Engl J Med* **332**: 305–11.

Marcelli, C., Yates, A.J.P.and Mundy, G.R. (1990) In vivo effects of human recombinant transforming growth factor beta on bone turnover in normal mice. *J Bone Miner Res* **5**: 1087–96.

Mayahara, H., Ito, T., Nagai, H. *et al.* (1993) In vivo stimulation of endosteal bone formation by basic fibroblast growth factor in rats. *Growth Factors* **9**: 73–80.

Mundy, G.R. (1990) Immune system and bone remodelling. *Trends Endocrinol Metab* **1**: 307–11.

Mundy, G.R. (1995a) Bone remodeling. In: *Bone Remodeling and Its Disorders*, Martin Dunitz, London.

Mundy, G.R. (1995b) No bones about fluoride. *Nature Med* **1**: 1130–1.

Noda, M. and Camilliere, J.J. (1989) In vivo stimulation of bone formation by transforming growth factor-beta. *Endocrinology* **124**: 2991–4.

Oursler, M.J., Osdoby, P., Pyfferoen, J. *et al.* (1991) Avian osteoclasts as estrogen target cells. *Proc Natl Acad Sci USA* **88**: 6613–17.

Pacifici, R., Rifas, L., Teitelbaum, S. *et al.* (1987) Spontaneous release of interleukin-1 from human blood monocytes reflects bone formation in idiopathic osteoporosis. *Proc Natl Acad Sci USA* **84**: 4616–20.

Pacifici, R., Rifas, L., McCracken, R. *et al.* (1989) Ovarian steroid treatment blocks a postmenopausal increase in blood monocyte interleukin-1 release. *Proc Natl Acad Sci USA* **86**: 2398–402.

Pak, C.Y.C., Sakhaee, K., Zerwekh, J.E. *et al.* (1989) Safe and effective treatment of osteoporosis with intermittent slow release sodium fluoride: augmentation of vertebral bone mass and inhibition of fractures. *J Clin Endocrinol Metab* **68**: 150–9.

Pak, C.Y.C., Sakhaee, K., Adamshuet, B. *et al.* (1995) Treatment of postmenopausal osteoporosis with slow-release sodium fluoride. Final report of a randomized controlled trial. *Ann Intern Med* **123**: 401–8.

Parfitt, A.M. (1979) Quantum concept of bone remodeling and turnover: implications for the pathogenesis of osteoporosis. *Calcif Tissue Int* **28**: 1–5.

Pfeilschifter, J. and Mundy, G.R. (1987) Modulation of transforming growth factor beta activity in bone cultures by osteotropic hormones. *Proc Natl Acad Sci USA* **84**: 2024–8.

Reeve, J., Meunier, P.J., Parsons, J.A. *et al.* (1980) Anabolic effect of human parathyroid hormone fragment on trabecular bone in involutional osteoporosis: a multicentre trial. *Br Med J* **280**: 1340–4.

Reeve, J., Davies, U., Arlot, M. *et al.* (1989) Parathyroid peptide (hPTH 1-34) in the treatment of osteoporosis. In: *Clinical Disorders of Bone and Mineral Metabolism*, (eds Kleerekoper, M. and Krane, S.M.), Mary Ann Liebert, New York, pp. 621–7.

Riggs, B.L., Seeman, E., Hodgson, S.F. *et al.* (1982) Effect of the fluoride/calcium regimen on vertebral fracture occurrence in postmenopausal osteoporosis. Comparison with conventional therapy. *N Engl J Med* **306**: 446–50.

Riggs, B.L., Hodgson, S.F., O'Fallon, W.M. *et al.* (1990) Effect of fluoride treatment on the fracture rate in postmenopausal women with osteoporosis. *N Engl J Med* **322**: 802–9.

Rodan, S.B., Wesolowski, G., Thomas, K. *et al.* (1987) Growth stimulation of rat calvaria osteoblastic cells by acidic fibroblast growth factor. *Endocrinology* **121**: 1917–23.

Rogers, M.J., Watts, D.J. and Russell, R.G.G. (1997) Overview of bisphosphonates. *Cancer* **80**: 1652–60.

Sato, M., Grasser, W., Endo, N. *et al.* (1991) Bisphosphonate action – alendronate localization in rat bone and effects on osteoclast ultrastructure. *J Clin Invest* **88**: 2095–105.

Schmidt, A., Rutledge, S.J., Endo, N. *et al.* (1996) Protein-tyrosine phosphatase activity regulates osteoclast formation and function: inhibition by alendronate. *Proc Natl Acad Sci USA* **93**: 3068–73.

Seyedin, S.M., Thomson, A.Y., Bentz, H. *et al.* (1986) Cartilage-inducing factor A: apparent identity to transforming growth factor beta. *J Biol Chem* **261**: 5693–5.

Seyedin, S.M., Segarini, P.R., Rosen, D.M. *et al.* (1987) Cartilage-inducing factor-B is a unique protein structurally and functionally related to transforming growth factor beta. *J Biol Chem* **262**: 1946–9.

Slovik, D.M., Rosenthal, D.I., Doppelt, S.H. *et al.* (1986) Restoration of spinal bone in osteoporotic men by treatment with human parathyroid hormone (1-34) and 1,25 dihydroxyvitamin D. *J Bone Miner Res* **1**: 377–81.

Sly, W.S., Hewett-Emmett, D., Whyte, M.P. *et al.* (1983) Carbonic anhydrase II deficiency identified as the primary defect in the autosomal recessive syndrome of osteopetrosis with renal tubular acidosis and cerebral calcification. *Proc Natl Acad Sci USA* **80**: 2752–6.

Soriano, P., Montgomery, C., Geske, R. *et al.* (1991) Targeted disruption of the c-src proto-oncogene leads to osteopetrosis in mice. *Cell* **64**: 693–702.

Stewart, A.F. (1996) PTHrP(1–36) as a skeletal anabolic agent for the treatment of osteoporosis. *Bone* **19**: 303–6.

Takahashi, N., Udagawa, N., Akatsu, T. *et al.* (1991) Deficiency of osteoclasts in osteopetrotic mice is due to a defect in the local microenvironment provided by osteoblastic cells. *Endocrinology* **128**: 1792–6.

Urist, M.R. (1965) Bone: formation by autoinduction. *Science* **150**: 890–3.

Vickery, B.H., Arnur, Z., Cheng, Y. *et al.* (1996) RS-66271, a C-terminally substituted analog of human parathyroid hormone-related protein (1–34), increases trabecular and cortical bone in ovariectomized, osteoperic rats. *J Bone Miner Res* **11**: 1943–53.

Wang, E.A., Rosen, V., Cordes, P. *et al.* (1988) Purification and characterization of other distinct bone-inducing factors. *Proc Natl Acad Sci USA* **85**: 9484–8.

Wiktor-Jedzrejzcak, W., Ahmed, A., Szczylik, C. *et al.* (1982) Hematological characterization of congenital osteopetrosis in op/op mouse. *J Exp Med* **156**: 1516–27.

Wozney, J.M., Rosen, V., Celeste, A.J. *et al.* (1988) Novel regulators of bone formation: molecular clones and activities. *Science* **242**: 1528–34.

Yoneda, T., Lowe, C., Lee, C.H. *et al.* (1993) Herbimycin A, a pp60c-src tyrosine kinase inhibitor, inhibits osteoclastic bone resorption *in vitro* and hypercalcemia *in vivo*. *J Clin Invest* **91**: 2791–5.

INDEX